Contents

W9-CZN-707

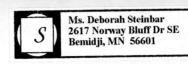

Thieme Clinical Companions

Dermatology

..

Wolfram Sterry, M.D.
Professor and Chairman
Department of Dermatology,
Venereology, and Allergy
Charité University Hospital
Berlin, Germany

Ralf Paus, M.D.
Professor
Department of Dermatology and Venereology
University Hospital Schleswig-Holstein
Luebeck, Germany

Walter Burgdorf, M.D.
Clinical Lecturer
Department of Dermatology
Ludwig Maximilian University
Munich, Germany

With contributions by

Heike Audring, Ulrike Blume-Peytavi, Guido Bruning, Peter von den Driesch,
Jorge Frank, Markus Friedrich, Christoph Garcia-Bartels, Sylke Gellrich,
Ina Hadshiew, Michael Hertl, Wolfgang Kimmig, Stefan Peker,
Andreas Plettenberg, Bertold Rzany, Peter Schulze, Wolfgang Schulze,
Ute Siemann-Harms, Hans Sperl, Eggert Stockfleth, Hans-Juergen Tietz,
Class Ulrich, Christiane Voit, Gerd Wolf, Margitta Worm, Torsten Zuberbier

345 illustrations

Georg Thieme Verlag
Stuttgart · New York

Library of Congress Cataloging-in-Publication Data

Sterry Wolfram.
  [Checkliste Dermatologie. English]
  Dermatology / Wolfram Sterry, Ralf Paus, Walter Burgdorf ; with contributions by Heike Audring ... [et al.].
    p. ; cm. -- (Thieme clinical companions)
  ISBN 1-58890-258-7 (alk. paper) -- ISBN 3-13-135911-0 (alk. paper)
  1. Dermatology--Handbooks, manuals, etc. 2. Skin--Diseases--Handbooks, manuals, etc.
  [DNLM: 1. Skin Diseases--therapy--Handbooks. 2. Dermatology--Handbooks. 3. Sexually Transmitted Disease--therapy--Handbooks. 4. Skin Neoplasms--Handbooks. WR 39 S838c 2006a] I. Paus, Ralf. II. Burgdorf, Walter H. C. III. Title. IV. Series.
  RL74.S81513 2006
  616.5--dc22   2006000851

1st German edition 1987	4th German edition 2000
2nd German edition 1992	5th German edition 2005
3rd German edition 1999	

Illustrator: Helmut Holtermann, Dannenberg, Germany

Important note: Medicine is an ever-changing science undergoing continual development. Research and clinical experience are continually expanding our knowledge, in particular our knowledge of proper treatment and drug therapy. Insofar as this book mentions any dosage or application, readers may rest assured that the authors, editors, and publishers have made every effort to ensure that such references are in accordance with **the state of knowledge at the time of production of the book.**

Nevertheless, this does not involve, imply, or express any guarantee or responsibility on the part of the publishers in respect to any dosage instructions and forms of applications stated in the book. **Every user is requested to examine carefully** the manufacturers leaflets accompanying each drug and to check, if necessary in consultation with a physician or specialist, whether the dosage schedules mentioned therein or the contraindications stated by the manufacturers differ from the statements made in the present book. Such examination is particularly important with drugs that are either rarely used or have been newly released on the market. Every dosage schedule or every form of application used is entirely at the users own risk and responsibility. The authors and publishers request every user to report to the publishers any discrepancies or inaccuracies noticed. If errors in this work are found after publication, errata will be posted at www.thieme.com on the product description page.

Some of the product names, patents, and registered designs referred to in this book are in fact registered trademarks or proprietary names even though specific reference to this fact is not always made in the text. Therefore, the appearance of a name without designation as proprietary is not to be construed as a representation by the publisher that it is in the public domain.

© 2006 Georg Thieme Verlag KG,
Rüdigerstraße 14, D-70469 Stuttgart
Germany

http://www.thieme.de

Thieme New York, 333 Seventh Avenue,
New York, NY 10001, USA

http://www.thieme.com

Typesetting by Götz, Ludwigsburg
Printed in Germany by Götz, Ludwigsburg

10-ISBN: 3-13-135911-0 (GTV)
13-ISBN: 978-3-13-135911-7 (GTV)
10-ISBN: 1-58890-258-7 (TNY)
13-ISBN: 978-1-58890-258-0 (TNY)

1 2 3 4 5 6

Preface

We are happy to present you with our new book *Dermatology* in the *Thieme Clinical Companions* series. A similar text has appeared in five German editions since 1987 and been highly successful. The goal of this book is to present everything one needs to diagnose and treat most cutaneous diseases in a compact, "one-stop" resource, carefully edited by three experienced dermatologists. The therapeutic options represent best practice internationally and reflect the diversified experience of three dermatologists, one of whom trained and worked in the USA for 20 years.

The contents have been extensively reviewed with the help of a number of colleagues listed on the title page. Some of them have provided additional input for the English version, including Drs. Peter von den Driesch, Bertold Rzany, Christiane Voit, and Margitta Worm. In addition, Dr. Maja Hoffmann helped with the differential diagnostic considerations in the last chapter. We would especially like to thank Dr. Gerd Wolf, who provided constructive criticism and detailed information on topical therapy.

Mr. Stephan Konnry at Thieme International guided the writing and production of this text. He was helped by Dr. Cliff Bergman and Dr. Christiane Brill-Schmid. We thank all three individuals for their cooperative spirit and valuable input.

We hope that you will enjoy reading this *Clinical Companion* as an introduction to dermatology and, moreover, that you find it helpful, if not indispensable, in your clinical training and practice. We are eager to hear from you, with complaints, constructive suggestions, or even praise.

Wolfram Sterry, M.D.
Ralf Paus, M.D.
Walter Burgdorf, M.D.

Contributors

Heike Audring, M.D.
Prof. Ulrike Blume-Peytavi, M.D.
Markus Friedrich, M.D.
Christoph Garcia-Bartels, M.D.
Sylke Gellrich, M.D.
Prof. Bertold Rzany, M.D.
Peter Schulze, M.D.
Hans Sperl, M.D.
Prof. Eggert Stockfleth, M.D.
Prof. Hans-Juergen Tietz, M.D.
Class Ulrich
Prof. Christiane Voit, M.D.
Prof. Margitta Worm, M.D.
Prof. Torsten Zuberbier, M.D.
Clinic and Polyclinic for Dermatology,
Venereology, and Allergy
Berlin, Germany

Ina Hadshiew, M.D.
Ute Siemann-Harms, M.D.
Wolfgang Kimmig, M.D.
Prof. Wolfgang Schulze, M.D.
Head and Skin Center
Clinic and Polyclinic for Dermatology
and Venereology
University Hospital
Hamburg-Eppendorf
Hamburg, Germany

Jorge Frank, M.D.
Professor
Afdeling Dermatologie
Academisch Ziekenhuis Maastricht
Maastricht, The Netherlands

Michael Hertl, M.D.
Professor and Chairman
Department of Dermatology and
Allergy
Phillips University
Marburg, Germany

Stefan Peker, M.D.
Private Dermatology Practice
Bad Segeberg, Germany

Guido Bruning, M.D.
Tabea Hospital Hamburg
Hamburg, Germany

Peter von den Driesch, M.D.
Professor
Bad Canstatt Hospital
Clinic for Dermatology
Stuttgart, Germany

Andreas Plettenberg, M.D.
Professor
Institute of Interdisciplinary
Infectiology and Immunology
(ifi-Medizin GmbH)
Hamburg, Germany

Gerd Wolf, M.D.
Pharmacist
Robert-Koch Pharmacy
Grafschaft-Ringen, Germany

Contents

Red Section: Therapy

1 Introduction to Skin Biology

1.1 Overview

The skin is not only the largest organ of your body, but also the heaviest: it has a surface of 1.5–2 m² and contributes $^1/_7$ to $^1/_6$ of body weight. The skin provides a fascinating "theater of life" in which—in contrast to all other organs—you can directly watch, dissect, and manipulate key principles of biology and pathology *in action*, and where the environment and an individual's way of life leave unmistakable traces for those who know how to read them.

Subjecting the skin to a professional examination, therefore, can reveal many invaluable clues about your patient's general well-being; internal disease; social, cultural, and eating habits; psychological disturbances; and occupation. All this provides medically very useful information, even when dermatology is not your main field of interest.

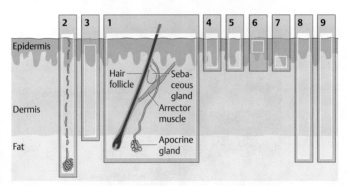

Fig. 1.**0** · Overview of skin, providing orientation for Figs. 1.**1–9**.

1.2 Functional Anatomy

The skin has many more crucial functions than we realize in daily life. It is therefore is not surprising that the loss of as little as 20% of your skin can condemn you to death. Architecturally, our skin is a constantly remodeled, intricately perfused and innervated three-layered structure (*epidermis, dermis, subcutis*). Specialized skin "appendages" protrude from the skin (*hair, nails*) or are embedded in it (*sweat and sebaceous glands*). Two special structures—*hair follicles* and *mammary glands* (derived from epidermis)—mark us as mammals. Figure 1.**0** provides an overview of the parts of the skin that are illustrated in the subsequent figures. Figures 1.**1**, 1.**2** are photomicrographs showing normal skin from a hair-bearing region and from the thickened palmar skin with sweat glands. Figure 1.**3** provides a three-dimensional view, showing how the epidermis and dermis interdigitate.

These basic skin layers are complemented and joined by three dense networks that link our skin to the rest of our body: *lymphatic system, blood vessels,* and *cutaneous nerves.* These networks provide proper nutrition, oxygen supply, and removal of toxic

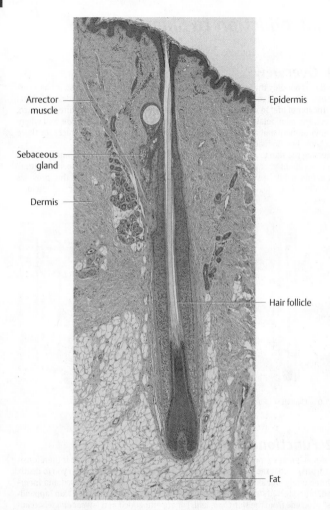

Fig. 1.**1** · Normal skin from hair-bearing area. Hematoxylin and eosin (H&E) stain.

products from our skin, and are vital for fluid balance, skin sensation, and proper skin immune responses. They also integrate the skin into very complex neuro-endocrine-immune networks essential for the organism's survival.

All organisms must have an outer covering that interacts with the environment, helping them to survive multiple exogenous threats while maintaining their structural integrity, be it the cell membrane of an amoeba or the skin of a human. Potential

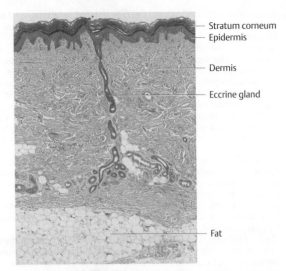

Fig. 1.**2** · Normal skin from palm. H&E stain.

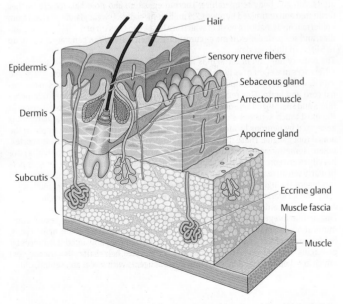

Fig. 1.**3** · Three-dimensional diagram of skin. Note how epidermis and dermis interdigitate.

dangers include UV radiation and free radicals which can damage DNA and cell membranes, dessication, overheating, mechanical trauma, infectious agents, toxins, and chemical irritants.

At the same time, this outer barrier must be flexible enough to allow for growth and movement of the organism it protects. In addition, it must also execute vitally important sensory functions by registering environmental signals (by the generation of pain and itch signals) so the organism can adequately respond to them (e.g. by flight reaction, shifting balance and position, striking out at an attacking force, or scratching away an unwelcome skin guest). This barrier also is vital for safeguarding the organism against the deadly loss or overaccumulation of heat and fluid. The skin is also the body's largest water storage site ($^1/_3$ of your total fluid is contained in the skin), and constitutes your major energy reserve (skin fat provides up to 40 days of energy reserve).

The gel-like, collagen-rich dermis, which underlies, supports, and nourishes the epidermis, is densely vascularized by two very extensive, interconnected, and well-innervated vascular networks: one at the border to the epidermis (*papillary plexus*), and one at the border of the subcutaneous fat (*reticular plexus*). These are complemented by a system of lymphatic vessels, whose inherited malformation or acquired malfunctioning results in massive skin edema due to an imbalance between fluid influx and efflux.

This very extensive skin perfusion system harbors about $^1/_4$ of your circulating blood (more than your brain!), and the total length of skin capillaries has been estimated as 240 km. This guarantees ample access of erythrocytes, nutrients, humoral blood components, and immune cells to the skin. This perfusion system is also critical for thermoregulation, since vasodilatation or vasoconstriction in a large area of skin rapidly alters skin and body temperature. Thermoregulation and fluid balance are further facilitated and optimized by about 2.5 million specialized sweat glands, derived from epidermal invaginations, most of which are located in the skin of the palms, soles, axillae, and scalp. Under extreme circumstances, their activity can generate a loss of up to 5 liters of fluid per day.

The sensory function of the skin is refined and sensitive. Our skin can discriminate differences in weight of as little as 0.005 g, react to temperatures between – 18 °C and + 44 °C, and send nerve impulses (action potentials) with a velocity of 2 m/s to the spinal cord and brain. This results from a dense network of interconnected free nerve fibers and specialized sensory receptors that populate the epidermis, most densely in the most touch-sensitive skin regions. This constantly remodeled neural network is generated by neurons located amazingly far away from the skin, for example in the dorsal root ganglia. These neurons feed skin-derived signals into the sensory cortex, where some individual skin regions (such as lips, fingers, tongue, genitalia) are heavily over-represented. Hair shafts with their generous neural supply serve as particularly sensitive touch receptors; just try slightly moving a hair and notice how you can record the lightest touch. Free nerve endings, specialized tactile organelles, intraepithelial Merkel cells and a plethora of receptors sensitive to pressure, heat, cold, and vibration complement the sensory armamentarium of the skin.

Finally, our integument serves as a crucial instrument of social and sexual communication, generates tools of defense, movement, and attack (hair, nails, claws, hoofs), and operates as an excretory organ: the skin removes unwanted substances by packaging them into dead cells (squames = corneocytes, hair shaft cells = trichocytes) which are then shed, and by excreting noxious agents with sweat and sebum.

1.3 Epidermis

The epidermis, a very thin but tough cornified (i.e. keratinized) avascular outer layer, provides the skin's direct interface with the environment (Fig. 1.**4**). It is composed primarily of keratinocytes along with smaller populations of two other resident cells—melanocytes and Merkel cells. In addition, there are migratory cells moving in and out of the skin, serving as outposts of the immune system (Langerhans cells, intraepidermal T cells) (Fig. 1.**5**, Table 1.**1**). When necessary, as during a bacterial infection, a rapid influx of (aggressive) neutrophils into the epidermis is triggered by the keratinocytes, thus producing pustules, and—not uncommonly—undesired neutrophil-induced tissue destruction alongside that of the insulting infectious agents.

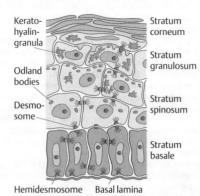

Fig. 1.**4** · Layers of epidermis.

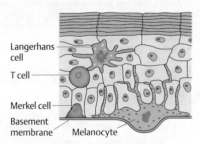

Fig. 1.**5** · Cells of epidermis.

The outermost layer of the epidermis is the *stratum corneum*. It is made up of terminally differentiated, dead keratinocytes (corneocytes). These are perfectly sculpted, flattened hexagons whose complex geometric shape allows for optimal packing. Corneocytes are nonvital epithelial cells that have lost and digested their nucleus, and are loaded with keratin filaments in an amorphous protein matrix, which is held together by the cornified envelope. They are glued together like bricks in a wall by a mortar rich in lipids (ceramides, cholesterol, free fatty acids). According to one estimate, a normal person sheds 50–60 billion corneocytes per day, supposedly adding up to a total annual loss of 4 kg; this amount is dramatically up-regulated in hyperproliferative skin diseases such as psoriasis. Many of these shed corneocytes end up as the "house dust" that settles in your home and work environments.

The stratum corneum is a semipermeable, hydrophobic layer that not only repels microorganisms, water, and chemicals, but also shields the layers of dividing keratinocytes deeper in the epidermis (basal cells) from UV light damage. It is covered with an acidic protective film generated by sweat, sebum, and decomposition products of the rich residential microflora which keeps the skin surface moist and smooth, and hinders the growth of pathogenic microorganisms. Additional defense against infection is provided by antimicrobial peptides (e.g. human β-defensins) that are generated by epidermal keratinocytes and stored in the stratum corneum. Thus, even in the absence of the key cellular protagonists of adaptive immunity (T cells, Langerhans cells), a healthy stratum corneum and its protective acidic film (pH 5.7) provide a tough penetration barrier to potential invaders, along with very effective innate immunity.

The process of terminal differentiation of epidermal keratinocytes originates in the basal layer of the epidermis, and ultimately in a pool of epithelial stem cells located in the bottom of the so-called *rete ridges*. The actual thickness of the epidermis varies widely, from 0.05 mm on the eyelid to 1.5 mm on the sole. Epidermal thickness is the net result of a carefully controlled equilibrium between keratinocyte proliferation in the basal layer, keratinocyte terminal differentiation in the stratum spinosum and granulosum, programmed epidermal cell death (keratinocyte apoptosis), and corneocyte shedding from the stratum corneum. Inherited or acquired deviations from the normal in any of these four parameters greatly disturb epidermal homeostasis and lead to scaling, thickening (lichenification), thinning (atrophy), or tumor formation (viral warts).

There are several types of cell junctions in the epidermis. Each plays an important pathophysiologic role in holding the cells together and allowing them to communicate.

► Desmosomes: many different proteins are involved in the complex structure. Among the most important are the desmogleins (Fig. 1.**6**). Antibodies against desmosomal proteins cause pemphigus (p. 229), while staphylococcal scalded skin syndrome (p. 75) with massive loss of epidermis is caused by a bacterial toxin damaging a desmoglein.

► Adherent junctions: connect actin filaments and help with signaling as well as adherence.

► Gap junctions: formed by connexins; create connecting pores which allow rapid transport of materials or signals between two cells; defects can cause deafness and skin diseases.

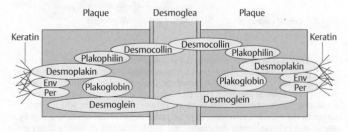

Fig. 1.**6** · Desmosome, showing complex way in which two keratinocytes are held together. Env = envoplakin; Per = periplakin (Image courtesy of Michael Hertl MD, Marburg, Germany).

Roughly one in ten cells in the basal layer of the epidermis is a melanocyte. These cells, derived from the neural crest, produce melanin, package it in organelles (*melanosomes*) and transfer it via long dendrites to epidermal and hair follicle keratinocytes so as to give color to the epidermis and hair. In both structures, melanin not only protects the skin against UV damage and serves as a free-radical scavenger, but also sends important social, psychological, and sexual communication signals to other members of the community. These are so important in human society that an entire industry caters to the modification of hair colors and to a lesser extent skin colors. Apocrine glands complement the social communication activities of the skin by sending invisible olfactory signals (pheromones) that, often only subconsciously, register as "very attractive" or "deeply repulsive." Never underestimate the profound impact a skin disorder can have on an individual's normal functioning in society and self-esteem, even if the disorder appears only trivial to you.

1.4 Hair

In most of our mammalian ancestors, the protective functions of the epidermis were further enhanced by a widespread, dense hair coat. These heavily melanized keratin fibers—being rigid and extremely resistant to wear and tear—provide additional protection against UV light and chemical damage, trauma, and attack; impede the access of airborne insects to the skin; and provide dramatically enhanced properties for skin insulation and thermoregulation (the latter so efficiently that we transform the hair shafts of other mammals into wool sweaters, or even wear fur coats). Furthermore, hair shafts disperse sebum, sweat, and odors over the skin surface, and transport cellular debris and resident parasites out of the follicular canal.

All of these functions of hair are still valid in humans today. The approximately 100 000 scalp hair follicles predominantly serve decorative and communicative functions. Our scalp and beard hairs send widely visible, immediately registered optical signals of social, sexual, cultural, psychological, or even political content to our fellow humans. Not surprisingly, therefore, sudden hair loss or excessive hair growth in cosmetically sensitive skin regions is often a catastrophic event, as the affected individual's psychological equilibrium, self-esteem, and well-functioning in society can be deeply threatened. Though this is often overlooked and underestimated, a similar argument can be made for abnormal nail growth and overactive sweat glands; discolored and misshapen nails, a sweaty shirt, and wet palms all send unwelcome signals and cause distress.

Moreover, we have recently come to understand that the pilosebaceous units that are distributed very irregularly and in strikingly different variants (e.g. vellus, terminal, pubic hair) throughout our entire integument—with very few notable exceptions such as palms and soles—not only tirelessly generate important epithelial skin products (hair shafts, sebum), but also are formidable endocrine factories. The most productive and versatile epithelial stem cells of skin also reside in a special region of the hair follicle's outer root sheath, the *bulge*. The entire epidermis can be regenerated from this source alone. In hair-bearing skin, the numerous hair follicles actually serve as the "bone marrow of the skin," from whose stem cell population skin regeneration (including skin repigmentation) begins. While epithelial stem cells in the epidermis and the hair follicle are the irreplaceable source of epidermal renewal and hair follicle cycling, they and their direct progeny also are subject to malignant degeneration—basal cell carcinomas are usually derived from follicle elements. Remarkably, most recent evidence suggests that the hair follicle epithelium even harbors stem cells derived from the neural crest, from which both neurons and melanocytes can be generated experimentally, while mesenchymal stem cells have been identified in the connective tissue sheath of the hair follicle.

1.5 Basement Membrane Zone

The ridge structure of the avascular epidermis is mirrored by and intertwined with a ridge-like counterpart (*papillary dermis*) in the underlying, much thicker, highly flexible and extremely elastic support layer, the dermis. This central layer of the skin bestows the remarkable mixture of structural firmness and flexibility that is so characteristic of mammalian skin, and is the chief component of leather used in clothes, shoes, and handbags. Together with the basement membrane that links epidermis and dermis, rete ridges and dermal papillae ensure good cohesion of the upper two skin layers, even under conditions of extreme stretch and shear.

The basement membrane zone (BMZ) has a surprisingly intricate architecture (Fig. 1.7). It is jointly generated by epidermal keratinocytes and dermal fibroblasts, and consists of extracellular matrix (type IV and type VII collagen, laminins, nidogen, glycosaminoglycans) and hemidesmosomal components (integrins, bullous pemphigoid antigens, plectin), various adhesion molecules, and a bewilderingly complex array of structural and signaling interactions between an ever-growing number of molecular players. This complexity may result from the fact that the BMZ serves as a very efficient attachment system for the epidermis, while still allowing it full access to nutrients, oxygen, antibodies, complement, and trafficking immune cells arriving via the dermis. Invading microorganisms (and topically applied therapeutic substances) must pass through the BMZ, while noxious products of epidermal metabolism and excess intraepidermal fluid must be removed into the circulation.

Thus, the BMZ represents an entire system of dermoepidermal anchorage, skin flexibility, and elasticity, as well as epithelial–mesenchymal communication and trafficking. Not surprisingly, it is in this dynamic, constantly remodeled dermoepidermal interface where most inflammatory skin diseases manifest themselves, and where defects in individual BMZ components result in a large array of therapy-resistant genodermatoses.

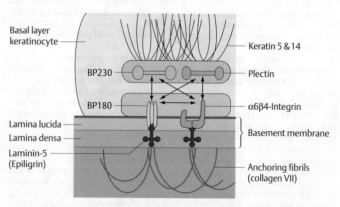

Fig. 1.7 · Basement membrane zone with hemidesmosome and extracellular matrix components (Image courtesy of Michael Hertl MD, Marburg, Germany).

1.6 Dermis

The adjacent dermis that underlies the BMZ is best viewed as a densely populated, well-hydrated, and exquisitely perfused mucopolysaccharide gel with added elastic properties (due to a network of interwoven elastic fibers, which degenerates with increasing sun damage and age), in which many interacting, different cell populations are suspended. Dermal fibroblasts are the key resident cells of the dermis. The location of the mesenchymal stem cells from which these fibroblasts originate is unclear. One likely possibility is the hair follicle connective tissue sheath, whose fibroblast populations may be quite important during cutaneous wound healing, as they may serve as a cell pool for the formation of granulation tissue.

The dermis harbors a rich network of nerves with free nerve endings in the epidermis, a generous network around hair follicles and specialized receptors (Fig. 1.**8**). In addition, the eccrine glands course through the dermis, before emptying sweat onto the epidermal surface. Finally there are complex networks of vessels (Fig. 1.**9**).

Fibroblasts are complemented by migratory immune cells, including the relatively sessile mast cells (preferentially located around skin nerves, blood vessels, and hair follicles), professional phagocytes (macrophages, also called histiocytes) and dermal dendrocytes (most of which may represent a subpopulation of Langerhans cells). These cells form yet another important line of defense against invading microorganisms, where innate and adaptive immunity meet. Mast cells and macrophages are also intimately involved in regulating fibroblast functions and thus fully participate in dermal remodeling under physiological and pathological conditions.

The abundant supply of resident dermal mast cells and macrophages offers additional, immediately operative, innate immune defenses once an infectious agent has trespassed the epidermal defenses, an insect bite has injected undesired material straight into the dermis, or skin trauma has torn an open pathway into the epidermal

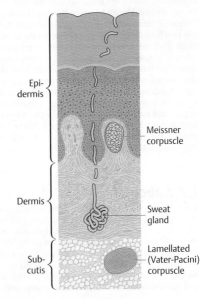

Epi-
dermis

Meissner
corpuscle

Dermis

Sweat
gland

Sub-
cutis

Lamellated
(Vater-Pacini)
corpuscle

Fig. 1.**8** · Specialized nerve receptors in the skin, shown along with an eccrine sweat gland.

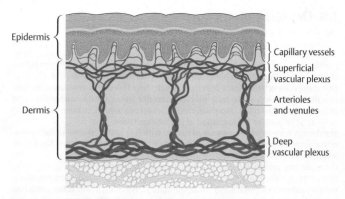

Epidermis

Capillary vessels

Superficial vascular plexus

Arterioles and venules

Dermis

Deep vascular plexus

Fig. 1.**9** · Vascular network of the skin.

immune defenses, suddenly exposing the much less well-defended dermis and sub-cutis to a hostile environment. These dermal mast cells and macrophages secrete a wide array of compounds that very rapidly up-regulate defensive (yet, often enough, also autodestructive) immune responses geared to contain and locally restrain invading infectious agents until the protagonists of specific immunity (Langerhans cells, T cells, and possibly dermal dendrocytes) have been called into action and have become fully operative, and/or until additional innate immune defenses (neutrophils, eosinophils) have been attracted from the skin vasculature.

Recent research shows, however, that the historical distinction between "innate" and "acquired" immunity, in real life and especially in the skin, is much more blurred than our love for simplistic categorization has led us to believe, and that both arms of the skin's immune system are intricately interwoven during essentially all major immune responses our skin can launch. A newly emerging related concept is that of the *dermal microvascular unit*, which consists of intimate and multidirectional interactions between endothelial cells, fibroblasts, smooth muscle cells, perivascular mast cells, and dermal dendrocytes with immune cells that exit from the cutaneous vasculature. This dermal microvascular unit is responsible for far more than the supply of oxygen and nutrients to the skin; it deeply influences immune cell trafficking, vessel tone, and many other aspects of normal skin function. It is here where many inflammatory skin diseases run through critical stages of their pathogenesis, and may be therapeutically targeted most effectively.

1.7 Subcutis

If you are not obese or anorectic, about 10% of your body weight is contributed by the third, deepest and usually thickest layer of your skin—the *subcutis* or subcutaneous fat. The predominant cells of the subcutis are *adipocytes*, highly specialized mesenchymal cells turned into a storage site for fat. The subcutis provides thermal insulation, serves as a crucial energy store, and acts as an important shock absorber for underlying organs and structures. This highly vascularized tissue is also a veritable hormone factory, where most steroid hormones can be metabolized or synthesized, and numerous neurohormones and neuropeptides are generated. Adipocytes also regulate food uptake, general energy metabolism, and resistance or sensitivity to insulin, primarily by the secretion of leptin and adipokines.

1.8 Neuroendocrine-immune Networking

These secretory activities of adipocytes lead us to one of the most fascinating aspects of skin biology: the full integration of our integument into the neural, immune, and endocrine networks that transcend and unite all of our individual organ systems and whose cooperation and coordination ultimately guarantee both our own survival as individuals and that of the human species.

How critical this level of full skin integration is for the entire organism has already been alluded to above, when we discussed the importance of skin as an organ of thermoregulation; sensation; energy, electrolyte and fluid balance; defense against infection; and social communication. Conversely, the skin cannot exist without adequate perfusion, nutrition, and oxygenation. We have learned that all this is largely accomplished by means of intricate vascular and neural networks that connect our skin to rest of the organism and serve as high-velocity, high-capacity conduits for oxygen, nutrients, toxins, mediators of anaphylaxis, neuropeptides, neurotransmitters, action potentials, immune cells, humoral immune components, antigens, hormones, eicosanoids, growth factors, cytokines, and excess fluid (among other things).

But our skin engages in more than networking via conduit systems. It also dispatches individual cells to distant organs, where they elicit responses in other defined cell populations, which then migrate into the skin to execute their characteristic functions. This is exactly what happens when allergic eczema develops in response to environmental antigens, or other type IV immune responses are launched (for example, against infectious agents): intraepidermal Langerhans cells take up, process, and present the antigen in question, and travel via skin lymphatics to the nearest regional lymph node, where they have the highest chances of encountering a T lymphocyte with just the right T-cell receptor that recognizes the antigenic peptide presented by the Langerhans cell's MHC class II molecule. If this most efficient of all antigen-presenting cells finds such a lymphocyte with a cognate T-cell receptor, and appropriate T-cell activation signals are provided (including so-called co-stimulatory ones), that T-cell proliferates, leaves the lymph node and eventually finds its way into the epidermal region that had dispatched Langerhans cells to call for help.

Similar trafficking and recruitment loops have been postulated for T-cell responses to skin tumor antigens, and numerous inflammatory skin diseases or inflammatory skin reactions are based on this basic immunocutaneous loop.

Over the past two decades, it has become clear that keratinocytes not only sport innate immune defenses of their own and are the site from whose midst the above loop originates: they also in crucial secretory activities that orchestrate cutaneous inflammation in response to, for example, allergens, irritants, microorganisms, and damage by UV radiation. By secreting a wide spectrum of agents from proinflammatory (TNF α, IL-1, chemokines, IFN-γ) to anti-inflammatory/tolerogenic (IL-10, TGFβ1, or IL-1RA) the skin epithelium thus profoundly influences whether a potent inflammatory response is triggered or suppressed, and which type of immune response is favored (e.g. type I or type IV). Other protagonists of the skin immune system, such as mast cells and macrophages, contribute to these long-neglected "unspecific" but important immunomodulatory controls that regulate immune responses within and far beyond the skin. Thus the skin has become appreciated as a central player even in systemic immunity, not just a passive battleground for the activities of T and B cells, as it had long been considered.

To complicate things further, immune responses in the skin and elsewhere in the body are also influenced by a plethora of additional, intracutaneously released or generated compounds that are not generally considered as primary immunomodulators. This includes the release of neuropeptides and neurotransmitters from skin nerve endings during neurogenic inflammation as well as the long unsuspected, yet powerful, endocrine and neuroendocrine activities of the skin. We now know that the skin, and most notably its pilosebaceous units, are active in the synthesis and metabolism of key steroid hormones such as androgens, estrogens, and vitamin D_3 derivatives. Moreover, they also generate hormones such as corticotropin releasing hormone (CRH), adrenocorticotropic hormone (ACTH), β-endorphin, cortisol, prolactin, and melatonin, and many other signaling molecules traditionally associated with extracutaneous functions of the nervous, hemopoietic, hepatobiliary and/or endocrine systems. Numerous cell populations in the skin are now known to also express functional, cognate receptors to all these secreted (neuro-) endocrine signals. This makes it much less of a mystery why psycho-emotional stress and hormonal changes can trigger so many skin diseases, change their course, or modulate their response to therapy.

To give one final example, it is now clear that the skin is an abundant source for nerve growth factors (neurotrophins). These are generated in quantity by the skin epithelium, not only in order to guide its own innervation during skin development and hair follicle cycling, but also to regulate its own growth, regeneration, and death in an autocrine and paracrine manner as well as to modulate the skin immune system (especially mast cell functions) and skin repair.

Thus, whatever happens in the skin immediately becomes part of wider neuroendocrine–immune networks, which can affect far-distant regions of our body and systemic response patterns. Conversely, numerous extracutaneous events, for better or worse, tightly link our integument via the above networks into what happens elsewhere. Moreover, the skin itself locally produces and uses classical signals of endocrine, neuroendocrine, neural, and immune communication to regulate its own growth, death, differentiation, repair, and/or metabolic activities.

1.9 Outlook

At the end of this brief introduction to the fascinating universe of skin biology, reflect a little longer on what we really know about the functions of our skin.

It is important to remember that we have come to understand these functions gradually, step by step, largely by observing what happens when normal skin functions are compromised or lost, are never fully acquired in the first place, or are overactive. For example:

▶ The skin's crucial role as a defense against infection system and an immune organ becomes evident in viral, bacterial, and fungal skin infections, as well as in allergic and autoimmune skin diseases.

▶ The skin's metabolic importance is demonstrated by the dire consequences of vitamin D deficiency due to inadequate sun exposure.

▶ The development of skin carcinoma as a result of excessive sun exposure or defective DNA damage repair systems highlights the role of the skin in protection against UV radiation.

▶ Vitiligo, albinism, and hair loss illustrate the consequences of changes in our social communication image.

▶ Chronic pruritus and peripheral neuropathy in diabetic patients point us to the sensory functions of skin.

► Skin ulcers, xerosis, excessive scaling, and disorders of keratinization such as the ichthyoses remind us of the crucial barrier function of our integument.

Yet, if our concepts of skin functions are essentially based on a "damage assessment strategy," we are likely to have missed many additional functions whose failure or absence does not cause easily apparent skin alterations. We still need to better comprehend the functional significance of the neuroendocrine–immune networking of the skin. Thus, the quest for understanding the full complexity of skin functions and skin physiology has only just begun.

And this is where *you* come in: When you use this book as your personal assistant to help you diagnose and treat defined skin diseases, do not miss the great opportunity that presents itself when you carefully look at, and reflect upon, the signals that the skin of your patient is trying to send you.

Remember: This is biology talking to you—just listen!

Table 1.1 · Cellular protagonists in the skin

Cell	Location	Function	Comments
Keratinocytes	Epidermis Hair follicle Nail apparatus	Barrier, UV protection, antimicrobial defense, secretion of enzymes and regulatory molecules, major endocrine and metabolic activity	Terminally differentiate into nonvital hexagonal corneocytes; epithelial stem cells located in bulge region of the hair follicle outer root sheath and epidermal rete ridges
Sebocytes	Dermis; usually associated with hair follicle ("pilosebaceous unit")	Sebum production, secretion of enzymes, regulatory molecules, major endocrine and metabolic activity	Derived from hair follicle keratinocytes; sebum production by holocrine secretion of sebocytes
Apocrine gland cells	Subcutis; usually associated with hair follicle ("folliculosebaceous-apocrine unit")	Production of apocrine sweat and pheromones	Derived from hair follicle keratinocytes, neural control: adrenergic; sweat production by "decapitation secretion"
Eccrine gland cells	Subcutis	Thermoregulation, excretion via eccrine sweat; many medications eliminated via sweat	Derived from epidermal keratinocytes; deeply coiled glands analogous to glomeruli in some ways
Myocytes	Arrector pili muscle, blood vessel smooth muscle	Contraction	Regulates blood flow, causes "goose bumps" by pulling hair erect
Granulocytes	Skin vasculature	Natural immunity	Neutrophils, basophils, eosinophils in normal, uninflamed skin almost exclusively in the blood vessel lumen
Vascular endothelial cells	Blood vessels	Formation, regeneration of blood vessels, perfusion	Interact with immune cells to further local immune response

Continued Table 1.1 ►

Table 1.1 · Continued

Cell	Location	Function	Comments
Lymphatic endothelial cells	Lymph vessels	Intracutaneous fluid balance, passageway for immunocyte trafficking and antigen transport, nutrition, removal of metabolic and other skin products	Dermal endothelial cells are an integral component of the dermal microvascular unit, where trafficking immune cells interact with endothelial cells, fibroblasts, smooth muscle cells, and perifollicular mast cells, macrophages and dermal dendrocytes
Erythrocytes	Skin vasculature	Oxygenation	In normal, uninflamed skin exclusively in the blood vessel lumen; amount and oxygenation status of erythrocytes in the papillary plexus is a key determinant of skin color
Merkel cells	Epidermis, hair follicle	Mechanosensory cell, (modulation of epithelial growth? neurosecretory functions?)	Origin disputed: epithelial or neural crest-derived?
Melanocytes	Epidermis, hair follicle	Protection from damage by UV light and reactive oxygen species; hair shaft pigmentation; other secretory activities	Neural crest-derived, dendritic cells that produce melanin and transfer it to keratinocytes and hair follicle cells
T lymphocytes	All skin compartments (but mainly epidermis and distal hair follicle epithelium)	Antimicrobial defense, tumor immunosurveillance, regulation of inflammatory responses	Invisible in routine histology of normal epidermis; preferred residence in epidermis (= epidermotropism) and distal hair follicle epithelium with dendritic morphology; traffic between epidermis, regional lymph node/spleen and circulation
Langerhans cells	Epidermis (dermis, distal hair follicle epithelium)	Chief antigen-presenting cell of the skin	Dendritic morphology; emigrate from epidermis to regional lymph node for antigen/allergen presentation to T cells; one dermal subpopulation of Langerhans cell-like cells is called dermal dendrocytes

Table 1.1 · Continued

Cell	Location	Function	Comments
Mast cells	Dermis, subcutis; preferential location around skin nerves, blood vessels and hair follicles	Major component of natural immunity: rapid defense against bacterial and parasitic infection; possibly involved in wound healing, angiogenesis, hair growth control	Mast cell degranulation leads to urticaria and angioedema; key role in neurogenic inflammation; "central switchboard" of inflammation and tissue remodeling
Neurons	Neuronal cell body of sensory neurons located in dorsal root ganglion or trigeminal ganglion; only axons project into the skin	Sensation, "trophic" functions, immunomodulation (e.g. neurogenic inflammation via induction of mast cell degranulation)	Intracutaneous nerve fibers have multiple different functions beyond sensation; autonomic fibers regulate blood vessel tone and sweat production
Glial cells (Schwann cells)	Sheath myelinated intracutaneous nerve fibers	Maintenance and modulation of nerve fiber function; release of "trophic" signals (nerve growth factors)	Important role during axonal regeneration during wound healing; rich sources of neurotrophins
Fibroblasts	Dermis, connective tissue sheath and dermal papilla of hair follicle	Secretion, organization, digestion, and remodeling of extracellular matrix (collagen and elastic fibers); generation and remodeling of basement membranes (together with epithelial cells)	Specialized fibroblasts of the hair follicle retain inductive/morphogenetic properties throughout life and dictate hair follicle size and growth activity; hair follicle connective tissue sheath contains mesenchymal stem cells, important for wound healing
Adipocytes	Subcutis	Thermal insulation, physical cushion/buffer function and energy store by fat accumulation; secretion of regulatory molecules, major endocrine and metabolic activity	Organized in well-vascularized fat lobules, separated by thin septae, which connect the subcutis to the underlying muscle fascia
Macrophages	Dermis, subcutis	Key phagocytes of the skin; regulate fibroblast functions	Also termed histiocytes; multiple macrophages coalesce to form multinucleated giant cells e.g. in foreign body, sarcoid, or tuberculoid granulomata

Dermatologic Diagnosis

2 Dermatologic Diagnosis

2.1 Components of the Dermatologic Evaluation

The diagnosis of skin diseases is not as difficult as it initially seems, so do not let yourself be intimidated. The keys to successful diagnosis are systemic and complete skin examination, an understanding of anatomy and physiology of the skin, and the use of basic dermatologic terminology.

► **Description of skin findings** (p. 7): Dermatology is a visual specialty. The careful morphologic description of cutaneous changes is at the center of dermatologic diagnosis. This skill must be learned, as it often leads to the correct diagnosis in itself, and cannot be replaced by laboratory examinations or other investigative procedures.

► **Simple clinical tests** (p. 22): One of the joys of dermatology is relative freedom from tracking down complex laboratory and imaging reports. On the other hand, a number of simple procedures carried out by dermatologists can rapidly indicate the correct diagnosis.

► **History** (p. 24): Although a dermatologic diagnosis can often be made without taking a history, relevant information should be collected to aid in the differential diagnostic process, to be aware of other medical conditions the patient is confronting, and to be aware of any medications the patient is taking.

2.2 Description of Skin Findings

The following tips will help improve your skills in diagnosing skin lesions:

► **Develop a logical and systemic approach to skin examination**: Approaching each patient in the same way, carefully examining the skin, and documenting your findings in a reproducible, legible fashion is the most reliable way to make correct diagnoses.

► **Try to examine the skin in a room with daylight.**

► **Examine the entire skin surface during the first dermatologic examination.** This should include:
  • Palms and soles, ears, submammary, interdigital, axillary, inguinal, genital, and perianal skin.
  • Adjacent mucosa including lips, mouth, conjunctivae, nasal mucosa, and in some instances anus.
  • Skin appendages (hair and nails) as well as scalp.
  • Screening for malignant melanoma (p. 396) and other skin malignancies (p. 419).
  • Assessment of general skin appearance (color, texture, dryness, hydration, odor).
  • Evidence for exposure to sunlight, nicotine, other noxious agents.

► **Match objective evidence to subjective complaints**; a patient who denies itch but has numerous excoriations may have an underlying psychosocial problem.

► A **total skin examination** should always be offered, although some patients may not consent. In the case of widespread rashes, it is mandatory. Consider this scenario—a patient presents with a skin problem on the hands and you fail to check the feet, where a fungal infection is obvious; you have made the entire diagnostic process slower.

▶ **Look with your fingers.** Many lesions, especially actinic keratoses, can be more easily felt or palpated than seen. Palpation also helps to determine the depth and consistency of a lesion, which may aid in the differential diagnosis.

▶ **Determine the anatomic location of the lesion:**
- Is it epidermal, dermal or subcutaneous?
- Are the skin appendages, blood vessels, or nerves involved?

▶ **Determine the primary symptom:** This often simplifies the diagnostic process.

▶ **Become skilled in using simple diagnostic aids:** The use of some of the procedures outlined below should be almost automatic. For example, if a rash is scaly, most dermatologists almost routinely do a potassium hydroxide (KOH) examination for fungi.

2.3 Primary and Secondary Lesions

Lesion morphology is the code language of dermatology. Using a surprisingly limited number of names for lesions and then a somewhat more complex series of modifiers, it is possible to describe everything one sees on the skin. Primary lesions (Table 2.**1**) are the basic elements of skin morphology; they can undergo a variety of changes to become secondary lesions (Table 2.**2**).

▶ Figure 2.**1** shows the primary and secondary lesions, while Figure 2.**2** demonstrates how the border of a lesion can vary.

Table 2.1 · Primary lesions

Lesion	Description
Flat; not palpable	
Macule	Localized change in color of the skin: "A blind man cannot find a macule."
	Possible colors and their common causes:
	Red: Hyperemia (erythema), telangiectases (small dilated vessels), leakage of blood (purpura, petechiae, ecchymosis, suggillation)
	Blue: Cyanosis, hematoma (black eye), dermal melanin
	Brown: Dermal and epidermal melanin, hemosiderin
	White: Anemia, vasoconstriction, loss of melanin
	Yellow: Carotenoids, bile, solar elastosis
	Gray-black: Epidermal melanin, heavy metals, tar, dithranol, foreign bodies
	Decorative tattoos can have many colors
Raised; palpable	
Papule	<5 mm in diameter, caused by increased thickness in epidermis, dermis, or both
Nodule	>5 mm
Plaque	Large flat slightly raised lesion, always >5 mm
Vesicle	<5 mm, filled with clear fluid (p. 702)
Bulla	>5 mm, filled with clear fluid (p. 704)
Pustule	Lesion filled with pus
Hive (urtica)	Transient papule or plaque caused by dermal edema (p. 706)

Dermatologic Diagnosis

Table 2.2 · Secondary lesions

Lesion	Description
Pustule	Pustules can be both primary, or develop secondarily from vesicles and bulla
Scale	Scales are visible aggregates of corneocytes, varying in size and color
Crust	Dried serum or exudate, often admixed with scale
Erosion	Superficial defect involving only epidermis
Excoriation	Defect extending into dermis, caused by scratching
Ulcer	Chronic defect extending into dermis or subcutaneous defect, which develops as a result of tissue necrosis and heals poorly
Scar	May be raised, flat (rarely) or atrophic; result of healing of skin defect
Cyst	Space lined by epithelium and usually filled with products of lining cells (keratin, sebum, mucin)
Necrosis	Dead tissue

2.4 Additional Descriptive Terms

Modifiers Used to Describe Lesions

▶ **Color:** Both name of color and its nature (uniform, irregular, patchy).
▶ **Form:** Configuration, border, and surface:
   • *Circinate:* arched or rounded border.
   • *Annular:* circular or ring-shaped.
   • *Discoid, nummular:* disk or coin-shaped.
   • *Serpiginous:* winding, twisting (snake-like).
   • *Iris* or *cockade* (target-like).
   • and many more, including *oval, finger-shaped, leaf-like, swirled,* or *starry.*
▶ **Border:** Sharp (well-circumscribed) or vague (blurred).
▶ **Surface:** Smooth, rough, warty, vegetating, glistening, dull.
▶ **Consistency:** Soft, doughy, hard, fluctuant, lobed, knotty, moveable, fixed, attached to ...

Patterns of Distribution

▶ **Linear:** Following a line.
▶ **Lines of Blaschko:** Following embryologic skin lines (Fig. 2.3).
▶ **Reticular:** Net-like.
▶ **Grouped.**
▶ **Herpetiform:** Arranged in clusters, grape-like.
▶ **Zosteriform:** Following a dermatome (p. 62).
▶ **Discrete:** Solitary.
▶ **Confluent:** Blending together.
▶ **Chessboard pattern:** Arranged in rectangular patterns.
▶ **Disseminated:** Randomly distributed.

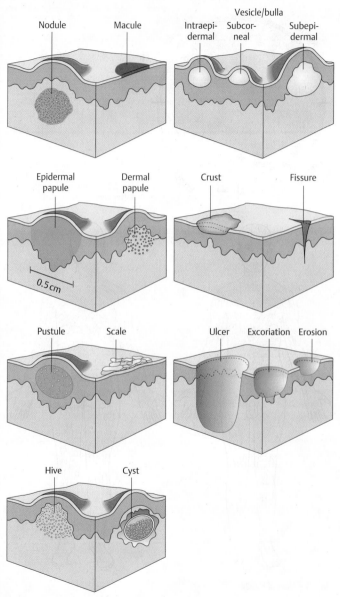

Fig. 2.**1** · Primary and secondary lesions.

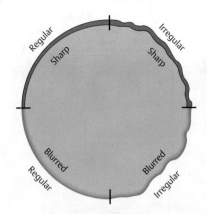

Fig. 2.2 · Borders of lesions (after Steigleder).

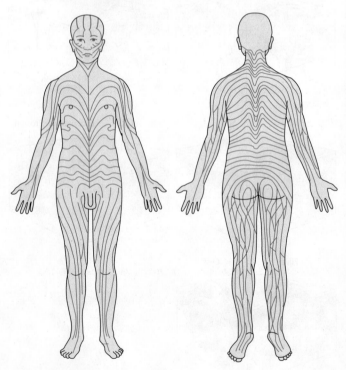

Fig. 2.3 · Lines of Blaschko.

Distribution Over the Skin Surface

► **Degree of spread:** Localized, regional, generalized (widespread), universal.
► **Limited to certain areas** (such as palms and soles or scalp).
► **Specific patterns** (p. 709): Symmetrical, asymmetrical, light-exposed skin, light-protected skin, intertriginous areas, seborrheic areas, pressure points, sites of pre-dilection.

Relation to the Skin Appendages

► Each lesion **centered about a hair**, producing a distinctive pattern.
► **Interfollicular:** Not involving hairs.
► **Palmoplantar:** Limited to palms and soles, thus not connected with hairs.
► Favoring regions with large concentrations of **sebaceous glands or sweat glands**.

Description of Complex Findings

► **Note:** The following terms are frequently used in dermatologic descriptions but are not traditionally considered primary or secondary lesions.
► **Atrophy:** Loss of substance of the skin.
► **Ecchymosis:** Large area of extravasation of erythrocytes.
► **Enanthem:** Abrupt appearance of mucosal lesions, similar to exanthem.
► **Erythema:** Redness of the skin (p. 707).
► **Erythroderma:** Diffuse redness of the entire skin, usually associating with scaling.
► **Exanthem:** Abrupt appearance of diffuse or generalized similar skin lesions (usu-ally represents viral infection or drug reaction).
► **Lichenification:** Response of skin to chronic rubbing, leading to thickening with accentuated markings.
► **Livedo:** Blue-red discoloration of skin due to passive congestion of vessels, often with net-like pattern.
► **Petechiae:** Tiny areas of extravasation of erythrocytes, usually pinhead-size.
► **Poikiloderma:** Combination of telangiectases, atrophy and pigmentary changes (p. 706).
► **Purpura:** General term for extravasation of erythrocytes into the skin.
► **Rhagade or fissure:** Linear split or defect, extending into dermis and often origi-nating from an orifice.
► **Sclerosis:** Hardening and thickening of skin, so that it is less freely moveable, often associated with contraction so that involved area lies below level of normal skin.
► **Sinus:** Tract lined with epithelium, often discharging secretions.
► **Suggillation:** Synonym for ecchymosis, also used for bruise or contusion.
► **Telangiectases:** Small, irreversibly dilated blood vessels (p. 706).

Description of General Skin Condition, Vascular Status, and Associated Findings

► **General terms:** Xerotic (dry), seborrheic (oily), ichthyotic (scaly), actinic damage, atrophic, thickened, abnormal texture, hyper-, hypo- or anhidrotic.
► **Vascular status:** Cyanotic, pale, cold, warm, edematous, with varicosities, necrotic.
► **Nature of wound healing:**
  • Central or peripheral healing, with scarring or atrophy.
  • Pigmentary changes, erosion or ulcer, crust, or scale.
► **Dynamics of lesion:** All lesions in same stage or lesions in different stages.
► **Associated findings:** Lymphadenopathy, fever, malaise, as examples.

Dermatologic Diagnosis

Simple Clinical Tests

These tests can be done during the initial examination.

► **Palpation:** Consistency, movability, adherence, borders, painful or tender, pulsation? Skin warm/cold, moist/dry? Peripheral pulses?
► **Remove crusts:** Bleeding, base of wound, extent of lesion.
► **Express secretions:** Nature, consistency, color, odor, amount.
► **Pull off scales or deposits:** Easily removed, firmly attached.
◘ *Note:* Scales mean epidermal involvement. Always remove scales or crusts; they may be "hiding" an underlying tumor.
► **Tug on hairs:** Easily breakable, readily removed, hair bulb visible.
► **Insert probe:** Can be used to explore sinus tract; used in the past to analyze tubercular lesions, which were relatively insensitive to such pressure.
► **Provocation tests:** Manipulate lesions by rubbing, pressing, applying heat or cold, having patient exercise.
► **Look for specific clinical signs:** Dermographism, pathergy (p. 257), Nikolski phenomenon (p. 230), Darier sign (p. 466).

2.5 Tools of the Trade

Spatula

► **Tongue blade:** Used to remove crusts and scales, test for dermographism, and examine mouth.
► **Glass spatula:** Used for diascopy. By pressing on the skin hard enough to exclude blood flow, one can eliminate purely vascular lesions and better appreciate dermal changes, such as the "apple jelly" color of many granulomatous infiltrates (tuberculosis, sarcoidosis).

Hand Lens

A hand lens or *loupe* is an essential instrument for anyone examining the skin. It allows a better view and easier appreciation of finer details.

Dermatoscopy

► **Synonyms:** Epiluminescence microscopy, dermoscopy.
► **Definition:** Method of observing superficial layers of skin using 10–100× magnification with oil immersion. Both hand-held and computer-assisted instruments are available.
► **Uses:**
  • *Differential diagnosis of pigmented skin lesions:* Separating melanocytic lesions from vascular lesions, basal cell carcinomas, dermatofibromas and others.
  • *Differential diagnosis of melanoma:* Using the dermatoscope, one can better distinguish between dysplastic or atypical melanocytic nevi and melanomas, increasing the diagnosis accuracy to around 90%. This approach is especially useful in patients with multiple atypical lesions and those at high risk of developing melanoma.
  • *Detailed examination of the skin:*
    – Proximal nail fold to look for abnormal vessels in connective tissue disorders.
    – Wickham striae as sign of lichen planus.

- Cauliflower surface with thrombotic capillary loops suggests verrucae.
- Scabies burrows (hang glider sign).
- On the scalp, cadaver hairs and exclamation point hairs suggest alopecia areata, loss of follicular openings indicates scarring alopecia, and follicular hyperkeratoses point towards lichen planus.

► **Procedure:**
- Apply appropriate oil (olive, peanut, immersion) or sonographic gel to the skin to improve the optic interface between skin and dermatoscope lens, which is gently pressed onto the skin.

🟣 *Caution:* When the skin surface is not relatively flat, dermatoscopy is less effective. This applies to nodular tumors and on mucosal surfaces. In curved areas, as between the digits, a smaller lens is available with some instruments.

► **Instruments:**
- *Dermatoscope:* 10× magnification, using achromatic lens and halogen or diode light source.
- *Stereomicroscope:* Allows 40–100× magnification.
- *Digital image processing:* When the optical system is connected to a computer, digital images can be processed and stored. Such a system allows rapid retrieval for later comparison and eliminates all the problems associated with storing many clinical slides. In addition, most systems have a computer-assisted analysis system, helping to distinguish between melanocytic nevi and melanomas. The main disadvantage is their high cost.

Wood's Light Examination

► **Definition:** UV radiation from a mercury-vapor source is passed through a nickel oxide filter, producing light at a wave length of about 365 nm.

► **Uses:**
- *Dermatophyte infection: Microsporum* species that infect hairs impart a green fluorescence. Wood's light can be used for screening or for control of therapy.

🟣 *Caution:* Both sebum and salicylic acid preparations may have blue-green fluorescence; also the scales do not fluoresce, just infected hairs. In addition, *Trichophyton* infections do not fluoresce.

- *Favus: Trichophyton schoenleinii* imparts a green fluorescence.
- *Erythrasma:* Coral red fluorescence.
- *Trichomycosis axillaris:* Orange fluorescence.
- *Tinea versicolor:* Orange fluorescence.
- *Pseudomonas:* Green fluorescence.
- *Porphyrin:* Red fluorescence of skin and teeth in some porphyrias; fluorescence of urine in others.
- *Pigment abnormalities:* Hypopigmentation can be distinguished from depigmentation, vitiligo more readily seen, ash leaf macules in tuberous sclerosis and café-au-lait macules in neurofibromatosis more easily found.
- *Tetracycline:* Can be identified in teeth, keratin plugs.
- *Contact allergens:* Some allergens fluoresce and can be found on the skin or in cosmetics; examples include halogenated salicylanilides and furocoumarins.
- *Mineral oil:* Remains in hair follicles and can be seen after washing (as in oil acne).
- *Miscellaneous:* Topical medications or protective creams can be labeled with fluorescent marker, allowing control of usage patterns.

Search for Parasites

▶ **Scabies:** Dermatoscopy can be very useful, showing the classic "hang glider" sign when the female is found at the end of the burrow. Another approach is to searched carefully for an intact burrow, cover it with immersion oil, unroof it carefully with a large-bore needle or fine scalpel blade, and search for mites and eggs under low magnification.

▶ **Lice:** Look carefully for moving objects on the hairs, adjacent skin and, in the case of pediculosis corporis, on the seams of the clothing. Pick them up with tweezers and fix to a slide with adhesive tape or xylol and then examine. In the same ways, nits can be separated from hair casts.

Other Diagnostic Procedures

Other tests and examinations are discussed as relevant under specialized topics such as diseases of hair, mycology, phlebology, and andrology.

2.6 History

Principles

The history is not as crucial to dermatologic diagnosis as it is in most other specialties, but it often provides valuable clues and should be taken carefully when the physical examination has not provided a diagnosis.

When allergic reactions, infections, exogenous damage, drug reactions, or cutaneous manifestations of systemic diseases are being considered, the history often is the only way to obtain the diagnosis. In addition, it is often essential in planning therapy.

Procedure

The most useful approach is to concentrate on a few **key questions**, which can be expanded upon depending on the clinical situation. The patient's answers also provide the framework for additional questions. Questioning should be direct, but not aggressive; preserving the doctor–patient relationship is more important than any single question.

▶ *When exactly did the skin changes start?*

⚠ Caution: Patients often gives misleading answers as they either have not noticed the early stages of their diseases or have ignored them.

▶ *Where exactly did the skin changes start?*

⚠ Caution: The first changes may have developed at a site where the patient could not easily observe them.

▶ *Are the lesions symptomatic?* (Do they burn, itch, feel tight, warm, cold?)

⚠ Caution: Symptoms such as itching or pain may turn out to be misleading. Do not ignore the possibility of scabies just because the patient says the lesions do not itch.

▶ *How did the lesions spread?*

▶ *How did the individual lesions first look and how have they changed?*

⚠ Caution: Patients often have a different understanding of morphologic terms than do physicians. Be sure to ask what is really meant by terms such as "pimple," "boil," "eczema,"or "sore."

► *What do you think started the problem? What makes it worse?*
► Ask what the patient was doing when the problem started. Some diseases are typically made worse by cold, exercise, or the like. Often the patient may provide valuable clues, but just as often their assessment of etiology or causality is very misleading—remain skeptical, without showing it.
► *How have you treated it so far?*
► Frequent washing or the use of a tincture may explain why an exanthem is very dry; use of an ointment in the groin may clarify the development of macerated lesions.

If the answer is still unclear, then take a complete medical, social and family history, as well as a detailed medication history.

Additional helpful questions include:
► *Have you ever had anything similar to this before?*
► *What was the diagnosis then?*
► *Do you have any skin problems elsewhere* (mouth, feet, nails, scalp, genital region, perianal region, groin, axillae, ears)?
► *What has been the influence of external factors* (sun, work, eating, drinking, cosmetics, stress, medications) or internal factors (menses, pregnancy, nursing, illnesses)?
► *What are the associated signs and symptoms?*
► *How do you feel otherwise* (malaise, fever, weight loss, night sweats)?
► *What medications are you taking?* Be sure to ask about tranquilizers, sleeping pills, vitamins, headache preparations, laxatives, appetite control pills and natural products. Patients often do not consider one or more of these categories as medications, and fail to report them.
► Lifestyle—drugs, alcohol, smoking, stress.
► Sexual practices, last time you had sex (when relevant).
► *Any systemic signs or symptoms before skin disease started* (prodrome)?
► *Any other illnesses?* Be sure to ask about cardiovascular, renal, hepatic, thyroid, rheumatologic diseases, HIV, diabetes mellitus.
► *Personal or family history of atopic dermatitis, hay fever or asthma?* Other allergies?
► Ethnic background.
► Foreign travel, especially to tropical regions.
► *How much does the skin disease influence daily function* (quality of life assessment)?
► Psychosocial situation—job, family, relationships, handicaps.

2.7 Histologic Diagnosis

Principles

► **Indications** for a histologic examination include:
  • All excised tumors and pigmented lesions.
  • Differential diagnostic questions.
  • Help with difficult or unclear diagnoses.
  • *Legal or cautionary reasons:* Sometimes, even though the diagnosis is clear, histologic proof is wise before embarking on potentially dangerous therapy.
► The choice of an **appropriate site and lesions**, the **care** with which the biopsy is taken, the **method** of fixation and processing, and the provision of **all relevant clinical data** all contribute greatly to the utility of a skin biopsy.

► **Importance of additional information:** The histological diagnosis of **tumors** can usually be made without a history, but is much easier and effective when historical data is available. In the case of **inflammatory dermatoses**, very few have a pathognomonic histological picture, so that the quality of the additional information almost directly correlates with the quality of the histological diagnosis.

Taking the Biopsy

► The biopsy must be large and deep enough.
► Avoid squeezing (crush artifact) by trying to pop out or lift out without a forceps.
► Place immediately in fixative; do not let the biopsy dry out.
► Intact lesions should be biopsied; ruptured blisters or excoriated papules provide little information.
► Punch biopsies should just include lesional skin, since they cannot be oriented during processing (Fig. 2.**4**). Punch biopsies in hair-bearing areas should be parallel to the direction of hair shafts (Fig. 2.**5**).
► If you are considering atrophy or cutaneous tissue changes, then an elliptical biopsy from the edge of the lesion including perilesional skin is helpful for orientation and comparison (Fig. 2.**6**).
► Only very small pieces of tissue (< 1 mm³) are needed for electron microscopy.

Fixation

► **Light microscopy:**
  • *Solution:* Standard is 10% buffered formaldehyde; when specimens are mailed, usually 4% is employed. Minimum fixation period is 24 hours.
  • Be sure there is enough solution; the ideal proportion is at least 10 times as much solution as tissue.
  • Formaldehyde solution is not well suited for molecular biological investigations.

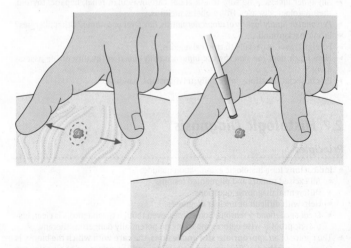

Fig. 2.**4** · **Punch biopsy.** Tension applied perpendicular to the skin tension lines will produce a more easily closed biopsy site.

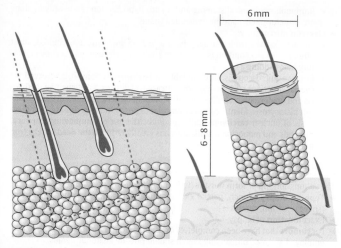

Fig. 2.**5** · **Scalp biopsy.** Angle of incision should be parallel to the hair shafts.

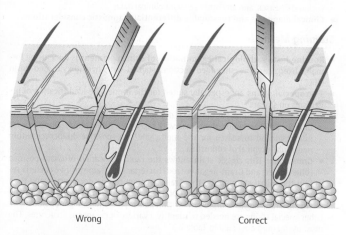

Wrong   Correct

Fig. 2.**6** · **Spindle-shaped excision.** The incision should be perpendicular to the skin surface, insuring a broad-based biopsy with an adequate sampling of the subcutaneous fat.

▶ **Immunofluorescence, immunohistochemical staining, and molecular biological studies:**
  • Check with the responsible laboratory for appropriate fixative. For immunofluorescence studies, special transport medium or freezing is usually chosen.
  • Frozen sections should be placed in a special plastic tube (perhaps filled with 0.9% NaCl solution), closed and immediately frozen in liquid nitrogen.

- Immunohistochemical staining and in-situ hybridization can usually be done on formalin-fixed, paraffin-embedded tissue.

▶ **Electron microscopy:**

- Special fixatives, which usually have a limited shelf life, are required; most often Karnovsky solution is used. Check with the electron microscopy laboratory before doing a biopsy.
- Electron microscopy is only available in larger institutions. It is reserved for special situations such as rapid identification of viruses, assessment of ichthyosis and epidermolysis bullosa, identification of Birbeck granules in Langerhans cell histocytosis, identification of vascular deposits in Fabry disease, and diagnosis of unclear carcinomas and sarcomas. The use of immunohistochemical methods and monoclonal antibodies has greatly reduced the need for electron microscopy.

Submission Slip

The submission slip or form must include the following information:

▶ **Type of biopsy** (punch, partial excision, total excision, re-excision, tangential (shave) excision, curettage).
▶ Exact **location** of biopsy.
▶ For **tumors** that have been completely excised, some system of marking should be employed and a accompanying sketch should provide anatomic details.
▶ **Important clinical details including:** duration of disease, age and type of lesion biopsied, size and distribution (for widespread disease), previous treatment, associated diseases, and any other relevant clinical data.
▶ **Clinical diagnosis and reasonable differential diagnostic considerations.**

Staining Methods

▶ **Routine histopathological examination of skin specimens** is done using formalin-fixed, paraffin-embedded sections stained with hematoxylin and eosin (H&E).
▶ Two **special stains** are especially suited for the immediate identification of organisms on smears:

- *Methylene blue stain:* Let the smear dry. Place in a dilute solution of methylene blue for 20–30 seconds, then rinse with tap water. Allow to dry. Observe with immersion oil to search for the methylene blue–positive diplococci within neutrophils typical of gonorrhea.
- *Gram stain:* This classic stain allows the rapid separation of Gram-positive (blue–violet) and Gram-negative (red) bacteria. The Gram-positive bacteria retain the initial stain, while the Gram-negative can be decolorized and then stained with a red counterstain. Commercial sets of dyes are used on a fixed smear. Gram-negative diplococci within neutrophils indicate gonorrhea.

▶ Other special stains are needed to identify a variety of cutaneous structures. The most useful ones are listed in Table 2.**3**.

Immunofluorescence

Principle:

- *Direct immunofluorescence* (DIF) staining labels a variety of antigens, antibodies, complement factors, fibrin, and other structures with fluorescent-labeled antibodies that can then be seen using a special microscope. Most commonly autoantibodies deposited during inflammatory reactions are identified in the

Table 2.3 · Common special stains

Stain	Used to identify:
Hematoxylin-eosin	(Routine)
Alcian blue	Mucin
Congo red	Amyloid
Fite	Mycobacteria
Fontana-Masson	Melanin
Giemsa	Mast cells
Hale (colloidal iron)	Mucin
Masson trichrome	Collagen
Methenamine silver	Fungi, basement membrane
Periodic acid–Schiff (PAS)	Fungi, glycogen, basement membrane
Silver nitrate	Melanin
Toluidine blue	Mucin
Von Kossa	Calcium
Verhoeff–van Gieson	Elastic fibers
Warthin–Starry	Spirochetes

patient's skin, using frozen tissue cut with a cryostat, to which antibodies are applied. DIF can also be used to identify microorganisms.

- *In indirect immunofluorescence* (IIF) the patient's serum is applied to normal skin or foreign issue (monkey esophagus, bladder epithelium, cultured cells). Any circulating antibodies that attach to target structures are then identified by a second application of labeled antibodies directed usually against antibody structures. The titer of serum that produces a positive response can be measured.
- ▶ **Uses:** Bullous autoimmune dermatoses, lupus erythematosus, other collagen–vascular disorders, lichen planus, and vasculitis. The diagnostic indications for immunofluorescence examination are shown in Table 2.**4**.

Immunohistochemical Methods

- ▶ **Principle:** Antibodies are available to identify a wide variety of antigens in both fresh and formalin-fixed tissue. The antibodies bind in a highly selective manner, often to small epitopes. They can be visualized with a variety of markers including enzymes and fluorescent dyes (Table 2.**5**).
- ▶ **Uses:** This technique is critical for the identification and classification of lymphomas as well as for the diagnosis of a wide variety of sarcomas and other tumors. In addition, the nature of inflammatory infiltrates can be assessed.
- ▰ *Caution:* Tumor cells may fail to express an antigen for their profile changes as they undergo mutations. One should not rely on a single antigen for diagnosis, but use a panel of markers to increase accuracy.

Table 2.4 · Diagnostic guidelines for immunofluorescence

Disease	Target antigen	Biopsy	Findings
Bullous dermatoses			
Pemphigus group			
1 Pemphigus vulgaris (suprabasal blisters)	Desmoglein 1,3 and plakoglobin	*HE:* Border of small fresh blister *DIF:* Perilesional intact skin or mucosa	*DIF:* 1, 3 IgG in intercellular spaces of epidermis, as well as C3, rarely IgM or IgA
2 Pemphigus foliaceus (subcorneal blisters)	Desmoglein 1	*IIF:* Serum	2 Intraepidermal IgG, C3
3 Paraneoplastic pemphigus (suprabasal blisters)	Plakin family: (desmoplakin 1,2, envoplakin, periplakin, plectin); desmogleins; BP-230		*IIF:* 1, 2 In 90%, circulating ABs 3 Wide variety of Abs labeling epidermal cells and basement membrane
Subepidermal blisters			
1 Bullous pemphigoid (also pemphigoid gestationis) (subepidermal blister)	Basement membrane BP-230	*HE:* Border of fresh blister *DIF:* Perilesional intact skin or mucosa; perilesional skin for split skin technique.	*DIF:* 1 Band of IgG and C3 or C3 alone along basement membrane; split skin blister roof
2 Linear IgA dermatosis (subepidermal blister in papillary tips)	BP-180	*IIF:* Serum; normal skin from triceps region for split skin	2 Linear IgA and also C3 along basement membrane 3 IgG and C3 along basement membrane; split skin blister floor
3 Epidermolysis bullosa acquisita (subepidermal blister)	Collagen VII		*IIF:* 1 In 50–70% circulating IgG against basement membrane; split skin blister roof 2 Negative 3 In 20–50% circulating IgG against basement membrane; split skin blister floor

Table 2.4 · Continued

Disease	Target antigen	Biopsy	Findings
Other bullous lesions			
Dermatitis herpetiformis (*Subepidermal* blisters concentrated in papillary tips)	Transglutaminase, endomysium	*HE:* Lesional skin *DIF:* Perilesional skin *IIF:* Serum	*DIF:* Granular IgA, C3 in papillary tips; rarely linear deposits of IgA
Cicatricial pemphigoid (subepidermal blisters)	BP-180, laminin 5, α6β4 integrin	*HE:* Lesional skin *DIF:* Perilesional mucosa *IIF:* Serum	*DIF:* Linear IgG and C3 at basement membrane, less often IgA and IgM Split skin: Varies with antigen *IIF:* Usually negative
Connective tissue disorders			
Lupus erythematosus		*HE:* Lesional skin *DIF:* Lesional, ideally non-sun-exposed skin; non-sun-exposed normal skin	Granular IgG, IgM, C3 along basement membrane In chronic cutaneous LE, only involved skin affected; in systemic LE, deposits in normal skin
Dermatomyositis		*HE:* Lesional skin *DIF:* Lesional, ideally non-sun-exposed skin; non-sun-exposed normal skin	Similar to LE, but often negative
Vasculitis			
Leukocytoclastic vasculitis Urticarial vasculitis Other forms of vasculitis		*HE:* Lesional skin *DIF:* Lesional skin; early lesion except for urticarial vasculitis when late lesion must be chosen	IgG, IgA, IgM or C3 around involved vessels; IgA common for Henoch-Schönlein purpura; DIF not required for diagnosis of vasculitis

AB = antibody; DIF = direct immunofluorescence; HE = hematoxylin-eosin; IIF = indirect immunofluorescence; LE, lupus erythematosus.

Table courtesy of Peter von den Driesch and Elke Knußmann-Hartig.

Table 2.5 · Common immunohistochemical stains

Stain	Identifies
Bcl2	Follicular B-cell lymphoma (negative in primary cutaneous follicular center lymphoma)
Bcl6	Follicular B-cell lymphoma
Carcinoembryonic antigen (CEA)	Eccrine, apocrine glands, Paget disease
CD3	T cells (T-cell receptor)
CD8	Cytotoxic T cells
CD10	B-cell and T-cell precursors
CD20	B cells
CD34	Stem cells, dermatofibrosarcoma protuberans
CD35	Follicular dendritic cells
CD45RO	Effector and memory T cells
CD68	Macrophages
CD79a	B cells
CD117	Mast cells
Cytokeratins	Epidermis, appendages, and related tumors
Desmin	Smooth and skeletal muscle
Epithelial membrane antigen (EMA)	Eccrine, apocrine, sebaceous glands and their tumors
Factor VIII	Endothelial cells, vascular tumors
Factor XIIIa	Dermal dendrocytes, dermatofibromas
HMB-45	Melanocytes, more often in melanoma than nevi
Ki-67	Proliferation marker
Leukocyte common antigen (LCA)	Leukocytes
MelanA	Melanocytes, nevi, melanomas
S-100	Melanocytes, neural cells, many others
Smooth muscle actin	Smooth muscle cells and myofibroblasts

2.8 Molecular Diagnostics

▶ **Principle:** Many new techniques involving molecular biological methods are available for dermatologic diagnosis. These new approaches have increased the sensitivity and specificity of diagnosis, and play a major role in diagnosing infectious diseases, tumors (primarily lymphoma and malignant melanoma), autoimmune disorders, and genodermatoses.

⚠ *Caution:* False-positive results are common; scrupulous attention to detail and use of appropriate controls are essential.

▶ **In situ hybridization:** A known nucleic acid, single stranded and usually labeled with radioactivity or fluorescence, is applied to prepared cells or histologic sections and annealing occurs in situ; purpose is to analyze the intracellular or intrachromosomal distribution, transcription, or other characteristics of the nucleic acids. In **fluorescent in situ hybridization (FISH)**, short sequences of DNA are labeled with florescent dyes and then allowed to hybridize to target DNA; useful for identifying specific mutations for which a probe is available.

▶ **Polymerase chain reaction (PCR)** provides the rapid amplification of specific DNA sequences using primers, leading to the identification of foreign nucleic acids present in very small amounts.

▶ **Reverse transcriptase PCR (RT-PCR)** demonstrates the transcription of a defined gene by generating cDNA from RNA.

▶ **Real-time PCR** allows quantification of either DNA or RNA.

▶ **Detection of immunoglobulin and T-cell receptor rearrangements:** Assessing clonality of B-cell or T-cell proliferation is essential in studying cutaneous lymphomas. PCR is widely used to study both the T-cell receptor (TCR) and IgH, having widely replaced Southern blotting.

▶ **DNA microarrays** contain many segments of DNA serving as probes mounted on a single chip. Messenger RNA is extracted from the specimen and applied to the chip. The expression of thousands of genes can be analyzed simultaneously, creating patterns of gene activity for various tumors.

2.9 Mycologic Diagnosis

Obtaining Culture Material

▶ **Dermatophyte infection:**
  • Generous amounts of material should be taken from the edge of the lesion, which is the site where fungi are most likely. The skin can be scraped with a sterile scalpel or curette; hairs should be epilated with a tweezers.
  • A bacterial smear obtained in the usual fashion is useless for diagnosing dermatophytes.
  • Disinfection is not needed if the material is to be cultured on media containing cycloheximide (directed against contaminating molds) and antibiotics (against bacteria). Strong disinfectant measures may destroy the suspected fungus.

▶ **Onychomycosis:**
  • Remove fine pieces of nail from the subungual area, after first cutting away markedly damaged nails.
  • If a superficial nail infection is suspected, scrape material from the surface of the nail using a scalpel.

▶ **Candida:**
  • Use bacteriological swabs to culture the mouth, intestinal tract, and vagina. The swabs are rolled over the surface of the culture medium.
  • If infection of the glans penis is suspected, the glans can be pressed directly on a culture plate.

Culture Conditions

▶ The usual culture medium is Sabouraud glucose agar (with cycloheximide for dermatophytes, without for yeasts) or Kimmig agar; in both instances antibiotics are added to the agar. Culture is at room temperature.

▶ Yeasts grow within a week and then are subcultured to rice agar for further differentiation (search for chlamydospores and pseudomycelia).

▶ The further identification of yeasts may require biochemical tests (uptake of sugar or nitrogen, fermentation of sugar). In unclear cases, PCR can be employed to identify the organism's nucleic acid fingerprint.

2.10 Diagnosis of Hair Disorders

Definitions

► **Alopecia:** Visible loss of hair, usually refers to scalp.
► **Color changes:** Canities = gray hair; poliosis = localized white hair.
► **Effluvium:** Increased daily hair loss; normal loss 25–100 hairs daily, so effluvium is loss of > 100 hairs daily.
► **Hair shaft anomaly:** Inherited or acquired structural hair shaft defect.
► **Hirsutism:** Increased hair growth in male pattern in a woman.
► **Hypertrichosis:** Increased hair growth in an area that is not normally rich in hairs.
► **Terminal hair:** Hair reaching into deep dermis or subcutaneous fat, 50–100 m in diameter, rich in pigment with medulla when examined microscopically.
► **Vellus hair:** Finer, more superficial hair, usually < 2 cm in length, < 30 m in diameter, with no pigment and no visible medulla when examined microscopically.

Approach to Alopecia and Effluvium

► **Careful history** (especially important when dealing with hair disorders).
  • *How long have you had hair loss?*
  • *Any associated problems*—nail changes, other skin problems, symptoms (scalp burning, pain pruritus), changes in general health?
  • *Personal history:* Endocrinologic disorders especially thyroid), underlying diseases (connective tissue disorders), operations, accidents, pregnancy and delivery, miscarriages, infections, severe acute illnesses in past year, diets (crash diets in recent months)?
  • *Any treatment? Did it help?*
  • *Allergies? Atopy?*
  • *Medication history:* Hair loss is listed a complication of many medications, but there are only a few medications that often cause the problem. They include chemotherapy agents, beta-blockers, thyroxine in excess dosages, antithyroid agents, and aromatase inhibitors. The list of medications that cause hypertrichosis is also small (p. 515).
  • *Hair problems in the family:* Similar to present illness? Others?
  ⚠ **Caution:** Patients generally deny the presence of male/female pattern baldness in their family; ask specifically about individual family members.
  • *Contact with animals:* Source of infection, especially for dermatophyte infections.
  • *Dietary habits:* Low protein or low iron diet? Zinc deficiency (especially in vegetarians and vegans, as zinc is found in meat and cheese)? Amphetamine misuse?
  • *Psychosocial history:* "Stress", anxiety, depression, other problems that could help explain a trichotillomania or overreaction to modest degree of hair loss.
► **Is there a pattern?**
  • *Male or female pattern baldness* (after Hamilton or Ludwig) indicates androgenetic alopecia (p. 500). Mixed patterns are common.
  • *Localized circular alopecia* without inflammation, and often with involvement of eyelashes or eyebrows, indicates alopecia areata (p. 503).
► **How much hair loss has really occurred?** Patients tend to overestimate the degree of hair loss. Try to confirm by looking at photos, such as on driver's license or credit card.

► **Check the hair shafts: RIB rule**.
  - **R**emoved easily: Think of alopecia areata, dermatophyte infections, anagen effluvium with acute poisoning or chemotherapy, severe systemic infections, telogen effluvium, loose anagen hair syndrome in young girls.
  - **I**rregularly spaced: Think of scarring alopecia, alopecia areata, traction alopecia.
  - **B**roken hairs: Think of alopecia areata, artifactual alopecia, dermatophyte infection (*Microsporum*) traction alopecia, hair shaft anomalies.

► **Check the scalp:**
  - *Erythema and scales?* → seborrheic dermatitis, psoriasis, atopic dermatitis, contact dermatitis, dermatophyte infection.
  - *Acneiform lesions?* → acne keloidalis nuchae, folliculitis decalvans.
  - *Papules, nodules, ulcers?* → adnexal tumors, nevus sebaceus, aplasia cutis congenita, basal cell carcinoma, epidermoid cyst, metastasis, sarcoidosis, nodular amyloidosis.
  - *Suggestion of scarring?* (missing follicles, irregular distribution of hairs, epidermal atrophy, sclerosis, telangiectases, pus, erosions, blisters) → chronic cutaneous lupus erythematosus (discoid), lichen planus, localized morphea, alopecia mucinosa, bullous diseases).
  - *Use dermatoscopy:* Cadaver and exclamation point hairs such alopecia areata, irregular distribution or loss of follicular orifices indicates scarring alopecia, follicular keratotic plugs point towards lichen planus.
  - 🗲 *Caution:* Urgent attention is required to **exclude scarring alopecia** because of the possibility of underlying disease and the likelihood of further scarring if no treatment is undertaken.

► **Total body examination:**
  - Check the distribution of *terminal and vellus hairs* (hypertrichosis, hirsutism, secondary sexual characteristics, alopecia universalis).
  - Check for other clues of associated diseases on the skin or mucosa.

► **Biopsy:** The best approach is to obtain three 6 mm punches from the border sampling areas where the scarring is most recent. Biopsies should be parallel to the adjacent hair shafts. Two biopsies are for routine histology, PAS, and Giemsa—one sectioned longitudinally and the other transversely. The third should be frozen for immunofluorescence and other special tests. Topical and systemic corticosteroids should be stopped for 2–4 weeks before biopsy and all other topical medications stopped for 3 days. Most patients are reluctant to have three biopsies, so compromises are the rule.

► **Laboratory studies:**
  - *Routine blood studies:* Complete blood count (CBC), sed rate, (C-reactive protein (CRP), antinuclear antibodies (ANA), glucose, HbA1c, serum protein electrophoresis, iron, ferritin, thyroid function tests, liver and renal parameters. If the history does not suggest hormonal problems, routine (expensive) hormonal analysis is not useful.
  - *When diffuse non-scarring alopecia is present:* Routine blood studies plus syphilis serology, serum zinc, HIV test; in addition in women, free testosterone, dehydroepiandrosterone sulfate (DHEAS), prolactin (improper drawing procedure may lead to false-positive values: blood should be drawn after patient has been lying down for 10–20 minutes, should be done on an empty stomach before 10 a.m. and with cigarette smoking not allowed beforehand).

Further Diagnostic Possibilities

► **Wood's light (p. 23):** Always use to exclude easily overlooked *Microsporum* infections.
► **Hair count:**
  • This test is easily done by the patient and helps to quantify the effluvium. Most patients dramatically overestimate the numbers of hairs they are losing.
  • The same test can be used to assess therapy and helps convince even skeptical patients.
  • Method:
    – Day 1: Wash the scalp vigorously and brush the hairs.
    – Days 2–4 or 5: Do not wash hair, comb hair once daily each morning, save all the hairs each morning, count them and place in a separate envelope that is dated and numbered.
    – In the office, transfer this data into the patient's record.
► **Diagnosis of hair shaft anomalies:** Made by cutting hairs off close to the scalp with as little tugging or trauma as possible. The hairs can be embedded in a standard medium and covered with a coverslip, then examined with routine and polarization microscopy. In special cases, scanning electron microscopy may be needed.
► **Toxicologic examination:** Often requested by patients, but only rarely helpful and frequently misleading. Many heavy metals and a variety of other substances are deposited in the hair shaft and thus excreted from the body. If poisoning is suspected, 20–30 hairs should be obtained and one should consult with legal medicine experts or law authorities to be sure appropriate tests and ordered and, if criminal poisoning is a possibility, that the chain of evidence is kept intact.

Hair Cycle, Trichogram, and Trichoscan

► **Hair cycle (Fig. 2.7):**
  • On the scalp, each hair bulb spends 2–6 years producing a hair shaft (*anagen* phase), and then rests for 3–5 months (*telogen* phase). The transition from anagen to telogen lasts 2–5 weeks and is known as *catagen*.
  ☐ *Note:* Anagen 1000 days; telogen 100 days; catagen 10 days.
  • With increasing age, the duration of the anagen phase decreases. The length of this phase is genetically determined and varies considerably from individual to individual. At the end of telogen, the hair separates itself from the follicle and falls out, either spontaneously with combing or brushing (< 100 hairs/day) or by hair washing (up to 300 hairs). A given hair follicles produces 10–12 hairs over a lifetime.
  • The proximal end of the hair shaft has a distinctive appearance during each phase. Telogen hairs have a club-like appearance that patients frequently fear is the root of the hair. Correcting this misconception alleviates much anxiety.
► **Trichogram:**
  • To be reproducible and useful, a trichogram must be done in a standardized way by an experienced individual. Problems include artifacts induced during removal of hairs, taking too few hairs, and errors in evaluating the hairs because of lack of understanding of the changes during the cycle.
  • The trichogram often has a positive psychological effect, in addition to quantifying the nature of the hair cycle. Patients sense that something is being done. A trichogram is not well-suited for monitoring therapy; the Trichoscan® is far superior for this purpose.

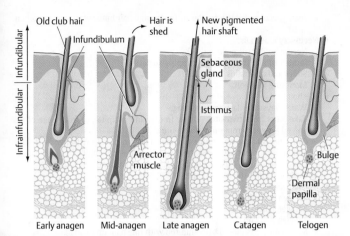

Fig. 2.**7** · Stages of the hair cycle.

- Method for analyzing the hair bulbs to identify in what stage hairs are being lost and thus to distinguish between different types of hair loss (Fig. 2.**8**):
  - *Shortened anagen phase:* Increased number of telogen hairs that can be recognized as bulged hairs without proximal pigment.
  - *Production of defective keratin:* Dysplastic hair bulbs with absent root sheath and proximal hair blub bent like a cane handle.

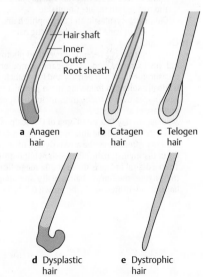

Fig. 2.**8 a–e** · Schematic representation of the hair bulbs during the physiologic hair cycle (**a**, **b**, **c**) as well as pathological findings (**d**, **e**) in trichogram.

- *Toxic effects on keratin synthesis*: Dystrophic hair bulbs with immature hair shaft.
- Necessary materials:
  - Needle holder (remove spring).
  - Rubber tubing (to cover the gripping surfaces).
  - Slides and coverslips.
  - Mounting solution.
- Method:
  - Wait 5 days after last hair washing.
  - Take hairs from two sites (either frontal and occipital, or from edge of involved area and from uninvolved site).
  - Grasp 60–80 (at a minimum 40) hairs 1 cm from scalp with needle holder and pull them out briskly in the direction of the hair shaft.
  - Fan the hairs on a glass slide, apply mounting solution and coverslip.
  - Evaluate under the microscope.
- Normal values:
  - Anagen hairs 80–95%.
  - Catagen hairs 0–5%.
  - Telogen hairs up to 20%.
  - Dysplastic hairs 20–30% (in children with fine hair, up to 50%).
  - Dystrophic hairs up to 2%.
  - Hair density on scalp: 250–450 hairs/cm^2.
  - Hair growth rate: 1 cm/month or 0.3 mm/day.
- Frequent mistakes:
  - Hair washing or aggressive combing before procedure reduces number of telogen hairs.
  - Poor epilation technique, such as removing too slowly or in the wrong direction, leads to increased number of dysplastic, pseudodystrophic, and broken hairs, as well as leaving more firmly adherent anagen hairs behind, making the trichogram results unreliable.
  - Confusing dysplastic and dystrophic hairs. Dystrophic hairs never have the fishhook or cane form of dysplastic hairs.

► **Trichoscan:**
- The Trichoscan is a recently-developed phototrichogram system that uses digital photography and an elegant computer program to provide objective measurements of hair density and hair follicle activity (anagen/telogen ratio). It is ideally suited to following these parameters during therapy. It offers many advantages over a trichogram including speed, painlessness, reproducibility, and ease of archiving.
- *Method:* On day 0, a small area of the scalp is shaved—about 1.8 cm^2—at a site about 2 cm behind the anterior hairline. This site can be easily covered by most patients. After 3 days, the area is dyed with a special dye, in order to make it easier to distinguish hair follicles showing regrowth from those without activity. Then a digital image is made at 20× magnification. The software then analyses the picture, measuring hair density and anagen/telogen ratio, as the anagen hairs are identified as having grown 0.3 mm/day.

3 Other Diagnostic Methods

3.1 Phlebologic Diagnosis

History, Inspection, and Palpation

▶ The **phlebologic history** searches for both predisposing factors and current problems. The most important points are shown in Table 3.1.

Table 3.1 · Phlebologic history and interpretation

History	Interpretation
Nature of pain: burning, lancinating, radiating	No correlation between nature of pain and phlebologic problem; often caused by orthopedic or neurologic problems
Calf cramps	Not common with varicose veins; more likely to reflect arterial disease, hypothyroidism, hypokalemia, osteoporosis, or spondylarthritis; often no cause found
History of fracture or injury to leg, especially with prolonged disuse.	Risk for phlebothrombosis; carefully exclude post-thrombotic syndrome
Family history of venous diseases, age of onset	Family history and early onset suggest disease is likely to be progressive and severe
Stationary job (standing/sitting)	Increased risk for varicose veins
History of thrombosis	Distinguish carefully between phlebitis and phlebothrombosis; patients often confuse the two
Allergies	Patients with chronic venous insufficiency at increased risk for allergic contact dermatitis
Heavy legs, tendency to swelling, warmth, pruritus	Unspecific complaints, but often associated with chronic venous insufficiency

▶ **Inspection:**
- The patient should be examined while standing.
- In thin patients, varicosities are easily visualized. Incompetent perforating veins are seen as a compressible, protruding nodule (blow-out vein).
- *Cutaneous manifestations of chronic venous insufficiency include:* Edema, corona phlebectatica paraplantaris (prominent small veins at edge of foot), starburst veins, dilated small veins (venectasia), pigmentary changes, stasis dermatitis, dermatosclerosis (hypodermitis), atrophie blanche, and ulceration (stasis ulcer). These features correlate with the severity of the venous stasis.
- Stages of chronic venous insufficiency (I–III) are based on Widmer's classification (p.555).
- Simply the location of a leg ulcer allows one to make an intelligent guess at the cause (Fig. 3.1).

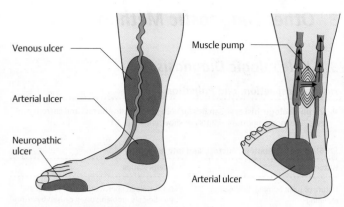

Fig. 3.1 · Location of leg ulcers.

▶ **Palpation:**
  • Palpation allows one to readily recognize edema, induration, and perforating veins. When incompetent perforating veins are palpated, a buttonhole defect in the fascia can often be detected; sometimes it is tender.
  • When the proximal great saphenous vein is palpated in the groin, one can detect an incompetent saphenofemoral junction valve as the patient coughs. Sometimes there is a permanent thrill if there is enough backflow.

Further Diagnostic Procedures

New diagnostic procedures such as Doppler ultrasonography and duplex ultrasonography have greatly reduced the important of phlebography. Functional testing with devices such as light reflection rheography, digital photoplethysmography, and venous occlusion plethysmography are less often employed. Clinical functional tests such as the Trendelenburg tests are of little more than historical interest.

Doppler Ultrasonography
▶ **Principle:**
  • Doppler ultrasonography is based on the observation by Doppler that an apparent change in frequency of waves results when the transmitter and receiver are in motion relative to one another. Shifts in frequency of emitted ultrasonic waves and their echoes are influenced by reflection of the blood flow. The change in frequency allows one to determine the direction of flow and measure the velocity.
  • Usually 4 MHz and 8 MHz devices are used to assess peripheral vessels. At these frequencies, shifts are audible. The 4 MHz unit is used for deep vessels, the 8 MHz for superficial vessels.
  ▣ *Note:* With increasing frequency, resolution improves but depth of penetration decreases.
  • *Indications:* Doppler ultrasonography is most useful for identifying nonfunctioning valves in both superficial and deep veins, as well as for assessing arterial flow. In most instances, it is not sensitive enough to diagnosis a thrombosis; one exception is detection of pelvic vein thrombosis.

► **Method:**
- *Subfascial system:* The patient lies on his back. First, the common femoral artery is identified in the groin. It should have a triphasic flow profile (peak–dip–peak). Then the receiver is placed over the various veins; the sound of the flow varies with breathing. When the Valsalva maneuver is performed, valvular incompetence can be identified by an audible reflux. The main causes of valvular insufficiency include previous phlebothrombosis, marked varicosities with secondary changes in deeper veins, and congenital absence of valves.
- The *popliteal space* is examined in the same way with the patient lying on their abdomen. The Valsalva maneuver is replaced by proximal and distal manual compression and distal decompression. The tibial arteries and veins are assessed in the same way.
- *Epifascial system:*
  - Reflux in the great and small saphenous veins is checked with the patient standing after distal compression. The extent of reflux is used to classify the degree of varicosities using the Hach scale (I–IV) (p. 554).
  - Incompetent perforating veins are best located with duplex ultrasonography. They can be identified with Doppler ultrasonography by applying a proximal tourniquet and then listening for distal reflux.

Duplex Ultrasonography

► **Principle:** Doppler ultrasonography is combined with conventional B-mode ultrasonography to show flow of blood within a vessel. The intravascular flow is color coded; colors differ depending on flow towards or away from the sound. Frequencies of 5.0–14.0 MHz are used.

► **Indications:** This technique allows one to also assess the nature of the vessel wall, the severity of a valvular defect, degree of recanalization, amount of collateral flow, and the speed of the reflux flow. Arterial narrowing and occlusion can also be assessed Perforating veins and the variable location of the junction of the small saphenous vein with the popliteal vein can be more accurately identified and marked on the skin (duplex mapping).

Compression Ultrasonography

► **Indications:** The main use is to detect phlebothrombosis. Doppler ultrasonography is only useful for pelvic vein thrombosis (loss of the breathing-modulated flow of the common femoral vein). Otherwise, compression ultrasonography is standard.

► **Principle:** The veins are compressed with the scanner, using B-mode ultrasonography. Compression should be slight; in the case of a thrombus, compression is more difficult. The sensitivity and specificity of this approach are over 95%, thus just as good as phlebography. The latter is reserved for cases where compression ultrasonography is unclear or cannot be performed.

Light Reflection Rheography and Photoplethysmography

► **Principle:** Light reflection rheography (LRR) and photoplethysmography (PPG) are indirect methods of measuring the return transport capacity of the venous system. The measurements are made with a measuring head that is fastened 10 cm above the medial malleolus. The head contains three sources of infrared light and one receiver. Light directed into the skin is reflected by local blood flow in the skin and redirected towards the receiver where they are captured by a photo element which then transmits electrical impulses that are recorded (Fig. 3.**2**).

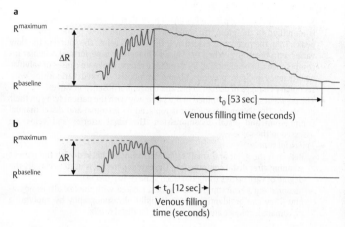

a

R^maximum

ΔR

R^baseline

t_0 [53 sec]

Venous filling time (seconds)

b

R^maximum

ΔR

R^baseline

t_0 [12 sec]

Venous filling
time (seconds)

Fig. 3.**2a,b** · LRR/PPG curves. **a** In a normal adult. **b** In a patient with venous insufficiency.

► **Indications:**
  • Estimation of the effectiveness of operations to remove incompetent saphenous veins or perforating veins.
  • Quantitate pumping capacity of calf muscles.
  • Although the method is simple and easily performed, it gives limited information that can only be used in conjunction with Doppler and duplex ultrasonography results.
► **Procedure:** First the calf muscles are used by performed dorsal flexion of the foot 10°. This reduces the degree of filling of the subpapillary veins. Then when the patient is still, the veins refill.
► **Interpretation:** The resulting curves allow one to determine two parameters:
  • *R-difference* (R), which reflects the difference in filling of the veins.
  • *Refilling time* (t_0):the time needed for the veins to refill. In normal individuals, this is around 25 seconds. A reduced refilling time results with deep or epifascial reflux, but also with perforator vein reflux alone.
► **Therapeutic consequences:** If the refilling time is shortened, surgery or sclerosing injections might lead to improvement both in this parameter and in venous stasis. Using a tourniquet, the great saphenous vein or an incompetent perforating vein can be compressed and then the refilling time measured again. If the refilling time is increased, then the chronic venous insufficiency is at least partially correctable and treatment is appropriate.

Plethysmography

► **Principle:** Plethysmography measures volume changes and thus arterial flow. Rapid volume changes in a limb can only be caused by changes in amount of blood.
► **Indication:** Diagnosis of leg and pelvic thromboses; monitoring of thrombosis therapy.
► **Other uses:** Demonstrating venous flow obstruction, measuring pump function of calf muscles, measuring the capillary filtration rate.

Strain-gauge Plethysmography

▶ **Principle:** Mercury in rubber tubes changes its resistance as the tubes are stretched. The strain-gauge tubes are placed around the extremity. Changes in circumference are reflected in changes in electric current, which can be recorded.

▶ **Example:**

- *Demonstration of obstructed venous return:* The leg is held at 45° with the knee joint flexed at 170°. The speed of the venous flow from the calf and foot is measured after compression has been applied and released.
- A strain-gauge tube is placed around the calf. A cuff with 80–85 mm Hg pressure is placed around the thigh.
- *Venous capacity:* The plethysmograph measures at minute intervals the increasing venous volume (= vein capacity in mL/100 mL).
- *Venous drainage:* The pressure cuff is released suddenly. The rate of drop in venous volume over 2 minutes is measured to reflect the degree of venous resistance (vein draining in mL/100 mL per minute).

▶ **Interpretation:**

- If there is an obstruction to venous flow proximal to the measuring device, venous capacity and venous drainage are reduced.
- Venous drainage values < 30 mL/100 mL per minute are abnormal.
- *⚠ Caution:* Dermatosclerosis or edema can also cause low values.

▶ **Reliability:** Leg vein thrombosis can be diagnosed with 90% accuracy when the veins are completely blocked and relatively high. The procedure is less helpful for calf and thigh thrombosis and in the postthrombotic syndrome.

Phlebodynamometry

▶ **Principle:** The venous pressure in the leg is measured directly.

▶ **Indications:** The main indication is in clarifying a postthrombotic syndrome, to see if surgical invention might be helpful. In addition, it offers the best way of quantifying the functional venous capacity.

▶ **Method:** A dorsal foot vein is cannulated with a butterfly needle. Then the venous pressure is measured with the patient standing using either a manometer or electronic device. The normal pressure varies with the height of the patient (distance from heart to foot vein). After the baseline pressure is established, the patient does 15 toe stands. Then the procedure is repeated with a tourniquet occluding the vein that is being considered for removal.

▶ **Interpretation:** Normally the pressure drops by 50%. The time for refilling is comparable to that with light reflection plethysmography. Less drop in pressure or a slower refilling time suggest postthrombotic syndrome. In the extreme situation, the pressure rises with exercise, indicating marked obstruction. If the parameters improve after the tourniquet is applied, then the compromised vein should be removed.

3.2 Allergy Testing

Patch Testing and Photopatch Testing

▶ **Principle:** In order to prove type IV contact sensitization, the potential allergen is applied to the skin under occlusion in a nontoxic concentration for 24–48 hours. In sensitized individuals, a localized dermatitic reaction occurs. In photopatch testing, the allergens are applied in parallel, and one set is irradiated.

► **Indications:**
- Allergic contact dermatitis (high sensitivity).
- Photoallergic or phototoxic reactions following UV light exposure.
- Fixed drug reaction (testing at site of reaction).
- Protein contact urticaria.
- Drug reactions and vasculitis (additional readings at 20 minutes and 6 hours, low sensitivity, use is controversial).

► **Procedure:**
- The test substances are applied to a 50 μL aluminum chamber or a patch (hence the name), which is attached to hypoallergenic tape.
- The allergens are usually diluted with white petrolatum or water; less often alcohol, olive oil, isopropyl myristate or acetone may be used.
- As a negative control, white petrolatum is usually chosen.
- The tape and aluminum chamber are firmly attached to the skin with additional wide strips of tape.
- The patches are applied to the upper $^1/_3$ of the back, or in special circumstances the triceps area.

► **Interpretation (Table 3.2):**
- The test substances are removed after 48 hours (some recommend 24 hours but we prefer 48 hours). After waiting 30 minutes to let local irritation subside, the reaction is read. The site is checked again after 72 hours and in some instances after 96 hours (in photopatch testing and if reactions are unclear).
- Sometimes it is wise to re-examine the site after several days, as some reactions, such as those to metals and corticosteroids, are notorious for appearing late.
- If contact urticaria is suspected, the site should be read after 20 minutes. These substances should be applied separately from the regular patches, as once the tape has been pulled off, even if it is re-applied, occlusion is compromised.

► **Side effects:**
- *Exaggerated dermatitis reaction:* Some patients with severe allergic contact dermatitis may experience a flare following patch testing. Treatment with topical corticosteroids usually suffices.
- Severe reactions, especially photopatch test reactions, can lead to postinflammatory *hyperpigmentation* that may be disturbing to the patient.
- Sensitization to a test substance occurs only very rarely.

Table 3.2 · Interpretation of patch tests

Symbol	Appearance	Interpretation
–	No reaction	Negative
?	Only erythema, no infiltrate	Allergic, irritant, or unclear
±	Few follicular papules	Allergic, irritant, or unclear
+	Erythema, infiltrate, discrete papules	Allergic reaction (1+)
++	Erythema, infiltrate, papules, vesicles	Allergic reaction (2+)
+++	Erythema, infiltrate, confluent vesicles	Allergic reaction (3+)
ir	Pressure changes, blisters, irritation from tape outside area of application	Irritant reaction
nt		Not tested

- *Anaphylactic shock:* In rare cases, exposure to a patch test allergen may cause anaphylaxis in a very sensitive individual. The risk is greatest with antibiotics. If the patient gives a history of a type I reaction, then patch testing should be done with care, with resuscitation equipment available.
- *Angry back syndrome:* Patients with active dermatitis often react to multiple allergens producing numerous false-positive reactions. After the dermatitis and the patch test reactions have calmed down, the patient should be re-tested for clinically relevant allergens. Any patient with more than seven positive reactions to non-cross-reacting allergens should be suspected of having angry back syndrome.
- *False-negative reactions:* Sometimes patients are truly allergic to a substance but patch testing fails to reproduce the clinical setting. For example, an individual may be sensitive to preservatives in eye drops, but may not react to the same material on the thicker skin of the back. The test area can be made more sensitive by repeated tape stripping, or a more sensitive site such as the temple can be chosen.
- ▣ *Note:* Patch testing should only be done when there is a reasonable clinical suspicion of allergic contact dermatitis. Since the allergen concentration is chosen so that some normal individuals react to the patch, a small number of false-positive reactions are built into the system. Thus every positive reaction should be viewed for its clinical relevance. Simply issuing an "allergy pass" listing all positive patch tests helps neither the patient nor future treating physicians.

Patch Test Series

▶ **Standard test series:** In Germany, the standard series is continually under modification but currently consists of 29 allergens that enable the identification of most common causes of allergic contact dermatitis. The current collection is shown in Table 3.**3**.

Photopatch Testing

▶ **Indication:** To confirm photoallergic reaction.
▶ **Method:** The standard series of photoallergens is applied in duplicate. After 24 hours, one set is removed and the area irradiated with 5–10 J/cm^2 or half the minimal erythema dose of UVA. Both sides are read after another 24, 48 and 72 hours.
▶ **Interpretation:** The same system is used as for regular patch testing. When the nonirradiated site is normal and the irradiated site shows a reaction, a photoallergic reaction has been shown.

Rub, Scratch, Prick, and Intracutaneous Testing

▶ **Indications:**
- *Acute allergic reaction* (type I reaction): Drug reactions, urticaria, food allergies, allergic rhinitis, allergic conjunctivitis, allergic asthma.
- Some instances of *delayed allergic reactions*, such as vasculitis and purpura, although the utility of this procedure is controversial.
▶ **Methods:**
- *Rub test:* The allergen is applied to the intact skin on the forearm. This is the least sensitive test for type I allergies, suited for very sensitive patients (those with severe reactions) and when testing native allergens.

Table 3.3 · Standard patch test series of the German Contact Allergy Group

No.	Substance	Concentration	Vehicle	24h	48h	72h	96h
1	Potassium dichromate	0.5%	WP				
2	p-Phenylene diamine	1.0%	WP				
3	Thiuram mix	1.0%	WP				
4	Neomycin sulfate	20.0%	WP				
5	Cobalt (II) chloride 6 H$_2$O	1.0%	WP				
6	Benzocaine (ethyl aminobenzoate)	5.0%	WP				
7	Nickel (II) sulfate 6 H$_2$O	5.0%	WP				
8	Colophony resin	20.0%	WP				
9	N-isopropyl-N′-phenyl-p-phenylene diamine	0.1%	WP				
10	Wool wax alcohol	30.0%	WP				
11	Mercapto mix without MBT	1.0%	WP				
12	Epoxide resin	1.0%	WP				
13	Balsam of Peru	25.0%	WP				
14	p-tert-Butyl phenol formaldehyde resin	1.0%	WP				
15	Formaldehyde	1.0%	Water				
16	Fragrance mix	8.0%	WP				
17	Mercury (II) amide chloride	1.0%	WP				
18	Turpentine	10.0%	WP				
19	(Chlor)-methylisothiazolinone (MCI/MI)	100 ppm	Water				
20	Paraben mix	16.0%	WP				
21	Cetyl stearyl alcohol	20.0%	WP				
22	Zinc diethyldithiocarbamate	1.0%	WP				
23	Dibromodicyanobutane + 2-phenoxyethanol	1.0%	WP				
24	Propolis	10.0%	WP				
25	Bufexamac	5.0%	WP				
26	Compositae mix	6.0%	WP				
27	Mercaptobenzothiazole (MBT)	2.0%	WP				
28	Lyral	5.0%	WP				
29	Dispersion mix blue 126/106	1.0%	WP				

WP = white petrolatum.

- *Scratch test:*
  - The skin of the forearm is scratched with a lancet, so that only the stratum corneum is damaged; no bleeding should occur. The allergen is applied as a solution.
  - Histamine (1 mg/mL) solution and normal saline are used as controls.
- *Prick test:*
  - About 3 µL of allergen in solution is applied to the skin of the forearm. Then the skin is pricked with a lancet or needle. The same controls are used as for scratch test.
- The prick test is better than the scratch test, as it is more sensitive and more reproducible. The scratch test is reserved for native allergens that are hard to dissolve, such as some foods and medications. The "prick in prick" test can also be used, where the lancet is first stuck into the allergen (for example, a nut) and then into the skin.
- *Intracutaneous test:* 0.02–0.05 mL of an antigen solution is injected superficially in the skin using a tuberculin syringe. The same controls are used as above.

▶ **Interpretation:** All these skin tests are read at 20 minutes, and if a delayed reaction is suspected, again after 6 and 24 hours.

- *20 minute reaction:* The allergen site is compared with the positive wheal from histamine and the negative wheal from the control. There is no standardized method of reading. We recommend measuring the wheal and the peripheral erythema; for example, $^5/_{12}$ means a 5 mm wheal with the erythematous ring measuring 12 mm. Positive reactions must be more than 50% of the size of the histamine wheal.
- *6 hour reaction:* The wheal and the erythema are once again measured.

Choosing the Right Test

▶ **The gold standard is the prick test.** The widest array of well-tested commercial allergens are designed for this procedure. The sensitivity of the test for inhalation allergens is high. In contrast, for food allergens, especially fruits and vegetables, the sensitivity is low. Thus, it is often necessary to use the foods themselves for testing. Since native allergens can lead to severe reactions, it is wise to do rub or scratch tests before doing prick tests.

▶ **The most sensitive in-vivo allergic test is the intracutaneous test.** Here the risk of a severe allergic reaction is the highest, and special sterile allergen solutions are required. Thus intracutaneous testing is reserved for special situations such as titrating the reaction in insect toxin allergies.

Provocation Tests

▶ **Indications:** If the skin tests are contradictory or do not fit with the history, the relevant allergen can be administered as a form of challenge, using a variety of routes.

🛈 *Caution:* All provocation tests are potentially dangerous and must be done in a setting where resuscitation measures are readily available.

▶ **Methods:**

- *Conjunctival provocation:*
  - *Principle:* The antigen is prepared in a sterile 0.09% NaCl solution. One drop is placed in the conjunctival sac.
  - *Reactions:* After about 2 minutes, the conjunctiva becomes reddened. The solution can also be irritating, so a control should be applied to the other eye.

- *Nasal provocation:*
  - *Principle:* The allergen extract is blown into the nose with a vaporizer.
  - *Reactions:* After about 10 minutes, sometime much sooner, the patient begins to experience sneezing, rhinorrhea, tearing and in severe reactions headache and bronchospasm.
  - *Interpretation:* The reduced nasal airflow or increased resistance can be quantified with a rhinomanometer. The identification of eosinophils in the nasal secretions also helps quantify the reaction.
- Bronchial provocation:
  - *Principle:* The allergen extract is inhaled.
  - *Reactions:* Bronchospasm.
  - *Interpretation:* Pulmonary function testing is used before and after exposure. A positive test is proven when the FEV_1 drops to $< 80\%$ of original value.
- *Oral provocation:*
  - *Principle:* Suspected medications or foods are given in capsules or concealed in foods with a intense covering taste; in Germany, blackcurrant juice is often used. Start with $1/10 - 1/100$ of the usual "dose." A placebo should be employed.
  - *Reactions:* Recurrence of the signs and symptoms described in the history, involving the skin, lungs, gastrointestinal tract, or other organs.
  - *Interpretation:* The gold standard for challenging patients with historically documented food allergies is double-blind placebo-controlled testing. Many patients are children; in this instance, the parents must also be blinded.

Factors Influencing Test Results

▶ **Site of testing:** Different areas of the skin react differently to challenge. For example, the upper back is more reactive than the lower back. The difference has been estimated as threefold. The back is also more sensitive than the forearm; under the same conditions, a wheal on the upper back will be twice as large as one on the forearm. The most sensitive area on the arm is the antecubital fossa. The ulnar aspect is more reactive than the radial.

▶ When testing with type I allergens there is a risk of a systemic anaphylactic reaction. This is especially true with tests for food allergens and insect toxins. In such instances, it is wiser to test on the forearm, as reactivity is lower and a tourniquet can be applied to reduce systemic spread, if needed.

▶ **Influence of medications:** Many medications can influence allergy testing, as shown in Table 3.**4**.

Serologic Tests

Identification of IgE

▶ **Principle:** The radio-allergosorbent test (RAST) identifies IgE antibodies directed against specific allergens.

▶ **Indications:** In-vitro diagnosis is a useful addition to the history and in-vivo tests. The sensitivity is comparable to prick tests and is also dependent on the quality of the allergen preparations.

▶ **Interpretation:**
- IgE values measured with ELISA, FAST, or radiochemical methods.
- Results are given in semi-quantitative fashion: RAST class 0 (negative); RAST classes 1–4 (positive).
- In the CAP test, the RAST class 4 is divided into CAP classes 4–6. CAP 1–3 correspond to RAST 1–3. The CAP test employs a different system of binding the antigen to a test surface.

Table 3.4 · Influence of medications on test reactions

Medication	Prick, scratch, intracutaneous tests	Patch tests	Provocation tests	Photopatch tests
Antihistamines				
Topical	↓ ↓ ↓	(↓)	0	(↓)
Systemic	↓ ↓ ↓	(↓)	↓	(↓)
Corticosteroids				
Topical	(↓)	↓ ↓ ↓	↓ ↓ ↓ [b]	↓ ↓ ↓
Systemic	↓ ↓	↓ ↓ ↓	↓ ↓	↓ ↓
B-mimetics	0	0	↓ ↓ ↓ [b]	0
Theophylline	0	0	↓ ↓ [b]	0
Indomethacin (NSAIDs)	0	0	0	↓
Cromoglycates	0	0	↓ ↓ ↓ [a,b]	0
Tranquilizers, antidepressants	↓	0	(↓)	0

a, conjunctival provocation; b, bronchial provocation.

Special Procedures

When a false-negative IgE test is suspected, the **basophil release test** can be employed. Basophils are challenged with the allergen and their release of histamine or leukotrienes quantified. In this way, bound IgE is also studied.

There are also many other tests including macrophage and leukocyte migration inhibition assays, as well as the lymphocyte transformation test (employed in some centers to study drug reactions). All of these tests are expensive and are not recommended for routine allergy testing. They should not be used to prove an allergy, either in a medical or medicolegal sense.

3.3 Light Testing

▶ **Indications:** Light testing (phototesting) is indicated whenever a skin disease is suspected of being caused by or aggravated by light. Phototesting is also used to determine the appropriate doses before starting UV therapy and to determine how light-sensitive an individual is.

▶ **Skin types:** An appreciation of the different skin types and their relative sensitivity to UV irradiation is essential before contemplating phototesting. Fitzpatrick and colleagues first described these types in Boston, based on 30 minutes sun exposure at mid-day in summer (Table 3.**5**).

Minimal Erythema Dose (MED)

▶ **Definition:** The amount of UV required to induce erythema in an irradiated site. The faintest erythema extending to the margins of the irradiated field is taken as a positive result (Table 3.**6**).

Table 3.5 · **Skin types (after Fitzpatrick)**

Skin type	Erythema	Pigment
I	Always	Never
II	Always	Sometimes
III	Sometimes	Always
IV	Never (Mediterraneans)	Always
V	Never (Asians, Indians)	Independent of sun exposure
VI	Never (Blacks)	Independent of sun exposure

⚠ *Caution:* Types V and VI can also develop sunburn after extreme exposures and darken.

Table 3.6 · **Interpretation of light testing**

Grade	Clinical Findings
0	No erythema
+/–	Recognizable but irregular erythema
+	Uniform faint erythema (used for MED)
++	Prominent erythema without edema
+++	Intense erythema with edema and pain
++++	Intense erythema and edema, marked pain, sometimes blister formation

► **Method:**
- The determination of the MED is done separately for UVA and UVB. The testing should be done with the same device with which therapy is planned, or at least with a device that emits the same quality of irradiation.
- Testing is carried out on previously nonirradiated skin, usually the buttocks. One can either use a plate with five holes, each about 1 cm², transmitting varying degrees of UV, or with a system where a light-impermeable shield has a number of small apertures that can be opened manually to increase the dose of light in a stepwise manner.
- UVB testing is read after 24 hours.
- For UVA testing, the MED is not applicable. Either immediate pigment darkening (IPD) can be assessed right after exposure or minimal tanning dose (MTD) can be determined after 24 hours.

Photo Provocation Testing

► **Principle:** Some skin diseases (lupus erythematosus, polymorphous light eruption) can be reproduced by exposure to repetitive UV light. In some instances, this is diagnostically useful when the clinical picture is unclear and other tests have failed to answer the question. In rare cares, provocation testing is done with visible light, as in some cases of light-induced urticaria.
► **Method:**
- The provocation fields should be 5 × 5 cm.
- *Visible light* (400–800 nm): exposure for 10 minutes, reading immediately and after 30 minutes.

- *UVA* (320–400 nm): exposure on four consecutive days: skin type I–II 60 J/cm², skin type III–IV 100 J/cm². Reading immediately, after 24 hours, and then after last exposure, readings also at 48 and 72 hours as well as 1 week (delayed reactions common in lupus erythematosus).
- *UVB* (280–320 nm): provocation testing rarely needed.
- *⚠ Caution:* There is a marked risk of sunburn.
- When a photoallergic or phototoxic reaction is suspected, caused either by ingested or topically applied agents, phototesting can be combined with exposure to agent to confirm the relation.

Minimal Phototoxic Dose (MPD)

▶ **Definition:** The MPD is the minimal UVA dosage that, combined with a standardized psoralen dosage, causes a barely visible uniform erythema. The MPD is used to assess the patient's sensitivity before starting PUVA therapy.
▶ **Method:**
- The patient receives a standardized, weight-adjusted dose of psoralen (p. 607). The same test area is used as for MED.
- For skin types I and II, doses of 0.5, 1.0, 2.0, 4.0, and 6.0 J/cm² are administered; for skin types III and IV, 1.5, 3.0, 6.0, 7.5 and 9.0 J/cm².
- The reaction is read after 72 hours, when a PUVA reaction is maximal. Thus it is ideal to irradiate on Friday and read on Monday.
▶ **Interpretation:** The light dose needed for a ± finding (Table 3.**6**) is the MPD.

3.4 Ultrasonography

Ultrasonography is discussed above in detail for phlebologic diagnosis, but it also has other uses in dermatology.

High-Frequency Cutaneous Ultrasonography

▶ **Principle:** A 20 MHz transducer with integrated gel stand-off pad and color coding is used.
▶ **Indications:** Measuring thickness of tumors before surgery, monitoring skin thickness, especially for scleroderma but also for psoriasis and in a variety of experimental settings.

Lymph Node and Soft Tissue Ultrasonography

Principle: A 7.5–14 MHz transducer is used with integrated water bath, along with color-coded duplex ultrasonography and power mode to show the perfusion pattern (central–peripheral).
Indications:
- Absolutely essential in the follow-up of malignant melanoma and other malignant skin tumors where there is a risk of nodal involvement, as the sensitivity is increased by at least 30%.
- Combined with fine needle aspiration to diagnosis melanoma metastases.
- Used preoperatively to assess the location of a tumor in relation to nerves, vessels, and other soft tissue structures.

Characteristic echo patterns:
- *Melanoma metastasis:* Echo-poor to echo-free, balloon-shaped structure with dorsal signal enhancement, especially when quickly growing hemorrhagic-necrotic metastases (length/width index < 2) are depicted.

- *Reactive lymph nodes:* Oval structure with echo-rich center and echo-poor periphery. When inflamed, echo-poor area increased (length/width index >2).
- *Lymphoma:* Large echo-poor structures, often irregular and confluent, with eccentric echo-rich centers, and typical branching of vasculature.
- *Other metastases:* Usually echo-poor, noncompressible structures with irregular vascular pattern.
- *Hematoma:* Early lesions are echo-poor structures with dorsal signal enhancement; later heterogenous, diffuse echo-rich interior structures as sign of organization.
- *Seroma/lymphatic cyst:* Well-circumscribed, echo-poor compressible structure with dorsal signal enhancement; later appearance of internal echo-rich structures suggesting septae.
- *Lipoma:* Circumscribed subcutaneous structure, varying from echo-poor to echo-rich, depending on degree of fibrosis, but with a sharp border.
- *Abscess:* Poorly circumscribed, echo-poor, compressible structure.

▨ *Caution:* All space-occupying lesions should be re-examined after 4 weeks. If they are progressing, then either fine needle biopsy or excision should follow.

▷ *Note:* Prospective studies have shown that the early identification of melanoma metastases with ultrasonography leads to a significant increase in the overall survival.

4 Viral Diseases

4.1 Overview (Table 4.1)

Table 4.1 · Overview of relevant dermatologic viral diseases and their causative agents

Virus group	Disease
Poxvirus	
Variola virus	Smallpox
Vaccinia virus	Vaccinia and related diseases
Cowpox/cat pox virus	Cowpox, cat pox
Paravaccinia virus	Milker's nodule
Parapoxvirus ovis (PPOV)	Orf (ecthyma contagiosum)
Molluscum contagiosum virus	Molluscum contagiosum
Herpesvirus	
Herpes simplex virus (HSV-1, HSV-2)	Herpes simplex
Varicella-zoster virus (VZV)	Varicella (chickenpox), zoster
Human cytomegalovirus (CMV)	Severe infections in immunosuppressed patients, neonates; Gianotti–Crosti syndrome
Epstein–Barr virus	Infectious mononucleosis (often with ampicillin/amoxicillin rash); Gianotti–Crosti syndrome
Human herpesvirus 6	Exanthem subitum
Human herpesvirus 8	Kaposi sarcoma
Picornavirus	
Coxsackieviruses	Hand-foot-and-mouth disease; herpangina; various exanthems
ECHO viruses	Various exanthems
Paramyxovirus	
Measles virus	Measles
Mumps virus	Mumps

Continued Table 4.1 ▶

Table 4.1 · Continued	
Virus group	**Disease**
Togavirus	
Rubella virus	Rubella (German measles)
Hepadnavirus	
Hepatitis B virus	Gianotti–Crosti syndrome
Flavivirus	
Hepatitis C virus	Co-factor in several disorders including porphyria cutanea tarda, cryoglobulinemia, and in some countries lichen planus
Parvoviruses	
Parvovirus B19	Erythema infectiosum
Papillomavirus	
Human papillomaviruses (HPV)	Warts, condylomata, cervical carcinoma
Retroviruses	
HIV-1, HIV-2	HIV/AIDS
HTLV-1	Adult T-cell leukemia lymphoma

▣ *Note:* The common childhood exanthems are considered under Dermatoses in Childhood (p. 571).

4.2 Poxvirus Infections

Introduction

▸ **Virology:** Poxviruses are complex DNA viruses and the largest viruses.
▸ **Primary hosts:** Humans, monkeys, cows, sheep, cats.
▸ **Major groups:**
  • Orthopoxviruses (smallpox, vaccinia, cowpox, monkeypox).
  • Parapoxviruses (milker's nodule, orf).
  • Miscellaneous (molluscum contagiosum).

Smallpox (Variola vera)

▸ **Definition:** Acute viral infection, highly contagious, with marked mortality.
▸ **Epidemiology:** Smallpox was declared extinct in the early 1980s by the World Health Organization. Since then, because of the discontinuation of vaccination and the lack of natural exposure, the overall resistance has become greatly reduced.

Laboratory accidents, spontaneous mutations in animal pox viruses, and acts of terrorism are all potential pathways for the reintroduction of this feared infection.

▶ **Clinical features:**
- Sudden onset of fever, chills, malaise and arthralgias.
- Rapid development of exanthem; initially macules, then blisters, pustules, and finally crusts and scars.
- All lesions are always in the same stage (synchronous development).
- Black pox refers to hemorrhagic lesions in the skin and mucosa, as well as in internal organs; frequently fatal.

▶ **Diagnostic approach:** History, identification of virus with electron microscopy (negative staining), viral culture, serology.

▶ **Differential diagnosis:** Chickenpox, cowpox, monkeypox, severe acute acne, meningococcal septicemia, acute generalized exanthematous pustulosis (pustular drug eruption).

▶ **Therapy:** Isolation of suspected cases, contact Centers for Disease Control or local public health officials; vaccinia immune globulin, semicarbazone derivatives, and symptomatic measures (topical antiseptics, supportive care).

▶ **Immunization:** Vaccines are available. Individuals with a high risk of exposure from terrorist activity (soldiers, emergency room workers) have been immunized in some countries; many developed countries have large stores of vaccines for use should smallpox break out.

▶ **Immunity:** Survivors are immune for many years.

Vaccinia

▶ **Definition:** Cutaneous complication of smallpox vaccination.

▶ **Epidemiology:** Since vaccination is used so little today, few problems are seen. Vaccinia is a relative of the smallpox viruses whose exact origins are unknown. It elicits a much milder disease but with cross-immunity.

▶ **Clinical features:**
- *Autoinoculation:* Vaccina virus transferred from vaccination site to other regions; grouped ulcerated or necrotic papules with erythematous base.
- *Transinoculation:* Virus is transferred to other individuals; appears similar to a vaccination reaction.
- *Eczema vaccinatum:* Severe widespread cutaneous disease following transfer of vaccinia virus to patients with atopic dermatitis, or less often, vaccination of affected patients. Widespread umbilicated pustules; lethality as high as 30%.

▶ **Diagnostic approach:** Identify virus (see smallpox).

▶ **Differential diagnosis:** Smallpox, eczema herpeticatum.

▶ **Therapy:** Vaccinia immune globulin, supportive care.

Cowpox and Cat Pox

▶ **Definition:** Infection following accidental transfer of cowpox/cat pox virus to humans.

▶ **Epidemiology:** Transfer from infected cows (farmers) or cats (pet owners); much more common in cats, despite the name.

▶ **Clinical features:** Crusted papules at inoculation site with fever and malaise; rarely disseminated pustular or hemorrhagic disease, but then life-threatening.

▶ **Diagnostic approach:** Identification of virus (see smallpox).

▶ **Therapy:** Supportive care.

Milker's Nodule

▶ **Definition:** Paravaccinia virus infection spread from cows to dairy farmers or veterinarians.
▶ **Epidemiology:** The infected cows (less often sheep or goats) have harmless warty growths on their udders (false pox); in contrast, cowpox causes mild clinical problems in the bovine hosts.
▶ **Clinical features:** Firm, dome-shaped nodules, several centimeters in diameter with an erythematous periphery, usually on the hands. They may trigger erythema multiforme or lymphangitis. Heal without scarring over weeks.
▶ **Diagnostic approach:** History, histology, identification of virus (not required).
▶ **Therapy:** Topical antiseptics. Lesions resolve spontaneously. If desired, cryotherapy or shave excision under local anesthesia can be employed.

Orf (Ecthyma Contagiosum)

▶ **Definition:** Parapoxvirus ovis infection spread from sheep or goats to contact persons.
▶ **Epidemiology:** The infected animals have a stomatitis, so infection requires contact other than milking. With sheep, those nursing the young lambs are at risk, as are the shepherds caring for sick animals.
▶ **Clinical features:** Identical to milker's nodule (Fig. 4.1).
▶ **Diagnostic approach:** History, histology, identification of virus (not required).
▶ **Therapy:** Supportive measures, see milker's nodule.

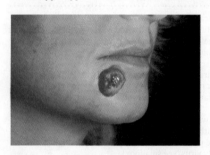

Fig. 4.1 · Orf.

Molluscum Contagiosum

▶ **Definition:** Multiple umbilicated papules or nodules caused by molluscum contagiosum virus; mollusca contagiosa (pl.).
▶ **Epidemiology:** Predisposing factors include atopic dermatitis, immune defects, immunosuppression, HIV/AIDS. Most patients are children.
▶ **Clinical features:**
  • Incubation period days to several months. Skin-colored, 1–5 mm umbilicated papules, often arranged in groups or linear fashion (Köbner phenomenon after autoinoculation) (Fig. 4.2 a).
  • Sites of predilection include face, neck, eyelids, axillae in children; genital region in adults; disseminated in atopic dermatitis or HIV/AIDS.
  • In patients with HIV/AIDS, giant molluscum contagiosum are possible, reaching 3–5 cm in size.

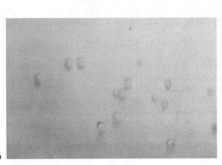
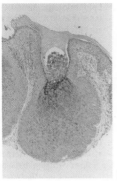

a   b

Fig. 4.**2** · **a** Mollusca contagiosa. **b** Histology of molluscum contagiosum, showing numerous inclusion bodies.

▶ **Diagnostic approach:** Clinical picture, histology (colorful giant molluscum bodies) (Fig. 4.**2 b**).
▶ **Therapy:**
  • Solitary lesions can be destroyed with curettage or a sharp tweezers; usually anesthesia is not needed but topical EMLA is useful in children (apply, occlude, wait 30–35 minutes).
  • Application of salicylic acid plasters is another approach.
  • Widespread disease, especially in children, may rarely require general anesthesia and then curettage of all lesions.
  • Always warn patient or parent to be alert for appearance of new lesions, as some may not be clinically apparent during treatment.
⚠ *Caution:* Mollusca contagiosa are contagious, and this point must be addressed. Infected children should avoid contact with other children with atopic dermatitis or immunosuppression. They should also avoid contact sports and shared wash clothes or towels.

4.3 Herpesvirus Infections

Herpes Simplex Virus Infections

▶ **Definition:** Diseases caused by infections with herpes simplex virus type 1 (HSV-1) or type 2 (HSV-2).
▶ **Pathogenesis:**
  • *Initial infection:* HSV enters via small defects in skin or mucosa and starts to replicate locally; then spreads via axons to sensory ganglia where further replication occurs. Through centrifugal spread via other nerves, affects wider areas. After resolution of the primary infection, the virus remains latent in the sensory ganglia.
  • *Recurrent infection:* Reactivation of virus by various stimuli (UV light, fever) as well as local or systemic immunosuppression leads to seeding of the virus into area served by the sensory ganglia and thus to local recurrences.

► **Epidemiology:** Almost everyone suffers from HSV-1 infection; the first infection is silent in 90%, non-specific in 9%, and clinically manifest in only 1%. Infection occurs in childhood. HSV-2 appears after start of sexual activity and affects 25–50% of population. Both viruses can be shed when patient is asymptomatic, easing transmission.

► **Clinical features:**
  • *Common findings:*
    – Incubation period 6–8 days.
    – Both HSV types can cause oral and genital infections; their clinical presentations are identical. In the genital area, the recurrence rate for HSV-2 infections is 10× greater than for HSV-1, while with orofacial infections, HSV-1 has a significantly higher recurrence rate.

► **Orofacial HSV infections:**
  • *Initial infection:* Herpetic gingivostomatitis. Usually in infants; extensive erosions with hemorrhagic crusts on lips and oral mucosa; difficulty feeding, foul smelling breath, systemic signs and symptoms.
  • *Recurrences:*
    – Small grouped blisters on erythematous base, rapidly become pustules and then eroded; often painful with dysesthesias and neuralgias.
    – Common sites: lips (*herpes labialis),* chin (Fig. 4.3 a), cheeks, periorbital region (Fig. 4.3 b).
  • *Eczema herpeticatum:* Patients with atopic dermatitis (p. 190) can develop extensive orofacial HSV infections which disseminate, especially favoring areas of active dermatitis (Fig. 4.3 c). Neck is most common site.

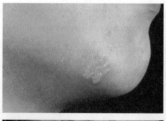
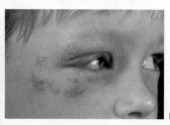
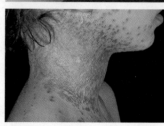

Fig. 4.3 · Herpes simplex. **a** Grouped vesicles on chin. **b** Multiple periorbital lesions. **c** Eczema herpeticum: disseminated HSV infection in atopic dermatitis.

► **Periungual HSV infection:** *Herpetic whitlow.* Most often affects doctors, dentists, and health personal; sharp reduction since more extensive use of gloves because of HIV. Periungual erythema, pain, and then vesicles.

🛈 *Caution:* Do not mistake for bacterial or candidal infection. No incision and drainage. Check for regional lymphadenopathy.

► **Genital HSV infections:**
- *Initial infection:*
  - Disseminated, rapidly eroded vesicles leading to small painful superficial ulcers as well as bilateral lymphadenopathy.
  - Burning or pain on urination common.
  - Cervix involved in 80% of women.
  - Systemic signs and symptoms; malaise, fever, headache.
  - Healing after 2–3 weeks.
- *Recurrences:* Grouped blisters or pustules on erythematous base (Fig. 4.4). Women often have minimal symptoms. In 80% of patients: HSV-2. Differential diagnosis includes all genital ulcers (see STD, p. 134).
- *Uncommon sites:* buttocks or upper thigh; anal or rectal involvement more painful with paresthesias, retention of urine or stool, impotence.

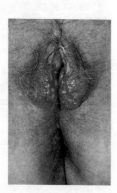

Fig. 4.4 · Chronic ulcerative genital HSV infection in immunodeficient patient (chronic lymphocytic leukemia).

► **Herpes gladiatorum**: Wrestling or other close contact sports (rugby : scrum pox) are ideal for transfer of HSV between team members, usually HSV-1 spread when beard is rubbed on trunk or neck of opponent. Widespread lesions in areas of body contact.

► **HSV encephalitis:** HSV is most common cause of viral encephalitis in adults. 95% HSV-1. Often no associated skin or mucosal lesions. Favors temporal lobes and limbic system. Quick diagnosis via MRI (sometimes brain biopsy) and aggressive antiviral therapy; mortality around 80%.

► **Neonatal HSV infections:**
- HSV-2 (and increasingly HSV-1) in birth canal with direct transfer to newborn and potential for HSV sepsis.
- Genital HSV recurrences in women are asymptomatic in 70% of cases, making diagnosis most difficult.
- Course of HSV in newborns tends to be severe because of incomplete immune response. Sepsis, encephalitis; 30% have no skin findings. If mother has genital herpes, cesarean section and antiviral therapy for newborn.

► **Herpetic keratitis:** Infection of cornea with HSV leading to erosions or ulcers. Often heals with scars, reducing visual acuity. Immediate ophthalmologic consultation at the slightest suspicion.

► **Postherpetic erythema multiforme:** Over 95% of patients with recurrent erythema multiforme have recurrent HSV as trigger (p. 281).

▶ **Diagnostic approach:**
- Clinical findings usually so typical that laboratory investigations not needed.
- *Most rapid approach:* Tzanck smear searching for multinucleated giant cells (Fig. 4.5).
- *Other possibilities:*
  - Identification of virus: immunofluorescent staining of smear with monoclonal antibodies, PCR, electron microscopy, culture.
  - Serology (ELISA): most useful for epidemiological studies.

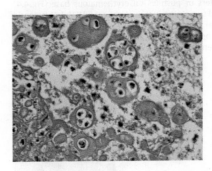

Fig. 4.5 · Herpes simplex, multinucleated giant cells.

▶ **Differential diagnosis:** Deciding between HSV and early zoster can be difficult, but zoster should be unilateral and not recurrent. HSV also develops more rapidly following immunosuppression than does VZV.

▶ **Therapy:**
- *Systemic treatment* with acyclovir, valaciclovir, or famciclovir.
- *Prophylaxis for recurrences:* If patient has more than six recurrences yearly, consider acyclovir 400 mg p.o. b.i.d. or valaciclovir 1000 mg p.o. daily. Use for 1 year; then vacation to check for improvement. Often used for many years. Same regimen can be employed for recurrent erythema multiforme.
- *Drying measures:* Zinc oxide lotion, calamine lotion.
- HSV vaccines are in development; most promising for HSV-2 in women.
- *Neonatal HSV:* Specific hyperimmune globulin and i.v. acyclovir.

Varicella (Chickenpox)

▶ **Definition:** Initial infection with varicella-zoster virus (VZV).

▶ **Clinical features:**
- Highly infectious childhood disease; in 30% clinically nonapparent.
- Incubation period 2–3 weeks.
- Typically starts with red maculae on trunk, oral mucosa and scalp, which rapidly become vesicular and pustular; later crusts (Fig. 4.6). As new lesions continue to appear, the rash is asynchronous with lesions in all stages and varying sizes present at once (in contrast to the synchronic rash of smallpox and eczema herpeticatum); "star map" appearance. Intensely pruritic. Palms and soles always spared.
- *Characteristic lesion:* 1–2 cm oval erythematous macule with central blister.
- Scalp involvement is very common and leads to nuchal lymphadenopathy.
- Scratching often leads to secondary infections and then scars.

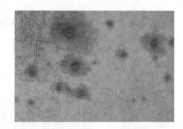

Fig. 4.**6** · Varicella (chickenpox).

- Children are usually not very ill, but adults often have systemic symptoms and even pneumonia.
► **Diagnostic approach:** Usually clinical; Tzanck smear, immunofluorescent staining of smear with monoclonal antibodies.
► **Therapy:** Drying lotions, antihistamines for itch, antibiotics (topical or systemic) for secondary infections. Systemic acyclovir is rarely used, but slightly reduces course of disease and may allow children to return to school or kindergarten sooner.
► **Immunization:** Varicella vaccine is a routine part of childhood immunizations.
► **Varicella in pregnancy:**
  - *1st and 2nd trimesters:* in 25–50% of cases transplacental transfer of VZV to fetus with risk of varicella embryopathy syndrome.
  - ⚠ *Caution:* Cooperate closely with gynecologist and pediatrician.
  - *3rd trimester:* Congenital varicella with poor prognosis.
  - *Therapy:* Pregnant patients with varicella should receive both varicella-zoster immune globulin and antiviral therapy (acyclovir).

Zoster (Herpes Zoster, Shingles)

► **Definition:** Segmental (dermatomal) painful skin disease caused by reactivation of VZV.
► **Epidemiology:** 10–20% of seropositive adults develop clinically apparent zoster. Peak age 50–70; in younger patients think of HIV and iatrogenic immunosuppression.
► **Pathogenesis:** Following the initial varicella infection, VZV persists life-long in the sensory ganglia of the spinal chord and cranial nerves. When reactivated, it follows the associated nerves into the skin; thus both the peripheral nerve and the skin of its dermatome involved (Fig. 4.**7**).
◪ *Note:* When patients know that the disease starts in a nerve, they seem to accept the dysesthesias and pain better.
► **Clinical features:**
  - *Prodromal phase:* dysesthesias or pain in distribution of the affected nerve without visible skin changes; may last up to 7 days. Typically burning or lancinating pain.
  - *Eruption* of grouped vesicles and then pustules on an erythematous base (Fig. 4.**8 a**), occasionally hemorrhagic or necrotic; also lasts about 7 days. Always respects the midline, and only few lesions are outside the involved dermatome and its two immediate neighbors (Fig. 4.**8 b**). More widespread disease suggests immunosuppression.
  - *Healing* with drying, crusting, and usually some scarring; also 7 days.

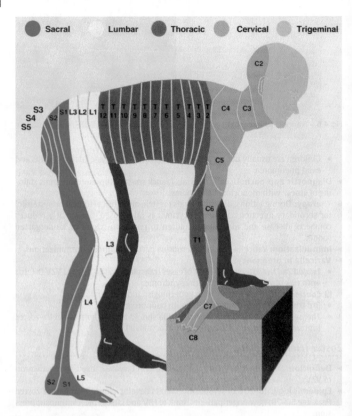

Fig. 4.7 · Dermatomes.

In the figure legend at top: Sacral · Lumbar · Thoracic · Cervical · Trigeminal

▶ **Complications:**

- *Ocular involvement:* When 1st branch of trigeminal nerve (opthalmic nerve) is involved (Fig. 4.8 c), 50% have ocular involvement, including keratitis, corneal erosions, conjunctivitis, iridocyclitis, secondary glaucoma, optic neuritis, impairment of muscles (double vision), facial paralysis. Vesicles on the tip of the nose (Hutchinson sign) indicate nasociliary nerve involvement and greater likelihood of eye involvement.

  ⚠ *Caution:* Always consult the ophthalmologist.

- *Otic involvement:* Involvement of inner ear when 8th cranial nerve is affected, leading to reduced hearing, vertigo, and zoster lesions of tympanic membrane and outer ear canal.

- *Ramsay Hunt syndrome:* Involvement of both 7th and 8th cranial nerves, leading to facial paralysis, hearing loss, vertigo, and zoster lesions of tympanic membrane and outer ear canal.

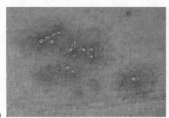 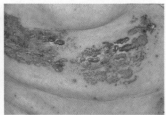

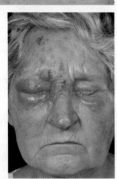

Fig. 4.8 · Zoster. **a** Early zoster with grouped vesicles on an erythematous base. **b** More severe zoster, clearly showing dermatomal limitation. **c** Zoster involving the first branch of the trigeminal nerve, with lid edema.

- Affected sacral ganglia can lead to retention of urine or stool.
- *Generalized zoster*: Usually in immunosuppressed patients, resembles varicella but starts in a dermatome before disseminating.
- ▣ *Note:* The clinical picture is more synchronous and uniform than in varicella.
- *Uncommon variants:* Zoster pneumonitis, encephalitis, nephritis, cystitis, and cholecystitis.
- *Postherpetic neuralgia*: Pain in the involved dermatome that lasts more than 6 weeks; the most dreaded complication of zoster.
- *Zoster in pregnancy:* No serious problems.
► **Diagnostic approach:** Clinical features, Tzanck smear, if questions exist, then immunofluorescent staining of smear with monoclonal antibodies. With trigeminal nerve involvement or any signs and symptoms of eye involvement, always get ophthalmologic consultation.
► **Differential diagnosis** (p. 704): HSV infection; in such a case, the immunofluorescent examination of a smear can readily separate VZV from HSV.
► **Therapy:**
  - *Acute zoster:*
    – Drying measures (zinc oxide lotion, calamine lotion).
    – In the case of severe infections or immunosuppressed patients, antiviral therapy is recommended (Table 4.2). Ideally should be started within 48 hours of presence of vesicles; most patients come to physician's attention much later.
  - *Postherpetic neuralgia*: Pain therapy is associated with a wide variety of side effects. Inexperienced physicians should work closely with a special pain clinic or physician.

Table 4.2 · Approved antiviral agents for zoster

Agent	Dose	Duration
Acyclovir i. v.[a]	Adults, infants < 3 months, children > 12 years: 5 mg/kg q. 8 hours Children 3 months–12 years: 250 mg/m² q. 8 hours	At least 5 days
Acyclovir p. o.	Adults 800 mg 5× daily	5–7 days
Brivudin[b]	Adults 125 mg daily in single dose	7 days; 10 days for severe cases
Famciclovir	Adults 250 mg t. i. d.	7 days
Valaciclovir	Adults 1000 mg q. 8 hours	7 days

a On the basis of our clinical experience, a dose of 5–10 mg/kg for adults or 250–500 mg/m² is recommended. Treatment should last 5–7 days. Immunosuppressed patients should receive the maximum dose for 10 days. Patients with severe disease should be treated with i. v. medication.
b Interactions with other drugs are common; check the manufacturer's recommendations.

- *Stage 1:* NSAIDs or similar agents (acetaminophen 1.5–4.0 g daily or ibuprofen 600–2400 mg daily).
- *Stage 2:* Add weak opiate analgesics such as tramadol 200–400 mg daily or codeine 120 mg daily; perhaps as combination products.
- *Stage 3:* Add strong central-acting opiate such as buprenorphine 0.6–1.6 mg daily or morphine 30–360 mg daily.
- When the pains are very neuralgic, consider adding carbamazepine 400–1200 mg daily to Stage 1 agents. Other possibilities include antidepressants (clomipramine 50–100 mg daily) or antipsychotic agents (methotrimeprazine 20–150 mg daily).
- Further possibilities include sympathetic nerve blockade, transcutaneous electric stimulation, and neurosurgical destruction of responsible pain pathways or centers.

Epstein-Barr Virus Infection

- ▶ **Causative agent:** Epstein–Barr virus (EBV) (human herpesvirus 4).
- ▶ **Pathogenesis:** EBV infects B cells and epithelial cells of the oro- and nasopharynx; capable of immortalizing cells and thus an effective carcinogen.
- ▶ **Clinical features:**
  - Most common disease is infectious mononucleosis, result of acute EBV infection. Patients have a pharyngitis and are often treated with ampicillin or amoxicillin. They then develop a characteristic morbilliform drug exanthem. Other less common acute findings include mucosal ulcerations and facial edema.
  - In small children. EBV is one of the triggers of Gianotti–Crosti syndrome (p. 574).
  - EBV is responsible together with HPV in oral hairy leukoplakia in HIV/AIDS patients (p. 161). In addition, usually found in CNS and primary effusion lymphomas in this patient group.
  - EBV is an important factor in both Burkitt lymphoma and nasopharyngeal carcinoma (primarily in East Asia); other co-carcinogens are likely to be involved.
- ▶ **Diagnostic approach:** Serology, peripheral smear.
- ▶ **Therapy:** Symptomatic therapy; antiviral agents are only minimally helpful.

Cytomegalovirus Infection

▶ **Causative agent:** Human cytomegalovirus (HCMV) (human herpesvirus 5); virus is so named because it induces megalocytes (large cells) in cell cultures. HCMV is preferred term because there are many animal CMVs.

▶ **Epidemiology:** HCMV is a common virus; 40–60% of adults show serologic evidence of infection, with higher numbers in sexually active individuals.

▶ **Clinical features:**
- Acute HCMV is usually asymptomatic but can mimic infectious mononucleosis and also have acute exanthem.
- Cutaneous manifestations of HCMV infections appear almost exclusive in immunocompromised patients (HIV/AIDS, posttransplantation, hematologic malignancies) or in newborns.
- Most important problem is HCMV retinitis in HIV/AIDS patients; prevalence dramatically reduced by HAART.
- Anogenital ulcerations are common in both HIV/AIDS patients (mistaken for severe HSV infection) and in immunosuppressed infants (overlooked as severe diaper dermatitis).
- Systemic infections in infants can lead to sepsis and extramedullary hematopoiesis with cutaneous nodules: blueberry muffin baby.
- ▣ *Note:* TORCH syndrome refers to transplacental infection with **t**oxoplasmosis, **o**ther agents, **r**ubella, **c**ytomegalovirus and **h**erpes simplex; mothers are often healthy but newborns critically ill; congenital leukemia, Langerhans cell histiocytosis, neuroblastoma, and mastocytomas can also appear similar.

▶ **Diagnostic approach:** Identification of virus with PCR, sometimes nuclear inclusions (owl eye cells) in skin biopsy.

▶ **Therapy:** For persistent cutaneous infections, valaciclovir, ganciclovir, cidofovir, or foscarnet can be employed.

4.4 Picornavirus Infections

Hand-Foot-and-Mouth Disease

▶ **Causative agents:** Coxsackievirus A (types 5, 9, 10, 16) and B (types 2 and 5), as well as enterovirus 71.

▶ **Epidemiology:** Usually children are affected; more common in summer.

▶ **Clinical features:**
- Incubation period 5–8 days.
- *Typical triad:*
  - Ulcerative stomatitis, especially on hard palate (lips, tonsils, and pharynx spared).
  - Small papules or papulovesicles on the hands and feet, including palms and soles.
  - Less often diffuse exanthem.
- Patients generally well; no serious complications.

▶ **Diagnostic approach:** Clinical findings; if questions, virus can be identified in oral rinsing; serological tests also available.

▶ **Differential diagnosis:** Often confused with herpes simplex but pattern is different and patient well. Oral lesions alone resemble herpangina and aphthae.

▶ **Therapy:** None needed; symptomatic mouth rinses.

Herpangina

▶ **Causative agents:** Coxsackievirus A (types 1–6, 8, 10 and 22); also some coxsackievirus B and ECHO viruses.
▶ **Epidemiology:** Usually children are affected; more common in summer.
▶ **Clinical features:**
  • Incubation period 3–4 days.
  • Patients are ill with sudden fever (up to 40.5 °C), malaise, headache, myalgias, sore throat. Lasts around 4 days.
  • *Oral lesions:* Characteristic tiny (1–2 mm) ulcerations on hard palate; rapidly ulcerate; often linear. Heal within a week.
▶ **Diagnostic approach:** Clinical findings; virus can be isolated from pharynx or stool; complement-fixing antibodies appear after 2 weeks.
▶ **Differential diagnosis:** Do not confuse with primary herpetic gingivostomatitis; patients are ill but oral findings much more discrete.
▶ **Therapy:** Supportive care; mouth rinses, antipyretics.

4.5 Cutaneous Manifestations of Hepatitis Virus Infections

Hepatitis B Infection

▶ **Causative agent:** Hepatitis B virus (HBV) is a hepadnavirus.
▶ **Epidemiology:** HBV is transferred parenterally (blood or blood products, contaminated instruments, injecting drug abusers), sexually (about 50%) or perinatally.
▶ **Dermatoses associated with HBV infection:**
  • Gianotti–Crosti syndrome.
  • Lichen planus.
  • Mixed cryoglobulinemia.
  • Erythema nodosum.
  • Pyoderma gangrenosum.
  • Polyarteritis nodosa.
  • Urticaria.
  • Leukocytoclastic vasculitis.
  • Serum sickness–like prodrome with urticaria, angioedema, arthritis, proteinuria, or hematuria.
  • Dermatomyositis-like syndrome.

Hepatitis C Infection

▶ **Causative agent:** Hepatitis C virus (HCV) is a flavivirus (RNA virus).
▶ **Epidemiology:** HCV is transferred parenterally in most cases; high prevalence in injecting drug abusers. Less often transferred by sexual intercourse or perinatally. Rarely causes jaundice, so infection often overlooked.
▶ **Dermatoses associated with HCV infection:**
  • B-cell lymphoma (lymphoplasmacytic lymphoma, Waldenström macroglobulinemia) associated with mixed cryoglobulinemia.
  • Leukocytoclastic vasculitis.
  • Polyarteritis nodosa.
  • Porphyria cutanea tarda.

- Lichen planus.
- Urticaria.

⚠ Caution: Many dermatoses formerly associated with HBV infection have turned out to be more often or exclusively associated with HCV. Thus, both of these lists should be viewed as working formulations.

4.6 Human Papillomaviruses

Introduction

▶ **Causative agent:** Human papillomaviruses (HPV) are a group of closely related DNA viruses. Over 100 subtypes have been identified, with differential epithelial preferences (skin vs. mucosa) and different clinical patterns (Table 4.3).

Table 4.3 · **Human papillomaviruses (HPV) and associated diseases**

Disease	HPV types	Oncogenicity
Plantar warts	1, 2, 4, 60, 63	0
Common, filiform, and plantar mosaic warts	1, 2, 3, 4, 7, 54	0
Plane warts, sometimes epidermodysplasia verruciformis	3, 10, 28 less often 2, 26–29,41	++
Macular and slightly raised lesions in epidermodysplasia verruciformis	5, 8, 14, 17, 20, 38	+++
Squamous cell carcinomas in immuno-suppressed patients	5, 8, 38	+++
Condylomata acuminata	6, 11 less often 16, 18, 31, 33	+
Bowenoid papulosis	16, 18	+++
Bowen disease (especially genital)	16, 18	+++
Carcinoma of the cervix	16 (60%), 18 (20%) rarely 11, 31, 33, 35	+++
Butchers' warts	7	?
Focal epithelial hyperplasia (Heck disease)	13, 32	?

+, low risk; ++, intermediate risk; +++, high risk.

▶ **Epidemiology:** 5–20% of all 15–49 year-old individuals have some form of HPV infection; children are very commonly infected. HPV-induced lesions can be transferred from site to site on host (finger to mouth) or from individual to individual (condylomata acuminata).

▶ **Oncogenic potential:** The demonstration that HPV 16 and 18 are the causative agents for human cervical carcinoma has had a great impact on the diagnosis and management of genital HPV infections in patients and their partners.

Common Warts

▶ **Synonym:** Verrucae vulgares.
▶ **Definition:** Hyperplastic tumors induced by HPV.
▶ **Clinical features:**

- Hyperkeratotic papillomatous tumors, usually 2–6 mm in diameter. Characteristic findings are loss of skin markings and intralesional hemorrhagic dots or streaks (Fig. 4.9 a).
- Most common sites are acral—hands, feet. On fingers, frequently periungual (Fig. 4.9 b).

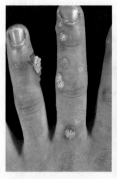
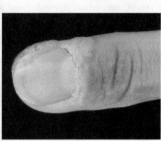

Fig. 4.9 · Common warts. **a** Common warts of hands with obvious papillomatous features. **b** Common periungual warts.

▶ **Diagnostic approach:** Clinical findings (punctate bleeding when pared), histology; identification of HPV type only essential for genital lesions with infected female or partner.
▶ **Differential diagnosis:** In children, molluscum contagiosum. In adults, actinic keratosis, seborrheic keratosis, stucco keratosis, keratoacanthoma.
▶ **Therapy:**

- ▣ *Cave:* Do no harm! Most common warts, especially in children, resolve spontaneously. Procedures that are extremely painful or cause scarring should therefore be avoided.
- All forms of therapy have at least a 50% recurrence rate.
- Small, not extremely hyperkeratotic lesions can be treated with cryotherapy; usually two freeze–spray cycles employed: repeated weekly.
- Application of salicylic acid plasters (every 2–3 days) or flexible gels (daily) followed by paring or curettage (1–2 × weekly by physician or aide).
- As the number of warts increases, the more painful the treatment becomes and the success rate drops.
- Laser destruction of individual resistant or painful lesions (especially periungual) may be useful.
- In resistant cases, imiquimod with aggressive removal of scale and occlusion (see condylomata acuminata below).

Plantar Warts

▶ **Synonym:** Verrucae plantares.
▶ **Definition:** Usually solitary endophytic, often painful, tumors of soles (and palms).
▶ **Clinical features:**
- Irregular papule with central loss of skin markings; usually at sites of mechanical pressure. Overlying reactive hyperkeratosis. Usually tender or painful (Fig. 4.10 a).
- May become quite large and, when therapy-resistant, may evolve into verrucous squamous cell carcinoma (epithelioma cuniculatum).
- Mosaic warts, caused by different HPV types, are diffuse sheets of small, relatively flat warts with lacy or mosaic pattern (Fig. 4.10 b).
▶ **Diagnostic approach:** Punctate hemorrhage, loss of skin lines, tenderness.
▶ **Differential diagnosis:** Clavus or corn is also located at site of pressure, usually over boney prominence; central plug but no punctate hemorrhage. Callus is reactive hyperkeratosis; larger more irregular lesion without central core or punctate hemorrhage.
▶ **Therapy:**
- Conservative approach with salicylic acid plaster or flexible gel, or simply occlusive tape (duct tape), followed by curettage or trimming; may require many treatments.
- Cryotherapy less effective than on other surfaces because of difficulty in raising a blister.
- *Resistant cases:* Laser destruction with CO_2 (risk of painful scars) or dye laser, or photodynamic therapy.
- Imiquimod can be used postoperatively, but is not effective as primary treatment because of the thickened stratum corneum.
- Controlling hyperhidrosis (p. 528) may be a useful adjunct.

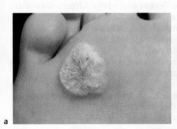
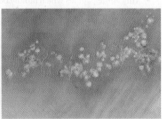
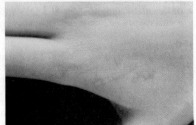

Fig. 4.**10** · Plantar warts. **a** Solitary. **b** Mosaic. **c** Plane warts.

Plane Warts

▶ **Synonym:** Verrucae planae.
▶ **Definition:** Small HPV-induced papules (plane as in flat, not as in plain or common).
▶ **Clinical features:**
  • 1–2 mm, skin-colored subtle papules, often not recognized as warts by patient (Fig. 4.**10 c**).
  • Most common sites are face and hands.
  • Frequently spread by autoinoculation, especially on face of men (less often legs of women) by shaving.
  • Most patients are children or young adults. Plane warts in older patients raise the question of immunosuppression.
▶ **Diagnostic approach:** Clinical findings, histology; HPV typing rarely needed.
▶ **Differential diagnosis:** On face, syringomas, xanthelasma; on chest, papular granuloma annulare and eruptive vellus hair cysts.
▶ **Therapy:** Therapy can easily cause lesions to spread; so "slow and gentle" are the magic words! Try imiquimod, topical retinoids, light cryotherapy, laser destruction.

Condylomata Acuminata

▶ **Synonym:** Genital warts.
▶ **Definition:** Sexually transmitted HPV infection of genital and perianal transition mucosa; most common STD.
▶ **Pathogenesis:** Most commonly caused by HPV 6 and 11 which are not oncogenic. Important to exclude infection with HPV 16 and 18 which are oncogenic. In affected women, HPV analysis of Pap smear may supplement cytology to assess risk.
▶ **Clinical features:**
  • Incubation period 4 weeks–6 months.
  • Tiny white papules which rapidly both spread and enlarge. Larger lesions often macerated. May be genital (Fig. 4.**11 a**) or perianal (Fig. 4.**11 b**).
  • *Infections in children:* Vertical transmission in utero or during birth can lead to infections which may appear with considerable time delay. Laryngeal papillomatosis is caused by HPV in infant's larynx.
  ⚠ *Caution:* Always think of potential sexual abuse when a child presents with condylomata acuminata. In boys, lesions usually perianal; in girls, more often vulvar or urethral.
▶ **Diagnostic approach:** Always examine sexual partner(s) and exclude other STDs. Painting with 5% acetic acid will unmask discrete lesions by turning them white. Be sure affected women have cervical examination. If lesions are recalcitrant, consider HPV typing.
▶ **Differential diagnosis:** Table 36.**3** (p. 548) discusses differential diagnosis of genital warts. Condylomata lata (secondary syphilis) sound similar, but are large broad-based moist lesions.
▶ **Therapy:**
  • Application of podophyllotoxin 0.5% solution by patient using various regimens (for example, b.i.d. for 4 days, then 3 days of rest; repeat as needed until clear). In some countries, 5–20% tincture of podophyllin is used; it must be applied by physician 1–2× weekly until clear.
  ⚠ *Caution:* The podophyllin tincture is more irritating and should not be applied to the urethra, internally, or during pregnancy. It also contains mutagenic and carcinogenic compounds and is, in our opinion, best avoided.

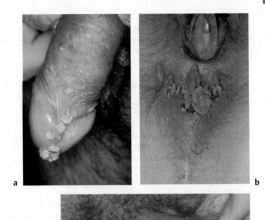

Fig. 4.11 · Condylomata acuminata. **a** Perianal. **b** Penile. **c** Bowenoid papulosis.

- Application of 50–85% trichloracetic acid tincture weekly; can be used during pregnancy.
- Cryotherapy (not anal or urethral).
- Imiquimod cream daily for 6 weeks; decrease frequency if irritating.
- Destruction with electrocautery, curettage, or laser.
- ⚠ *Caution:* Fumes are infectious and must be properly evacuated; masking is essential, to avoid any chance of inhalation.
- Adjuvant therapy with IFN-α (intralesional or systemic) may improve response in immunocompetent patients but has not been proven to reduce recurrence rate; expensive and associated with systemic side effects.
- *Adjuvant measures:*
  - Always refer patients with perianal disease for proctologic examination. Most have anal disease which serves as source of re-infection and in homosexuals as favored site of transmission.
  - Correct predisposing factors (maceration, intertrigo, vaginal discharge, phimosis, immunosuppression, sources of mechanical damage).
  - With widespread penile disease, circumcision is sometimes required.

Bowenoid Papulosis

- ▶ **Definition:** Genital carcinoma in situ, histologically resembles Bowen disease (p. 418) but may regress.
- ▶ **Pathogenesis:** Bowenoid papulosis was originally described as a pseudomalignancy, because the tendency of individual lesions to regress; HPV studies have shown it is early carcinoma in situ. Typically affects young patients.

▶ **Clinical features:** Multifocal pigmented macules or papules on the genital skin and mucosa; often involve perineum or penile shaft (Fig. 4.11 c).
▶ **Diagnostic approach:** Histological diagnosis; should be followed by HPV typing, evaluation of cervix and rectum, and partner check.
▶ **Differential diagnosis:** Closely resemble seborrheic keratosis, but these are not expected on genital skin.
▶ **Therapy:** Same as for condylomata acuminata; larger lesions can be excised.

Epidermodysplasia Verruciformis (EDV)

▶ **Synonym:** Lewandowsky–Lutz disease.
▶ **Definition:** Rare chronic HPV infection with specific autosomal recessive immune defect (MIM code 226400). Two different mutations in *EVER1* and *EVER2* genes on chromosome 17q25 which code for membrane proteins of the endoplasmic reticulum.
▶ **Pathogenesis:** Patients are infected by a series of different HPV types, some of which are carcinogenic.
▶ **Clinical features:** In childhood patients develop multiple warts and large flat lesions resembling tinea versicolor, with no tendency to spontaneous regression. Later Bowen disease and squamous cell carcinoma develop, primarily in sun-exposed skin.
▶ **Diagnostic approach:** Clinical findings; HPV typing and genetic studies essential.
▶ **Differential diagnosis:** Widespread warts in immunosuppressed individuals, such as posttransplantation or HIV/AIDS.
▶ **Therapy:** All the measures discussed above can be tried; careful monitoring and compulsive use of sunscreens; both imiquimod and topical 5-FU may be helpful; systemic retinoids for prophylaxis. Carcinomas treated in standard fashion.

5 Bacterial Diseases

5.1 Introduction

Some common cutaneous bacterial diseases are listed in Table 5.1.

Table 5.1 · Common cutaneous bacterial diseases

Group	Bacteria	Diseases
Staphylococcia	*Staphylococcus aureus* *Staphylococcus epidermidis*	Folliculitis, furuncle, furunculosis, carbuncle, impetigo, cellulitis, paronychia, toxin-mediated diseases (staphylococcal scalded skin syndrome)
Streptococci[a]	*Streptococcus pyogenes* (group A, β-hemolytic) *Streptococcus viridans*	Erysipelas, impetigo (less often), scarlet fever, ecthyma, lymphangitis, necrotizing fasciitis, purpura fulminans
Corynebacteria	*Corynebacterium minutissimum* *Corynebacterium tenuis* *Corynebacterium diphtheriae*	Erythrasma Trichomycosis axillaris Cutaneous diphtheria
Borrelia	*Borrelia burgdorferi*	Lyme borreliosis including erythema migrans, lymphadenosis cutis benigna, acrodermatitis chronica atrophicans
Treponemes	*Treponema pallidum* *Treponema pertenue* *Treponema carateum*	Syphilis Yaws Pinta
Mycobacteria	*Mycobacterium lepra* *Mycobacterium tuberculosis* *Mycobacterium bovis* *Mycobacterium avium-intracellulare* *Mycobacterium marinum* *Mycobacterium buruli*	Leprosy Tuberculosis Tuberculosis Chronic infections in HIV/AIDS Swimming pool granuloma Buruli ulcer
Actinomycetales	*Actinomyces israelii* *Nocardia brasiliensis*	Actinomycosis Nocardiosis
Gram-negative bacteria		Gram-negative folliculitis, gram-negative toe web infection, mixed infections, pyoderma in immunosuppressed patients
	Haemophilus ducreyi *Haemophilus influenzae*	Chancroid Facial cellulitis in childhood
	Pseudomonas aeruginosa	Nail fold infections, toe web infections, sepsis
	Klebsiella pneumoniae	Mixed infections

Continued Table 5.1 ▶

Table 5.1 · Continued

Group	Bacteria	Diseases
Gram-negative bacteria (Continued)	*Salmonella typhi*	Typhoid fever
	Escherichia coli	Mixed infections
	Yersinia enterocolitica	Yersiniosis, erythema nodosum
	Yersinia pestis	Plague
Chlamydia	*Chlamydia trachomatis*	Lymphogranuloma venereum
Neisseria	*Neisseria gonorrhoeae*	Gonorrhea
	Neisseria meningitidis	Meningococcal meningitis, pneumonia

a Infections with staphylococci and streptococci are usually referred to as pyodermas.

5.2 Gram-positive Bacteria: Staphylococci

▶ Staphylococci can be divided into two clinically relevant groups:
- Coagulase-positive staphylococci (*Staphylococcus aureus*) producing both invasive and toxin-mediated infections.
- Coagulase-negative staphylococci (*Staphylococcus epidermidis*), causing variety of hospital infections.

Folliculitis

▶ **Definition:** Hair follicle infection or irritation. The most common forms are caused by invasive staphylococci, but other bacteria, viruses, and fungi may also be responsible. Yet other forms (eosinophilic folliculitis in HIV/AIDS) are noninfectious. Mechanical irritation is also a factor, such prolonged sitting (*truck driver folliculitis*) or tight clothes (*blue jean folliculitis*); exposure to cutting oils is another factor.

Superficial Folliculitis
▶ **Synonyms:** Bockhart impetigo.
▶ **Clinical features:**
- Tiny pustules with erythematous border localized in superficial aspect (infundibulum) of follicle (Fig.5.**1 a**).
- *Localization:* In children, usually scalp; in adults, trunk, buttocks, thighs, beard area.
▶ **Therapy:** Topical antiseptics or antibiotics (fusidic acid or erythromycin). If lack of response, systemic antibiotics (penicillinase-resistant penicillins or first-generation cephalosporin for 7–10 days).

Furuncle

▶ **Clinical features:**
- Deep follicular infection that starts as firm red nodule which rapidly becomes painful and then, after a few days, fluctuant (Fig. 5.**1 b**). Heals with scarring over weeks. In some individuals, chronic-recurrent.
- *Localization:* Neck, face, axillae, groin, upper back.
- ⚠ *Caution:* There is a risk of sepsis in immunosuppressed patients.

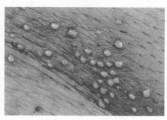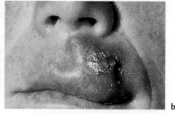

Fig. 5.1 · **a** Superficial folliculitis. **b** Furuncle on upper lip with massive edema.

▶ **Therapy:** (p. 675).
- Avoid manipulation; topical antiseptics, systemic antibiotics (penicillinase-resistant penicillin or first-generation cephalosporin for 7–10 days).
- *Solitary furuncle:* Systemic antibiotics; incision and drainage after several days when fluctuant.
- *Recurrent furuncles* (furunculosis): Systemic antibiotics (often clindamycin 300 mg q.i.d. for 7–10 days), search for predisposing factors (diabetes mellitus, immunosuppression, perineal or nasal carriage of *Staphylococcus aureus*—see below, careful skin hygiene.

Carbuncle

▶ Large indurated plaque resulting from confluence of multiple furuncles; same treatment as for furuncles.

Bullous Impetigo

▶ **Epidemiology:** In Germany most impetigo is caused by streptococci; in the USA, most caused by staphylococci. Bullous lesions suggest staphylococcal origin, but lack of blister is not diagnostically helpful.
▶ **Pathogenesis:** Staphylococci in phage group II produce a toxin, exfoliatin, coded by the phage virus, which is capable of splitting the epidermis in the stratum granulosum (acting on desmoglein 3). This action produces large superficial blisters or more diffuse superficial skin loss.
▶ **Clinical features:**
- Most patients are neonates (neonatal pustulosis) infants, or small children.
- Sudden appearance of small blisters that rapidly enlarge; little associated erythema. Soon form yellow crusts.
▶ **Diagnostic approach:** Bacterial culture; see if siblings have similar lesions.
▶ **Therapy:**
- Topical antiseptics or fusidic acid.
- Systemic antibiotics (penicillinase-resistant penicillins or first-generation cephalosporins) may slightly speed course of healing.

Staphylococcal Scalded Skin Syndrome (SSSS)

▶ **Definition:** Widespread superficial skin loss caused by exfoliation.
▶ **Clinical features:**
- Most patients are newborns or small infants.

- Rapid onset (sometimes with prodrome) of diffuse erythema and fever. After 12 hours, Nikolski phenomenon positive—stratum corneum can be pushed over underlying layers.
- Problems with temperature and fluid control because of widespread skin loss.

► **Diagnostic approach:** The organism usually cannot be cultured from the skin, but often from pharynx or other sites. Biopsy with frozen section.

► **Differential diagnosis:** In SSSS, the skin biopsy shows a very superficial epidermal split, whereas in toxic epidermal necrosis, there is full-thickness epidermal necrosis.

► **Therapy:**
- Topical antiseptics or fusidic acid.
- Place on bed covered with nonadherent sheeting.
- Attention to fluid replacement, electrolytes, temperature control.
- Systemic antibiotics (penicillinase-resistant penicillins or first-generation cephalosporins; as soon as possible, culture and sensitivity-directed choice of agents).
- Search for staphylococcal carrier among parents or especially nursing personnel in case of nursery epidemics.

  ⚠ *Caution:* Systemic corticosteroids are not effective in SSSS and should be avoided.

► **Prognosis:** Rapid healing with therapy; less than 5% mortality.

Staphylococcal Scarlet Fever

► Exanthem resembling scarlet fever produced by exfoliation. In contrast to true streptococcal scarlet fever (p. 573), pharyngitis, strawberry tongue, and oral lesions are all absent. Treatment same as for bullous impetigo.

Staphylococcal Sepsis

► **Pathogenesis:** *Staphylococcus aureus* is a common cause of community-acquired sepsis, whereas *Staphylococcus epidermidis* is the major cause of Gram-positive nosocomial sepsis. Major causes are intravenous access lines, dialysis lines, CNS shunts, artificial joints.

► **Clinical features:** Skin findings include pustules, subcutaneous abscesses, areas of purpura with pus.

◨ *Note:* Skin findings may be the first clue to a life-threatening infection.

► **Diagnostic approach:** Blood culture.

► **Therapy:**
- Systemic antibiotics; choice of agent directed by local hospital patterns as well as culture and sensitivity.
- Remove offending line or medical device.

Staphylococcal Carriage

► **Clinical features:** About 20% of individuals carry *Staphylococcus aureus* in their nares, a lesser number in the perineum. Up to 60% may transiently be carriers. The bacteria at these sites serve as a source for recurrent furunculosis, for other endogenous infections and for wound infections (with inadequate handwashing by patients or medical personnel).

► **Therapy:**
- Meticulous attention to handwashing and other personal hygiene.
- Disinfectant soaps and shampoos, used daily.

- Mupirocin ointment applied b.i.d. for 5 days, and then twice weekly, is the most effective prophylactic measure.
- Various systemic antibiotic regimens, using agents such as clindamycin and clofazimine, can be tried in consultation with infectious disease consultants.

Methicillin-resistant Staphylococcus aureus

▶ With increasing and sometimes inappropriate use of antibiotics, methicillin-resistant *Staphylococcus aureus* (MRSA) has become a major problem in hospitals, accounting for 20–30% of hospital infections. Community-based MRSA is also becoming more common. In the ambulatory setting, dermatologic patients have relatively high carrier rates, presumably because of dermatitis with barrier defects aiding colonization. Nursing home inhabitants are more likely to bring MRSA to the hospital than to take it home. Hospital staphylococcal infections can be endogenous or exogenous, in which case the hands of medical personnel are the usual culprits for transfer from one patient to another.

▶ Patients with MRSA must be isolated immediately; the single most important measure is to stop the spread of MSRA to other patients and to avoid a chronic "colonization" of the medical care facility. If MSRA is identified in cultures from outpatients, they should not be admitted unless absolutely essential. The usual antibiotic agent is vancomycin, although, disturbingly, reports of resistance to this antibiotic are also appearing.

5.3 Gram-positive Bacteria: Streptococci

There are many schemes for classifying streptococci. *Streptococcus pyogenes* (group A, β-hemolytic streptococci) account for 90% of infections. *Streptococcus viridans* (α-hemolytic streptococci) and *Streptococcus pneumoniae* are other important members of the group.

Impetigo

▶ **Definition:** Superficial skin infection.

▶ **Epidemiology:** Most patients are children. Infections usually in late summer and fall; more common under poor hygienic conditions.

▶ **Pathogenesis:** In Europe most impetigo is caused by group A streptococci (*Streptococcus pyogenes*), as well as by mixed infections with *Staphylococcus aureus*.

▣ *Note:* It is impossible to distinguish between staphylococcal and streptococcal impetigo on clinical examination. Furthermore, many infections are mixed.

▶ **Clinical features:** Crusts that develop from tiny blisters and superficial pustules. Usually on face or hands (Fig. 5.**2**).

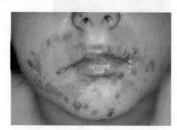

Fig. 5.**2** · Impetigo with honey-colored crusts.

- ▶ **Complications:** Glomerulonephritis is very common; rheumatic fever almost unheard of.
- ▶ **Diagnostic approach:** Culture usually reveals mixed infection. Antistreptolysin (ASL) and antistreptodornase-B (ADB) titers elevated. Check urine status at start of therapy and after 6 weeks.
- ▶ **Therapy:** Topical therapy with disinfectants or fusidic acid ointment is satisfactory for mild cases. Crusts should be removed with disinfectant soaps. Systemic antibiotics, usually penicillin, may speed healing and will reduce spread to contacts.
- ◨ *Note:* Avoid contact with other children, as well as shared washclothes and towels.

Ecthyma
....

- ▶ **Definition:** Ulcerative infection usually caused by group A streptococci.
- ▶ **Epidemiology:** Patients often show immunosuppression, inadequate nutrition, poor hygiene (homeless, drug abusers). Also common in tourists following visits to the tropics.
- ▶ **Clinical features:** Punched-out ulcers, usually on legs, presumably at sites of minor trauma (Fig. 5.**3**). Typically 0.5–3.0 cm with peripheral erythema. Healing is slow and with scarring.
- ▶ **Diagnostic approach:** Culture and sensitivity.
- ▶ **Therapy:**
  - Address predisposing factors; compression therapy may be needed.
  - Topical disinfectants or fusidic acid ointment; in difficult cases, mupirocin ointment.
  - Culture-directed systemic antibiotics.

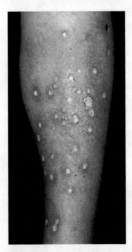

Fig. 5.**3** · Ecthymata.

Erysipelas
....

- ▶ **Definition:** Acute superficial cellulitis involving dermal lymphatics; caused by group A streptococci.

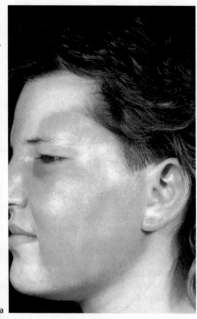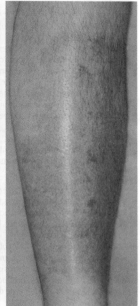

Fig. 5.4 · **Erysipelas. a** Facial. **b** On the leg.

▶ **Pathogenesis:** There is usually a portal for entry. On the face, it is often herpes simplex; on the legs, interdigital tinea with maceration. The streptococci come from nasal or perineal carriage, or from respiratory tract infections.

▶ **Clinical features:**
- Bright red, sharply demarcated, rapidly spreading erythematous patch. On the face, usually symmetrical involving the cheeks (Fig. 5.4 **a**). On the legs, unilateral with associated swelling (Fig. 5.4 **b**).
- Fever, chills, malaise.

▶ **Complications:**
- Recurrent infections lead to lymphatic damage and then lymphedema. Facial: swollen lip or lid edema; leg: *elephantiasis nostra*.
- Glomerulonephritis.
- ⚠ *Caution:* In immunosuppressed patients, there is a risk of sepsis, necrotizing fasciitis, or shock if treatment is not prompt.

▶ **Diagnostic approach:** Lesion very difficult to culture; can attempt aspirates from edge. Elevated white blood cell count, sed rate and C-reactive protein; ASL and ADB titers raised.

▶ **Therapy:** (p. 675).
- High-dose penicillin i.v.; raise limb; cool compresses.
- Later attempt to address portal of entry; consider compression, prophylactic antibiotics.

Cellulitis

▶ **Definition:** Deep infection involving dermis and subcutaneous fat, and often extending to muscles or bones.

◩ *Note:* In English, erysipelas refers only to superficial streptococcal disease, but in German it also includes superficial forms of cellulitis.

▶ **Pathogenesis:** Staphylococci and streptococci are the most common causes, but many other organisms may be involved including *Clostridium* (gas gangrene), *Haemophilus influenzae* (facial cellulitis), Gram-negative bacteria, and often mixed infections. Often a history of trauma or impaired circulation.

▶ **Clinical features:** Localized deep erythematous process usually associated with systemic signs and symptoms.

▶ **Therapy:**
  • Culture-directed systemic antibiotic therapy.
  • Incision and drainage may also be needed.

Necrotizing Fasciitis

▶ **Synonyms:** Necrotizing or gangrenous erysipelas.

▶ **Definition:** Fulminating infection of the subcutaneous fat and muscle.

▶ **Pathogenesis:** Usually caused by group A streptococci; less often by MRSA or Gram-negative bacteria.

▶ **Clinical features:** Usually involves legs. Often cutaneous lesion is entry portal. Starts with erythema, edema, and warmth. After 2–3 days red-blue color, blisters, and widespread dermal necrosis with vessel thrombosis. Spreads to involve the deep fascia and muscles, producing compartment syndrome (Fig. 5.5). The toxic bacterial products and necrotic debris trigger a massive destructive inflammatory reaction.

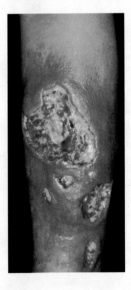

Fig. 5.**5** · Necrotizing fasciitis.

► **Diagnostic approach:** Clinical features, imaging, sonography to exclude deep vein thrombosis; ADB titer rises out of proportion to ASL titer.
► **Therapy:** Immediate generous débridement, even with just clinical suspicion, as diagnosis is notoriously difficult. Adequate drainage. Initially high-dose penicillin G (30 million IU daily) i.v. or broad spectrum coverage, switching to culture and sensitivity-directed agents as soon as possible (p. 675).

Perianal Streptococcal Dermatitis

► **Epidemiology:** Persistent perianal infection by group A β-hemolytic streptococci. Usually in children, especially boys.
► **Pathogenesis:** Patients usually have the same bacteria in their pharynx although they are asymptomatic. Presumed hand transfer. No explanation for perianal location.
► **Clinical features:** Children may complain of pain on defecation, or pruritus. Often subtle erythematous band around anus.
► **Diagnostic approach:** Culture; warn laboratory that streptococci are expected, otherwise they will only look for enteric organisms.
► **Differential diagnosis:** Psoriasis, candidiasis, pinworms, inflammatory bowel disease, child abuse.

Subacute Bacterial Endocarditis

► **Pathogenesis:** α-Hemolytic streptococci account for 60% of cases, staphylococci 20%; Gram-negative bacteria and fungi 10%; other rare causes, especially in immunosuppressed patients; in 10% no organism is cultured.
► **Clinical features:**
  • The cutaneous findings may be the first clue to the life-threatening cardiac infection.
  • Petechiae present on extremities, upper thorax, conjunctivae, gums.
  • *Subungual splitter hemorrhages:* Small red streaks seen subungually at distal end of nail. Can also be produced by chronic trauma (manual laborers).
  • *Janeway spots:* Small hemorrhagic macules on palms and digits.
  • *Osler nodes:* Small 2–3 mm tender erythematous papules on tips of digits, less often more centrally; represent septic microemboli.

Purpura Fulminans

► **Definition:** Life-threatening special form of disseminated intravascular coagulopathy (DIC).
► **Epidemiology:** Most cases follow a streptococcal infection such as scarlet fever; some may appear during the recovery period; on occasion, other infectious triggers.
► **Clinical features:**
  • Skin findings include massive ecchymoses with irregular borders, almost always starting on the legs. The intravascular thromboses lead rapidly to gangrene.
  • Patients are critically ill with fever, shock, anemia, and tachycardia. Consumptive coagulopathy leads to dramatic reduction in platelets.
► **Diagnostic approach:** CBC, platelet count, coagulation parameters.
► **Differential diagnosis:** Waterhouse–Friderichsen syndrome (meningococcal sepsis) is similar, but lesions are more widespread and CNS findings prominent.
► **Therapy:** Intensive care, high-dose penicillin, anticoagulation, perhaps high-dose corticosteroids.
► **Prognosis:** High mortality rate.

Therapy of Streptococcal Infections

▶ **Principles:**
- Culture and sensitivity for serious manifestations.
- Antibiotic of choice is penicillin G; in case of penicillin allergy, rely on local sensitivity guidelines.
- If mixed infection with staphylococci is suspected, then penicillinase-resistant penicillin, perhaps combined with ampicillin.
- Therapy for at least 10 days.

▶ **Mild infections (impetigo, scarlet fever, mild erysipelas):**
- Procaine penicillin (penicillin G) 600,000 IU i. m. 1–2× daily.
- Penicillin V 250 mg p. o. 4–6× daily.
- If mixed staphylococcal infection is suspected, dicloxacillin 500–1000 mg p. o. q8 h.
- *Penicillin allergy:* Erythromycin 500 mg p. o. q.i.d. or clindamycin 150–300 mg p. o. t.i.d.

▶ **Severe infections (widespread erysipelas, necrotizing fasciitis):**
- Hospital admission, culture and sensitivity, infectious disease consultation.
- Penicillin G 10 million IU i. v. q. 8 hours.
- If mixed staphylococcal infection is suspected, nafcillin 500–1000 mg i. v. q4–6 h (infusion over 1 hour to avoid irritation) or flucloxacillin 1 g i. v. q. 8 hours.
- If penicillin allergy suspected, cephalothin 500–1000 mg i. v. q4–6 h or cefazolin 500–1000 mg i. v. q6–8 h.
- If penicillin allergy certain, vancomycin 1.0–1.5 g i. v. daily.

▶ **Anticoagulation:** All patients receive low-dosage heparin (500 IU fractionated heparin subq. daily) while in hospital.

▶ **Chronic recurrent erysipelas:** After finishing the therapy for an acute flare, then long-term prophylaxis with benzathine penicillin 1.2 million IU i. m. monthly for 6 months. Alternative regimens include erythromycin 1.0 g p. o. daily and/or co-trimoxazole 800 mg b.i.d. for 5 days every 4–6 weeks.

▶ **Follow-up:** Because of the risk of cardiac and renal complications, the patient should be followed for at least 6 weeks. If the ASL level remains elevated or the urine sediment is abnormal, treatment should be continued until the values normalizes or nephrology consultation obtained. Follow-up electrocardiogram at 6 weeks. Always look for signs of subacute bacterial endocarditis.

Toxin-mediated Syndromes

▶ Both staphylococci and streptococci secrete a wide variety of toxins. Hallmark features are:
- Distant infection (such as streptococcal pharyngitis) causes cutaneous findings (scarlet fever). The bacteria are usually not found in the skin.
- Often actual infection is mild or limited, but secondary effects of toxins are severe. Often the toxins act as superantigens and trigger a cytokine storm.

▶ Table 5.**2** summarizes the toxin-mediated reactions, some of which are discussed in more detail above. Kawasaki disease (p. 256) may be a superantigen-mediated disorder.

Table 5.2 · Toxin-mediated reactions		
Bacteria	Toxin	Disease
Streptococcus pyogenes	Pyrogenic toxins	Scarlet fever
		Streptococcal toxic shock syndrome
Staphylococcus aureus	TSST-1	Toxic shock syndrome
	Exfoliatins	Bullous impetigo
		Staphylococcal scalded skin syndrome
		Staphylococcal scarlet fever
		Recalcitrant erythematous desquamating disorder (REDD syndrome)

5.4 Gram-positive Bacteria: Corynebacteria

Erythrasma

▶ **Definition:** Common superficial bacterial infection of intertriginous areas caused by *Corynebacterium minutissimum*.
▶ **Clinical features:** Red-brown superficial patches with fine scale, often overlooked by patients, located in intertriginous areas (groin, axillae (Fig. 5.6), interdigital).

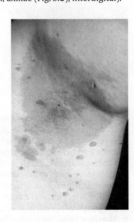

Fig. 5.**6** · Erythrasma.

▶ **Diagnostic approach:** Clinical suspicion, coral-red fluorescence on Wood's light examination. Microscopy is difficult; culture is impossible.
▶ **Differential diagnosis:**
  • *Tinea inguinalis:* Patches more infiltrated and with active border.
  • *Candidiasis:* Patches more macerated, with satellite pustules.
  • *Interdigital:* Tinea pedis, Gram-negative toe web infection.
▶ **Therapy:** Topical erythromycin solution or cream; topical imidazoles; meticulous hygiene. If resistant, then erythromycin 250 mg p. o. q.i.d. for 5–7 days.

Trichomycosis Axillaris

- ▶ **Definition:** Axillary hair infection with *Corynebacterium tenuis*.
- ▶ **Clinical features:** The axillary hairs are coated by tiny bacterial colonies (Fig. 5.7); their orange-brown color (secreted by the corynebacteria) suggests that the hairs have been dusted with a colored powdered sugar. Unpleasant odor. Pigment also found on underwear.
- ▶ **Diagnostic approach:** Clinical appearance, unpleasant odor, coral-red fluorescence in Wood's light examination; microscopic examination.
- ▶ **Differential diagnosis:** Both nits (p. 126) and hair casts (p. 513) can be excluded on microscopic examination.
- ▶ **Therapy:** Shaving of axillary hairs, deodorants, antibacterial soaps, disinfectant solutions.

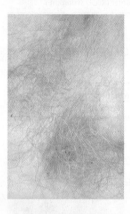

Fig. 5.7 · Trichomycosis axillaris.

Cutaneous Diphtheria

- ▶ **Definition:** Primary cutaneous infection with *Corynebacterium diphtheriae*.
- ▶ **Epidemiology:** Cutaneous diphtheria is common in the tropics; usually children are infected. Introduction via tourists is possible. In the USA, pockets of endemicity among homeless people, especially in Seattle, Washington.
- ▶ **Clinical features:** Initial blisters, then necrosis and development of shaggy, dirty ulcer that is slow to heal. Initially no generalized symptoms.
- ▶ **Complications:** Risk of nasal or pharyngeal diphtheria, production of toxins and then neurological and cardiac complications.
- ▶ **Diagnostic approach:** Skin or throat culture, immune status.
- ▶ **Therapy:** Penicillin G 1.2 million IU i.m. daily for 3 weeks or erythromycin 500 mg p.o. 3–4× daily for 3 weeks. If there is any suspicion of classic respiratory tract diphtheria, then also antitoxin and infectious disease consultation.

5.5 Gram-negative Bacterial Infections

Acute Meningococcal Sepsis

▶ **Definition:** Life-threatening infection caused by *Neisseria meningitidis*.
▶ **Clinical features:**
- General signs and symptoms include headache, neck stiffness, nausea, vomiting, myalgias.
- *Skin findings:*
  - Multiple tiny petechiae, usually on limbs, palms, soles; sometimes mucosa.
  - Larger areas of hemorrhage and necrosis are poor prognostic signs.
- *Waterhouse–Friderichsen syndrome:* Maximal variant with disseminated intravascular coagulation and adrenal infarcts. Usually in small children.
▶ **Diagnostic approach:** Immediate spinal puncture and blood cultures; intra- and extracellular paired diplococci in CSF.
▶ **Differential diagnosis:**
- *Neisseria meningitidis* causes about 50% of bacterial meningitis in adolescents and 30% in adults; consult infectious disease textbooks for other common organisms.
- The main cutaneous differential considerations are purpura fulminans (usually from streptococci) in severe cases, as well as subacute bacterial endocarditis, leukocytoclastic vasculitis, and viral exanthems for milder forms.
▶ **Therapy:** Isolate patient on suspicion of meningococcal meningitis. Infectious disease consult. For uncomplicated cases, ceftriaxone 2.0 g b.i.d. and ampicillin 2.0 g q.i.d. for 2 weeks. For complicated cases (ENT infection, trauma, nosocomial infection), contact public health officials. Tracking of contacts; prophylaxis with rifampicin or ciprofloxacin.

Chronic Meningococcal Sepsis

▶ **Definition:** Frequently overlooked chronic *Neisseria meningitidis* infection involving skin and joints.
▶ **Epidemiology:** Uncommon, but occurs in epidemics in university dormitories, army basic training camps.
▶ **Clinical features:**
- Slow onset of variety of signs and symptoms including fever, headache, myalgias, arthralgias. Recurrent bouts of fever.
- Skin changes often located near affected joints. Tiny papules or pustules, petechiae, sometimes hemorrhage, less often erythema nodosum.
▶ **Diagnostic approach:** Blood culture, skin biopsy.
▶ **Differential diagnosis:** Similar to disseminated gonococcal disease, but more chronic.
▶ **Therapy:** Same as for acute meningococcal sepsis; some recommend shorter duration.

Pseudomonas Infections

Pseudomonas aeruginosa causes a wide variety of cutaneous infections, ranging from harmless to life-threatening.

Pseudomonas Paronychia

▶ **Definition:** Infection of nail apparatus with *Pseudomonas aeruginosa*.
▶ **Clinical features:** Patients usually have prolonged exposure of hands to water and lack an intact cuticle. Painful erythematous swelling of nail fold with green-gray discoloration of nail.

▶ **Diagnostic approach:** Wood's light examination as *Pseudomonas aeruginosa* produces a green fluorescent pigment; bacterial and fungal cultures.
▶ **Differential diagnosis:** All forms of paronychia, especially candidal.
▶ **Therapy:**
- Drying measures, topical antiseptics, acetic acid (vinegar soaks, followed by blow drying).
- Correct predisposing factors.
- If mixed infection with *Candida albicans*, also treat with imidazole solution or systemic fluconazole.
- In rare circumstances, systemic antibiotic therapy; check with public health for patterns of resistance of organism.

Gram-negative Toe Web Infection
▶ **Definition:** Acute infection of the interdigital spaces of the feet; most common cause is *Pseudomonas aeruginosa*, but other Gram-negative organisms can be found, often in combination.
▶ **Clinical features:** Weeping, macerated, foul-smelling interdigital infection, usually associated with hyperhidrosis and occlusion. Major problem among US soldiers in Viet Nam. Often chronic tinea pedis survives as portal of entry.
▶ **Diagnostic approach:** Bacterial and fungal cultures; KOH examination.
▶ **Therapy:**
- Drying measures; topical disinfectants; treat fungal infection with topical or systemic imidazoles.
- Quinolones (ciprofloxacin) are probably best agent; follow culture results. Cotrimoxazole also effective, but increasing Gram-negative resistance.

Hot Tub Folliculitis
▶ Recurrent folliculitis caused by *Pseudomonas aeruginosa*; hot tubs become colonized by the bacteria and users then develop superficial, usually follicular infections. Little risk of severe disease.

Wound and Burn Infections
▶ **Clinical features:** *Pseudomonas aeruginosa* is a common colonizer of burns and extensive wounds, imparting a green color and sweet-sour smell to the exudate.
▶ **Diagnostic approach:** Culture and sensitivity; the wounds can be screened with Wood's light, as the green bacterial pigment fluoresces.
▶ **Therapy:** Most patients have superficial infections which can be treated with wet dressings using disinfectants.
🗲 *Caution:* Risk of pseudomonas sepsis, especially in patients with diabetes mellitus or immunosuppression.

Pseudomonas Sepsis
▶ **Definition:** Life-threatening infection with *Pseudomonas aeruginosa*, which can sometimes be diagnosed early on the basis of skin findings.
▶ **Epidemiology:** Predisposing factors include immunosuppression, diabetes mellitus, malignant tumors, and long-term antibiotic therapy.
▶ **Clinical features:**
- Initially hemorrhagic vesicles and blisters, solitary or grouped, and widespread. Tendency towards ulceration in flexural areas. Also widespread hemorrhagic lesions. Known as *ecthyma gangrenosum*.
- Advances to subcutaneous abscesses and cellulitis gangrenosa, which resembles decubital ulceration but not localized at sites of pressure.

▶ **Diagnostic approach:** Suspect in acutely ill patient with risk factors and cutaneous hemorrhage or ulceration; Gram stain of smear; tissue for culture and histology.
▶ **Differential diagnosis:** Almost any organism can cause sepsis in immunosuppressed patients. Possibilities include meningococcal sepsis and purpura fulminans.
▶ **Therapy:** Broad-spectrum antibiotic coverage based on culture and sensitivity results; initial therapy with tobramycin, perhaps combined with broad-spectrum penicillins or cephalosporins.
⚠ *Caution:* Tobramycin is ototoxic and nephrotoxic. Do not mix aminoglycosides with penicillin in the same bottle, as the aminoglycosides are inactivated.

Haemophilus influenzae Infections

▶ **Clinical features:** Invasive *Haemophilus influenzae* infections used to be most common in infants, causing most meningitis in this age group, as well as cellulitis and other infections. The cellulitis typically follows upper airway infections; it is usually facial. The availability of immunization has dramatically reduced this problem. Noninvasive (noncapsulated) *Haemophilus influenzae* causes community-based pneumonia in adolescents and adults, as well as less serious airway infections.
▶ **Diagnostic approach:** Culture of nose or pharynx.
▶ **Therapy:** Broad-spectrum antibiotics, such as second-generation cephalosporins, amoxicillin/clavulanic acid; alternatives include co-trimoxazole or ciprofloxacin.

Salmonella Infections

▶ **Definition:** *Salmonella typhi* and the related paratyphi cause systemic infections including typhoid fever, whereas the other forms of salmonella cause primarily gastroenteritis.
▶ **Epidemiology:** 60% of *Salmonella typhi* infections have skin findings; with other species, fewer and less specific changes.
▶ **Clinical features:**
  • Severe illness with fever, chills, respiratory symptoms and hepatomegaly. Enteritis may be present at start, but usually resolved before patient becomes so ill.
  • *Typhoid roseola or rose spots:* Subtle grouped 2–3 mm pink papules that blanch with diascopy; almost always on abdomen, appearing later in course of disease. Resolve with hyperpigmentation; new lesions can continue to appear.
  • Other skin findings include ulcerative vulvitis or proctitis, hemorrhagic exanthems, erythema nodosum.
▶ **Diagnostic approach:** Stool culture.
▶ **Therapy:** Ciprofloxacin 500 mg b.i.d. or ceftriaxone 2 g i. v. daily for 10–14 days.

Gram-negative Pyoderma

▶ **Definition:** Therapy-resistant pyodermas often occurring after visits to the tropics, following long-term antibiotic therapy, or in immunosuppressed patients.
▶ **Epidemiology:** Culture results confusing, as both staphylococci and streptococci may be isolated, as well as a spectrum of aerobic and anaerobic Gram-negative bacteria. Host immune response may also be exaggerated.
▶ **Clinical features:** There are several clinical patterns:
  • *Tropical ulcers:* Punched-out, dirty ulcers following a visit to the tropics.
  • *Chancriform pyoderma:* Aggressive widely undermined ulcers, often genital, confused with pyoderma gangrenosum (p. 251).

- *Blastomycotic pyoderma:* Same as chancriform pyoderma but with epithelial reaction resembling lesions of blastomycosis.
- *Noma:* Destructive orofacial ulceration seen in malnourished children in poor countries; may represent an extreme variant on this theme.
▶ **Diagnostic approach:** Culture of smear and tissue biopsy under aerobic and anaerobic conditions.
▶ **Differential diagnosis:** Ecthyma is similar but by definition only caused by streptococci. Overlaps exist.
▶ **Therapy:** Culture and sensitivity-directed choice of agents; often metronidazole 400 mg t.i.d. combined with ciprofloxacin.

Bartonella Infections

▶ Bartonella are small Gram-negative bacteria that are difficult to culture and classify. They overlap with Rickettsiae. The main organisms are:
- *Bartonella henselae:* Causes cat scratch fever, a zoonotic infection considered below.
- *Bartonella quintana:* Responsible for *trench fever*, a louse-transmitted disease but with humans as the reservoir; a major problem in World War I.
- *Bartonella bacilliformis*: Found in the Andes and transmitted by sandflies. Causes an acute infection (*Oroya fever*) and chronic self-healing verrucous vascular tumors (*verruga peruana*).

Bacillary Angiomatosis
▶ **Definition:** Chronic infection with *Bartonella henselae* or *Bartonella quintana* resulting in vasculogenesis; usually in patients with HIV/AIDS.
▶ **Clinical features:** Erythematous papules and plaques, often on face, which rapidly increase in number and coalesce. May also involve liver (peliosis), spleen, and bone marrow (common cause of osteomyelitis in HIV/AIDS).
▶ **Diagnostic approach:** Skin biopsy shows large numbers of bacteria positive on Warthin–Starry stain; confirmation with PCR.
▶ **Differential diagnosis:** Kaposi sarcoma, atypical mycobacterial infection, vast range of other possibilities in immunosuppressed patients.
▶ **Therapy:** Long-term erythromycin 500 mg q.i.d. or other macrolides; local destructive measures such as CO_2 laser or cryotherapy.

5.6 Miscellaneous Bacterial Infections
In this section we consider unusual infections, special clinical settings, and infections at selected sites.

Hidradenitis

▶ Hidradenitis or infections of the sweat glands are surprisingly uncommon; presumably the flushing action of sweating reduces the risk of infection. An acute abscess in an area rich in sweat hairs is difficult to define clinically; in the axillae, for example, most lesions are folliculitis or acne inversa. Chronic hidradenitis suppurativa is a misnomer; it is almost always acne inversa, involving hair follicles.
▶ Eccrine sweat ducts may be occluded; this is known as *miliaria*. Typical causes are high external temperatures, increased sweating, and occlusive clothing or bedding. Miliaria are common in newborns, as they adjust to a drier environment. Most miliaria are clear (*miliaria crystallina*), but when inflammation occurs, the

term *miliaria rubra* is applied. Such lesions look like a bacterial infection, but usually are not.
▶ A similar process occurs with *neutrophilic eccrine hidradenitis*. Eccrine sweat is responsible for eliminating many chemotherapeutic agents. Sometimes the sweat glands are damaged by these chemicals, producing a sterile pustular response. Similar lesions may occur on the palms and soles of children, perhaps representing a deep miliaria variant.

Ocular Infections

The lids and periocular region are predisposed to several bacterial infections that are similar in appearance:
▶ **Hordeolum:** Acute usually staphylococcal infection of glands of eyelid; also known as *stye*.
  • *External hordeolum* involves margin of lid and may effect glands of Zeis (modified sebaceous glands) or glands of Moll (modified apocrine glands).
  • *Internal hordeolum* involves Meibomian glands (modified sebaceous glands in the deeper tarsal plate). Can only be identified when conjunctiva is everted; often associated with edema or cellulitis.
▶ **Chalazion:** Chronic granulomatous inflammation of Meibomian gland; usually presents as painless, sometimes cystic nodule, in upper lid.
▶ **Blepharitis:** Inflammation of lid margin; most common cause is seborrheic dermatitis; always look for signs of erythema and scaling in other typical sites (hair line, behind ears). *Rosacea* (p. 535) may also cause blepharitis with dryness and pain. When staphylococci cause blepharitis, there is almost always associated conjunctivitis. Also look for nits and consider allergic contact dermatitis to ophthalmologic products.

Infections of the Fingers

In addition to bacterial and candidal paronychia, there are deeper bacterial infections of the digits requiring prompt attention. They are discussed in conjunction with diseases of the nails (p. 520).

5.7 Zoonotic Infections
▶ **Definition:** Infections transmissible from animals to humans under natural conditions.

Anthrax

▶ **Epidemiology:** *Bacillus anthracis* is a Gram-positive rod that forms spores which can live in the soil for decades. Anthrax occurs in a variety of wild and domestic animals; it has traditionally been a disease of veterinarians, farmers, and those in the leather and fur industries. Today feared as a biological weapon; a notorious incident was the sending of anthrax spores via the mail in the USA in 2002.
▶ **Clinical features:** Two major types of anthrax:
  • *Cutaneous anthrax:* Spores enter the skin through a minor injury, producing red papules that become edematous, then vesicular, and ulcerate; later a firm dark eschar develops and heals with little scarring. Although the lesion is called a malignant pustule, pus is uncommon. Surprisingly asymptomatic. May have associated lymphadenopathy (ulceroglandular form); if untreated, can lead to sepsis.

- *Pulmonary anthrax:* Spores are inhaled; initially flu-like symptoms with fever, as well as widened mediastinum (necrotizing mediastinitis) on radiograph, then fulminant course with death in 1–2 days. Intestinal anthrax is rare, but may develop when spores are ingested; also usually fatal.
▶ **Diagnostic approach:** History, bacteriologic studies, determine sensitivity to penicillin.
▶ **Differential diagnosis:** Furuncle (painful), orf, milker's nodule, tularemia, plague.
▶ **Therapy:** Treatment of choice is ciprofloxacin 500 mg p.o. b.i.d. or doxycycline 100 mg p.o. b.i.d. for mild disease below the neck. If severe, marked edema, or facial, then i.v. use of the same agents is recommended. If the bacillus is sensitive to penicillin, then a switch to amoxicillin or high-dose i.v. penicillin is appropriate. Intravenous corticosteroids may be needed for edema.
◨ **Note:** Treatment does not influence the skin lesions. It must be continued for 60 days to offer effective prophylaxis against pulmonary anthrax.
▶ **Prophylaxis:** Either ciprofloxacin or doxycycline can be used following possible exposure.
▶ **Immunization:** Two vaccines are available, but they are short-acting and of questionable efficacy. US military immunizes all soldiers.
▶ **Prognosis:** Pulmonary anthrax is almost always fatal; most cutaneous anthrax can be treated.

Erysipeloid

▶ **Epidemiology:** *Erysipelothrix rhusiopathiae* is a Gram-positive rod that infects a variety of animals including pigs, saltwater fish, and poultry. Risk groups include butchers and fishermen. Infections more common in summer.
▶ **Clinical features:** Incubation period 2–8 days. Livid or red plaque with central healing, usually on finger or hand. Usually mild course; rarely joint involvement, or in immunosuppressed patients sepsis or endocarditis.
▶ **Diagnostic approach:** History, culture usually from biopsy material.
▶ **Differential diagnosis:** Despite name, not easily confused with erysipelas. *Seal finger* is clinically similar, but occurs following contact with seals, as it is caused by a marine mycoplasma. *Vibrio vulnificus* is found is shallow or marshy seawater; injuries handling crabs or lobsters may produce such lesions, especially in immunosuppressed patients.
▶ **Therapy:** Penicillin G 1.2 million IU i.m. daily or b.i.d. for 10 days. With penicillin allergy, erythromycin or tetracycline.

Rickettsial Diseases

▶ **Definition:** Rickettsia are small Gram-negative bacteria, with cell walls, that multiple only within host cells Examples are listed in Table 5.**3**.
▶ **Epidemiology:** Rickettsia live within the gut of arthropods and are transferred to humans by bites. Often the natural host is a rodent; the human is an incidental host. Geographic and hygienic factors play a major role, as demonstrated by outbreaks of epidemic typhus during wars and following natural disasters. After an infection, there is long-standing immunity.
▶ **Clinical features:**
  - Headache, nausea, chills, and high fever 1–3 weeks after bite. Typical is a necrotic papule at the site of bite (eschar). Rocky Mountain spotted fever (RMSF) may have lymphadenopathy; typically absent in typhus.
  - Soon after the fever, macular to maculopapular exanthems appear on the trunk; they may become hemorrhagic. In RMSF, first lesions are on palms and soles. Epidemic typhus may also have a thrombotic vasculitis.

Table 5.3 · Rickettsia

Organism	Disease	Vector
Rickettsia rickettsii	Rocky Mountain spotted fever	Ticks
Rickettsia prowazekii	Endemic typhus	Lice
Rickettsia typhi	Epidemic typhus	Lice, fleas
Rickettsia conorii	Mediterranean tick bite fever	Ticks
Rickettsia akari	Rickettsial pox	Mites

▶ **Diagnostic approach:** The classic Weil–Felix test is first positive after 2 weeks and does not help identify the species of rickettsia. Microimmunofluorescence or immunoblot tests are usually used; the same immunofluorescence antibodies can be applied to skin biopsies.
▶ **Differential diagnosis:** Exanthems are not clinically specific; history and presence of eschar help.
▶ **Therapy:** Doxycycline 100 mg b.i.d. for 5–7 days for mild disease; severely ill patients should be hospitalized for i.v. medications. Many different alternatives; consult infectious diseases books.
▶ **Prophylaxis:** Doxycycline 100–200 mg in single dose sometimes employed after tick bite in endemic region, but little supporting data. Aggressive control of vectors.

Tularemia

▶ **Definition:** *Francisella tularensis* is a Gram-negative rod present in a variety of small mammals in Europe and primarily North America.
▶ **Epidemiology:** Spread is usually via direct contact, such as in hunters, but spread by vectors is also possible.
▶ **Clinical features:** Four clinical forms:
  • *Ulceroglandular form:* Most common, often in hunters who skin rabbits. Organisms enter skin, cause small pustules after 2–10 days, rapid advance to dirty ulcers. Regional lymphadenopathy. Less than 5% fatality.
  • *Oculoglandular form:* Similar, but entry via conjunctiva.
  • *Pulmonary form:* Direct lung infection.
  • *Typhoidal form:* Fever without local findings.
▶ **Diagnostic approach:** Usually clinical diagnosis; immunofluorescence antibodies available for tissue detection, as usual stains difficult; lymph nodes have typical histology (zonal necrosis); serology takes several weeks to become positive.
▶ **Therapy:** Streptomycin 1–2 g i.m. daily for 7–14 days or gentamicin 5 mg/kg i.v. daily; numerous alternatives; see infectious disease texts.

Cat Scratch Fever

▶ **Definition:** Self-limiting infection with *Bartonella henselae*, a small Gram-negative rod.
▶ **Epidemiology:** Most patients are children or adolescents; transmission is via cat scratch or other contact.

▶ **Clinical features:**
- Incubation period 3–14 days.
- Primary lesion at site of scratch; papule that evolves into pustule and then nodule; usually on hand or arm, resolves over 1–2 months; only occurs in 50% of patients.
- Regional lymphadenopathy, usually unilateral, often fluctuant and painful, resolves after 1–2 months.
- Systemic signs and symptoms including fever, chills, malaise, myalgias, arthralgias; both erythema multiforme and erythema nodosum may be seen. Rare complications include retinitis, encephalitis, and Parinaud syndrome (sterile conjunctivitis plus unilateral lymphadenopathy).

▶ **Diagnostic approach:** Very difficult, causative organism confirmed in past decade; usually a clinical decision confirmed by PCR.

▶ **Differential diagnosis:** Tularemia, sarcoidosis, tuberculosis.

▶ **Therapy:** Often no therapy needed, but azithromycin 250 mg p.o. daily appears to be agent of choice.

Animal Bites

Bites account for about 1% of emergency room visits in the USA. All patients should be assessed for the risk of rabies and need for tetanus immunization. Bites from different sources have different features:

▶ **Dog bites:** Most injuries are from crushing or chewing; risk of infection is greatest on distal extremities. Only about 20% become infected. Common organisms include staphylococci, streptococci, *Pasteurella multocida*, and a number of pathogens unique to canines, including *Capnocytophaga canimorsus* (which may cause sepsis in splenectomized individuals). Usually treated with amoxicillin/clavulanic acid. Nonfacial or older wounds generally not closed.

▶ **Cat bites:** Felines are more likely to inflict puncture wounds; deeper structures more easily reached than by dog bites. At least 50% of bites become infected. *Pasteurella multocida* is most common cause; amoxicillin/clavulanic acid once again appropriate.

▶ **Exotic bites:** Always check Internet to see what is known; for example, swans transmit *Pseudomonas aeruginosa*; there was an epidemic of monkeypox in USA transmitted by pet ground squirrels.

▶ **Human bites:** The worst bite of all. The "inadvertent" bite when a clenched fist contacts the teeth (in other words, a punch) often leads to tendon and joint infections in the aggressor. Most infections are mixed, with anaerobic species usually admixed. Amoxicillin/clavulanic acid is usually appropriate; hand injuries should be referred promptly to hand surgeon.

5.8 Borreliosis

▶ **Synonyms:** Lyme borreliosis or Lyme disease.

▶ **Definition:** Infection with *Borrelia burgdorferi*, transferred by ticks. Stage I and stage II represent early disease; stage III, late (Fig. 5.**8**).

▶ **Epidemiology:** *Borrelia burgdorferi* is a spirochete; three different species have been identified:
- *Borrelia burgdorferi sensu stricto*.
- *Borrelia garinii*.
- *Borrelia afzelii*.

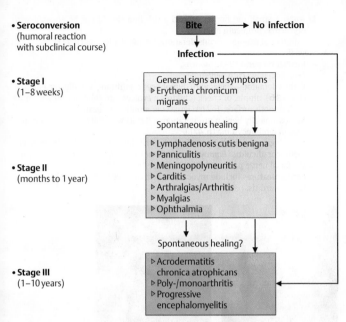

Fig. 5.8 · Stages of borrelial infection (after Orfanos and Garbe).

► All three are found in Europe, but only *Borrelia burgdorferi sensu stricto* is found in USA. *Borrelia afzelii* is more likely to cause neurologic disease and acrodermatitis chronica atrophicans, perhaps explaining the paucity of these problems in the USA. The initial cases of borrelial arthritis were described along the Lyme River in Connecticut, leading to the name Lyme disease.

► The natural hosts are ticks; in endemic areas, over 90% may be infected. The main vectors are *Ixodes ricinus* (Western Europe), *Ixodes scapularis* (Eastern USA), and *Ixodes pacificus* (Western USA). Both adult ticks and small nymphs transfer the bacteria by bites; in 50% of cases not noticed as the bites are painless. The risk of infection is estimated at 1–5/100 bites, depending on how endemic the disease is. Transmission in the first 36 hours is rare, as the organism must be activated in the tick following attachment. Antibodies are developed, but provide no protection against reinfection (p. 679).

► **Clinical features:**
  ● *Stage I:*
    – Incubation period 1–8 weeks.
    – *Erythema chronicum migrans* (ECM): Red papule develops on trunk or limb at site of bite. Slowly a spreading annular erythema evolves as the papule fades (Fig. 5.9 a). Often pruritic. Variants include multiple lesions and complex intersecting lesions.
    – Associated headache, malaise, or joint pain. Resolution after about 10 weeks with or without treatment.

▶ *Note:* A small red border around a tick bite should not be equated with erythema chronicum migrans.

– Differential diagnostic considerations for annular lesions (p. 711).

• *Stage II:*

– Incubation period 2–12 months.

– *Lymphadenosis cutis benigna:*

– Early edematous stage with lymphocytic infiltrate, usually on ear lobe (Fig. 5.**9 b**), nipple, or cheek (children); evolves into solid red-brown tumor with smooth surface, 1–2 cm large over months to a year.

– Microscopically benign proliferation of B cells with follicles; most common type of lymphocytoma (p. 471).

– Neurologic manifestations include meningoencephalitis, lymphocytic meningoradiculitis (*Bannwarth syndrome*), radicular pains, peripheral paresis (facial nerve palsy and others); pleocytosis of CSF.

– Cardiac features include myocarditis with atrioventricular block, pericarditis, pancarditis.

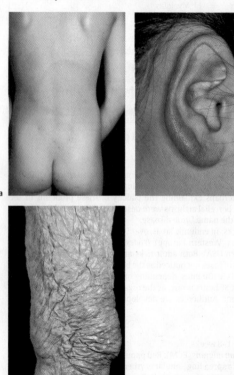

Fig. 5.**9** · **a** Erythema chronicum migrans. **b** Lymphadenosis cutis benigna (lymphocytoma). **c** Acrodermatitis chronica atrophicans.

- Rheumatologic manifestations include arthralgias, myalgias, oligoarthritis (often knee), more common in USA.
- Other findings include lymphadenopathy, inflammatory ocular disease, renal involvement.
- *Stage III:*
  - *Acrodermatitis chronica atrophicans:* Most dramatic change with development of very atrophic skin (*cigarette paper skin*) over the distal extremities (ankles, knees, Fig. 5.**9** c). Initially puffy vague erythema which over years becomes atrophic with loss of subcutaneous fat so that underlying vessels can be easily visualized.
  - *Juxtaarticular nodules:* Fibrous proliferations over the elbows and knees; when the lesion is linear extending down the forearm, known as *ulnar streak*.
  - Some cases of lymphadenosis cutis benigna may evolve into cutaneous marginal zone B-cell lymphoma, which sometimes responds to antiborrelial therapy.
  - Systemic features include peripheral neuropathies, encephalomyelitis, chronic arthritis.

▶ **Diagnostic approach:**
- Dermatologic, neurologic, rheumatologic, and cardiologic evaluation, depending on stage and clinical features.
- Serological studies include ELISA and Western blot demonstration of antibodies; in stage I 20–50% (usually IgM); stage II 70–90% (initially IgM, then IgG); stage III 100%.
- **🗹 Caution:** False-positive IgM titers arise in syphilis, some malignancies, autoimmune diseases, and acute Epstein–Barr virus infection. IgG titer alone does not prove active infection.
- Other signs of infection: complement ↓ , sed rate ↑ , C-reactive protein ↑ .
- Active neuroborreliosis diagnosed on basis of CSF pleocytosis with increased lymphocytes and intrathecal antibody product (CSF/serum quotient).
- Histology for lymphocytoma, acrodermatitis chronica atrophicans.

▶ **Therapy:**
- Stage-adjusted therapy as shown in Table 5.**4**. Adequate therapy is essential to avoid the complications associated with later stages; on the other hand, therapy should not be administered on a prophylactic basis or when the diagnosis is not certain.

Table 5.4 · **Treatment of cutaneous borreliosis**

Stage I	Stage II	Stage III
Doxycycline 100 mg p. o. b.i.d. for 14–21 days	Doxycycline 100 mg p. o. b.i.d. for 21 days or ceftriaxone 2 g i. v. daily for 14 days	Ceftriaxone 2 g i. v. daily for 14 days
Alternatives: Tetracycline, ampicillin, oral cephalosporins	Alternative: Penicillin G 5–10 million IU i. v. t.i.d. for 21 days	Alternative: Penicillin G 5–10 million IU i. v. t.i.d. for 21 days
Children/pregnancy: Ampicillin, amoxicillin, erythromycin	Children/pregnancy: Ampicillin, amoxicillin, erythromycin	

Bacterial Diseases

⚠ Caution: It is especially important to avoid treating patients with positive IgG titers for borrelial antibodies and vague symptoms for chronic borreliosis.
- If titers remain elevated and clinical findings persists, re-treatment with ceftriaxone i. v. should be considered.

▶ **Prophylaxis:**
- Avoid exposure in endemic areas; avoid woods as much as possible, use insect repellents; check carefully for ticks 1–2 × daily.
- Removal of tick in first 24 hours is the single most important measure.

5.9 Mycobacterial Infections: Tuberculosis

Overview
....

▶ **Causative agent:** Mycobacteria are small, nonmotile, slightly curved acid-fast rods. *Mycobacterium tuberculosis* causes >95% of human tuberculosis; *Mycobacterium bovis* is responsible for the rest.

▶ **Epidemiology:**
- Only 10% of individuals with normal immune status who are infected with *Mycobacterium tuberculosis* develop active tuberculosis.
- Factors that decrease host resistance include:
  - Malnutrition, immunosuppression, malignancies, other major illnesses.
  - *Age:* Children <3 years of age have a more severe course; 3–12 year-olds almost always have spontaneous healing. Later, resistance drops with increasing age.
  - *Pulmonary silicosis:* Increased risk for tuberculosis; always ask in history.
- Today in Europe drug abusers, patients with HIV/AIDS, lymphoma, leukemia, and iatrogenic immunosuppression are all at great risk for tuberculosis. In some situations, such as prisoners in some parts of Eastern Europe, the problem is epidemic.
- Immigration of patients from countries where tuberculosis is endemic is another factor in the surge of cases in developed countries.
- *Mycobacterium bovis* has become uncommon as cattle tuberculosis has almost been eliminated in most developed countries.

▶ **Resistance:**
- The number of strains resistant to single agents or to multiple drugs is continuing to increase. Factors include inappropriate single drug therapy and inadequate duration of therapy, both leading to selection of resistant strains. Strict combination regimens, perhaps administered under direct observation, are considered the only effective public health measure.
- ▣ **Note:** Patients with HIV/AIDS and multidrug resistant *Mycobacterium tuberculosis* are currently the major sources of infection.

▶ **Diagnostic approach:**
- *Microscopic examination:* Staining with Ziehl–Neelsen stain or auramine fluorescence staining can be used to examine tissue sections or bodily fluids. Rapid, but only sensitive when large numbers of organisms are present (10^3–10^4/mL).
- *Culture:* Both species grow slowly on special media (Löwenstein–Jensen) under anaerobic conditions. Initial growth takes 3–10 weeks, followed by differentiation and determination of drug sensitivity, lasting total of 2–3 months. BACTEC method with radiometric measurement of metabolites takes 7–10 days.

- *Other possibilities:* PCR for *Mycobacterium tuberculosis* DNA in skin biopsies; this technique has become important because it is so difficult to culture the organisms in skin.

▶ **Pathogenesis**.
- *Primary infection:*
  - The usual site of infection is the lungs following droplet spread. A nonspecific leukocyte-rich inflammatory response develops, known as a *tubercle*. From there the bacteria move to regional lymph nodes (*primary complex* or *Ghon complex*). Then the bloodstream is invaded, so that the mycobacteria can be spread throughout the body.
  - After 2–4 weeks a specific cell-mediated immunity develops and the host is usually able to bring the infection under control. Healing occurs with fibrosis and calcification.
- *Endogenous reactivation:* Organisms that have been spread about the body during the primary infection can survive in different organs for years. If the host immune response diminishes, then the bacteria can once again cause active disease. If the resistance is modest, the disease will remain localized; with sharp diminution in resistance, disseminated disease occurs.
- *Secondary infection:* Secondary infections are uncommon with specific immunity and good resistance, but they can occur.

Clinical Forms of Cutaneous Tuberculosis

The clinical expressions of cutaneous tuberculosis all reflect an interplay between the virulence of the bacteria and the variations in host resistance and previous exposure. There is a bewildering list of names; we have picked just a few examples. All are rare today, but may increase in prevalence if the current increasing trend in pulmonary tuberculosis continues.

Primary Cutaneous Tuberculosis (Inoculation Tuberculosis)
▶ **Definition:** Lesion resulting from direct introduction of *Mycobacterium tuberculosis* or *Mycobacterium bovis* into skin of previously unexposed host.
▶ **Epidemiology:** Uncommon; most patients are children.
▶ **Clinical features:** At first small papules develop at inoculation site; they expand into a painless ulcer several centimeters across: *primary lesion* (analogous to tubercle in lung). Then after 3–8 weeks, regional lymphadenopathy appears: *primary complex* (analogous to Ghon complex). Healing within a year, usually with scarring.
▶ **Diagnostic approach:** Culture and biopsy.
▶ **Therapy:** Systemic therapy; (p. 100).

Tuberculosis Cutis Miliaris Disseminata
▶ **Clinical features:** Hematogenous dissemination in infants or immunosuppressed individuals; many skin lesions, as well as systemic lesions, and a very poor prognosis.

Tuberculosis Mucosae et Cutis Ulcerosa
▶ **Synonym:** Orificial tuberculosis.
▶ **Clinical features:** Patients with a high load of *Mycobacterium tuberculosis* and poor resistance develop mucosal lesions, usually ragged, painful oral ulcers. Prognosis is dismal.
▶ **Therapy:** Systemic therapy; (p. 100).

Tuberculosis Cutis Colliquativa

▶ **Synonyms:** Scrofuloderma.

▶ **Definition:** Subcutaneous tuberculosis with development of cold abscesses and spread to skin.

▶ **Epidemiology:** Patients are usually young children or elderly people.

▶ **Pathogenesis:**

- *Scrofuloderma:* Spread of subcutaneous tuberculosis into subcutaneous fat and then skin from infected lymph node, bone, or other tissue.
- *Tuberculous gumma:* Hematogenous spread of mycobacteria with multiple liquefying cold abscesses that break though to the skin.

▶ **Clinical features:**

- Usually the lymph nodes of the neck and submandibular region are involved. They are infected from the primary pulmonary tuberculosis or directly infected from the tonsils (in the past when milk infected with *Mycobacterium bovis* was ingested).
- Initially indolent blue-red nodules (cold abscesses) that enlarge and break down. The ulcers are bizarre, undermined, and tend to form fistulas (Fig. 5.10 a). Healing occurs after years, with typical strands of scarring.
- Hematogenous lesions involve the trunk and extremities, often with simultaneous lesions in bones (fingers, sternum, ribs).

▶ **Diagnostic approach:** Histology of edge shows typical tubercles; culture or PCR of discharged materials.

▶ **Differential diagnosis:** Syphilitic gumma, deep fungal infections, acne conglobata, acne inversa.

▶ **Therapy:** Systemic therapy (p. 100).

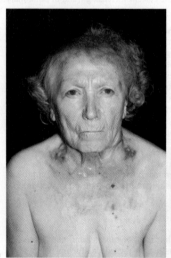
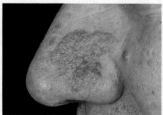

Fig. 5.**10** · **a** Tuberculosis cutis colliquativa. **b** Lupus vulgaris.

Lupus vulgaris

► **Definition:** Chronic dermal infection with *Mycobacterium tuberculosis* or *Mycobacterium bovis*.
► **Epidemiology:** Most patients are elderly; women are affected twice as often as men. Most common form of cutaneous tuberculosis in Europe.
► **Pathogenesis:** Lupus vulgaris is usually the result of endogenous reactivation; the mycobacteria reach the dermis by direct spread from lymph nodes, or by hematogenous or lymphatic spread.
► **Clinical features:**
  • Large red-brown atrophic patches or plaques with telangiectases (Fig. 5.**10 b**). Sites of predilection include face (especially nose and ears), breasts, and thighs. Crusts, ulceration, and destruction of adjacent tissue (cartilage of ear or nose) lead to mutilation.
  • Classic lesion is the *lupus nodule,* 2–3 mm slightly elevated papule at periphery. On diascopy, characteristic "apple jelly" color surrounded by pale border. When one presses on a lupus nodule with a sound, one can break through with little pain: *sound phenomenon.* The histologic equivalent of a lupus nodule is a tubercle.
  • 40–50% of patients have tuberculosis in other organs. Pulmonary tuberculosis is 10-fold as common as in general population. Other sites include lymph nodes, mucosa, joints, bones.
► **Diagnostic approach:**
  • Biopsy; very few organisms present so PCR more useful than Ziehl–Neelsen stain. Microscopic picture reveals granulomas with classic three-zone pattern of tuberculosis: central necrosis, band of epithelioid macrophages and Langhans giant cells, rim of lymphocytes.
  • Culture and sensitivity.
  • Complete examination to identify tuberculosis elsewhere and search for signs of impaired immune response.
► **Therapy:** Systemic therapy; (p. 100).

Tuberculosis Cutis Verrucosa

► **Definition:** Exogenous reinfection in individual with intact specific immune response; very uncommon.
► **Pathogenesis:** Two sources of infection:
  • *Infected human material:* Injuries during autopsies or other medical services, known as *prosector's wart.*
  • *Infected cows:* Now very rare, but used to be common in slaughterhouse workers and butchers.
► **Clinical features:** Solitary verrucous papule or nodule, no lupus nodules, central clearing.
► **Diagnostic approach:** Biopsy, PCR; organisms otherwise hard to identify.
► **Differential diagnosis:** Butcher's warts are usually multiple; erysipeloid is more inflammatory; atypical mycobacterial infection (swimming pool granuloma).
► **Therapy:** Systemic therapy; (p. 100).

Tuberculids

► **Definition:** In the past tuberculid was defined as a reaction to *Mycobacterium tuberculosis* without direct infection; it included many diseases with granulomatous histology but no connection to tuberculosis, such as rosacea. As tuberculosis became more rare, it became clear that the connections were tenuous. Examples include:

- *Tuberculids with some evidence of relationship to* Mycobacterium tuberculosis: Lichen scrofulosorum, papulonecrotic tuberculid, erythema induratum.
- *Tuberculids unlikely to be infection-related:* Lupus miliaris disseminatus faciei, rosacea-like tuberculid, acneiform tuberculid.

Therapy

▶ **Overview:** The World Health Organization has issued very specific guidelines for treating tuberculosis (Table 5.5). The goals are to effectively arrest the disease in the patient, to decrease transmission, and to avoid selecting drug-resistant strains. Treatment plans all have two phases: an initial phase (more aggressive daily therapy; usually for 2 months) and a continuation phase (less aggressive, often 3× weekly, for 4–6 months). Crucial points are:

- Use of multiple agents, often in combination to avoid resistance.
- Direct observation of patients where possible.
- Minimum of 3× weekly dosing; otherwise peaks and troughs not adequate.

Table 5.5 · **WHO essential drugs for tuberculosis**

	Drug	Dosage (mg/kg)
	Daily	3 × weekly
Isoniazid	5	10
Rifampicin	10	10
Pyrazinamide	25	35
Streptomycin	15	15
Ethambutol	15	30
Thiacetazone[a]	2.5	2.5

a Not recommended when ethambutol is available.

▶ **Treatment of cutaneous disease:** There are few guidelines addressing the treatment of extrapulmonary tuberculosis, since from a public health point of view most patients require treatment for their pulmonary disease. Rifampicin appears to be the single most important agent. A typical regimen for lupus vulgaris or other primarily cutaneous tuberculosis might include:

- *Phase I:* isoniazid + rifampicin + ethambutol or pyrazinamide, all daily for 2–3 months.
- *Phase II:* Same drugs as above, but only 3× weekly for 4–6 months; ethambutol can be eliminated or dose lowered.
- *Alternative:* isoniazid 300 mg daily + rifampicin 600 mg daily for 6 months.
- Immunosuppressed patients should be treated longer. Four-agent scheme with streptomycin may be indicated.
- Follow-up after 6 and 12 months.

5.10 Mycobacterial Infections: Leprosy

Overview

▶ **Definition:** Chronic infection with *Mycobacteria lepra*.
▶ **Epidemiology:**
  • Found primarily in tropical and subtropical countries.
  • 2–3 million individuals are infected worldwide, most in the Indian subcontinent.
  • Has disappeared or been eliminated in temperate countries, but cases continue to be introduced by immigration from countries with endemic disease.
  • Aggressive public health measures have dramatically reduced the incidence, but strains resistance to dapsone and rifampicin have started to appear.
  • Infection usually occurs in childhood. The incubation period is 2–10 years; most patients develop adequate immunity so that relatively few patients develop clinical findings. Chronic exposure also appears essential; tourists almost never acquire leprosy, although longer-term visitors occasionally become infected.
▶ **Pathogenesis:** Just as with tuberculosis, leprosy reflects an interplay between the immune status of the patient and the virulence of the mycobacteria. Didactically useful to think of two poles (Table 5.**6**), although many patients lie somewhere between these extremes.

Table 5.6 · **Comparison of the two poles of leprosy**

Form	Tuberculoid	Lepromatous
Resistance	High	Low
Number of organisms	Low	High
Clinical symmetry	Asymmetrical	Symmetrical
Lesion border	Sharp	Vague
Histology	Granulomas	Diffuse infiltrates

▶ **Clinical features:**
  • *Indeterminate leprosy:* The initial cutaneous manifestations of leprosy are subtle and not specific. Initially erythematous patch, which in darker-skinned individuals appears pale; most cases resolve, some advance into more severe disease. Differential diagnostic considerations include vitiligo, nevus anemicus, nevus depigmentosus, postinflammatory hypopigmentation, pityriasis alba, tinea versicolor.
  • *Tuberculoid leprosy:*
    – *Skin findings:* One or multiple erythematous or scaly, well-circumscribed macules or patches; usually hypo- or anesthetic (Fig. 5.**11a**). Differential diagnostic considerations include lupus vulgaris, chronic cutaneous lupus erythematosus (discoid), tinea corporis.
    – All patients have nerve involvement. Inflammation of Schwann cells leads to thickening of peripheral nerves.
    – Course generally benign.
  • *Borderline leprosy:* More lesions, more widespread and less sharply defined than in tuberculoid form. Usually symmetrical on trunk but may be asymmetric on face. Less likely to have scale. Nerve involvement less prominent.

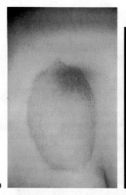 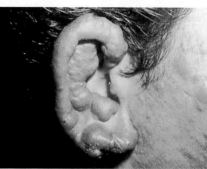

a   b

Fig. 5.**11** · **Leprosy. a** Tuberculoid. **b** Lepromatous (Images courtesy of Juan J. Ochoa MD, Chihuahua, Mexico).

- *Lepromatous leprosy:*
  – Papular and nodular lesions symmetrically distributed. Often start on nose and ears, later involve hands, arms, buttocks (Fig. 5.**11b**). Facial lesions can be markedly swollen (*leonine facies*) with loss of eyebrows (*Lucio sign*). In Mexico and Central America, *leprosy bonita* (pretty leprosy) refers to the initial loss of wrinkling in some patients with diffuse disease. Glossitis may occur. Later, destruction of the nasal cartilage with mutilation.
  – Nasal secretions rich in organisms.
  – Complications include orchitis, facial mutilation, neurotrophic ulcers, flexion contractures of hands, foot drop.
  – Differential diagnostic considerations include myxedema, neurofibromatosis, post-kala-azar dermal leishmaniasis.
- ▶ **Diagnostic approach:**
  - Skin biopsy; histological examination; Ziehl–Neelsen works well in lepromatous leprosy. For paucibacillary forms, PCR is available, but has not been as effective as hoped.
  - Nasal smear or scraping from tissue fluid from ear in lepromatous leprosy reveals numerous organisms on Ziehl–Neelsen stain.
  - Neurological examination (anesthetic patches, enlarged nerves).
  - *Lepromin test (Mitsuda test):* Injection of an extract from lepromatous tissue; positive response is development of nodule after 3–4 weeks in tuberculoid leprosy.
  - False-positive serological tests for syphilis in lepromatous leprosy.
- ▶ **Therapy:**
  - Many different agents available for treating leprosy. Current WHO recommendations:
    – *Tuberculoid leprosy:* Dapsone 100 mg daily and rifampicin 600 mg monthly for 6–9 months.
    – *Single lesion (tuberculoid or indeterminate):* Dapsone 600 mg, ofloxacin 400 mg, and minocycline 100 mg as single dose.
    – *Lepromatous leprosy:* Dapsone 100 mg daily; clofazimine 150 mg, and rifampicin 600 mg monthly for 12–18 months.

◪ *Note:* After the first dose, patients are no longer infectious to others.
- In case of questions or poor response, always consult responsible public health officials.

Leprosy Reactions

▶ **Definition:** Acute inflammation that appears suddenly during treatment.
▶ **Clinical features:**
- *Type I reaction (reversal reaction):*
  - Increase in cell-mediated (type IV) immunity with flaring of nerve or skin involvement.
  - Therapy: systemic corticosteroids (prednisone 20–60 mg daily).
- *Type II reaction (vasculitic reaction):*
  - Increased in circulating immune complexes with vasculitis.
- *Two clinical forms:*
  - *Erythema nodosum leprosum*: Erythematous nodules on legs and arms (in contrast to true erythema nodosum).
  - *Lucio phenomenon*: Necrotizing small vessel vasculitis.
▶ **Therapy:** Thalidomide 100–200 mg daily.

5.11 Atypical Mycobacterial Infections

Swimming Pool Granuloma

▶ **Definition:** Infection with *Mycobacterium marinum*.
▶ **Pathogenesis:** *Mycobacterium marinum* is an aquatic species that causes tuberculosis-like disease in fish. It can enter the skin following injuries in swimming pools, natural bodies of water, or home aquariums.
▶ **Clinical features:**
- Incubation period 3 weeks.
- Site of entry minor injuries on hands, knees.
- Usually verrucous papules or nodules (Fig. 5.**12**); sometimes associated with sporotrichoid lymphangitic spread (p. 713).
- Spontaneous healing over years.
▶ **Diagnostic approach:** Culture from homogenized skin biopsy, at 31–33 °C. Always warn laboratory when diagnosis is suspected. Photochromogen that grows out in 7–10 days.
▶ **Differential diagnosis:** Common wart, tuberculosis cutis verrucosa, squamous cell carcinoma; if lymphangitic, sporotrichosis.

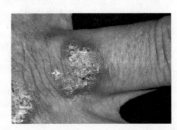

Fig. 5.**12** · Swimming pool granuloma.

► **Therapy:**
  • Small lesions can be excised.
  • Doxycycline 100 mg b.i.d. for 8–12 weeks.
  • Local heat application (hand warmer or similar device).
  • If not responsive, then rifampicin 150 mg t.i.d. and ethambutol 400 mg t.i.d. until clinically responsive, following culture and sensitivity studies.

Buruli Ulcer

► **Epidemiology:** Infection with *Mycobacterium buruli*, which is found primarily in tropical Africa and Australia. Associated with moist environments.
► **Pathogenesis:** *Mycobacterium buruli* is the only mycobacterium that produces a highly tissue-destructive toxin.
► **Clinical features:** Initially subcutaneous nodules develop at the site of injury or inoculation, usually on limbs. These progress rapidly to large undermined ulcers extending down to the fascia, which are surprisingly asymptomatic considering their size and depth. Healing with scarring occurs spontaneously after years.
► **Therapy:**
  • Surgical debridement and then skin grafting.
  • Supplemental heat therapy (infrared radiation).
  • Rifampicin perhaps in combination with co-trimoxazole or clarithromycin appears to be the most effective agent.

Mycobacterium avium-intracellulare

► Group of slow-growing bacteria that are ubiquitous, so that avoidance is impossible.
► Rare cause of primary inoculation or pulmonary lesions in healthy individuals.
► Prior to HAART, major problem in HIV/AIDS affecting at least 40 % of patients with disseminated infection contributing to wasting syndrome. Today, more likely to cause localized disease such as soft tissue abscesses or lymphadenitis (p. 160).
► Therapy is complex; multiple agents are always required for long periods of time. The standard regimen is clarithromycin (or azithromcin), ethambutol and rifabutin for at least six months.

5.12 Actinomycosis

► **Definition:** Chronic, slowly spreading infection with *Actinomyces israelii*, an anaerobic, Gram-positive bacterium.
► **Pathogenesis:** *Actinomyces israelii* is part of the normal flora of the mouth, airways, and gastrointestinal tract. Infections are endogenous, following tissue injury which favors anaerobic growth. Patients are not infectious. Secondary mixed infections, especially with *Actinobacillus actinomycetemcomitans*, are common.
► **Clinical features:** Three classic forms:
  • *Cervicofacial:* Most common form (> 50 %); usually follow dental work or periapical inflammation; induration of chin or neck with sinus tracts and drainage of pus; no lymphadenopathy.
  • *Thoracic:* Pulmonary lesions often with drainage to overlying skin; usually follow aspiration.
  • *Gastrointestinal:* Chronic inflammation and drainage, following infection (appendicitis) or bowel injury. A possible variant is pelvic actinomycosis, associated with use of an intrauterine contraceptive device.

▶ **Diagnostic approach:** Histology, direct identification of yellow granules (*sulfur bodies* = clumps of bacteria) in discharge, anaerobic culture.
▶ **Therapy:**
  • Surgical excision of injected areas with antibiotic coverage.
  • Treatment of choice for cervicofacial form is amoxicillin 30 mg/clavulanic acid 3 mg/kg t.i.d. for 2 weeks.
  • The standard treatment of high-dose penicillin G (10–20 million IU i. v. daily for 4–6 weeks) fails to consider the many secondary bacteria and is not as effective.
  • In case of penicillin allergy, then clindamycin or tetracyclines.
  • For gastrointestinal and thoracic forms, infectious disease consultation. Choice of regimen dictated by nature of secondary infection.

5.13 Nocardiosis

▶ **Definition:** Infection caused by *Nocardia asteroides* or *Nocardia brasiliensis*, Gram-positive filamentous bacteria.
▶ **Pathogenesis:** *Nocardia* are found in soil and plants material worldwide. More likely to cause disease in immunosuppressed individuals.
▶ **Clinical features:**
  • *Nocardia asteroides* causes pulmonary disease and brain abscesses in those with reduced resistance.
  • *Nocardia asteroides* and *Nocardia brasiliensis* can cause cutaneous disease following inoculation, producing local abscesses or a sporotrichoid pattern.
  • *Nocardia brasiliensis* is one of the common causes of mycetomas (p. 118).
▶ **Diagnostic approach:** Slow-growing and difficult to culture; always warn laboratory that *Nocardia* are being considered so they can employ correct approach.
▶ **Differential diagnosis:** Sporotrichoid pattern (p. 713).
▶ **Therapy:** Co-trimoxazole for at least 6 weeks; longer in immunosuppressed patients.

6 Fungal Diseases

6.1 Nomenclature

Classification

The most useful clinical classification of fungi is:

► Dermatophytes.
► Molds.
► Yeasts.
► Subcutaneous mycoses.
► Systemic or deep mycoses.

6.2 Dermatophytes

Overview

Dermatophytes (Table 6.1) live as parasites in tissue containing keratin. They can be divided into:

► *Anthropophilic:* found in humans.
► *Zoophilic:* found in animals.
► *Geophilic:* found in soil.
► **Clinical picture:** Determined by the nature of the dermatophyte, by the tissue it invades, and by the degree of host response. Infections with dermatophytes are usually called *tinea*; for further description, the anatomical site is added, such as tinea capitis for scalp disease. The clinical infection usually starts from an inoculation site and spreads peripherally; thus annular lesions with an active border. In nonmedical jargon, the diagnosis is often "*ringworm*".
► Most common cause of fungal infections in Europe is *Trichophyton rubrum*.
☐ *Note:* Zoophilic and geophilic infections always elicit a more intense immune response and thus appear more aggressive.
► **Id reactions:** The immune response to dermatophyte infections can also cause disease at distant sites where no fungi are present. Most typical picture is dyshidrotic dermatitis.
► **Diagnostic approach:**
  • *Taking specimen:* Disinfect site first to reduce contamination. Use a sterile instrument (scalpel blade, curette, scissors) to obtain tissue from border zone between normal and involved tissue (where concentration of organisms is usually highest).
  • *Microscopic examination:* Hyphae or spores are identified after dissolving the keratin in a 10–15% solution of potassium hydroxide (*KOH examination*). Dyes (chlorazol black E) or fluorochromes (for fluorescent microscopy) can be added. Examination is made at 200–400×.
  • *Culture:* Many standard culture media are available; usually two cultures are made, one on a media containing cycloheximide (for dermatophytes) and one without (yeasts and molds). Hairs can be placed directly on the culture media; fragments from the underside of the nail should be used.

Table 6.1 · Important dermatophytes

Species	Host	Clinical features	Frequency
Trichophyton			
Trichophyton rubrum	Humans	Tinea pedis, tinea manuum, tinea corporis, onychomycosis	Common
Trichophyton mentagrophytes			
var. *interdigitale*	Humans	Tinea corporis, tinea faciei, tinea barbae, tinea capitis	Common; often in children
var. *granulosum*	Mice, guinea pigs		
Trichophyton erinacei	Hedgehogs	Tinea corporis, tinea manuum	Rare
Trichophyton verrucosum	Cows, horses	Tinea corporis, tinea barbae, tinea capitis (often kerion)	Common
Trichophyton violaceum	Humans	Tinea capitis, tinea barbae, tinea corporis	Common in Mediterranean region
Trichophyton tonsurans	Humans	Tinea capitis (black dot), tinea corporis	Common in North and Central America
Trichophyton schoenleinii	Humans	Tinea capitis (favus), onychomycosis	Uncommon; endemic areas
Epidermophyton			
Epidermophyton floccosum	Humans	Tinea inguinalis, tinea pedis, tinea corporis; almost never hair or nail disease	Uncommon
Microsporon			
Microsporon canis	Dogs, cats	Tinea capitis, tinea corporis	Common
Microsporon gypseum	Soil	Tinea capitis, tinea corporis	Common
Microsporon audouinii	Humans	Tinea capitis	Common (uncommon in North America)

▶ **Note:** Wood's light examination is useful for *Microsporon* species and *Trichophyton schoenleinii*; a negative Wood's light examination does not exclude a fungal infection.

▶ **Therapy:** The standard therapy includes both topical (p. 594) and systemic agents (p. 622). All are covered in detail elsewhere and only alluded to under the different disease forms in this chapter.

Tinea Corporis

▶ **Definition:** Dermatophyte infection of the skin of the trunk and extremities, excluding the palms, soles, and inguinal region.

▶ **Pathogenesis:** Wide variety of dermatophytes can be responsible.
▶ **Clinical features:** Round or polycyclic circumscribed scaly areas with central clearing. Variable degree of inflammation, in some instances with pustule formation, depending on nature of dermatophyte and host response.
▶ **Differential diagnosis:** Psoriasis, lichen simplex chronicus, nummular dermatitis, pityriasis rosea, tinea versicolor, parapsoriasis, mycosis fungoides.
▶ **Therapy:** Topical antifungal agents b.i.d. for 1 month; for more widespread disease, following culture confirmation, systemic agents.

Tinea Capitis

▶ **Definition:** Infection of the scalp by dermatophytes with hair shaft involvement.
▶ **Pathogenesis:** Various clinical forms develop, based on host response and nature of hair involvement. Most common causes in USA are *Trichophyton tonsurans* and *Microsporon canis* (very infectious).
▶ **Clinical features:**
  • *Ectothrix infection:* Spores coat outer surface of hair. Areas of hair loss with stubble of varying size (Fig. 6.1 a). Hairs may fluoresce green under Wood's light. Scarring rare. Epidemic tinea capitis is the most common form of ectothrix; caused by *Microsporon canis*, *Microsporon audouinii*, or *Microsporon gypseum*. Responsible for epidemics among schoolchildren. Usually multiple round areas of hair loss; inflammation varies (marked with *Microsporon canis*, while *Microsporon audouinii* produces fine scales with little erythema). Wood's light examination may be positive.
  • *Endothrix infection:* Spores grow into the hair shaft, making it more breakable. Thus, hairs usually end at skin surface, leaving black dots (*Trichophyton ton-*

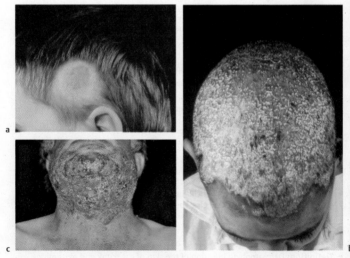

a
c
b

Fig. 6.1 · **a** Tinea capitis. **b** Favus. **c** Tinea barbae with marked inflammation, caused by *Trichophyton verrucosum* in a farmer.

surans or *Trichophyton violaceum*). Differential diagnosis includes chronic cutaneous lupus erythematosus (discoid), pseudopelade.

- *Kerion:* Intense inflammatory reaction to zoophilic fungus in previously unexposed host, such as young farmers with first exposure to milking cattle; usually *Trichophyton verrucosum* or *Trichophyton mentagrophytes.* Painful inflammatory plaque or nodule with pus draining from follicular openings and honeyyellow crusts (kerion is Greek for honeycomb). Heals with scarring (Fig. 6.1 b).
- *Favus:* Infection with *Trichophyton schoenleinii*; relatively common in Middle East, South Africa, and Greenland, otherwise rare. Foul smell (mouse urine). Marked inflammation, large (1–2 cm) adherent crusts that may cover entire scalp, heal with scarring (scarring alopecia). Same clinical picture rarely produced by *Trichophyton violaceum* or *Microsporon gypseum.*

▶ **Therapy:** Topical therapy ineffective; systemic antifungal agents for 1–2 months, until culture is negative. Only griseofulvin officially approved for children, but others all safe and effective. In case of kerion with secondary infection, add systemic antibiotics based on culture and sensitivity.

Tinea Barbae

▶ **Definition:** Dermatophyte infection in beard region of men.
▶ **Pathogenesis:** Similar to kerion; *Trichophyton verrucosum* or *Trichophyton mentagrophytes.*
▶ **Clinical features:** Patients usually farmers with close animal contact. Develop erythematous plaques with follicular pustules, drainage and crusts (Fig. 6.1c). Surprisingly painless. Heals with scarring.
▶ **Differential diagnosis:** Staphylococcal infection with multiple furuncles (*sycosis barbae*); usually painful.
▶ **Therapy:** Topical therapy ineffective; systemic antifungal agents for 1–2 months.

Tinea Faciei

▶ **Definition:** Facial dermatophyte infection.
▶ **Pathogenesis:** Usual cause is sleeping with a pet with zoophilic infection. Infection may be transmitted by close personal contact or spread from other sites to face. Extensive tinea faciei may be sign of immunosuppression.
▶ **Clinical features:** Erythematous, often scaly patches; often not annular because of facial configuration. Pruritic; may worsen with light exposure.
▶ **Differential diagnosis:**
- *Chronic cutaneous lupus erythematosus (discoid):* Slower to develop and more persistent; prominent follicles, may be painful.
- *Psoriasis, impetigo,* less often *rosacea, polymorphous light eruption.*
▶ **Therapy:** Topical antifungal agents for mild disease; otherwise systemic agents.

Tinea Pedis

▶ **Definition:** Dermatophyte infection of feet and toes.
▶ **Synonym:** Athlete's foot.
▶ **Epidemiology:** Most common fungal infection; 30–50% of adults affected.
▶ **Pathogenesis:** Most common agents are *Trichophyton rubrum, Trichophyton mentagrophytes,* and *Epidermophyton floccosum.* Infections favored by poor hygiene, increased sweating, occlusive footwear; perhaps by impaired peripheral circulation. Swimming pools, community showers, and saunas are likely sources of infection.

► **Clinical features:** Pattern varies greatly with causative dermatophyte:
- *Hyperkeratotic type:* Also known as moccasin type; diffuse fine scale (Fig. 6.2 **a**), rarely symptomatic, often overlooked or mistaken for palmoplantar keratoderma. First noticed with nail involvement. Usually caused by *Trichophyton rubrum.*
- *Chronic interdigital type:* Typically involves space between more lateral toes; macerated epidermis is white and fissured (Fig. 6.2 **b**). May spread to soles, but rarely top of foot. Usually caused by *Trichophyton mentagrophytes* var. interdigitale.
- *Dyshidrotic type:* Recurrent attacks of pruritic vesicles and pustules, identical to dyshidrotic dermatitis. Same principle as fungal id reaction, but organisms (usually *Trichophyton mentagrophytes* var. *interdigitale*) can be found.

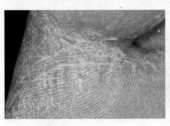 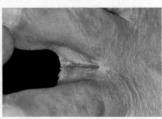

a

Fig. 6.2 · Tinea pedis. **a** With fine scale. **b** Interdigital, with fissures.

► **Complications:** Gram-negative toe web infections, entry site for erysipelas, predisposing factor for postcoronary bypass cellulitis.

► **Differential diagnosis:**
- *Candida infection:* May also produced macerated appearance, but rare.
- *Gram-negative toe web infection:* usually associated with tinea pedis, search for both.
- *Juvenile plantar dermatosis:* Bilateral, symmetrical, associated with atopy.
- *Dyshidrotic dermatitis.*
- *Palmoplantar pustulosis.*
- *Allergic contact dermatitis.*

► **Therapy:**
- Topical antifungal agents; in severe cases, systemic antifungal agents for 1–3 months.
- Treatment of associated onychomycosis and continued prophylactic use of topical agents are essential to reduce the relapse rate.
- In the case of macerated forms, keep area dry, wear absorbent socks, use sandals in summer.
- Shoes should be disinfected with antifungal sprays to reduce likelihood of reinfection.
- ▣ *Note:* Tinea pedis is very common and very difficult to eradicate. It can be viewed as a parasite that is simply too well adapted to the host. The older the patient, the less the likelihood of cure.

Tinea manuum

▶ **Definition:** Dermatophyte infection of the palms.
▶ **Pathogenesis:** Causative agents include *Trichophyton rubrum, Trichophyton mentagrophytes* var. *interdigitale*, less often *Trichophyton violaceum* and *Trichophyton erinacei*. Either primarily inoculation (handling hedgehogs or infected farm animals) or secondary to tinea pedis.
▶ **Clinical features:** Most often dry hyperkeratotic form (Fig. 6.3a); then always check the feet; peculiar but not so rare variant is *"one hand, two feet disease"*. If caused by zoophilic fungus, more localized and inflamed.
▶ **Differential diagnosis:** Hand dermatitis in all its variants.
▶ **Therapy:** Topical antifungal agents usually inadequate; systemic therapy required.

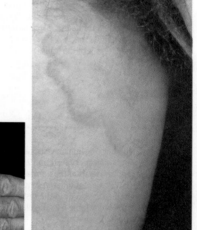

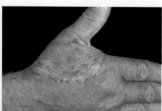

Fig. 6.3 · **a** Tinea manuum. **b** Tinea inguinalis.

Tinea Inguinalis

▶ **Synonym:** Sometimes incorrectly called *tinea cruris* (but cruris refers to lower leg in Latin); eczema marginatum.
▶ **Definition:** Dermatophyte infection in groin or genital region.
▶ **Pathogenesis:** Most common causative agents are *Epidermophyton floccosum* and *Trichophyton rubrum*; often associated with tinea pedis or onychomycosis. Old saying, "Put on your socks before your underwear" to avoid spread. More common in men.
▶ **Clinical features:** Pruritic circumscribed patches with sharp border favoring the medial thigh; may extend to buttocks or perianal region; rarely involves scrotum (Fig. 6.3 b).

▶ **Differential diagnosis:** Candidiasis (more common in women, satellite lesions), erythrasma (Wood's light positive), inverse psoriasis (look for psoriasis elsewhere), contact dermatitis, Hailey-Hailey disease. Intertrigo is a superficial irritation which arises when skin folds touch each other, as in the groin, under the breasts or in abdominal folds. It is most often seen with obesity. The occlusion and retention of moisture leads to maceration which may predispose to any of the diseases lists above. We view intertrigo more as a description than as a disease entity.

▶ **Therapy:** Topical antifungal agents usually sufficient. Drying measures (absorbent powders, astringent solutions, blow dry area after washing, then apply medication).

◨ *Note:* Check for associated onychomycosis or tinea pedis, which would require systemic antifungal agents.

Onychomycosis

▶ **Definition:** Infection of nail fold and nail plate with dermatophytes (*Trichophyton rubrum*, *Trichophyton mentagrophytes*, *Epidermophyton floccosum*) as well as molds (*Hendersonula toruloidea*, *Scopulariopsis brevicaulis*), and yeasts (*Candida albicans*, other *Candida* species). Refers only to a dermatophytic nail infection.

▶ Covered under Diseases of the Nails (p. 522).

6.3 Yeasts

Overview

▶ **Pathogenesis:**

- Almost all pathogenic human yeasts are from the genus *Candida*. The major species is *Candida albicans* types 1 and 2 (formerly known as *Candida stellatoidea*). *Candida albicans* is part of the normal flora of the mouth, gastrointestinal tract, and vagina; it is present in limited numbers, waxing and waning. It is not normally found on the skin or in the respiratory tract. The potentially pathogenic yeasts are shown in Table 6.2. The old terms *Monilia* and moniliasis are incorrect and should be avoided.

Table 6.2 · Yeast species

Species	Diseases
Candida albicans	Cutaneous candidiasis, esophagitis, vulvovaginitis, endocarditis, and many more
Candida krusei	Cutaneous candidiasis, esophagitis, endocarditis, vaginitis
Candida parapsilosis	Endocarditis, paronychia, otitis externa
Candida pseudotropicalis	Vulvovaginal candidiasis
Candida tropicalis	Onychomycosis, vaginitis, meningitis, respiratory infections
Torulopsis glabrata (*Candida glabrata*)	Part of normal flora but in immunosuppressed patients may cause life-threatening systemic disease including fungemia and meningitis

- Skin and mucosal infections are caused by candidal mycelia; systemic candidiasis is usually caused by blastospores (budding yeasts).
- The host–organism interplay with *Candida albicans* is very complex and poorly understood; experts disagree on the significance of the yeast in the stool, for example. Some feel that gastrointestinal candidal colonization or quantitative increases in yeasts may be associated with diseases such as atopic dermatitis or urticaria. Treatment with nonabsorbable oral anticandidal agents such as nystatin occasionally produces improvement, but we remain skeptical.
- Patients with very specific immune defects tend to have extremely persistent infections (*mucocutaneous candidiasis*).

► **Epidemiology:**
- *Candida albicans* causes disease in young, old, or immunosuppressed individuals; exceptions are vulvovaginitis and balanitis, which affect patients with intact immunity.
- Over 90% of infections are caused by *Candida albicans,* but other species cannot be overlooked; often difficult to identify and typically more resistant to therapy.
- ☐ *Note: Candida* infections are often a sign of immunosuppression (diabetes mellitus, HIV/AIDS, long-term antibiotic therapy, hematologic malignancies). Patients with recurrent or refractory disease should be evaluated for such risk factors.

► **Clinical features:** *Candida albicans* infections are known as candidiasis; usually involve the skin or mucous membranes but can be systemic in immunosuppressed patients (Table 6.2). Rich clinical spectrum: intertriginous and anogenital candidiasis, onychomycosis, paronychia, oral candidiasis in many forms, intestinal candidiasis, systemic candidiasis, mucocutaneous candidiasis.

► **Therapy:**
- *Polyene antifungal agents* such as nystatin, amphotericin B, and natamycin are old standbys but still effective; they form complexes with ergosterol in the plasma membrane and thus inhibit growth. Nystatin is not absorbed and thus often used for treating oral and intestinal infections.
- *Imidazoles,* both topical and systemic, are also highly effective. They are available as lozenges for oral and gastrointestinal disease, as well as for vaginal use.
- ☐ *Note:* It is critical to correct the predisposing factors, ranging from occlusion and maceration to weight loss, control of diabetes, or avoidance of long-term antibiotic usage.

Oral Candidiasis

....

► **Clinical features:** A variety of clinical forms that vary greatly in appearance:
- *Acute pseudomembranous candidiasis (thrush):* The classic form, known to every mother; thick, cottage-cheese-like plaques that can be easily scraped off, revealing an erythematous base (Fig. 6.4a). Most common in infants. Common sites include buccal mucosa, tongue, palate.
- *Acute atrophic candidiasis:* Often painful, flat erythematous areas; typically involves tongue and is secondary to long-term antibiotic usage.
- *Chronic hyperplastic candidiasis:* Thick persistent white plaques, usually in men; not easily removed. Differential diagnosis: other forms of leukoplakia (p. 490).
- *Chronic atrophic candidiasis:* Most often affects denture wearers; atrophic dusky erythematous area confined to area under denture; often confused with allergic or irritant reaction.

- *Angular cheilitis (perlèche):* Painful rhagades at corner of mouth; predisposing factors: drooling (infants and elderly), eating disorders (malnutrition and forced vomiting), poorly fitting dentures. Often combined infection with *Candida albicans* and bacteria.
- *Median rhomboid glossitis:* Erythematous rhomboid patch without papillae on the midline of the dorsal surface of the tongue at the transition from middle to the posterior portion; long thought to represent an embryologic fusion defect, but now considered another form of candidiasis.

► **Therapy:**
- Nystatin or imidazole lozenges t.i.d.–q.i.d. for 5–10 days; easier to use than direct application of medications.
- In the case of angular stomatitis, protective imidazole pastes are helpful.
- In resistant cases, consider 10 days of oral nystatin to reduce bowel load.
- ▣ *Note:* Correct the predisposing factors.

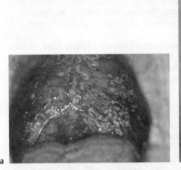
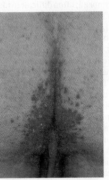

a   b

Fig. 6.4 · Candidal infection. **a** Of oral mucosa with easily removed white coating. **b** Intertriginous, with typical satellite lesions.

Intertriginous Candidal Infections

► **Clinical features:**
- Any moist intertriginous area can be infected; examples include submammary, inguinal, perianal, and occasionally axillary disease. Lesions typically macerated with fissures and satellite lesions, often pustules (Fig. 6.**4b**).
- In addition, candidal vulvovaginitis and balanitis are common.
- Most diaper dermatitis is irritant, but then rapidly colonized by *Candida albicans*; the presence of satellite lesions is a good clue to this. Problem worse when topical corticosteroids are applied. *Granuloma gluteale infantum* refers to reactive red-brown inflammatory nodules that develop in this setting.

► **Therapy:** Drying measures usually suffice. Dye solutions are effective and economical but messy. In Europe, methylrosaniline chloride and eosin solutions (p. 592) are still used. Topical nystatin or imidazole products are also widely used. Oral nystatin is also safe. For vulvovaginitis, vaginal suppositories usually highly effective; if not or with recurrent disease, then oral imidazoles (usually fluconazole) is recommended.

Chronic Mucocutaneous Candidiasis

► **Definition:** Heterogenous group of congenital immune defects featuring severe and persistent candidal infections.
► **Clinical features:** The classification of chronic mucocutaneous candidiasis (CMC) is shown in Table 6.3. Patients have persistent cutaneous, mucosal, and nail infections, usually with *Candida albicans*. Some forms are associated with endocrinologic disturbances.

Table 6.3 · **Forms of chronic mucocutaneous candidiasis (CMC)**

CMC type	Inheritance	MIM code	Onset
Familial CMC with endocrine disturbances	AR	212050	Childhood
	AD	114580	Childhood
Familial CMC with hypothyroidism	AD		Childhood
Autoimmune polyendocrinopathy candidiasis ectodermal dystrophy (APECD)	AR	240300	Childhood
Chronic localized candidiasis	Unknown		Childhood
Candidiasis with hyper-IgE syndrome	AR	24370	Childhood
CMC with thymoma	Unknown		Adult
Familial chronic nail candidiasis with ICAM-1 deficiency	AR	607644	Childhood
CMC with chronic keratitis	Unknown		Adult
Chronic oral candidiasis	Unknown		Adult

AD = autosomal dominant; AR = autosomal recessive.

► **Diagnostic approach:** Persistence, age of onset, and associated features usually lead to diagnosis; exact immunologic evaluation and in some instances, genetic evaluation.
► **Therapy:** Fluconazole has become the standard therapy; usually 200–800 mg daily. Higher doses needed when *Torulopsis glabrata* identified. In resistant cases, voriconazole (200–400 mg daily) is promising.

Tinea Versicolor

► **Synonym:** Pityriasis versicolor.
☐ *Note:* The European term *pityriasis versicolor* is preferable as this disorder is not a dermatophyte infection and therefore not a "*tinea*.".
► **Definition:** Common superficial yeast infection causing hypo- or hyperpigmentation.

▶ **Pathogenesis:** Causative agent is *Malassezia furfur*, which is the pathogenic form of the commensal cutaneous yeasts *Pityrosporon ovale* and *Pityrosporon orbiculare*. Because the causative agent is part of the normal flora, it is impossible to eradicate and thus recurrences are common. Mechanisms of pigmentary change are unclear; darkening is a result of hyperkeratosis, but lightening may reflect an umbrella effect as well as a direct effect on melanocytes.

▶ **Clinical features:**

- Typical sites are the upper chest and back; much less often the neck, upper arms, and face. The scalp is the most abundant reservoir of *Pityrosporon*.
- In fair-skinned individuals, the lesions are typically hyperpigmented, tan 1–3 cm oval patches, often confluent. When scraped lightly, they are very scaly; a good diagnostic clue, as few other disorders release so much scale. After tanning or in dark-skinned individuals, the lesions tend to be light. Versicolor refers to the variable colors (Fig. 6.5 a,b).

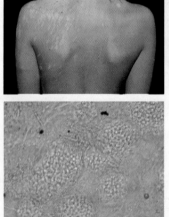
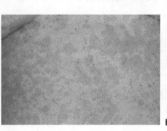

Fig. 6.5 · Tinea versicolor. **a** Hypopigmented form. **b** Hyperpigmented form. **c** KOH examination showing hyphae and spores (spaghetti and meatballs).

▶ **Diagnostic approach:** KOH examination reveals hyphae and spores (spaghetti and meatballs, Fig. 6.5 c). Another approach is stripping with clear adhesive tape, staining with methylene blue for 5 seconds, rinsing, and examining under the microscope. Culture not possible.

▶ **Differential diagnosis:**

- *Hypopigmented lesions:* Vitiligo, pityriasis alba.
- *Hyperpigmented lesions:* Ephelides, lentigines, café-au-lait macules.
- *Erythematous lesions:* Tinea corporis, pityriasis rosea, secondary syphilis, seborrheic dermatitis.

▶ **Therapy:**

- Standard approach is to use either imidazole shampoo (ketoconazole) or selenium sulfide shampoo. Scalp and entire body surface to the groin should be lathered up and then rinsed after a few minutes. Initially, the treatment daily for 7–10 days.

☒ Caution: Always treat the scalp; it is the major reservoir for the yeasts.
- Recurrences are common; patients can simply use the medicated shampoo 1–2× weekly indefinitely.
- In stubborn cases, a short course of itraconazole or fluconazole can be employed; some recommend 1 tablet weekly for prophylaxis.

6.4 Subcutaneous Mycoses

The subcutaneous mycoses are not a biological family, but a group of clinical problems all caused by direct inoculation of the organism into the skin and subcutaneous tissue. They are more common in tropical and subtropical regions, presumably because of both enhanced growth of fungi in the soil and on plants and increased likelihood of injury (going barefoot, less protective clothing).

Sporotrichosis
....

▶ **Definition:** Subcutaneous and occasionally systemic mycosis caused by *Sporothrix schenckii.*
▶ **Epidemiology:** Although *Sporothrix schenckii* is found worldwide, sporotrichosis is primarily seen in North and Central America; famous epidemic among South African miners.
▶ **Pathogenesis:** The fungus is inoculated through injuries, usually from wood or plants; a classic injury is from a rose thorn.
▶ **Clinical features:**
- *Localized sporotrichosis:* Verrucous papules and plaques develop following inoculation. Then spread with firm subcutaneous nodules appearing along the path of lymphatic drainage. In the USA, diseases that spread in this fashion (nocardiosis, atypical mycobacterial infections, plaque, and many others) are referred to as *sporotrichoid* (p. 713).
- *Superficial ulcerated sporotrichosis:* In this form, many spores are inoculated by abrasion. The classic setting is a gardener or farmer carrying bales of sphagnum moss that rub on his abdomen.
- *Systemic sporotrichosis:* Rare; involves lungs, muscles, bones, and even CNS.
▶ **Diagnostic approach:** Occasionally cigar-shaped yeasts can be seen on biopsy with periodic acid–Schiff (Pas) stain; *Sporothrix schenckii* is dimorphic; culture at 25 °C reveals a mold and at 37 °C, a yeast.
▶ **Therapy:**
- Itraconazole 400–600 mg p. o. daily for 6–8 weeks. With systemic involvement, amphotericin B also is a possibility.
- Localized lesions can be treated with either cryotherapy or hyperthermia to speed healing.

Chromomycosis
....

▶ **Synonym:** Chromoblastomycosis, verrucous dermatitis.
▶ **Definition:** Chronic infection, usually involving foot or leg, following inoculation injury with soil-borne fungi.
▶ **Epidemiology:** Most common in rural areas of tropical and subtropical countries.
▶ **Causative agents:** Many dematiaceous fungi including *Phialophora verrucosa, Fonsecaea pedrosoi, Fonsecaea compactum, Cladosporium carrionii, Rhinocladiella aquaspersa.*

▶ **Clinical features:** Over weeks to months, verrucous nodules and plaques develop at the site of injury (*mossy foot*). Sporotrichoid spread along lymphatics is possible, but systemic spread rare.

▶ **Diagnostic approach:**
- Histology reveals subcutaneous granulomas containing small (5–15 µm) brown bodies that divide by equatorial splitting, not budding. They have many names: copper pennies, sclerotic bodies, Medlar bodies.
- *Culture:* Slow-growing dark filamentous colonies at 20–25 °C; speciation based on microscopic findings.

▶ **Differential diagnosis:** Chromomycosis and mycetoma often confused.

◳ **Note:** Chromomycosis grows outwards (raised verrucous lesions) whereas mycetoma grows inwards (sinus tracts).

▶ **Therapy:**
- Small lesions should be excised.
- Systemic antifungal therapy is difficult; itraconazole and voriconazole are least toxic; flucytosine may be more effective but quite toxic. Systemic amphotericin B is not recommended; intralesional may be effective but is extremely painful.
- Cryotherapy and hyperthermia may also be of supplemental value.

Mycetoma

▶ **Synonym:** Madura foot (from the Indian state of Madura).

▶ **Definition:** Chronic soft tissue infection caused by a wide variety of fungi and bacteria; placed under fungal infections for convenience.

▶ **Pathogenesis:** The list of causative agents is long. All cause disease in the same way—they are inoculated into the skin via an injury and then proliferate in the subcutaneous tissue, extending to fascia, muscles, and bones. Two types:
- *Eumycetoma:* Caused by fungi in the genera *Aspergillus, Exophiala, Madurella, Pseudallescheria,* and others.
- *Actinomycetoma:* Caused by bacteria in the genera *Actinomadura, Actinomyces, Nocardia,* and *Streptomyces.*

▶ **Clinical features:** Initial finding is a soft tissue swelling, usually involving the foot. The process develops to involve deeper structures but also to form abscesses and draining sinuses with discharge of colored granules (colonies of organisms).

▶ **Diagnostic approach:** The granules have different colors (white, yellow, black), which give clues to the organisms; microscopic examination and culture needed to confirm diagnosis.

▶ **Differential diagnosis:** Chromomycosis with verrucous exophytic lesions.

▶ **Therapy:** Culture-directed antibiotic or antifungal therapy, the latter usually with amphotericin B. The bacterial forms are relatively therapy-responsive; the eumycetomas are often so resistant that amputation is the most reasonable approach.

6.5 Systemic Mycoses

Overview

▶ **Pathogenesis:** The systemic mycoses are caused by dimorphic fungi that live as a yeast or a mold, depending on environmental conditions. They often cause asymptomatic infections in healthy individuals, but are frequently more aggressive in weakened individuals. Risk factors include HIV/AIDS, cancer chemotherapy, solid organ transplantation, and long-term intensive care treatment. Depending on what organisms are locally common, a variety of prophylactic regimens are employed in high-risk patients.

▶ **Epidemiology:** In Europe the two most common infections are cryptococcosis and aspergillosis. To avoid diagnostic errors, it is important to know where the various deep fungal infections are common.

▶ **Diagnostic approach:** In all causes, histologic examination of skin lesions can reveal the causative organisms. Final confirmation is made via culture. Infectious diseases texts should be consulted for more advanced diagnostic techniques including serological studies.

▶ **Therapy:** Systemic therapy is always required.

Cryptococcosis

▶ **Epidemiology:** Found worldwide; first described in Berlin, Germany.

▶ **Pathogenesis:** *Cryptococcus neoformans* is presumably spread from bird droppings. Initial infection via the lungs; dissemination seen only in immunosuppressed individuals.

▶ **Clinical features:**
- Cutaneous fadings are uncommon; they reflect dissemination and indicate a critically ill patient. In HIV/AIDS, the disseminated papules closely resemble molluscum contagiosum.
- Cryptococcal meningitis is the most feared complication. Renal and bone disease is also common, but less catastrophic.

▶ **Therapy:** Previous mainstays of therapy were amphotericin B and flucytosine. Fluconazole appears effective for meningitis; voriconazole also shows promise.

Aspergillosis

▶ **Pathogenesis:** The usual pathogen is *Aspergillus fumigatus,* although occasionally other species are isolated. All have a worldwide distribution. The usual home of aspergillus is the lungs, where it may cause a fungal ball (*aspergilloma*) or allergic reaction. Invasive pulmonary disease is usually the starting point in immunosuppressed patients. Local inoculation, usually with *Aspergillus flavus,* may occur in burn patients or leukemia patients (via contaminated tape or at venous access sites).

▶ **Clinical features:**
- Locally destructive skin disease following inoculation, with red-violet color, central necrosis, and ulceration. Other forms of local disease may involve ear or eye.
- As part of disseminated disease, septic emboli blocking vessels, causing necrosis and eschar formation.
- Main clinical risk in disseminated disease is aspergillus meningitis, which is almost always fatal; endocarditis is a problem in cardiac transplantation.

▶ **Therapy:** Many agents available including voriconazole, caspofungin, and combinations of the standard agents, amphotericin B, flucytosine, and itraconazole. Regimen depends on immune status and organ pattern.

Blastomycosis

▶ **Epidemiology:** *Blastomyces dermatitidis* is a soil fungus, found primarily in the central USA.

▶ **Pathogenesis:** Initial infection is pulmonary and usually asymptomatic. The organism can later cause pulmonary cavitation or spread to involve most often bone or prostate, as well as skin. The causes of reactivation are poorly understood; blastomycosis is not a problem in HIV/AIDS.

▶ **Clinical features:** The cutaneous lesions are typically verrucous, slowly spreading nodules or plaques (Fig. 6.**6**). They are almost always the result of dissemination, not local inoculation. They may be confused with a basal cell carcinoma, tuberculosis cutis verrucosa, or halogenoderma.

▶ **Therapy:** Itraconazole is usually the treatment of choice; in severe cases, amphotericin B may be employed.

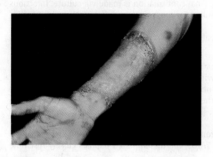

Fig. 6.**6** · Blastomycosis (Image courtesy of Robert H. Schosser MD, Greenville, North Carolina, USA).

Histoplasmosis

▶ **Epidemiology:** *Histoplasma capsulatum* var. *capsulatum* is also most common in the central USA, but also found in South America, Asia, Australia, and Africa. *Histoplasma capsulatum* var. *duboisii* causes African histoplasmosis.

▶ **Pathogenesis:** Primary infection is in the lungs. Reactivation occurs after many years, causing chronic pulmonary disease. An aggressive course may be seen in children or in HIV/AIDS with widespread involvement.

▶ **Clinical features:**

- Skin involvement is uncommon in disseminated disease; less than 10% have papules or nodules following hematogenous seeding. Oral infiltrates and ulcers are more common.
- Major systemic problems are hepatosplenomegaly, bone marrow infiltrates with pancytopenia, endocarditis, and meningitis.
- In African histoplasmosis, cutaneous nodules and abscesses are common; they can be excised.

▶ **Therapy:** Itraconazole or ketoconazole are used for non-life-threatening cases. In immunosuppressed patients, initial control must be obtained with amphotericin B. In HIV/AIDS, once the infection is under control, then lifelong prophylaxis with itraconazole.

Other Uncommon Fungal Infections

Other uncommon infections are listed in Table 6.**4**.

Table 6.4 · Other uncommon fungal infections

Disease	Causative agent	Comments	Treatment
Superficial infections			
Tinea nigra	*Exophiala werneckii*	Dark patch on sole; mistaken for pigmented lesion	Topical antifungal agents, perhaps with keratolytics or curettage
Piedra alba	*Trichosporon beigelii*	Black nodules attached to hairs; usually scalp; common in Gulf States of USA	Shaving; imidazole or ciclopirox olamine lotions
Piedra nigra	*Piedraia hortae*	White nodules attached to hairs; usually pubic or axillary; common in Asia, South Pacific	Shaving; imidazole or ciclopirox olamine lotions
Tinea imbricata (tokelau)	*Trichophyton concentricum*	Disease of Pacific islands; large concentric scaly rings; so common that initially diagnosed as genodermatosis	Systemic antifungal agents
Subcutaneous infections			
Zygomycosis (mucormycosis)	Fungi of the Zygomycetes class (*Mucor*, *Rhizomucor*, *Rhizopus*, and others)	Immunosuppressed or diabetic patients; cutaneous inoculation or sinus infections which can extend to the CNS	Amphotericin B plus debridement
Subcutaneous zygomycosis	*Basidiobolus ranarum*	Subcutaneous granulomas in non-immunosuppressed children; Indonesia, India and Africa.	Amphotericin B
Lôbo disease (keloidal blastomycosis)	*Loboa loboi*	Keloidal or verrucous plaques; Central and Northern South America; no systemic disease	Excision
Deep infections			
Coccidioidomycosis	*Coccidioides immitis*	Deserts of southwestern USA, northern Mexico. Usually pulmonary disease; often presents with erythema nodosum. Disseminated lesions resemble molluscum contagiosum. Severe problem in HIV/AIDS and pregnancy	Fluconazole, amphotericin B for life-threatening disease
Paracoccidioidomycosis (South American blastomycosis)	*Paracoccidioides brasiliensis*	Usually pulmonary disease; skin findings include crusted periorificial nodules resembling leishmaniasis	Itraconazole, fluconazole, or amphotericin B

7 *Other Infectious Diseases*

7.1 *Leishmaniasis*

Overview

▶ **Epidemiology:** An estimated 10 million people around the world have leishmaniasis, with 400 000 new infections yearly. Although leishmania have a worldwide distribution, absent only in Australia, there are pockets where various forms of the disease are endemic. In Europe, increasing tourism in the Mediterranean basin and Middle East has made cutaneous leishmaniasis one of the more common exotic diseases. Recent military actions in the Middle East mean that many Western soldiers and civilian employees are at risk of acquiring leishmaniasis.

▶ **Pathogenesis:** Leishmania are flagellate protozoans; there are approximate 30 species, a good number of which are pathogenic. The species are identified on the basis of geographic distribution and disease forms. A simplified scheme (Table 7.1) recognizes four complexes of species, each responsible for a clinical symptom complex. This scheme is an oversimplification; current references should be sought by those few who require more information on speciation of protozoans.

▶ A wide variety of mammals, in most cases rodents, are the natural hosts. Infected patients with widespread or systemic disease are another source of infection. All forms are transferred by sandflies (*Phlebotomus* in Old Word, *Lutzomyia* in New World). Individuals who are infected develop a lifelong immunity, but this may be of limited utility as it is restricted to a given species or even subspecies.

▶ **Diagnostic approach:** Clinical features, smear or scraping, biopsy. Microscopic examination reveals intense lymphocytic infiltrate; Giemsa stain may make it easier to find the intracellular parasites (2–5 µm). Speciation is based on the polymerase chain reaction (PCR).

Table 7.1 · **Leishmania complexes**

Complex	Disease
Leishmania tropica	Old World cutaneous leishmaniasis
Leishmania mexicana	New World cutaneous leishmaniasis
Leishmania viannia (brasiliensis)	New World cutaneous and mucocutaneous leishmaniasis
Leishmania donovani	Visceral leishmaniasis

Old World Cutaneous Leishmaniasis

▶ **Synonyms:** Hundreds of synonyms reflecting the many cities in the Middle East where one can become infected: Baghdad boil, Aleppo boil, Jericho boil, or simply Oriental boil.

▶ **Definition:** Cutaneous infection with *Leishmania tropica* complex.

▶ **Epidemiology:** Found in Mediterranean basin, Middle East, and sub-Saharan highlands.

▶ **Pathogenesis:** The normal host for *Leishmania tropica* is rodents, as well as infected humans in endemic areas. Sandflies are low-flying (3 meters) nocturnal insects; tourists living in the upper stories of hotels are at much less risk than those on the ground floor. After inoculation, the organisms undergo a complex life cycle in humans.

■ *Note:* The incubation period is extremely variable, ranging from a few days to several years; the average is 2–4 weeks.

► **Acute cutaneous leishmaniasis:**
- Following the bite, a papule develops, then rapidly enlarges and breaks down in the center. The ulcer usually has a rolled border and may become secondarily infected (Fig. 7.1).
- The lesion heals over about a year, leaving a distinctive depressed hyperpigmented scar.

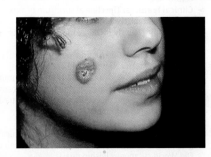

Fig. 7.1 · Cutaneous leishmaniasis in American college student recently returned from visit to the Middle East.

- Typical sites are exposed areas such as the cheeks and arms.
- In some classifications three types are recognized, each with different vectors and causative species:
  - *Dry or urban:* Classic form with single lesion as described above (*Leishmania tropica*).
  - *Wet or rural:* More acute infection with multiple lesions (*Leishmania major*).
  - *Ethiopian:* More chronic and less severe (*Leishmania aethiopica*) but may lead to diffuse cutaneous leishmaniasis.

■ *Note:* Always suspect leishmaniasis when confronted with a facial nodule or ulcer in someone who has lived in or visited the endemic areas. It is frequently confused with lymphoma.

► **Leishmaniasis recidivans:** A form of either wet or dry leishmaniasis, characterized by chronic course, central healing, and development of serpiginous lupoid nodules at the periphery.

► **Diffuse cutaneous leishmaniasis:** Rare form in patients who are relatively anergic and develop disseminated disease, with both local and hematogenous spread to produce nodular lesions resembling lepromatous leprosy, as well as mucosal disease. Also called *anergic cutaneous leishmaniasis.* Caused by *Leishmania aethiopica* and several New World species.

► **Differential diagnosis:** Infected bites and stings, bacterial pyoderma, subcutaneous fungal infections, basal cell carcinoma, squamous cell carcinoma. Leishmaniasis recidivans resembles lupus vulgaris; diffuse cutaneous leishmaniasis is similar to lepromatous leprosy.

► **Therapy:**
- Spontaneous healing is the rule, so often no therapy is needed for acute cutaneous leishmaniasis.

- Standard treatment is intralesional injection of sodium stibogluconate (Pentosan) diluted 1:3 with a local anesthetic; 1–2 × weekly for 2–4 weeks.
- Cryotherapy or surgical excision of small lesions is also appropriate.
- Recent literature suggests using ketoconazole, itraconazole, or allopurinol.
- Topical paromomycin 15% with 10% urea can be applied b.i.d. for 3 weeks.
- Leishmaniasis recidivans and diffuse cutaneous leishmaniasis require systemic therapy (see below).

New World Cutaneous Leishmaniasis

▶ **Definition:** Cutaneous infection with *Leishmania mexicana* or *Leishmania viannia* complexes.
▶ **Clinical features:** The clinical spectrum of New World cutaneous leishmaniasis is wide. In general, the lesions are more likely to be multiple, ulcerative, destructive, and chronic than their Old World counterparts. A number of colorful terms have been applied:
- *Chiclero ulcer:* Destruction of the ear cartilage in forest workers (chicleros harvest chicle, a ingredient in chewing gum).
- *Uta:* Variant in Andean highlands; limited number of lesions.
▶ Members of the *Leishmania viannia* complex cause both persistent ulcerative cutaneous disease and mucocutaneous leishmaniasis. Several species can cause diffuse cutaneous leishmaniasis (see above).
▶ **Diagnostic approach:** See above.
▶ **Differential diagnosis:** Depending on the clinical form, lepromatous leprosy and yaws may also come into consideration, as well as the diseases discussed under Old World cutaneous leishmaniasis.
▶ **Therapy:** Systemic therapy is indicated because of the likelihood of multifocal or chronic disease and the risk of both mucocutaneous (for many species) and diffuse cutaneous disease. The mainstay of therapy is systemic pentavalent antimony compounds—either sodium stibogluconate or meglumine antimonite. Liposomal amphotericin B and pentamidine are also effective. Public health officials should be consulted for exact therapeutic guidance; speciation of the leishmania may be important in choosing the agent.

Mucocutaneous Leishmaniasis

▶ **Synonym:** Espundia.
▶ **Definition:** Infection with *Leishmania viannia* complex.
▶ **Epidemiology:** Most common in the jungles of Brazil and Peru. Most common species in the complex is *Leishmania brasiliensis*.
▶ **Clinical features:** Following facial infection, the leishmania spreads via blood vessels or lymphatics to the nasopharyngeal mucosa. After an interval of months or years, the feared destructive starts, usually in the nasal septum, but spreading to involve lips, palate, pharynx, and even larynx.
▶ **Differential diagnosis:** Paracoccidioidomycosis, lepromatous leprosy, and destructive carcinomas.
▶ **Therapy:** Systemic therapy is always required (see above).

Visceral Leishmaniasis

▶ **Synonyms:** Black fever, Dumdum fever, kala-azar.
▶ **Definition:** Infection with *Leishmania donovani* complex.
▶ **Epidemiology:** Primarily seen in India and the Sudan, but also occurs in South America, China, other parts of Africa, even the Mediterranean basin.

► **Clinical features:** A completely different disease than the other forms. Patients have disseminated disease with leishmania in their reticuloendothelial system (liver, spleen, bone marrow, lymph nodes); they suffer from fever, chills, malaise, and anemia; over a period of time their skin acquires a gray shade. Untreated, generally fatal in 1–2 years.

► **Complications:** Those patient who survive may develop *post-kala-azar dermal leishmaniasis*; this happens to about 20% of patients in India, but is rare in other regions. Years after successful treatment or spontaneous cure, they acquire hypopigmented or erythematous facial (and sometimes truncal) macules that progress to papules and nodules. Clinical picture resembles lepromatous leprosy.

► **Diagnostic approach:** The protozoan can be found in the bone marrow or lymph nodes. Serological diagnosis is possible, but often false-negative in immunosuppressed patients. In the unfortunate with both visceral leishmaniasis and HIV/AIDS, the organisms are seen in the buffy coat. In post-kala-azar dermal leishmaniasis, skin biopsy is diagnostic.

► **Differential diagnosis:** Consider hematologic malignancies, subacute infections (such as brucellosis, malaria, tuberculosis), and other diseases associated with hepatosplenomegaly.

► **Therapy:** Liposomal amphotericin B is the treatment of choice. Antimony compounds are used for post-kala-azar dermal leishmaniasis.

7.2 Other Protozoan Infections

There are surprisingly few other protozoan diseases with cutaneous manifestations (Table 7.2).

Table 7.2 · Protozoan infections with cutaneous manifestations

Disease	Organism	Comments
Amebiasis	*Entamoeba histolytica*	Patients with hepatic or intestinal disease develop ulcers, either perianal, or via direct extension to overlying skin; jagged painful ulcers with undermined borders
Chagas disease	*Trypanosoma cruzi*	Transmitted by reduviid bugs. Site of bite is chagoma; periorbital edema known as Romaña sign; later cardiac, gastrointestinal, and CNS disease
Toxoplasmosis	*Toxoplasma gondii*	One cause of TORCH syndrome (p. 65)
Trichomoniasis	*Trichomonas vaginalis*	Sexually transmitted disease; vaginal burning and discharge; urethritis and ascending infections
Trypanosomiasis (African sleeping sickness)	*Trypanosoma brucei*	Only skin change is nodule at site of tsetse fly bite; primary problem CNS disease

7.3 Pediculosis

Overview

▶ **Definition:** Lice (*Pediculus* spp.) are blood-sucking, wingless, ectoparasitic insects that infest their victims for long periods of time with a high degree of host specificity.
▶ **Disease transmission:** Lice transmit a number of important diseases:
- Epidemic typhus (*Rickettsia prowazekii*).
- Relapsing fever (*Borrelia recurrentis*).
- Trench fever (*Bartonella quintana*).

Pediculosis Capitis

▶ **Synonym:** Head lice.
▶ **Definition:** Infestation with *Pediculus humanus capitis*.
▶ **Epidemiology:** Often seen in epidemics among kindergarten and grade school children; also common in homeless people.
▶ **Pathogenesis:** Lice live on the scalp and suck blood there. They firmly attach their eggs (nits) to the hair shaft just at the skin surface.
▶ **Clinical features:** Pruritic eruption on back of scalp and nape (Fig. 7.2 a,b); often with excoriations and secondary infections (lice dermatitis). The hairs may become matted from repeated scratching (*plica polonica*).
◪ *Note:* Always think of pediculosis capitis when confronted with dermatitis of the nape.

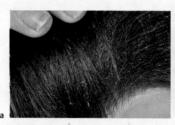 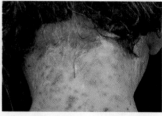

Fig. 7.2 · **Pediculosis capitis. a** With multiple nits on hairs. **b** With typical nuchal dermatitis.

▶ **Diagnostic approach:** Look for nits on the hair shafts, as well as for lice on the scalp.
▶ **Differential diagnosis:** Hair casts look similar to nits, but form an encompassing cylinder whereas the nits are attached at an angle. *Piedra* is much less common and consist of clumps of bacteria or fungi.
▶ **Therapy:**
- Resistance of head lice to pediculicides has become a problem. Check for local resistance pattern.
- All agents should be applied twice, 7–14 days apart. Recommendations vary regarding length of application, including overnight use, but all appear effective when used for 10–30 minutes and rinsed.
- Malathion 0.5% lotion is most effective, but there is resistance in France and the UK.

- Pyrethrins and the synthetic permethrin have fair action and a reasonable resistance profile.
- Lindane (gamma benzene hexachloride) is still widely used, but relatively ineffective for this indication and with marked resistance.
- The nits are always a problem; many schools have rules banning children returning as long as nits are present. Best solutions following treatment are soaking with vinegar and water (50:50) and using a fine-toothed nit comb.

Pediculosis Corporis

▶ **Definition:** Infestation with *Pediculus humanus corporis*.
▶ **Epidemiology:** Pediculosis corporis is primarily a disease of the unwashed. It is common in homeless people and during wars (trench fever) and other disasters.
▶ **Pathogenesis:** The lice feed on the body, but live in the clothing and tend to lay their eggs along the seams.
▶ **Clinical features:** Presents with marked pruritus, lack of personal hygiene, and secondarily infected, excoriated dermatitis on trunk (*vagabond skin*).
☐ *Note:* Look for the lice and nits on the clothing, not on the skin.
▶ **Differential diagnosis:** All pruritic dermatoses, especially scabies.
▶ **Therapy:**
- Disinfection of clothing and bedding (boiling, hot ironing, fumigation).
- Attempt to change living conditions.
- Same pediculicides as for *Pediculus humanus capitis* can be used, but less important.
- In mass epidemics, usually insecticidal dusting powders employed.

Pediculosis Pubis

▶ **Definition:** Infestation with *Phthirus pubis*.
▶ **Epidemiology:** Usually transmitted by sexual contacts.
▶ **Clinical features:** Patients usually identify moving lice on their pubic hairs (*crabs*). Also complain of pruritus. Nits usually on pubic hair, but occasionally elsewhere (axillary or body hairs; eyelashes, eyebrows). The feeding sites turn into distinctive blue-gray hemorrhagic macules (*maculae ceruleae* or *taches bleuâtres*).
▶ **Diagnostic approach:** Identification of lice or nits.
▶ **Therapy:**
- Permethrin cream or shampoo or lindane lotion or shampoo applied for 10 minutes; repeat in 1 week.
- Ivermectin p.o. is also effective for resistant cases (see scabies).

7.4 Scabies

▶ **Definition**: Intensely pruritic infestation with the mite *Sarcoptes scabiei*.
▶ **Epidemiology:** Worldwide distribution. In some areas, such as certain Caribbean islands, it is endemic with virtually everyone infested. In the past, it typically appeared in cycles (*seven year itch*), but this is no longer the case. In recent years, epidemics in homes for the elderly have become a problem.
▶ **Pathogenesis:** *Sarcoptes scabiei* is a mite that lives only on humans. It does not transfer any diseases. Transfer is by close personal contact, such as mother–child, siblings, or sexual partners. Female mites burrow in the epidermis just below the stratum corneum, depositing eggs and feces as they move along. The first infestation remains asymptomatic for a period of weeks, until an immune response

develops and pruritus results. Upon re-infestation, the symptoms appear in a matter of days.

► **Clinical features:**

- *Burrows:* Fine slightly raised, sometimes erythematous, irregular lines with a terminal swelling where the female mite can be found. Typical sites (Fig. 7.3) include interdigital spaces, sides of the hands and feet, flexural surface of the wrist, anterior axillary line, penis, nipples (Fig. 7.4 a,b).
- *Intense pruritus:* Few skin diseases itch as much as scabies; usually worst at night.
- *Dermatitis:* Immune reaction (type IV) to mites leads to both pruritus and diffuse exanthem. Typical sites are thighs, buttocks, trunk.
- *Variations:*
  - *Pyoderma:* Pruritus leads to excoriations and erosions which become secondarily infected. In some areas, there is a vicious cycle of scabies → impetigo → glomerulonephritis.
  - *Scabies incognita:* Patients with meticulous personal hygiene (*scabies of the cleanly*) or those using topical corticosteroids may completely mask the findings of scabies, complaining only of pruritus.
  - *Nodular scabies:* Persistent papules usually in infants, favoring the groin, axillae, and genitalia. Occasionally seen in adults once again genitalia most

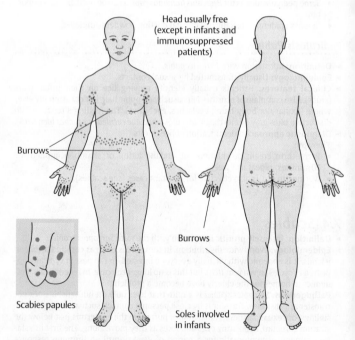

Head usually free
(except in infants and
immunosuppressed
patients)

Burrows

Burrows

Scabies papules

Soles involved
in infants

Fig. 7.3 · Sites of predilection for scabies.

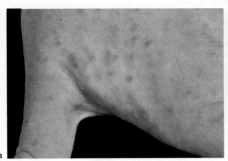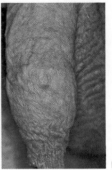

Fig. 7.**4** · **Scabies. a** With burrows and inflammatory papules in interdigital spaces. **b** Burrow on penis.

common. On biopsy, lymphocytic infiltrate. Remain for months after elimination of all mites; blamed on "antigen persistence".

- *Crusted scabies (Norwegian scabies):* Massive scabies infestation with crusted hyperkeratotic, psoriasiform lesions, as well as subungual lesions. Seen in debilitated patients, sometimes in Down syndrome; increasingly common in HIV/AIDS patients.
- *Animal scabies:* There are over 40 different forms of animal scabies, including those involving cats, dogs, and birds. These mites cannot reproduce on humans. They tend to bite at sites of contact (hands, arms, face if sleeping with pet), cause pruritus without any incubation period, and then die.

► **Complications:** Acarophobia: fear of persistent infection following cure; major psychological problem (p. 580).

► **Diagnostic approach:** Identification of mite; look at ends of burrows (dermatoscopy can help; *hang glider sign*); unroof with fine scalpel and examine under microscope.

▣ *Note:* Suspect scabies in any unexplained pruritic disease which is worse at night or also present in family members or other contacts.

► **Differential diagnosis:** All pruritic diseases; the issue is always to include scabies in the differential diagnosis.

► **Therapy:**
- Permethrin 5% cream has the best safety record and the least reports of resistance. It should be viewed as the agent of choice. Apply at night, wash in morning; repeat after 1 week.
- Lindane lotion is the worldwide standard, but not as effective as permethrin. It should be used in the same way.
- ▨ *Caution:* Lindane should not be used in pregnancy or in infants. It is potentially neurotoxic and there are several alternatives.
- A warm bath prior to application will increase the efficacy of treatment; remember that with eroded areas, absorption is increased.
- Bedding and clothing should be washed in hot cycle of washing machine; under normal conditions no other precautions are needed.
- For resistant cases, epidemics or crusted scabies, ivermectin 150–400 µg/kg p.o. administered on days 1 and 14 is highly effective.

7.5 Other Epizoonoses

Arthropod Assault Reaction

▶ **Definition:** Pruritic nodule resulting from bite or sting of arthropod.
▶ **Epidemiology:** Knowledge of local factors and seasonal variation is required to accurately guess at source of arthropod assault.
▶ **Pathogenesis:** The term "insect bite" reaction is an oversimplification, as many arthropods, both insects and arachnids (spiders, ticks, mites, and scorpions), can inflict injury. Bites are inflicted by the mouth parts, while stings are administered by other body parts, such as the tail stinger of a scorpion. The resulting lymphocytic infiltrate, often rich in eosinophils, may be the result of retained body parts, injected toxins, or injected microbes (as in borreliosis, p. 92).
▶ **Clinical features:** Typically there are one or more erythematous papules or nodules. They are on exposed skin, often grouped, and sometimes stopping at a point where clothing causes constriction, such as a sock or belt line. The diagnosis of arthropod assault is an awkward one; patients often say something like "It can't be a sting or bite, I would never come to the doctor for that." Some convincing talk is usually required. There may be unique patterns such as bullous reactions (more common in infants, immunosuppressed, especially patients with chronic lymphocytic leukemia).
▶ **Histology:** The microscopic picture is a mixed lymphocytic infiltrate, usually with eosinophils. In the case of tick bites, the mouth parts will sometimes be retained, easing the diagnosis.
▶ **Diagnostic approach:** If the pattern is common in your area, then the clinical diagnosis usually suffices. Biopsy may be helpful in puzzling cases.
▶ **Differential diagnosis:** Insect bite reactions were formerly called pseudolymphomas. We do not like this term and have avoided it. The classic well-accepted examples of an insect bite reaction are nodular scabies and the reaction surrounding molluscum contagiosum, but any bite or sting can induce a persistent nodule. Lymphadenosis cutis benigna in borreliosis occurs later and not necessarily at a bite site, but has a similar histologic pattern. Another cause of erythematous nodules with a dense lymphocytic infiltrate (and mucin) is lupus tumidus. Finally, many low-grade B-cell lymphomas were formerly identified as pseudolymphoma.
▶ **Therapy:** Topical or intralesional corticosteroids; on rare occasions, excision.
▶ **Prophylaxis:** Avoiding outdoor activity. The best insect repellents are those containing diethyltoluamide (DEET). When extensive exposure is anticipated, choose the product with the highest DEET concentration.

Cimicosis

▶ **Synonym:** Bedbug bites.
▶ **Pathogenesis:** *Cimex lectularius* or bedbug is 0.5 cm flattened bug that lives in furniture or crevices in the bedroom, is active at night, and feeds on humans by obtaining blood. Bedbugs are uncommon in both Germany and the USA, but can be seen; often patients return from vacations with bites.
▶ **Clinical features:** Bedbug bites are painless, but soon itch intensely and are quite persistent. They often follow a line and are grouped (breakfast, lunch, and dinner).
▶ **Diagnostic approach:** History of night-time bites, linear arrangement.
▶ **Therapy:** Symptomatic measures (antipruritic agents or topical corticosteroids, systemic antihistamines); call the exterminator.

Pulicosis

- **Synonym:** Flea bites.
- **Pathogenesis:** Fleas are 1–3 mm insects capable of jumping quite far; they have limited host specificity and often transfer from household pets or other animals to humans.
- Human pathogens include:
  - *Pulex irritans:* Human flea; relatively uncommon.
  - *Ctenocephalides felis* or *C. canis:* Cat and dog fleas; common.
  - *Xenopsylla cheopis:* Rat flea, worldwide distribution; transmit endemic typhus and plague.
  - *Ceratophyllus gallinae:* Chicken flea; common.
- **Clinical features:** Multiple tiny pruritic papules, often with central hemorrhagic punctum. Surprisingly, often one family member will be extensively involved, and the others spared or minimally affected.
- ▣ *Note:* A typical feature of flea bites is that when a new bite occurs, the older lesions also begin to itch again.
- **Diagnostic approach:** Clinical features and appropriate exposure.
- **Therapy:** Symptomatic therapy; veterinary examination of suspected domestic animals.

Trombiculiasis

- **Epidemiology:** Trombiculidae mites are scattered around the world. They are sometimes known as *harvest mites* because they so often infect grains, but they are also seen in gardens and forested areas. They are indiscriminate, attacking birds, mammals, and humans. In East Asia they transmit *Rickettsia tsutsugamushi*, the causative agent of scrub typhus.
- **Pathology:** The most common agent in Europe is *Trombicula autumnalis*. Larval forms of the mites, known as chiggers, attach themselves to passers-by and then use enzymes to create a hole in the epidermis through which they can receive nutrients. The chemicals they employ cause intense pruritus.
- **Clinical features:** Intensely pruritic small red papules on exposed areas; typically on the legs just above the sock line or on the trunk just above the belt line.
- **Diagnostic approach:** History, clinical findings.
- **Therapy:** Symptomatic therapy with topical corticosteroids or antipruritic agents. The best approach is regular use of insect repellents.

7.6 Worms

There are many worm infestations that cause tremendous public health problems in developing countries. They are seldom seen in developed countries, except among tourists. In almost all cases, elevated eosinophil levels are seen, so any patient with unexplained hypereosinophilia, perhaps associated with pruritus or urticaria, should be checked for the presence of parasitic worms.

Cutaneous Larva Migrans

- **Synonym:** Creeping eruption.
- **Definition:** Infestation of human skin by larva that are unable to complete their life cycle in the skin.

Other Infectious Diseases

▶ **Epidemiology:** The most common cause of cutaneous larva migrans is infestation by the dog and cat hookworm, *Ancylostoma braziliense*. Tourists to the Caribbean islands are a high-risk group.

▶ **Pathogenesis:** The larval worms are deposited in moist soil via stool. They enter their accidental host via the skin, and wander about creating complex burrowing patterns. Many other worms also migrate through the skin. They include the animal parasites *Ancylostoma caninum* (dog hookworm), *Uncinaria stenocephala* (pig hookworm), and *Gnathostoma spinigerum* (fish nematode), as well as the human parasites *Necator americanus* (human hookworm) and *Strongyloides stercoralis*. The human parasites enter via the skin but rapidly get to their target organs. In the case of *Strongyloides stercoralis*, if the larva mature rapidly in the bowel, they can penetrate the perianal skin causing *larva currens*.

▶ **Clinical features:** After a few hours, the entry site begins to itch and a red papule develops. After a few days, the larva begins to migrate in the skin, creating bizarre erythematous curved lines.

▶ **Diagnostic approach:** Classic clinical picture.

▶ **Therapy:**
- The nonhuman worms will die after a few months, but few patients are willing to wait.
- Cryotherapy is often endorsed, but the worms can live for at least 5 minutes at −25 °C, so it is probably not efficacious.
- Topical thiabendazole is the treatment of choice. No commercial product is available but it can be easily compounded (p. 699). Apply t.i.d. for 1 week, or apply 1× daily under plastic wrap (Saran, cling-film) occlusion for 1 week.
- If not responsive, then systemic therapy with thiabendazole 500 mg b.i.d. for 3–4 days, albendazole 400 mg daily for 3 days, mebendazole 100 mg b.i.d. for 3 days, or ivermectin 200 µg/kg in single dose, which can be repeated weekly for 2 weeks.

Other Diseases Caused by Worms

▶ **Myiasis:** Many different fly larvae (*maggots*) can invade human flesh. Usually they need an entry site, such as a chronic ulcer or wound. Most maggots only eat necrotic debris, although some attack healthy tissue. Specially bred sterile maggots are used in wound débridement. Some maggots may migrate below the skin surface (*myiasis migrans*). Individual maggots must be extracted or excised; many tricks are recommended to ease the process, such as covering the entry tunnel with oil or attaching a piece of bacon to attract the parasites.

▶ **Enterobiasis:**
- Worldwide infection caused by *Enterobius vermicularis*, the pinworm. Most common in young children; frequently brought home from day nurseries or kindergarten.
- Life cycle is simple; eggs are ingested; after developing in gut, female wanders out of anus at night and lays eggs on perianal skin. If not treated, cycle repeats itself every 4–6 weeks following reingestion of eggs.
- Main complaint is pruritus ani, worse at night. Complications include chronic urticaria, vulvovaginitis (direct spread), and a fertile ground for human papillomavirus and molluscum contagiosum infections.
- Diagnosis made by clear adhesive tape stripping of perianal region. Stool examination also positive.
- Always consider when confronted by perianal pruritus or dermatitis in children.
- Treatment includes pyrantel pamoate (10 mg/kg), mebendazole 100 mg or albendazole 400 mg in single dose; perhaps repeated in 2 weeks.

▶ **Onchocerciasis:**

- Caused by *Onchocerca volvulus* and transmitted by *Simulium* flies. The main endemic areas are in equatorial Africa and Yemen, as well as foci in Central and South America.
- The larvae (microfilariae) migrate through the skin, causing pruritus and itching, as well as frequent postinflammatory hypopigmentation. Some patients have very few organisms but an intense edematous inflammatory reaction (*sowda* in Yemen, *coastal erysipelas* in the Americas).
- The mature female and her much smaller partner coiled together in a subcutaneous nodule (*onchocercoma*); she releases many new microfilariae.
- The main problem with onchocerciasis is involvement of the eyes (*river blindness*). The microfilariae wander through the eyes and trigger a destructive inflammatory response.
- Diagnosis is based on identifying the organisms in the eye or in skin snips. Serologic studies are also available.
- The treatment of choice is ivermectin 150 µg/kg in a single dose. In endemic areas, an extensive World Health Organization campaign is underway to completely eliminate onchocerciasis. Here the entire population receives a single dose of ivermectin once yearly, as only microfilariae are killed and one must wait for the adult worms to die.

▶ **Schistosomiasis:**

- Schistosomiasis is a major public health problem in the world. Infections with several different *Schistosoma* flukes cause chronic bladder and bowel disease, including bladder cancer. The distribution includes Africa, Middle East, Asia, and Central America.
- The eggs are excreted via urine or stool into water; snails serve as intermediate hosts. The free-swimming cercariae are the form that re-enter humans.
- The migrating cercariae cause a pruritic dermatitis. A few weeks later a severe allergic reaction occurs (*Katayama fever*). Then later, as the female releases eggs, some may wind up in the skin where they cause a granulomatous dermatitis. The must common sites are the anogenital and periumbilical regions.
- The diagnosis is based on finding eggs in the urine or stool, as well as on serological tests. Eggs can also be found in skin biopsy from granulomatous lesions.
- Praziquantel is the treatment of choice; either 40 mg/kg in a single dose or 20 mg/kg q8 h × 3. Programs with population-based use of praziquantel, as well as attention to sanitation measures, are under way.
- *Swimmer's itch:* There are many non-human flukes involving, for example, water birds. When humans swim in shallow infested water, the cercariae may penetrate their skin, causing pruritic red papules and nodules. The animal parasites cannot complete their life cycle in humans, so there is no risk of internal involvement. This problem is common in both North America and Europe. Treatment is symptomatic.

8 Sexually Transmitted Diseases

8.1 Overview

▶ **Terminology:** The term *sexually transmitted disease* (STD) is being replaced in some circles by *sexually transmitted infection (STI)*. We see little advantage in the change. The older term *venereal disease* refers in a more limited way to diseases such as gonorrhea that are almost exclusively transferred by sexual contact, whereas STDs include diseases that are also acquired by nonsexual means. The most common STDs are shown in Table 8.1.

Table 8.1 · **Common sexually transmitted diseases**

Classic venereal diseases (covered in this chapter)	Other sexually transmitted infections
Syphilis	HIV/AIDS
Gonorrhea	Candidal balanitis and vulvovaginitis
Chlamydia infections	Condylomata acuminata
Chancroid	Herpes genitalis
Lymphogranuloma venereum	Cytomegalovirus
Granuloma inguinale	Hepatitis B and hepatitis C
Bacterial vaginosis	Pediculosis pubis
	Scabies

▶ **Public health considerations:** Every country has public health regulations of varying degrees of complexity, indicating which infectious diseases (both STDS and other infections such as tuberculosis deemed to be community threats) must be reported, who must report them (treating physician, laboratory), and how patient confidentiality is to be treated. The AIDS epidemic has put entirely new constraints on the system; in Germany, the reporting of cases of HIV infection is entirely anonymous.

▶ **Tracking contacts:** Only if public health authorities have the name of the patient can they assist the practicing physician in identifying and treating contacts of the patient, thereby interrupting the chain of transmission. The treating physician's rule is to win the patient's confidence so that this effort is as successful as possible.

▶ **Treatment guidelines:** There are many well-known guidelines for the treatment of STDs. We have used those of the Germany STD Society, published in 2001.

8.2 Syphilis

Overview

▶ **Synonym:** Lues.
▶ **Definition:** Chronic infection caused by *Treponema pallidum* and almost exclusively transferred by sexual intercourse. The early stages are primarily cutaneous and mucocutaneous; after decades, untreated syphilis affects the cardiovascular and nervous systems.
▶ **Epidemiology:** The epidemiology of syphilis would fill a book in itself. After the advent of penicillin, many predicted the demise of syphilis, but in the past two decades it has made a discouraging resurgence, fuelled by the increasing incidence of HIV/AIDS and the breakdown of many social systems in the former Soviet Union.
▶ **Pathogenesis:** *Treponema pallidum* is a spirochete 6–20 µm long and 0.1–0.2 µm wide with 10–20 spirals. The generation time is long, > 30 hours; this plays an important role in therapy. The organism is very sensitive and scarcely survives in the environment. Transmission is by close tissue contact with entry through minor points of injury.

Clinical Classification

The stages of syphilis are shown in Table 8.2.
▶ **Early syphilis:** All disease manifestations and the subsequent latent period during the first 2 years after the infection:
  • *Primary syphilis:* About 3–8 weeks after the primary infection, inflammation arises at the site of inoculation and the regional lymph nodes.
  • *Secondary syphilis:* Around 9 weeks (between 6 and 12 weeks) after the infection, bacteremia, generalized exanthem, systemic signs and symptoms, and production of antibodies. Rarely, this stage may be prolonged by inadequate antiobiotic therapy.
  • *Latent syphilis:* Symptom-free period following secondary syphilis; only recognized by positive serological tests. Can be caused by subcurative antibiotic dosages, often given for other infections, when syphilis is overlooked.
  ▣ *Note:* Be careful not to confuse latent syphilis, which is untreated or improperly treated syphilis, with positive seroreactions in appropriately treated patients.
▶ **Late syphilis:** Syphilis occurring more than 2 years after primary infection. Granulomatous inflammation with few organisms and marked cellular immune response, which causes most of the trouble. Organs most often involved include skin, bones, cardiovascular system, and CNS.
▶ **Congenital syphilis:** Also known as *syphilis connata*. Follows transplacental transmission of *Treponema pallidum*.

Table 8.2 · Stages of syphilis		
Stage	**Time after infection (years)**	**Disease**
Early syphilis	0–2	Primary syphilis
		Secondary syphilis
		Latent syphilis (seropositive)
Late syphilis	> 2	Tertiary syphilis
		Quaternary syphilis
		Latent syphilis
		(seronegative)

Sexually Transmitted Diseases

Primary Syphilis

▶ **Clinical features:**

- Dark red nodule develops at site of entry about 3 weeks after contact; it becomes eroded and then ulcerated.
- *Chancre (ulcus durum):* Firm, 1 cm, circumscribed ulcer; base is ham-colored while periphery is more red (Fig. 8.1). On palpation, firm, compared to button or small coin. The size of ulcers varies greatly (larger when herpes genitalis is entry site). Heals spontaneously over 3–8 weeks.

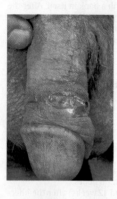

Fig. 8.1 · Primary syphilis: chancre.

- **Location:**
- ▶ *Note:* Any location is possible.
  - *Men:* Prepuce, glans, sulcus, less often shaft. In homosexuals, perianal region or rectum.
  - *Women:* Vagina or cervix (often overlooked), labia majora or minora, clitoris, posterior commissure, perianal region, rectum.
  - *Extragenital lesions:* Lips, tongue, palate, finger.
- Most chancres are asymptomatic; about 50% are either overlooked or not clinically appreciable. Rectal and anal lesions more likely to be painful. Occasionally chancre coupled with marked edema of foreskin and secondary phimosis. Sometimes with mixed infections, inflammation is so extreme that the foreskin must be split to avoid penile gangrene.
- *Regional lymphadenopathy:* Appears 1–2 weeks after chancre; usually unilateral; 1–2 cm firm, nontender lymph nodes without inflammation of overlying skin.

▶ **Diagnostic approach:**

- *Darkfield examination: Treponema pallidum* cannot be seen with usual stains such as Gram stain; darkfield microscopy is the most convenient way to identify the organism.
  - Clear secretions from the ulcer are needed.
  - *Treponema pallidum* shows three characteristic motions: rotation on the long axis, sharp folds, and minimal motion forward and backwards.
  - Secretions can be dried on a slide which is then studied with the fluorescent treponemal antibody (FTA) technique; can be mailed to referral laboratory.
  - Lesions that are usually positive include chancres, early congenital syphilis, condylomata lata, and other secondary lesions where secretions can be extracted.

- Darkfield of limited utility for mucosal lesions as there are many normal spirochetes in the mouth.
- *Obtaining secretions:* Considerable mechanical irritation and pressure is needed to obtain clear lymphatic fluid for a darkfield examination.
  - Cotton gauze soaked in physiological saline is used to rub ulcer (painful!) until clear fluid appears.
  - Pick up fluid with coverslip; apply to one drop of physiologic saline on glass slide.
- *Serologic testing:* FTA-IgM is positive 2 weeks after initial infection. If clinical suspicion exists, but the darkfield and serology are negative, the patient should be rechecked in 1–2 months.

▶ **Differential diagnosis:**
- *Herpes genitalis:* Usually multiple erosions and painful lymphadenopathy.
- *Traumatic ulcers:* Painful and not firm or button-like.
- *Chancroid:* Painful, soft, undermined ulcer.
- *Lymphogranuloma venereum:* Little or no ulceration, but fluctuant lymphadenopathy.
- *Erythroplasia of Queyrat (mucosal squamous cell carcinoma in situ):* Chronic, histology decisive.
- *Plasma cell balanitis of Zoon:* Chronic, histology decisive.
- *Fixed drug eruption:* Erosion, no ulcer; no lymphadenopathy; usually helpful drug history.

Secondary Syphilis

▶ **Clinical features:**
- There are an incredible number of exanthems and enanthems associated with secondary syphilis. Syphilis was formerly known as the great imitator. The rashes in secondary syphilis are known as syphilids. All reflect local inflammation caused by *Treponema pallidum* during its bacteremic phase. The role of circulating immune complexes is unclear.
- ▣ *Note:* The rashes of secondary syphilis usually do not itch and are only rarely bullous; anything else is possible.
- *Macular syphilid:* The most common finding, initially pale irregular pink macules (*syphilitic roseola*) typically on side of chest, later spreading to involve trunk, palms, and soles with typical red-brown color (Fig. 8.2 a). Marked individual variation. Nonpruritic, nonscaling, blanchable with diascopy.
- *Variations:*
  - *Papular syphilid:* Sometimes firm red-brown papules evolve in varying numbers. Multiple small papules known as *lenticular syphilid* (Fig. 8.2 b).
  - *Annular or circinate syphilid:* Spread of papules with central clearing and peripheral growth.
  - *Corymbose syphilid:* Many small papules surrounding a single larger lesion.
  - *Corona venerea:* Papules along anterior hair line.
  - *Palmoplantar syphilid:* Papules on palms and soles with red-brown color and scale (*clavi syphilitici*) (Fig. 8.2 c).
  - ▣ *Note:* Always suspect syphilis when confronted with an acute palmoplantar rash.
  - *Lichen syphiliticus:* Tiny follicular papules, resembling milia; rare and occurs late.
  - In immunosuppressed patients, especially HIV/AIDS, larger lesions may be ulcerated (*malignant syphilid*, Fig. 8.2 d) or crusted (*rupial syphilis*).

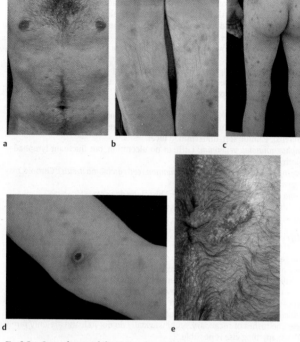

Fig. 8.2 · **Secondary syphilis. a** Maculopapular exanthema. **b** Syphilis on soles. **c** Papular exanthem. **d** Ulcerated nodule. **e** Condylomata lata.

- *Syphilitic leukoderma:* Any of the secondary lesions can heal with postin-flammatory hypopigmentation; most common on the nape; usually resolves.
- *Condylomata lata:* Eroded genital papules teeming with spirochetes (Fig. 8.2 e). Sometimes similar lesions inter digitally.
- *Syphilitic alopecia:* Moth-eaten hair loss; usually numerous small, poorly circumscribed areas of incomplete hair loss (never complete loss as in alopecia areata).
- Mucosal changes:
  - *Mucous plaques:* Small papules on oral mucosa, which rapidly become eroded.
  - *Opaline plaques:* Later stage with glossy gray membranous covering.
  - *Plaques fouée:* Dark red plaques on tongue.
  - *Syphilitic angina:* Involvement of tonsils by spirochetes with swelling and dusky erythema; usually unilateral. In German, known as specific angina (because in the early days of dermatology, everything that was not syphilis was not specific).

- *Other systemic changes:*
  - *Generalized lymphadenopathy:* Most regular feature—painless firm lymph-adenopathy involving antecubital, axillary, nuchal, preauricular, and other nodes. In the famous *syphilitic handshake*, the physician slid his hand up the arm to palpate the patient's antecubital nodes; sometimes known as the father-in-law check.
  - *Liver:* Acute hepatitis.
  - *Kidneys:* Acute glomerulonephritis with deposition of immunoglobulins and complement.
  - *Spleen:* Enlarged in almost 100% of cases.
  - *CNS:* Meningitis or meningoencephalitis; 25% have CSF abnormalities. Perhaps more common in HIV/AIDS.
- *Musculoskeletal abnormalities:*
  - *Periostitis:* Most commonly involves bones close to skin surface; typical sites tibia, sternum, and medial end of clavicle; pain worse at night.
  - Polyarthritis (immune complex disease).
  - Tenosynovitis.
▶ **Diagnostic approach:** Serology (100% positive; one has only to think of the possible diagnosis); dark field of eroded lesions.
▶ **Prognosis:** Even in the absence of treatment, all lesions resolve and many patients never develop further manifestations.

Latent Syphilis

▶ **Definition:** Seropositive latent syphilis is the phase following the resolution of secondary syphilis where the patient looks and feels normal but has a positive serology.
▶ **Diagnostic approach:**
- If the FTA-IgM test is positive in an asymptomatic patient, a complete examination is needed.
- The following steps are essential:
  - CSF examination and neurological evaluation.
  - Assessment of aorta (ultrasonography or imaging techniques).
  - Ophthalmologic consultation.

Tertiary Syphilis

▶ **Cutaneous manifestations:** Sometimes referred to as late benign syphilis, as these changes are much less serious and much more responsive to therapy than the other late manifestations.
- *Tuberous syphilid:*
  - Grouped red-brown papules and nodules (1–2 cm) that clear centrally and expand peripherally over years. Often annular or curved pattern (*tuberoserpiginous syphilid*).
  - Can occur anywhere, but more often on upper arms, back, or face.
- *Gumma:*
  - Firm 1–3 cm subcutaneous nodules that are painless and usually solitary, but frequently ulcerate discharging a rubbery (gum-like) substance.
  - Typical sites include palate (perforation), nose (collapse causing *saddle nose*, scalp, and face. May also involve liver, bone, or testes.
▶ **Musculoskeletal disease:**
- *Periosteitis:* Continuation of process starting in secondary syphilis.
- *Osteolysis* sometimes progressing to sclerosis of the entire marrow cavity: *ivory bones.*

- *Gummata* involving bone.
- *Juxtaarticular nodes:* Gummata that tend not to liquefy.

► **Cardiovascular disease:**
- About 10% of untreated patients develop cardiovascular syphilis.
- *Treponema pallidum* involves the vaso vasorum (vessels nurturing the aorta) and leads to aneurysm formation and aortic insufficiency.
- Diagnosis is based on standard ultrasonography and imaging procedures to measure aorta and then monitor changes.
- ☑ *Note:* 80% of patients with syphilitic aortic disease die from this problem, despite both antibiotic therapy and surgery.

► **CNS disease:** In late syphilis, most neurological symptoms are caused by chronic vessel inflammation. Spontaneous resolution can occur during the tertiary inflammatory phase, but not in the quaternary phase.
- *Asymptomatic neurosyphilis:* CNS involvement is only detected by examination of CSF; no signs or symptoms.
- *Meningovascular neurosyphilis:* Main finding in meningeal inflammation, usually with prominent headache. Also numerous CNS thromboses cause a variety of neurological and psychiatric symptoms. Gummata may also caused focal defects.
- Diagnosis based on CSF examination for cells and protein, serology (blood and CSF) and neurologic examination.

Quaternary Syphilis

The most devastating complications of syphilis are the late parenchymal problems, which are not generally reversible.

► **General paresis:**
- Formerly known as general paresis (or paralysis) of the insane; before the advent of antibiotic therapy, syphilitic patients kept mental institutions filled.
- About 2% of untreated patients advance to this stage; onset of signs and symptoms is 20–25 years after initial infection. Primary damage is to the gray matter of the anterior lobes, causing a wide spectrum of neurological and psychiatric disease.

► **Tabes dorsalis:** About as common as general paresis. Changes involve the dorsal roots and posterior columns of spinal cord. Divided into three stages:
- *Anesthetic stage:* Hypesthesia especially on the feet leads to neurotropic ulcers *(mal perforant);* lancinating abdominal and extremity pain, and paralysis of ocular nerves. *Argyll Robertson pupil* describes a pupil that is miotic and responds to accommodation effort but not to light.
- ☑ *Note:* Pupil abnormalities must be present for the diagnosis of tabes dorsalis.
- *Ataxic stage:* Uncoordinated movements with typical locomotion (*slap walk*) and positive *Romberg sign* (unable to stand steady with eyes closed).
- *Pseudoparetic stage:* Patient also develops signs and symptoms of paresis.

► **Diagnostic approach:** Same as for tertiary neurosyphilis.

Congenital Syphilis

► **Definition:** Syphilis in utero from mother to fetus. Two subtypes:
- *Early congenital syphilis* (*syphilis connata praecox*): Lesions occur during the first 2 years of life (analogous to primary syphilis).
- *Late congenital syphilis* (*syphilis connata tarda*): Lesions occur after 2 years of life (analogous to secondary syphilis).

▶ **Pathogenesis:** The degree of fetal damage depends on the time of infection in the mother (Table 8.3) and, more importantly, on whether or not she is treated promptly and appropriately.

Table 8.3 · **Relationship between time of untreated maternal infection and manifestations of congenital syphilis**

Time of maternal infection	Consequences for fetus
Before pregnancy	
> 2 years (late syphilis)	Little risk
< 2 years (early syphilis)	Intrauterine death or early congenital syphilis
During pregnancy	
1st half	Intrauterine death or early congenital syphilis
2nd half	Mild congenital syphilis, or child is normal at birth but develops late congenital syphilis (and mother, secondary syphilis)

▶ **Early congenital syphilis:**
- The fetus's immature immune response allows syphilis to run a rapid and damaging course. Prognosis is especially poor if signs and symptoms are present at birth.
- Clinical findings include:
  - *Present at birth:* Low birth weight, abnormally large placenta, hepatosplenomegaly, blisters and erosions mainly on palms and soles (*pemphigus syphiliticus*), osteomyelitis—mortality rate 50%.
  - *Developing in first months in untreated infants: Snuffles* (chronic runny nose, often bloody), periorificial rhagades, pemphigus syphiliticus may also appear here in delayed fashion, periosteitis and osteochondritis involving mainly long bones with so much pain that infants do not move limbs (*Parrot pseudoparalysis*), CNS disease (50%), glomerulonephritis with nephrotic syndrome.

▶ **Late congenital syphilis:**
- Resembles late syphilis, but cardiac involvement is uncommon.
- Clinical findings include:
  - *Interstitial keratitis:* Affects about 10%, usually bilateral; appears at age 10–30. Initially iritis, then corneal neovascularization and clouding. Treatment is topical corticosteroids, not antibiotics, which cause a flare; sometimes corneal transplantation needed.
  - Salt and pepper retina.
  - *Sensory deafness:* Develops at 10–20 years of age in 10–30%; usually bilateral.
  - *Neurosyphilis:* Late onset but affects 30–50%.
  - *Cutaneous findings:* Analogous to late syphilis (gummata and tuberous lesions).

▶ **Stigmata:** Clinical lesions that develop secondary to congenital syphilis, even after treatment. One or more is almost always present. Findings include:
- Saddle nose (75%).
- Frontal bossing (hot cross bun or buttocks skull).

- Maxillary hypoplasia (85%).
- *Higouménaki sign:* Thickening of medial end of clavicle.
- Saber shins.
- *Clutton joints:* Effusions into large joints.
- Gothic palate (high arched palate): 75%.
- Periorificial furrowed scars (*Parrot lines*).
- Dental changes:
  - *Hutchison incisors:* Incisors shaped like tip of a screwdriver, often notched; 65%.
  - *Mulberry molars:* First molars with complex surface; 65%.
  - ▣ *Note:* The *Hutchinson triad* consists of Hutchison incisors, sensory deafness, and interstitial keratitis.

Serologic Diagnosis of Syphilis

Overview

There are a number of serologic tests for syphilis. They are used to make the diagnosis, to confirm the effectiveness of therapy, and to monitor patients for recurrence. An overview of the available tests and their use is given in Table 8.**4**. Two screening tests and two confirmatory tests suffice for almost all circumstances; not all the tests listed in the table are described in detail. There are two basic categories of tests:

▶ **Nontreponemal tests:** Identify antibodies against phospholipids such as lecithin or cardiolipin.
▶ **Treponemal tests:** Identify antibodies against *Treponema pallidum*.

The former are cheaper and more sensitive; the latter, more specific.

Table 8.4 · **Serologic tests for syphilis**

Screening test	TPHA test
	VDRL test
	RPR card test
	IgG-ELISA test
Confirmatory test	FTA-ABS test
	VDRL titers
Need for therapy	IgM-FTA-ABS test
	19S-IgM-FTA-ABS test
	IgM-ELISA
	Cardiolipin test
Follow-up	Cardiolipin test
	VDRL test
	19S-IgM-FTA-ABS test
	IgM-ELISA test

Treponema pallidum Hemagglutination Test (TPHA Test)

▶ **Basis:** Sheep erythrocytes coated with *Treponema pallidum* antigens are incubated with patient serum; if antibodies are present, the red cells agglutinate.
▶ **Indications:** Screening.
▶ **Evaluation:** Highly specific; false positive under 0.1%; becomes positive in third week and remains positive for life of patient.
▶ **Advantages:** Easy to do.
▶ **Disadvantages:** Standardized reagents not available so reproducibility varies; expensive.

Venereal Disease Research Laboratory Test (VDRL Test)

► **Basis:** Flocculation test. Nonspecific antibodies that react with both *Treponema pallidum* cell wall phospholipids and cardiolipin are identified. The patient's serum is mixed in a colloidal solution of cholesterol, lecithin, and cardiolipin. If antibodies are present, a precipitate occurs. The serum is diluted and the level at which a reaction still occurs (for example 1:64) is noted. After treatment, the titer will drop over months.

► **Indications:** Screening and monitoring of therapy.

► **Evaluation:** Highly sensitive nontreponemal test, 100% positive in secondary syphilis.

► **Advantages:** Cheap, reproducible, worldwide usage, ability to titrate makes it quantitative.

► **Disadvantages:** 10–20% false-positive results; a positive VDRL test must always be confirmed.

► **False-positive reactions:** Diabetes mellitus, cirrhosis, autoimmune diseases (lupus erythematosus, systemic sclerosis, rheumatoid arthritis), pregnancy, viral diseases (HIV, measles, mumps, even herpes genitalis), advanced systemic malignancies, multiple blood transfusions, advanced age, i.v. drug abuse.

Fluorescent Treponema pallidum Antibody Absorption Test (FTA–ABS Test)

► **Basis:** A slide is coated with *Treponema pallidum*. Patient's serum is absorbed with nonpathogenic treponemes and then applied to slide. Antibodies bound to *Treponema pallidum* are identified with immunofluorescence.

► **Indications:** Confirmatory.

► **Evaluation:** Becomes positive in fourth week and remains so forever.

► **Advantages:** Very sensitive and specific.

► **Disadvantages:** Standardized reagents not available so reproducibility varies.

IgM–FTA–ABS Test

► **Basis:** Same as FTA–ABS test, but only labeled anti-IgM antibodies are used to determine if patient has IgM antibodies against *Treponema pallidum*.

► **Indications:**
  - *Early diagnosis:* IgM antibodies are the first to be produced; they can be found at 2 weeks, before a chancre appears.
  - *Assessing disease activity:* IgM production continues as long as living *Treponema pallidum* are present in body, so one can determine if latent phase is present or not.
  - *Evaluating therapy:* The IgM–FTA–ABS test usually turns negative 1 month after therapy; always within 1 year.
  - *Diagnosis of congenital syphilis:* IgM cannot cross the placenta, so if the infant has IgM antibodies, *Treponema pallidum* has crossed the placenta.
  - *Recognition of second infection:* Increase in IgM antibodies coupled with VDRL titer increase suggests second infection without clinical signs.

► **Advantages:** Very sensitive and specific.

► **False-positive reactions:** Rheumatoid factor is an IgM antibody whose Fc portion is directed against IgG. If the patient has a positive rheumatoid factor and treated syphilis, then persistent IgG antibodies will bind to treponemes on the slide; rheumatoid factor molecules bind to them and are identified by the labeled anti-IgM.

19S–IgM–FTA–ABS Test

► **Basis:** If a patient has a large amount of IgG antibodies against *Treponema pallidum* and only a small amount of IgM, then the IgG can block the test treponemes on the

slide, giving a false-negative test for IgM. To correct this, the 19S fraction of serum where IgM is found is separated out and only this portion used for testing.
► **Indications:** Negative IgM–FTA–ABS test but appropriate history.

Evaluation of Serologic Tests
► **Confirmation of infection with** *Treponema pallidum*: Two positive tests with *Treponema pallidum*-specific tests. Blood should be re-drawn for the confirmatory testing. An endemic treponematosis must be excluded.
► **Assessing degree of activity:** IgM–FTA–ABS becomes negative when *Treponema pallidum* has been eliminated. VDRL titer > 1:64 also suggests active disease.
► **Second infection:** New appearance of IgM antibodies, and rapid increase in VDRL titer by 2 dilutions or more.

CSF Serologic Diagnosis
► **Absolute indications:**
  • Confirmed and treated early syphilis with delayed drop in titer (IgM still present 1 year after therapy).
  • Confirmed early or late syphilis (treated or not) and development of neuropsychiatric signs and symptoms.
  • Patient with newly discovered positive serology, no previous documentation, and neuropsychiatric signs and symptoms.
  • Follow-up examination after positive CSF examination, 1 year after therapy.
  • HIV infection.
► **Relative indications:**
  • Any early syphilis except primary syphilis.
  • Latent syphilis without suitable history and documentation.
► **Technique:** The CSF tests are analogous to the blood tests. At the same time, the CSF is analyzed in routine fashion for cells and protein.

Therapy

► **Overview:**
  • The therapeutic recommendations of the German STD organization are shown in Table 8.**5**.
  • Therapy first after diagnosis is completely confirmed (identification of *Treponema pallidum* or confirmatory serological testing).
  • Syphilis is a reportable disease in most countries.
  • HIV serology.
  • Examination of sexual partners; then treatment or follow-up.
  • No sexual contacts until treatment is completed.
► **Penicillin therapy:**
  • Penicillin G remains the treatment of choice; still no evidence of resistant *Treponema pallidum*.
  • Therapeutic serum, level of 0.03 IU/mL must be maintained for 7 days. Because of the serious nature of tertiary syphilis, it is generally recommended to treat for 2–3 weeks.
  • Intramuscular injections are preferred to oral therapy, because of both unreliable patients and unreliable absorption.
  ☐ *Note:* Do not combine with bacteriostatic agents; penicillin interferes with cell wall production and is only effective against growing spirochetes.
  • *Complications:* Allergic reactions common; each patient must be asked about penicillin allergy and emergency equipment must be available.
  • *Penicillin allergy:* Doxycycline is the usual choice; if tetracyclines cannot be used, then erythromycin may be employed.

Table 8.5 · Treatment of syphilis

	Agent	Dose	Duration
Early syphilis			
Standard	Benzathine penicillin	2.4 million IU i.m. (1.2 million IU in each buttock)	Single dose
Alternatives			
	Doxycycline	100 mg b.i.d. p.o.	14 days
	Erythromycin	500 mg q.i.d. p.o.	14 days
Late syphilis			
Standard	Benzathine penicillin	2.4 million IU i.m.	Days 1,8,15
Alternatives	Procaine-benzylpenicillin	1.2 million i.m. daily[a]	21 days
	Doxycycline	200 mg b.i.d. p.o.	28 days
	Erythromycin	2.0 g i.v. daily	21 days
Neurosyphilis	Penicillin G	5 million IU 6x daily	14–21 days
Congenital syphilis	Penicillin G	50,000 IU/kg i.v. × 2 50,000 IU/kg i.v. × 3	Days 1–7[b] Days 8–10

a Procaine-benzylpenicillin 0.9 million IU and benzylpenicillin 0.3 million IU.
b Days of life.

▶ **Treatment during pregnancy:**
  • Penicillin is employed exactly as in nonpregnant patients.
  • In the case of penicillin allergy, use erythromycin. Since erythromycin crosses the placenta poorly, the infant should be treated with penicillin after birth.
▶ **HIV infection:** Always check CSF if the time of initial infection cannot be precisely identified (frequent second infections) or is more than 1 year in the past. If this cannot be clarified, then treat as neurosyphilis for at least 14 days.

8.3 Endemic Treponematoses

The endemic treponematoses are important both because they infect large numbers of people and because they cause false-positive reactions for syphilis; even the *Treponema pallidum* specific tests cannot help separate the diseases. The diseases go through stages parallel to syphilis, but with significant differences in organ involvement.

Yaws

▶ **Synonym:** Frambesia.
▶ **Definition:** Endemic treponematosis caused by *Treponema pertenue*.
▶ **Epidemiology:** Previously widespread in equatorial Africa and South America; today, small endemic areas in South America, occasional cases in Africa. Transmitted by close contact during childhood.

► **Clinical features:**
- *Incubation period:* 3–6 weeks.
- *Primary stage:* Verruciform nodule at site of inoculation; mother yaws, which resembles a raspberry (framboise in French); heals spontaneously.
- *Secondary stage:* Disseminated cutaneous lesions, sometimes worse in occluded or moist areas. Palmoplantar fissuring and keratoses known as *crab yaws.* Bone pain common, especially in tibia.
- *Tertiary stage:* Gummata develop but no CNS or cardiovascular disease.

► **Diagnostic approach:** Same as for syphilis.
► **Therapy:** Benzathine penicillin 2.4 million IU once.

Pinta

► **Definition:** Endemic treponematosis caused by *Treponema carateum.*
► **Epidemiology:** Limited to remote areas of southern Mexico, Central America, and northern South America. Transfer by direct contact.
► **Clinical features:**
- *Incubation period:* 3–6 weeks.
- *Primary stage:* Smooth papule, usually on extremity. Sometimes grouped papules, persists for months.
- *Secondary stage:* Disseminated papules (*pintids*), often appear before primary lesions is resolved. Resolve with hypopigmentation. May continue to appear for years.
- *Tertiary stage:* No bone, CNS, or cardiovascular disease.

► **Diagnostic approach:** Same as for syphilis.
► **Therapy:** Benzathine penicillin 2.4 million IU once. Totally depigmented lesions not influenced.

Endemic Syphilis

► **Definition:** Endemic treponematosis caused by *Treponema pallidum* var. *endemicus.*
► **Epidemiology:** Occurs mainly in dry regions of Middle East and North Africa; previously endemic in Bosnia but eradicated by mass treatment program in 1960s. Spread by direct contact and perhaps drinking vessels.
► **Clinical features:** Primary lesion usually oral and overlooked. Secondary lesions include mucous patches and bony lesions. Tertiary disease consists primarily of gummata and bony changes; CNS or cardiovascular disease extremely rare.
► **Diagnostic approach:** Same as for syphilis.
► **Therapy:** Benzathine penicillin 2.4 million IU once.

8.4 Gonorrhea

Overview

► **Definition:** Common sexually-transmitted infection caused by *Neisseria gonorrhoeae,* affecting mucosa and transitional epithelium; typically leading to urethritis in men and to an often asymptomatic cervicitis in women.
► **Epidemiology:**
- Peak ages: 18–25; more than 50% are under 25 years of age.
- Always sexually transmitted except for blennorrhea in newborns and some cases of vulvovaginitis in prepubertal girls.

- After intercourse with an infected women, 35% of men become infected. In the reverse setting, 60–90% of women become infected after contact with an infected man.
- Most men develop signs and symptoms within 3–4 days. Asymptomatic infections, often persistent and usually in women, are a significant reservoir.
- Development of resistant strains is a worldwide problem.

▶ **Pathogenesis:**
- *Neisseria gonorrhoeae* is a Gram-negative diplococcus (paired coccus), typically coffee-bean shaped; also known as *gonococcus*.
- Initially mucosal surfaces are infected: urethra, rectum, endocervix, pharynx, conjunctiva. Later, there may be regional complications and systemic spread.
- Gonococci have a variety of variable surface antigens. The most important are the thread-like pili that help the bacteria anchor to epithelial cells or even sperm. The main subunit, pilin, has antigenic variation that makes development of an immunization an as yet unmet challenge.

Local Infections

▶ **Genital gonorrhea in men:**
- *Urethritis:* Incubation period 3–4 days. In 70–85%, dysuria and pus-laden discharge, which cannot be clinically separated from other urethritides. 15–30% asymptomatic. Without treatment, resolution in days to weeks.
- *Regional complications:* Acute epididymitis, chronic prostatitis.

▶ **Differential diagnosis:** Nongonococcal urethritis.

▶ **Genital gonorrhea in women:**
- *Urethritis:* Incubation period 5–8 days. Often overlooked or misdiagnosed as cystitis; 80% of cases asymptomatic.
- *Cervicitis:* Also usually asymptomatic, mild cloudy discharge and erythematous ostium.
- *Regional complications:*
  - *Salpingitis:* Gonococci attach to sperm and can infect the fallopian tubes; more common around menses.
  - *Peritonitis:* Most common site for peritoneal infection after exiting tubes is perihepatic *(Fitz-Hugh–Curtis syndrome)*. May cause adhesions.
  - *Pelvic inflammatory disease:* Infection involving fallopian tubes, ovaries, and peritoneum; *Neisseria gonorrhoeae* is common cause. Leads to chronic abdominal pain, dyspareunia, infertility, and tubal pregnancy.
  - *Vulvovaginitis in children:* The vagina is more sensitive and easily infected in prepubertal girls. Thus *Neisseria gonorrhoeae* can cause a purulent vulvovaginitis, which is usually the result of sexual abuse. Differential diagnostic considerations include other bacterial infections (often spread from perianal region, herpes simplex, foreign bodies, irritating bubble baths).

  🗹 *Caution:* Always consider sexual abuse when confronted with vaginal discharge in a prepubertal girl. Culture for gonococci.

▶ **Gonococcal blennorrhea:**
- Infection occurs by direct spread of bacteria during passage through birth canal; less often in adults by direct contact.
- Erythema and swelling of the lids, conjunctivitis, and pus-laden discharge. Risk of corneal ulceration.
- Uncommon because of prophylaxis (see therapy).

▶ **Anorectal gonorrhea:**
- Present in 40–50% of women with cervical or urethral gonorrhea; higher percentage of male homosexuals.

- Often overlooked clinically; usually asymptomatic (85%) or mistaken for normal discharge.
► **Pharyngeal gonorrhea:**
  - Disease of women and male homosexuals; not clinically distinctive.
  - Asymptomatic in 90% of cases; otherwise mistaken for "sore throat".

Disseminated Gonococcal Infection (Gonococcal Sepsis)

► **Epidemiology:** Disseminated gonococcal infection (DGI) is rare, occurring in 1–3% of infections. At greatest risk are menstruating females who are asymptomatic carriers.
► **Pathogenesis:** Strains of *Neisseria gonorrhoeae* that cause DGI are usually exquisitely penicillin-sensitive.
► **Clinical features:**
  - *DGI triad:*
    - Polyarthralgia without arthritis.
    - Tenosynovitis.
    - *Dermatitis:* Tiny tender grey pustules on erythematous base, often over joints; histologically, septic vasculitis.
    - Patients usually have systemic signs and symptoms: fever, chills, malaise.
  - *Gonococcal arthritis:* At start, polyarthritis (knee, ankle, hand); later monoarthritis (almost always knee); diagnosis based on isolating *Neisseria gonorrhoeae* in joint aspirate.
  - Other rare systemic findings include endocarditis (EKG abnormalities) and meningitis.

Diagnostic Approach

► *Direct smear:* Urethral or cervical smear with Gram or methylene blue stain (p. 28).
► *Indirect identification:* Dried smear (can be mailed) labeled with immunoassay (Gonozyme); not suited for pharyngeal or rectal smears.
► *Culture:*
  - Take material with Dacron or calcium alginate-tipped applicator or platinum loop.
  - Can culture urethra, cervix, rectum, or pharynx. Also first-catch urine sediment following centrifugation.
  - Plate immediately on selective medium (Thayer–Martin) at 37 °C with CO_2 enrichment; commercial products include TransGrow. Transport media available but less desirable.
  - The colonies appear after 24–36 hours; they stain dark with dimethyl-*para*-phenylene diamine (*oxidation reaction*). Positive microscopy and oxidation reaction together are more than 99% accurate.
  - Simple test available for β-lactamase formation using chromogenic cephalosporin (Cefinase).

Therapy

► **Overview:**
  - Important factors include increased numbers of penicillinase-producing *Neisseria gonorrhoeae* (PPNG) strains in different parts of the world, as well as multiresistant strains.
  - 🚩 *Caution:* Be aware of local resistance patterns and of where your patient's infection was acquired.

- Frequent chlamydial coinfection (25–50%); many countries recommend always adding antichlamydial therapy to any regimen for gonorrhea.

► **Uncomplicated urethral gonorrhea:**
- *Intramuscular:* Spectinomycin 2.0 g or ceftriaxone 250 mg, each as single dose.
- *Oral:* Cefixime 400 mg, ciprofloxacin 500 mg, ofloxacin 400 mg, or azithromycin 1.0 g, each as single dose.
- Azithromycin also covers chlamydial infection; otherwise add either doxycycline 100 mg b.i.d. for 7 days or azithromycin 1.0 g in a single dose.

► **Pharyngeal gonorrhea:** Intramuscular ceftriaxone is preferred but oral quinolones are acceptable (dosages as above).

► **Anal gonorrhea:** Intramuscular therapy is preferred.

► **Complicated/disseminated gonorrhea:**
- Ceftriaxone 1–2 g i.m. or i.v. 1 × daily for 7 days (b.i.d. if meningitis or endocarditis).
- Cefotaxime 1.2 g i.v. t.i.d. for 7 days.
- Alternatives for β-lactam allergy:
  – Spectinomycin 2 g i.m. b.i.d. for 7 days.
  – Erythromycin 500 mg i.v. q.i.d. for 7 days.
- If epididymitis is present, add prednisolone 30 mg daily and NSAIDs.

► **Mixed infections:** Because of the high likelihood of coexistent chlamydial or anaerobic infections, most regimens for pelvic inflammatory disease offer broader coverage. Examples include:
- Second-generation cephalosporin and metronidazole or doxycycline.
- Clindamycin and gentamicin.

► **Pregnancy:** Erythromycin 500 mg i.v. q.i.d. for 7 days.

► **Blennorrhea:**
- *Adults:* Ceftriaxone 1 g i.m. (single dose usually suffices).
- *Infants:* Ceftriaxone 25–50 mg/kg i.v. or i.m. (single dose usually suffices).
- Rinse eyes with physiological saline.
- Children:
  – Ceftriaxone 25–50 mg/kg i.v. or i.m. 1x daily for 7 days (10–14 days if signs and symptoms persist).
  – Cefotaxime 25 mg/kg i.v. or i.m b.i.d. for 7–14 days.
  – If > 50 kg, adult dose.

► **Additional measures:**
- Always treat sexual partners; risk of overlooked gonorrhea is high. If treatment not possible, then culture and follow-up.
- Rule out accompanying syphilis or HIV infection.
- Follow-up culture 4–7 days after therapy.
- Rectal culture on all women with gonorrhea.
- Rectal and pharyngeal cultures on all homosexual men with gonorrhea.
- *Recurrent gonorrhea:* Culture and treat all sexual partners (no exceptions), rectal and pharyngeal cultures.

8.5 Other Sexually Transmitted Diseases

Chlamydial Infections

► **Epidemiology:** *Chlamydia trachomatis* (serotypes D–K) is a common cause of STD and the most usual cause of nongonococcal urethritis.

▶ **Clinical features:**
- **Men:**
  - *Urethritis:* Incubation period 1–3 weeks. Discharge (often minimal) and dysuria. In smear, >5 WBC per oil immersion field without gonococci. Without treatment, spontaneous resolution but recurrences possible. In 25–50% of cases, accompanying gonorrhea.
  - *Epididymitis:* Usually unilateral; swelling and induration of testes; very painful with fever. Usually accompanied by urethritis. Smear as above.
  - *Reiter syndrome* (p. 275): Urethritis, arthritis, conjunctivitis, psoriasiform skin changes; chlamydia are established trigger (along with bowel flora).
  - *Proctitis:* Usually male homosexuals; rectal pain, discharge, diarrhea; negative gonococcal culture; neutrophils in rectal smear.
- **Women:**
  - *Cervicitis:* Usual site, pus-laden or watery vaginal discharge with cervical erosions.
  - *Salpingitis (PID):* Most common cause of acute infection.
  - *Urethritis:* Dysuria, without hematuria or urge; often associated with cervicitis.
- **Children:**
  - *Pneumonia:* Acquired in birth canal, often with permanent lung damage.
  - *Conjunctivitis:* Common, but long-term sequelae rare.

▶ **Diagnostic approach:**
- Smear and methylene blue stain; >4 WBC/oil immersion field and no gonococci; fluorescent-labeled monoclonal antibodies (Micro Trac) also available.
- *Method of choice:* PCR or ligase chain reaction (LCR) of cervical smear (women) or first urine (men); almost 100% specificity and over 80% sensitivity; two products available (PCR–Amplicor; LCR–LCx); both easily transported; also can be used for ejaculate or conjunctival discharge.
- Cultures and serologic procedures not necessary for routine practice.

▶ **Therapy:**
- Doxycycline 100 mg b.i.d. for 7 days or azithromycin 1 g in single dose.
- *Alternatives:* Tetracycline 500 mg q.i.d. for 7 days, erythromycin 500 mg b.i.d. for 14 days, erythromycin 500 mg q.i.d. for 7 days, or ofloxacin 300 mg b.i.d. for 7 days.
- In pregnancy, erythromycin.
- With chronic disease, longer courses (10–14 days).
- *Epididymitis:* Hospitalize, prednisolone 30 mg daily and NSAIDS.
- *PID:* Hospitalize, treat with minocycline and ciprofloxacin.
- Always treat partner.

Chancroid

▶ **Synonym:** Ulcus molle.
▶ **Definition:** Acute STD with painful genital ulcers and lymphadenopathy caused by *Haemophilus ducreyi*.
▶ **Epidemiology:** Endemic in many parts of Africa, South-east Asia and Central America, where it is one of the most common STDs. Focal endemic areas in USA; most recently in Jackson, Mississippi. In Europe, usually in tourists. Male:female ratio 5:1.
▶ **Pathogenesis:** *Haemophilus ducreyi* is a Gram-negative, thermolabile anaerobic rod. Transmission is almost always by sexual intercourse.

▶ **Clinical features:**
- *Incubation period:* 3–5 days (very variable, range 1–35 days).
- *Ulcer:*
  - Starts as small red papule that rapidly becomes pustular and then ulcerates (2–3 days). Sometimes several papules. Ulcers jagged, undermined and painful; mirror image (kissing) ulcers common.
  - Painful, especially when splashed with urine.
  - *Location:* Men: glans penis, inner aspect of foreskin, frenulum. Women: labia, perianal region, cervix.
- *Lymphadenopathy:* Acute painful, usually unilateral; develops in 50% after 1–2 weeks. Typically forms abscesses that rupture forming fistulas.
- *Course:* Spontaneous healing after 4–6 weeks in men, many months in women.

▶ **Diagnostic approach:**
- Clinical features (painful soft ulcer); smear (Gram-negative rods grouped like a "school of fish"; both relatively inaccurate.
- Culture requires special media and methods; check with local lab. In best hands, 75% sensitivity. Ideally PCR confirmation.

▶ **Differential diagnosis:**
- *Primary herpes simplex:* 50% also have lymphadenopathy; starts with blisters; often systemic signs and symptoms that are not seen with chancroid.
- *Syphilitic chancre:* Firm ulcer; lymphadenopathy never fluctuant or draining.
  🛈 *Caution:* Always rule out mixed infection. Test for syphilis and HIV.
- *Lymphogranuloma venereum:* Ulcer smaller, often overlooked; lymphadenopathy occurs after ulcer is healed; bilateral and nontender.
- *Other possibilities:* Granuloma inguinale, chancriform pyoderma, traumatic ulcer.

▶ **Therapy:**
- Azithromycin 1 g p.o. single dose.
- Ceftriaxone 250 mg i.m. single dose.
- Erythromycin 500 mg p.o. q.i.d. × 7 days (preferred in HIV infections).
- Ciprofloxacin 500 mg p.o. b.i.d. × 3 days.
- Pregnancy: Erythromycin or ceftriaxone.
- Examine and treat partners.

Lymphogranuloma Venereum

▶ **Synonym:** Durand–Nicolas–Favre disease.
▶ **Definition:** STD caused by *Chlamydia trachomatis* serovars L1–L3 with acute lymphadenopathy and late fibrosis.
▶ **Epidemiology:** Lymphogranuloma venereum (LGV) is becoming less common in its endemic regions in Latin America, Africa, India, and South-east Asia. Foci in some European port cities (Amsterdam, Hamburg), as well as in Houston, Texas and some other southern areas of USA. Recently an upsurge in homosexual men with primarily diarrhea and proctitis.
▶ **Pathogenesis:** *Chlamydia trachomatis* is an obligate intracellular pathogen, which is transferred in this setting almost exclusively by sexual contact.
▶ **Clinical features:**
- *Incubation period:* 3–30 days (usually 10–14 days).
- *Genital infection:*
  - Primary lesion is 5–8 mm painless erosion, usually overlooked, which heals over days.

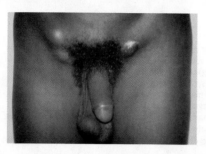

Fig. 8.3 · Lymphogranuloma venereum with massive lymphadenopathy (Image courtesy of Peter J. Kohl MD, Berlin, Germany).

- Lymphadenopathy is prominent, bilateral, and both above and below inguinal ligament (*crease sign*, Fig. 8.**3**). The enlarged nodes become adherent and often rupture with fistula formation. Without treatment, healing occurs in 2–3 months.
- Late complications include destruction of lymphatics with elephantiasis of the penis, scrotum, or vulva, accompanied by fistulas.
- *Rectal infection:* More common in women and homosexual men. Bloody discharge with pain; late complications include fistulas, structures, and elephantiasis (*esthiomène*).
- *Oral infection:* Enlarged cervical nodes, later axillary and thoracic nodes involved; differential diagnosis is lymphoma.
- *Systemic symptoms:* During the acute phase, patient usually ill with fever, headache, myalgias; may even get aseptic meningitis or hepatitis. Skin findings include erythema nodosum, exanthems, and photosensitivity.

▶ **Diagnostic approach:**
  - Most reliable approach is serology to identify 4-fold increase in antichlamydial titers. Not serovar specific.
  - Direct identification of organisms in smear with fluorescent-labeled monoclonal antibodies.
  - Culture on McCoy cell line followed by identification with labeled antibodies.
  - PCR possible but also not serovar specific.
  - Lymph nodes show microabscesses with granulomatous inflammation and epithelioid giant cells.

▶ **Differential diagnosis:** Syphilis, herpes genitalis, granuloma inguinale, chancroid, acne inversa, other causes of anal and rectal inflammation and fistula formation (e.g., Crohn disease).

▶ **Therapy:**
  - Doxycycline 100 mg b.i.d. for 21 days or tetracycline 500 mg q.i.d. for 21 days.
  - Alternatives include erythromycin 500 mg q.i.d. for 21 days or sulfamethoxazole/trimethoprim 800/160 mg b.i.d. for 21 days.
  - Erythromycin is preferred in pregnancy.
  - Partners should be treated.
  - Late complications require surgical management.

Granuloma Inguinale

▶ **Synonym:** Donovanosis.
▶ **Definition:** Chronic granulomatous destructive STD caused by *Calymmatobacterium granulomatis*.

▶ **Epidemiology:** Main endemic areas are India and New Guinea; occasionally seen in other tropical areas and imported into Western countries. Men are more often infected than women.

▶ **Pathogenesis:** *Calymmatobacterium granulomatis* is a Gram-negative intracellular rod, transmitted almost exclusively by sexual intercourse.

▶ **Clinical features:**
- *Incubation period:* 1–12 weeks.
- Initial lesion is papule in anogenital region that rapidly ulcerates with juicy red granulation tissue (Fig. 8.4). Spreads locally or by auto-inoculation.
- Sites include penis, labia, and perianal region.
- Complications include deep ulcers, massive scarring causing pseudo-lymphadenopathy, lymphedema and elephantiasis. Chronic lesions are at risk of development of squamous cell carcinoma. Rare hematogenous spread.
- Spontaneous healing may occur, but often persistent and destructive infection.

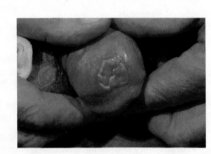

Fig. 8.4 · Granuloma inguinale (Image courtesy of Peter J. Kohl MD, Berlin, Germany).

▶ **Diagnostic approach:**
- No reliable, sensitive method.
- Direct identification of *Calymmatobacterium granulomatis* in crush preparation of curetted tissue; classic finding is *safety pin sign*—bipolar staining bacteria within macrophages.
- Histology shows granulomas in which the organisms can sometimes be identified with Giemsa or silver stains.
- Culture very difficult; can be tried on McCoy cell lines.

▶ **Differential diagnosis:** Lymphogranuloma venereum, chancriform pyoderma, pyoderma gangrenosum; late stages, verrucous squamous cell carcinoma, acne inversa.

▶ **Therapy:**
- Many alternatives available: azithromycin 1 g weekly for 3 weeks; erythromycin 500 mg q.i.d. for 21 days, norfloxacin 400 mg b.i.d. for 21 days, ciprofloxacin 750 mg b.i.d. for 21 days, doxycycline 100 mg b.i.d. for 21 days or sulfamethoxazole/trimethoprim 800/160 mg b.i.d. for 21 days.
- Erythromycin or azithromycin used in pregnancy.
- Treat patterns.

Additional Sexually Transmitted Diseases

Nongonococcal Urethritis (NGU)

▶ **Definition:** Commonly used but less than ideal term for infectious urethritis not caused by *Neisseria gonorrhoeae*.

▶ **Pathogenesis:** The most common causes are:
- *Chlamydia trachomatis*, serovars D–K (40–60%).
- *Ureaplasma urealyticum* and other mycoplasma (30–40%).
- *Trichomonas vaginalis* (1–2%).
- Herpes simplex virus, *Candida albicans* (very rare).

▶ **Clinical features:** Burning and pain on urination. Gonococcal urethritis has a much more purulent discharge than the others, but clinical identification is impossible. Mixed infections are common.

▶ **Diagnostic approach:**
- *Examination of urine sediment:* > 4 WBC per high power field.
- Direct examination and culture for *Neisseria gonorrhoeae*.
- Identification of chlamydia.
- Not necessary to search for other causes on initial encounter.

▶ **Therapy:** See chlamydial infections (p. 149).

Bacterial Vaginosis

▶ **Definition:** Vaginal inflammation caused by increased concentration of anaerobic bacteria in vaginal flora (dysbacteriosis—alternation in normal balance, rather than true infection).

▶ **Pathogenesis:** Most common organism identified is *Gardnerella vaginalis*, small Gram-negative cocci.

▶ **Clinical features:** Thin, gray, vaginal discharge with classic fishy odor; little inflammation.

▶ **Diagnostic approach:** Examination of discharge: fishy odor enhanced when KOH is added (*whiff test*), pH > 4.5, *clue cells* (vaginal epithelial cells coated with cocci).

▶ **Therapy:**
- Metronidazole 500 mg bid for 7 days (or 1 g daily for 7 days).
- In pregnancy or when metronidazole is otherwise contraindicated: ampicillin 500 mg q.i.d. for 7 days.
- Rapid response, but also check for other infections. Sometimes necessary to remove intrauterine device.

9 HIV Infection and AIDS

9.1 Overview

Definition

▶ **HIV infection:** Epidemic infection with the human immunodeficiency virus HIV-1 or HIV-2.
▶ **AIDS:** *Acquired immunodeficiency syndrome*—advanced stage of HIV infection which is defined by the presence of AIDS-defining illnesses and reduction in CD4 cells (CD4+ T cells).

Causative Agent

▶ HIV-1 and HIV-2 are retroviruses in the lentivirus group. They are single-stranded RNA viruses employing reverse transcriptase with an affinity for CD4 cells which exert cytopathic and cytolytic effects.
▶ In the course of the infection, new mutations in HIV appear. Causes are the extremely high spontaneous mutation rate associated with reverse transcriptase copying and the selection pressure from antiretroviral agents.

Epidemiology

▶ HIV-1 began to spread in the 1970s. It presumably arose from monkey retroviruses in Africa, with initial human infections occurring in Africa, the Caribbean, and the USA.
▶ Groups with high seropositivity for HIV-1 include:
  • Male homosexuals with multiple partners (initial major risk group).
  • Intravenous drug abusers.
  • Recipients of HIV+ blood or organs (now very low risk; but in early days of epidemic, devastating affect on hemophiliacs).
  • Sexual contacts of HIV+ individuals.
  • Infants born to HIV+ women.
▶ HIV-2 started in West Africa in the 1980s and spread to India in the 1990s; does not play a role in Western Europe or USA.
▶ AIDS has switched from a disease of male homosexuals in Western countries to a devastating disease of heterosexuals in sub-Saharan Africa, India, South-east Asia, and now appears to be established in China.
▶ At the end of 2004, around 40 million people worldwide were infected with HIV, with 5 million new infections yearly. There were 3 million deaths from AIDS in 2004.
▶ **Methods of transmission:**
  • *Sexual intercourse:* Most common; men more likely to infect women than vice versa; male homosexuals still a risk group.
  • *Perinatal:* During birth or in the perinatal period by nursing; tremendous problem in developing countries.
  • *Blood inoculation:* Shared needles among drug abusers; improper sterilization of needles; injuries to health care workers and laboratory personnel (usually needle stick; other routes unlikely).
  • *Transfusions:* Risk of receiving HIV-infected blood very small when proper screening procedures used.

- *Organ transplantation:* Risk also very small.
- *Saliva:* Controversial; risk extremely low, if any.
- *No transmission* by close personal contact or insects.

Centers for Disease Control (CDC) Staging

HIV infection is divided into three clinical categories (A, B, C) and three levels of CD4 cells (Table 9.1). Once the infection has reached a given stage, there is no upgrading, even in the face of clinical improvement or increasing CD4 counts.

▶ **Category A:** Documented HIV infection but none of the conditions listed in B or C:
- Asymptomatic HIV infection.
- Persistent generalized lymphadenopathy (lasting > 3 months in at least two extrainguinal locations).
- Acute primary HIV infection: resembles infectious mononucleosis with lymphadenopathy, fever, malaise, and a truncal exanthem (Fig. 9.1).
▶ **Category B:** Documented HIV infection; accompanying illnesses which are not AIDS-defining (category C) but suggest immunodeficiency:
- Bacillary angiomatosis.
- Candidiasis, oropharyngeal (thrush).
- Candidiasis, vulvovaginal; persistent, frequent or poorly responsive to therapy.
- Cervical dysplasia or carcinoma in situ.
- Constitutional symptoms (fever > 38.5 °C or diarrhea for > 1 month).
- Zoster involving multiple dermatomes or recurrent.
- Idiopathic thrombocytopenic purpura.
- Listeriosis.
- Pelvic inflammatory disease, especially with complications.
- Oral hairy leukoplakia.
- Peripheral neuropathy.
▶ **Category C:** Documented HIV infection; AIDS-defining illness.
- Candidiasis of bronchi, trachea, or lungs.
- Candidiasis, esophageal.
- Cervical carcinoma, invasive.
- Coccidioidomycosis, disseminated or extrapulmonary.
- Cryptococcosis, extrapulmonary.
- Cryptosporidiosis, chronic (> 1 month).

Table 9.1 · CDC classification of HIV infections			
CD4 category	Clinical category		
	A	**B**	**C**
	Asymptomatic, acute HIV infection, persistent lymphadenopathy	Neither A nor C	AIDS-defining illness
1 (CD4 > 500/l)	A1	B1	C1
2 (CD4 200–500/l)	A2	B2	C2
3 (CD4 < 200/l)	A3	B3	C3

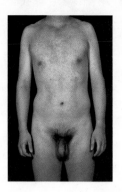

Fig. 9.1 · Exanthem with acute HIV infection.

- Cytomegalovirus (CMV) infection (other than liver, spleen, or lymph nodes).
- CMV retinitis (with loss of vision).
- Encephalopathy, HIV-related.
- Herpes simplex virus infection: chronic (>1 month) ulcers or herpetic bronchitis, pneumonia, or esophagitis.
- Histoplasmosis, chronic (>1 month).disseminated or extrapulmonary.
- Isosporiasis, chronic (>1 month).
- Kaposi sarcoma.
- Lymphoma (Burkitt lymphoma, primary effusion lymphoma, or CNS lymphoma, as well as others).
- *Mycobacterium avium-intracellulare* or *Mycobacterium kansasii* infections, disseminated or extrapulmonary.
- *Mycobacterium tuberculosis*, any site.
- *Mycobacterium*, other or unidentified species, disseminated or extrapulmonary.
- *Pneumocystis carinii* pneumonia (main signs and symptoms: dry cough, dyspnea, fever).
- Pneumonia, recurrent.
- Progressive multifocal leukoencephalopathy (JC virus).
- Salmonella septicemia, recurrent.
- Toxoplasmosis of brain (main signs and symptoms: focal neurologic findings, headache, loss of consciousness, seizures, fever).
- Wasting syndrome (HIV cachexia).

▶ Patients in subcategories A3, B3, and C3 meet the immunologic criteria for AIDS; those in C1, C2, and C3 meet the clinical criteria.

9.2 Cutaneous Manifestations

Overview
....

The possibility of HIV infection should be suggested by the appearance of skin diseases in atypical age groups, with atypical localization or morphology and with a prolonged or severe course. Figure 9.**2** correlates the various cutaneous manifestations with the stage of HIV/AIDS when they usually appear. Possible differential diagnoses are listed in Table 9.**2**.

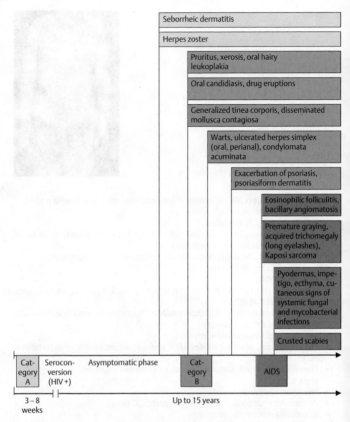

		Seborrheic dermatitis		
		Herpes zoster		
			Pruritus, xerosis, oral hairy leukoplakia	
			Oral candidiasis, drug eruptions	
			Generalized tinea corporis, disseminated mollusca contagiosa	
			Warts, ulcerated herpes simplex (oral, perianal), condylomata acuminata	
			Exacerbation of psoriasis, psoriasiform dermatitis	
			Eosinophilic folliculitis, bacillary angiomatosis	
			Premature graying, acquired trichomegaly (long eyelashes), Kaposi sarcoma	
			Pyodermas, impetigo, ecthyma, cutaneous signs of systemic fungal and mycobacterial infections	
			Crusted scabies	
Category A	Seroconversion (HIV +)	Asymptomatic phase	Category B	AIDS
3–8 weeks		Up to 15 years		

Fig. 9.2 · Skin and mucous membrane changes in HIV infection.

Infections

▶ **Fungal infections:**
- Candida infections of the oral mucosa; appearance in adult life without explanation or with ulceration—think of HIV.
- Heartburn in an HIV-positive patient is candidal esophagitis until proven otherwise.
- Severe seborrheic dermatitis; *Malassezia* species play a role in immunodeficient patients (p. 276).
- Onychomycosis (Fig. 9.3 a), tinea pedis or disseminated tinea corporis.
- Cutaneous cryptococcosis (nodules resembling molluscum contagiosum).

▶ **Bacterial infections:**
- Acneiform exanthems triggered by *Staphylococcus aureus* (superficial folliculitis) or *Malassezia* species; occasional no causative agent is found.

Table 9.2 · Differential diagnosis of skin changes in HIV infections

Type of lesion	Possible diagnoses
Papules, nodules	
Any site	Common warts, plane warts, bacillary angiomatosis, nodular scabies, disseminated deep fungal infections (coccidioidomycosis, cryptococcosis, histoplasmosis), Kaposi sarcoma, basal cell carcinoma, squamous cell carcinoma
Facial	Mollusca contagiosa, common warts, plane warts, disseminated deep fungal infections, Kaposi sarcoma, bacillary angiomatosis, basal cell carcinoma, squamous cell carcinoma
Anogenital	Mollusca contagiosa, condylomata acuminata, squamous cell carcinoma in situ or invasive, nodular scabies, Kaposi sarcoma
Crusted	Impetigo, ecthyma (caused by mycobacteria or gram-positive bacteria), ecthyma-like infections with varicella-zoster virus (painful), persistent herpes simplex virus infections, especially perianal with ulcers, disseminated deep fungal infections, Kaposi sarcoma, basal cell carcinoma, squamous cell carcinoma
Vesicles, bullae, pustules	
Grouped	HSV or VZV infections; all rules are off—recurrent, crusted, chronic, disseminated, atypical
Multiple	Bullous impetigo, erythema multiforme/toxic epidermal necrolysis, Reiter syndrome, pustular psoriasis, eosinophilic folliculitis, ecthyma gangrenosum, infectious endocarditis
Erosions, ulcers	
Any site	HSV, VZV, CMV, ecthyma, nocardiosis, mycobacterial infection, fixed drug eruption, basal cell carcinoma, squamous cell carcinoma
Anogenital	HSV, CMV, foscarnet-induced ulcers, squamous cell carcinoma
Acneiform	Acne, rosacea, perioral dermatitis, eosinophilic folliculitis, papular eruption of AIDS, rarely disseminated deep fungal infections
Folliculitis	*Staphylococcus aureus*, *Candida albicans*, *Malassezia* species, eosinophilic folliculitis, papular eruption of AIDS
Erythematosquamous	Psoriasis, severe seborrheic dermatitis, Reiter syndrome, tinea corporis, xerosis
Acute exanthem	Primary HIV infection, other infectious exanthems (childhood exanthems may recur), drug eruptions (very common)

Continued Table 9.2 ▶

Table 9.2 · Continued	
Type of lesion	**Possible diagnoses**
Purpura	Idiopathic thrombocytopenic purpura, leukocytoclastic vasculitis, infectious endocarditis, drug eruptions
Pruritus	Xerosis, atopic dermatitis, scabies, eosinophilic folliculitis, papular eruption of AIDS, drug reaction
Nail and nailbed lesions	Tinea unguium (often white, superficial), candidal parony-chia and onychomycosis, herpetic and *Staphylococcus aureus* whitlows, marked psoriatic changes (pits, ony-cholysis, subungual debris), yellow nail syndrome, zidovudine hyperpigmentation, ingrown nails and parony-chia from protease inhibitors
Drug reactions	Exanthems (almost 100% for sulfamethoxazole/trimetho-prim, for example), often severe; nail discoloration from zidovudine, ingrown nails and paronychia from protease inhibitors, lipodystrophy from protease inhibitors

Modified from Johnson RA, Dover JS. Cutaneous manifestations of human immunodeficiency virus disease, Table 215–4, in Fitzpatrick TB et al. (eds) *Dermatology in General Medicine*, 4th edition, New York, McGraw-Hill, 1993.)

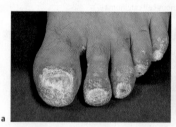
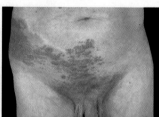

Fig. 9.3 · **a** Massive onychomycosis in HIV infection. **b** Severe herpes zoster in HIV infection.

- Pyoderma, ecthyma.
- Mycobacterial infections: *Mycobacterium avium-intracellulare*.
- Bacillary angiomatosis (caused by *Bartonella*; differential diagnosis Kaposi sarcoma, pyogenic granuloma).
- Exanthems associated with variety of infections.
- All STDs are more common (syphilis, chancroid, herpes genitalis).

▶ **Viral infections:**
- Ulcerated persistent (usually perianal) herpes simplex.
- Zoster; appearing at young age, often recurrent (Fig. 9.3 **b**).
- Condylomata acuminata; recurrent, therapy-resistant, widespread).
- Common and plane warts; widespread, therapy-resistant.
- Mollusca contagiosa; numerous, occasionally giant.
- Kaposi sarcoma (see below).
- Oral hairy leukoplakia (see below).

Other Skin Diseases Associated with HIV/AIDS

▶ Xerosis, acquired ichthyosis, pruritus.
▶ Psoriasis, Reiter syndrome; overlaps with severe seborrheic dermatitis.
▶ Pityriasis rubra pilaris.
▶ Anal dermatitis.
▶ Eosinophilic folliculitis, papular dermatitis of AIDS (perhaps identical).
▶ Increased number of drug reactions.
▶ Alopecia.
▶ Elongated eye lashes (acquired trichomegaly).
▶ Nail changes include yellow nail syndrome, leukonychia, splitter hemorrhages; linear hyperpigmentation secondary to antiretroviral therapy.
▶ Vasculitis, such as polyarteritis nodosa or leukocytoclastic vasculitis.
▶ Telangiectases, cherry angiomas.
▶ Scabies, often crusted scabies.
▶ Idiopathic thrombocytopenic purpura.
▶ Aphthae.

Kaposi Sarcoma

▶ Kaposi sarcoma (p. 460) is a vascular tumor caused by human herpesvirus 8, probably infecting lymphatic vessels. It classically affects elderly men in Europe, but affects children in Africa and is seen with both HIV infection and iatrogenic immunosuppression. Although the skin is most often involved, Kaposi sarcoma can affect the gastrointestinal tract and other internal organs.
▶ Typical lesions are red-brown macules or papules, usually initially following skin lines; lesions may wax and wane as CD cell count varies. Later nodules and ulcerated plaques. Oral involvement is particularly common in HIV/AIDS.
  ▣ *Note:* If Kaposi sarcoma is identified in a young patient, or occurs on the face or in the mouth, always think of HIV/AIDS.

Oral Hairy Leukoplakia

▶ One of the most sensitive clinical signs for HIV/AIDS, and a poor prognostic sign.
▶ Fine filamentous strands are found on the lateral edges of the tongue. They are asymptomatic but firmly adherent and not easily removed with a tongue blade or toothbrush.
▶ The primary cause is Epstein–Barr virus, but the lesions frequently contain human papillomavirus (thought to be a co-factor) and are colonized by *Candida albicans*.
▶ Usually improves or resolves with highly active antiretroviral therapy (HAART); specific systemic antiviral therapy is not warranted. Topical retinoids may produce improvement.

9.3 Extracutaneous Manifestations

Almost every organ can be involved in HIV/AIDS; extensive knowledge of all possible manifestations is required to manage such patients. Common and troublesome complications include pulmonary infections, retinal CMV infection with risk of sudden blindness, neurological and psychiatric problems, chronic diarrhea, several unusual lymphomas, and a broad spectrum of drug side effects including life-threatening toxic epidermal necrolysis.

Diagnostic Approach

► **History:**
  • *Travel:* Southeast Asia, Africa.
  • *Sexual practices:* Homo-, bi-, heterosexual; number of partners; unprotected sexual intercourse; contact with prostitute, members of risk groups or individuals known to have HIV/AIDS.
  • *Sexually transmitted infections:* Syphilis, gonorrhea, others.
  • *Other infectious diseases:* Hepatitis B, hepatitis C, zoster, candidiasis, tuberculosis, histoplasmosis, coccidioidomycosis.
  • History of intravenous drug use, blood transfusions or other blood product replacement, organ transplantation, injuries with contact with infectious materials (health care workers).
  • Other diseases with intrinsic or iatrogenic immunosuppression.

► **Clinical examination:**
  • Inspection of entire skin surface and accessible mucosa.
  • Close search for skin infections that are common in HIV/AIDS.
  • Evaluation of lymph nodes with documentation.
  • Weight.
  • Auscultation and percussion of lungs.
  • Palpation of abdomen (liver, spleen, other masses).
  • Neurological status.
  • Retinal examination (CMV retinitis).

► **Laboratory:**
  • CD4 absolute count and CD4/CD8 ratio.
  • CBC.
  • Hepatic and renal function tests.
  • *Serology:* Antibodies against hepatitis A, B, and C, syphilis, toxoplasmosis, CMV, Epstein–Barr virus.

Diagnosis of HIV

► **Legal aspects:** HIV testing can only be done with the written permission of the patient. The physician must counsel patient, obtain written permission, and document this in the chart. In Germany, if the permission is not granted, the physician can refuse to treat nonemergency problems.

► The results of the testing are absolutely confidential. Positive tests are reported for national statistical purposes using a code that insures anonymity. The confidentiality can legally be broken to protect others at risk of HIV/AIDS, such as sexual partners or a health care worker exposed to patient's blood or serum.

► **Technical aspects:** ELISA test is used for screening; confirmation with Western blot. Two different blood specimens (*not two different tests*) must be positive before the patient is considered HIV-positive.

► **Meaning of a positive test:**
  • An HIV infection is present; this does not equate to AIDS.
  • HIV is in the patient's cells and can be transferred to others. Blood, organs and sperm are infectious and should not be "transferred".
  • Pregnant patients can transfer HIV to their offspring.
  • The prognosis of an HIV infection cannot be stated at the time of first diagnosis; there are too many variables.

► **Meaning of a negative test:**
  • The possibility of an HIV infection acquired in the past 3–6 months is not excluded.

- If risk-taking behavior has occurred in the past 3 months, the test must be repeated in 6–12 weeks.
- More sensitive tests searching for HIV RNA in the blood or lymphatic system can greatly reduce the chances of a false-negative test.

▶ **Further testing:**
- *Viral load:* Quantification of HIV load. Several techniques are used: RNA–PCR, branched DNA signal amplification assay (b-DNA-SA) or nucleic acid sequence based amplification (NASBA). In order to allow the viral load tests to be compared, results are expressed in copies/mL.
- *HIV resistance analysis (genotypic):* Should be carried out before switching retroviral therapy when a patient shows clear signs of viral replication while under treatment. The value of such testing before starting therapy is disputed, but there is at least 10% primary resistance among new infections in Europe.

Therapy

🛈 *Caution:* The treatment of HIV infection with retroviral agents is one of the most rapidly changing and complex areas of medicine. Physicians should be familiar with the most recent national or international therapeutic guidelines.

▶ **Therapeutic principles:**
- Current therapeutic recommendations are available from many Internet sources including www.aidsinfo.nih.gov, www.cdc.gov.hiv/treatment, www.aids.org, www.aidsnews.org. The World Health Organization site (www.who.int/hiv/en) contains extensive statistics and news, but little on therapeutic issues.
- Only physicians with extensive experience should manage patients receiving antiretroviral therapy.
- The success of the various HAART regimens means that many patients with newly diagnosed HIV infections will not die from their disease. In each individual case, one of the determining factors for life or death is the skill with which the antiretroviral drugs are administered.
- The first regimen prescribed should be highly active and contain multiple agents. The quicker the viral load is reduced, the longer the treatment is likely to be effective. Multiple agents are required to minimize the development of resistant strains.
- More than 20 agents are approved worldwide for antiretroviral therapy, so the number of possible regimens is almost unlimited. In each case, individual decisions should be based on methods of administration, side effects and cross-reactions, as well as associated diseases.
- Advice on therapeutic problems, such as a lack of response or drug interactions, should be obtained from an expert.
- Lymphocyte subpopulations and HIV load should be measured every 3 months. Routine blood work including CBC, liver, and kidney function should be checked every 4–6 weeks initially, and then less often as indicated.
- In the case of therapy failure, resistance analysis should be carried out. If protease inhibitors are employed, their blood levels should be measured.

▶ **Therapeutic agents:** Three classes of therapeutic agents are available (Table 9.**3**):
- *Fusion inhibitors* block the entry of HIV into cells.
- *Reverse transcriptase inhibitors* (RTI) block the translation of viral RNA into DNA. Three subcategories are available: nucleoside analogs (NRTI) and one nucleotide analog (NtRTI), and nonnucleoside inhibitors (NNRTI).
- *Protease inhibitors* (PI) block the maturation and discharge of new viral particles.

Table 9.3 · Antiretroviral therapy

Drug types	Drugs available in Germany in 2004
Reverse transcriptase inhibitors	
Nucleoside analogues (NRTI)	Zidovudine, stavudine, didanosine, emtricitabine, lamivudine, abacavir, zalcitabine
	Combinations: Zidovudine + lamivudine, zidovudine + lamivudine + abacavir
Nucleotide analog (NtRTI)	Tenofovir
Nonnucleotide reverse transcriptase inhibitors (NNRTI)	Nevirapine, efavirenz, delavirdine
Protease inhibitors	Saquinavir, indinavir, ritonavir, atazanavir, saquinavir, nelfinavir, amprenavir, fosamprenavir
	Combination: Lopinavir + ritonavir
Fusion inhibitor	T20

▶ **Indications:**
  • The optimal time for the initiation of antiretroviral therapy has not yet been decided. The tendency is to treating as soon as the diagnosis is made, but most recent guidelines should be followed.
  • Patients in stage A1 are the source of controversy. Patients with a reduced CD4 cell count or manifestations of disease are generally treated. In A1 patients, both the CD4 cell count and viral load are weighed in determining the need for therapy.
▶ **Therapeutic approach:**
  • Treatment is usually started with 2 NRTI combined with a NNRTI or a PI.
  • An effective response is indicated by a 10–100-fold reduction in the viral load in the first 2–4 weeks. A less rapid drop suggests suboptimal therapy. After 3 months, the viral load should be below measurable levels.
  • Opportunistic infections are treated as indicated by infectious disease guidelines and consultation. The use of HAART has reduced the need for prophylaxis, but after the occurrence of an infection, prophylactic measures should be reviewed.
▶ **Treatment of Kaposi sarcoma:**
  • *Cosmetically or functionally disturbing stable lesions:* Excision, cryotherapy, intralesional injection of vinblastine (0.2 mg/mL), ionizing radiation (single dose 800 cGy or fractionated up to 1300 cGy).
  • *Disseminated nonpulmonary disease with CD4 cell count > 200 μL:* HAART plus IFN-α (9 million IU subq. daily for 12 weeks, then 3× weekly for 6–9 months).
  • *Disseminated progressive disease with CD4 cell count < 200 μL:* HAART plus liposomal doxorubicin 20 mg/m² i. v. over 30–60 minutes every 2–3 weeks.

Prevention

▶ No efforts should be spared in AIDS prevention. Education of all at-risk groups, widespread availability of condoms, consideration of needle exchange programs for drug abusers, and screening of prostitutes are all measures which have reduced the transmission of HIV. The politics of their implementation is a major social issue in many countries.

▶ Although there are many programs devoted to developing an HIV vaccine, no effective productive is currently available.

Occupational Injury with Possible HIV Exposure

▶ **Needle stick injuries**, both working directly with a patient and transferring blood in a laboratory, are capable of transmitting HIV to a health care worker.

▶ **Every patient and their bodily products** should be regarded as potentially carrying HIV (*universal precautions*).

▶ **If an injury with contamination occurs**, let the wound bleed freely if possible and then disinfect.

▶ **Prophylactic medications:**
- Always take the first round of medications; then one can carefully consider all the options, assess the patient, and check the latest guidelines.
- Inquire as to patient's HIV and hepatitis status; draw blood for confirmatory testing.
- Usual recommendation is two NRTIs and two PI, often available as combination products. Check latest guidelines.
- In pregnancy, there is insufficient data on PI and efavirenz is contraindicated.
- Report the incident *without fail* to occupational health authorities.
- The risk of acquiring hepatitis B and hepatitis C from a needle stick injury or other contact is considerably greater than that of acquiring HIV. Do not overlook this possibility.
  - All health care workers should be immunized against hepatitis B; if this is not the case and the patient is positive, then both active and passive immunization in the first 48 hours is recommended.
  - No immediate treatment for hepatitis C is recommended; exposed individual should be followed; those who do not develop clinical hepatitis but harbor the virus are at high risk of being carriers and should be treated with ribavirin and IFN-α.

10 Allergic Diseases

10.1 Basic Mechanisms

Allergy

▶ **Definition:** An acquired exaggerated or potentially harmful immune response to harmless exogenous substances, known as *allergens*. The immune reaction has two phases—the *sensitization phase* and the *effector phase*. During sensitization, the body acquires the ability to recognize an antigen as an allergen. Once this ability is present, subsequent exposures can lead to an allergic reaction—the effector phase.

▶ **Gell and Coombs classification:** Gell and Coombs identified four forms of "allergic reactions" with different immune mechanisms for tissue injury:

- *Type I reaction (immediate hypersensitivity):* A type I reaction occurs within seconds to minutes after exposure when allergen combines with IgE on mast cells and causes degranulation and release of mediators. Typical reactions include urticaria, allergic rhinitis, conjunctivitis, or extrinsic asthma, and anaphylactic reactions. After about 6 hours, the late phase of the acute reaction can kick in; this may explain both the delayed appearance of urticaria or asthma and the lesion morphology in atopic dermatitis.
- *Type II reaction (antibody-mediated hypersensitivity reactions):* Antibodies recognize allergens bound to cell surfaces. Included in this group are complement-dependent lysis, antibody-dependent cell-mediated cytotoxicity, and phagocytosis induced by opsonizing antibodies. Reactions occur 6–12 hours after exposure. Typical clinical reactions include some forms of hemolytic anemia and many drug reactions.
- *Type III reaction (immune complex–mediated hypersensitivity reactions):* Here circulating immune complexes activate the complement cascade; reactions occur after 6–12 hours and include serum sickness, some forms of vasculitis, and many aspects of lupus erythematosus.
- *Type IV (cell-mediated or delayed hypersensitivity reaction):* This reaction appears first after 24 hours or longer; sensitized T cells either release mediators or steer T-cell cytotoxicity; examples include allergic contact dermatitis, tuberculosis, rejection of allografts, and graft-versus-host disease.

  ▷ *Note:* In any immune reaction, one must distinguish between the highly specific reactions between antigens (allergens) and T-cell receptors or immunoglobulin chains on B-cells, and all the nonspecific responses that accompany this interaction. In addition, most allergic disorders exhibit several mechanisms contributing to the inflammatory response.

Pseudoallergy

▶ **Definition:** Hypersensitivity reactions to exogenous substances that clinically mimic allergic reactions but are not mediated by specific immunologic sensitization.

▶ **Pathogenesis:** Although the mechanisms are poorly understood, they may include direct release of mediators, other intrinsic pharmacologic properties, and perhaps unexplained host response mechanisms. Common examples include release of histamines by certain pharmacologic agents or food components, as well as aspirin intolerance.

▶ **Diagnostic approach:** The diagnosis of pseudoallergy is always difficult, as there are no reliable skin or blood tests. In almost all cases, elimination followed by provocation challenge is required to confirm the suspected diagnosis.

10.2 Urticaria

Definition

▶ **Urticaria** (hives) is a group of inflammatory disorders characterized by wheal and flare type skin reactions (urtica, erythema) and pruritus resulting from the release of histamine and other mediators by activated skin mast cells. Similar reactions in the subcutaneous tissue or mucosa feature primarily swelling and are known as *angioedema*.

▷ *Note: Urticaria* refers to a disease, *urtica* (wheal, hive) to its primary lesion.

Pathogenesis

▶ Urticaria symptoms are mast cell–dependent and their induction requires mast cell activation (degranulation) by specific or nonspecific triggers. Mast cells are key effector cells in the immune response. Specific triggers of mast cell degranulation include stimulation of mast cell surface IgE by selected allergens or drugs as well as physical stimuli (cold, friction, pressure) in physical urticaria disorders. Nonspecific triggers such as stress are relevant to all urticaria disorders. In addition, modulators of mast cell activation and/or degranulation (ambient temperature, alcoholic drinks, fever, emotions, hyperthyroidism, and other endocrine factors) can modify the induction of symptoms and the course of urticaria.

Clinical Features

▶ The basic lesion in urticaria is a hive or wheal (Fig. 10.**1 a,b**). Wheals vary greatly in size and configuration but have three unifying features:
  • Central swelling surrounded by reflex erythema.

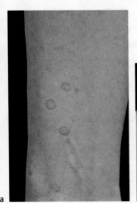
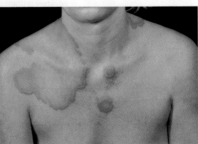

Fig. 10.1 · Urticaria. **a** Typical lesions. **b** Giant lesions.

- Marked pruritus.
- Transitory nature with individual lesions lasting 1–24 hours.
- ☑ *Note:* The time course of urticaria is essential to describing and investigating the disease:
  - *Acute urticaria* lasts < 6 weeks; individual lesions are short-lived but the patient has urticaria daily for up to 6 weeks.
  - *Chronic urticaria* lasts > 6 weeks.
  - In general, patients with acute urticaria are evaluated with history alone and then treated; those with chronic urticaria are extensively investigated searching for a treatable underlying cause.
- ▶ The released mediators may cause associated signs and symptoms such as diarrhea, tachycardia, or respiratory problems, but they are not usually of major clinical significance.

Histology

▶ The key features are dilated upper dermal vessels with marked tissue edema. Depending on the duration of the lesion, a mixed perivascular infiltrate can be seen, as well as eosinophils. Urticaria is biopsied only to exclude vasculitis, bullous pemphigoid, and other urticarial lesions, as the diagnosis can best be made clinically.

Classification

▶ Urticaria is classified on the basis of both course and triggers (Table 10.1). The categories are not mutually exclusive, as physical urticaria can be chronic.

Table 10.1 · **Classification of urticaria**

Group	Subgroup
Idiopathic urticaria	Acute urticaria (< 6 weeks)
	Chronic urticaria (> 6 weeks)
Physical urticaria	Dermographism (urticaria factitia)
	Cold contact urticaria
	Solar urticaria
	Delayed pressure urticaria
	Heat contact urticaria
	Vibratory urticaria/angioedema
Other urticaria disorders	Cholinergic urticaria
	Contact urticaria
	Aquagenic urticaria
	Exercise induced urticaria/anaphylaxis
	Associated disorders

Differential Diagnosis

▶ The main differential diagnostic consideration is deciding which form of urticaria is present. Urticarial drug reactions must also be excluded, as well as serum sickness, early lesions of bullous pemphigoid (especially when dealing with elderly patients), and arthropod assaults (often difficult to determine if lesions are multiple bites and stings, or a few bites and secondary urticaria). The lesions of bullous pemphigoid clinically resemble urticaria but are highly inflammatory with numerous eosinophils and sometimes histologically show early subepidermal blister formation.

▣ *Note:* Some disorders that carry the name urticaria are not "urticaria disorders." For example, "Urticaria pigmentosa" is a form of cutaneous mastocytosis and "urticarial vasculitis" is a vasculitis, as is "familial cold urticaria."

Idiopathic Urticaria

▶ Most common group of urticaria disorders. Up to 25% of individuals develop idiopathic urticaria at one time in their life. In almost all cases remission occurs within 6 weeks (acute urticaria); in some patients symptoms persist (chronic urticaria), usually for months to years. Urticaria develops spontaneously (out of the blue) and usually cannot be induced.

Acute Urticaria

▶ **Pathogenesis:** The underlying cause remains unknown in most cases. The most common triggers include food components, drugs (NSAIDs), infections, and infestations.

▶ **Diagnostic approach:** No routine testing recommended, unless the history strongly indicates a need.

▶ **Therapy:** Nonsedating antihistamines are the mainstay of therapy; sedating agents can be used in the evening if desired. A short course of prednisolone (50 mg p. o. daily × 3 days) may be helpful, but controlled studies are lacking. Topical treatment is not effective; if patient insists, a topical anesthetic (polidocanol) or distractor (menthol cream or lotion) may be tried (p. 674).

Chronic Urticaria

▶ **Pathogenesis:** The three most common underlying causes (Table 10.2) of chronic urticaria are:
- Autoreactivity or expression of circulating mast cell secretagogues including autoantibodies (autoimmune urticaria).
- Chronic infections.
- Intolerance to food components.

▶ Note that all of the factors listed in Table 10.2 can also induce acute urticaria. They are emphasized here because patients with chronic urticaria are more likely to be subjected to detailed investigations.

▶ **Diagnostic approach:**
- *History:* Establish clinical course; associated angioedema; ask specifically about possible triggers including stress, drugs (analgesics, penicillin, laxatives, oral contraceptives), food components (preservatives, food colorings, foods rich in histamine), and any relation to certain eating situations (certain restaurants); exclude physical triggers (often overlooked by patients), especially when delayed); family history of urticaria or angioedema.
- *Laboratory:* Guided by history, test for underlying causes such as autoreactivity (autologous serum skin test, thyroid function and autoantibodies, antinuclear antibodies); screen for chronic infections (sed rate, aspartate aminotransferase [AST], *Helicobacter pylori* testing, stool for ova and parasites); exclude dental and ENT inflammatory foci.

Table 10.2 · Possible causes of chronic urticaria

Type	Cause	Eliciting factor[a]	Pathomechanism (MC activating signal)
Autoreactivity	Autoreactivity	Unknown	Circulating MC secretagogues
	Autoimmunity	Unknown	Anti-$Fc_\varepsilon RI$-AAb, anti-IgE-AAb
	Others	Unknown	Unknown
Chronic infection	Chronic infection	Unknown	Unknown[b]
Intolerance	Intolerance	Foods, drugs, others	Unknown
	Pseudoallergy	Pseudoallergens	Unknown[c]
	Others	Others	Unknown
Other causes	Type I allergy	Allergens	IgE and antigen via $Fc_\varepsilon RI$
	Internal disease	Unknown	Gammopathy
	Others	Unknown	Unknown
Idiopathic	Unknown	Unknown	Unknown

AAb = autoantibody; CU = chronic urticaria; MC = mast cell.

a Specific eliciting factors only; unspecific eliciting factors (e.g. stress) impact on disease activity of all CU subtypes.

b Potential candidates include: (1) pathogen-derived signals (e.g. toxins, LPS); (2) pathogen–host interaction (e.g. immune complexes, pathogen specific IgE); (3) host-derived signals (e.g. complement, neuropeptides).

c Potential mechanisms include activation by neuropeptides and/or complement of MCs that exhibit pseudoallergen-mediated reduction of activation thresholds.

- *Test for intolerance to food components:*
  - Pseudoallergen-free diet for 3 weeks.
  - Oral provocation testing in patients who have benefited from pseudoallergen-free diet. Requires hospitalization. Provocation tests are carried out either using capsules containing small amounts of suspected agents or foods that contain potentially relevant components such as those listed in Table 10.**3**.
- Exclude less common causes such as allergies (specific IgE, prick testing) and underlying internal diseases (systemic lupus erythematosus).

Table 10.3 · Possible food allergens

Dyes	Quinoline yellow, yellow-orange S, azorubin, amaranth, erythrosine, Ponceau 4R, patent blue, indigo carmine, brilliant black, ferric oxide red, cochineal, tartrazine
Preservatives	Sorbic acid, sodium benzoate, sodium metabisulfite, sodium nitrate
Antioxidants	Butyl hydroxyanisole (BHA), propyl gallate, butyl hydroxytoluol (BHT), tocopherol
Taste enhancers	Monosodium glutamate
Natural substances	Salicylic acid, biogenic amines, *p*-hydroxy benzoic acid esters, fragrances

▶ **Therapy:** The only real treatment is to find the underlying trigger. Nonsedating H1 antihistamines are first-line treatment; consider dosing them higher than recommended, alternating two or more agents and adding H2 antihistamines. Ketotifen and doxepin are also occasionally effective. Immunosuppressive drugs such as cyclosporine A and corticosteroids should not be chosen for long-term use because of unavoidable severe side effects.

Physical Urticaria

Physical urticarias are conditions in which one specific physical trigger is required to induce urticaria symptoms. Two or more forms of physical urticaria may be present in one patient, and patients with chronic idiopathic urticaria may also have physical urticaria. In some patients a combination of two or more physical triggers may be required to induce urticaria.

▶ **Dermographism:**
- *Definition:* The development of urticarial lesions when the skin is stroked or written on (Fig. 10.**2**); caused by shearing pressure applied to the skin, but the mechanisms of mast cell activation are unclear.
- *Diagnostic approach:* Write on the skin, using a tongue blade or reverse end of a pen. Standard is a 10 cm line. The reaction is read after 5–10 minutes and in 4–6 hours, as late reactions occasionally occur.
- *Therapy:* Nonsedating antihistamines; sometimes higher dosages are needed.

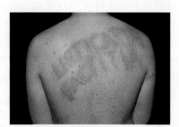

Fig. 10.**2** · Urticaria factitia, as written on the patient's back, is a synonym for dermographism.

▶ **Cold urticaria:**
- Hives are triggered by varying degrees of cold exposure. In some patients, only a slight drop in room temperature is sufficient; others require contact with ice cubes.
- *Diagnostic approach:* Apply 4 °C (ice cube, TEMPTest) for 5 minutes, reading after 10 minutes and after 2 hours if delayed reaction suspected Some forms can only be triggered by cold water bath or cold breeze; if available, place patient in cold chamber at 4 °C.
- Determine the threshold for cold urticaria (small glasses filled with water or TEMPTest at 4 °C, 8 °C, 12 °C, and 16 °C, applied consecutively starting with warmest to inner aspect of forearm for 5 minutes.
- ⚠ *Caution:* Only carry out extensive cold testing when resuscitation facilities are available.
- *Laboratory:* Cold agglutinins, cryoglobulins, cryofibrinogen, borrelial serology.
- *Differential diagnosis:* Familial cold urticaria is a rare type of periodic fever inherited in an autosomal dominant manner featuring arthralgias, fevers, and vasculitis; intensely pruritic erythematous macules and sometimes hives are seen.

- *Therapy:*
  - Warn the patient about sudden exposure to cold (swimming, ice cream/cold drinks, cold i. v. infusions); jumping into a cool pool or lake can be fatal.
  - Oral antibiotics for 3 weeks (penicillin V 500 mg q.i.d. or doxycycline 100 mg b.i.d.) has about a 40% cure rate. The mechanism is unclear.
  - Careful conditioning with cold baths or showers may help, but must be continued indefinitely.
  - Nonsedating antihistamines; sometimes higher dosages are needed.

▶ **Solar urticaria:**
  - Rarely, various wavelengths of UV or visible light may trigger urticaria. The cause remains unidentified in most cases.
  - *Diagnostic approach:* Incremental increase in light (p. 49), using both UV light and visible light of various wavelengths.
  - *Therapy:* Light avoidance or protection; light conditioning, nonsedating antihistamines; sometimes higher dosages are needed.

▶ **Other types:** Less frequent forms of physical urticaria include delayed pressure urticaria, heat contact urticaria, and vibratory urticaria/angioedema, which are diagnosed on the basis of provocation tests using the specific physical trigger (i.e. pressure, heat, vibration). As in other physical urticarias, the underlying mechanisms remain largely unknown, which limits therapeutic options to conditioning and nonsedating antihistamines.

Other Forms of Urticaria

This group includes urticarias that can be induced by triggers other than physical stimuli.

▶ **Cholinergic urticaria:**
  - Triggered by an increase in body temperature (exercise, emotional stress, passive heat exposure).
  - Tiny, transient, pruritic urticarial lesions appear promptly with increased temperature.
  - ◨ *Note:* The skin findings are not typical of hives, so most patients simply describe an itchy rash, in contrast to other forms, where they say "I have hives."
  - Cholinergic urticaria is often combined with other forms.
  - *Diagnostic approach:* Physical activity (running stairs, stationary bicycle) or warm bath (40 °C); test is only valid when body temperature rises more than 0.5 °C (confirm with electronic thermometer).
  - *Therapy.* An antihistamine with a strong cholinergic effect such as cetirizine should be used. Conditioning can be effective.

▶ **Contact urticaria:**
  - Caused by a type I allergy to contact allergens or by an intolerance to substances that come in contact with the skin. Triggers include allergens as well as toxins, pseudoallergens, and mast cell activators (Table 10.**4**).
  - *Diagnostic approach:* Prick and patch testing; reading after 20 minutes.
  - ◨ *Note:* Patch testing for contact urticaria should be done separately from the usual batteries of patch tests. If the other patches are removed after 20 minutes, they may not re-adhere for the desired 24 or 48 hours.
  - *Therapy:* Avoidance of the eliciting agent; nonsedating antihistamines.

▶ **Other forms:** Less frequent types of urticaria conditions include aquagenic urticaria (trigger: skin contact with water) and exercise-induced urticaria/anaphylaxis (trigger: physical exercise). Diagnosis is made with provocation tests. Once again, nonsedating antihistamines are the treatment of choice.
  - ◨ *Note:* Sometimes antihistamines can be taken 1–2 hours before the anticipated exposure or activity, with good effect.

Table 10.4 · **Causes and triggers of contact urticaria**

Cause	Common triggers
Allergic reaction (type I allergen)	Plants (latex, cornmeal, pollen, mahogany, teak, roses, wheat flour)
	Animal proteins (fish, milk, meat, silk; saliva, dander, blood)
	Vegetables, spices, and fruits (potato peels, pitted fruits, oranges)
	Medications (bacitracin, cephalosporins, chloramine, chlorhexidine)
	Industrial materials (ammonia, formaldehyde, acrylic acid)
Nonallergic reaction (toxin, pseudoallergen, mast cell secretagogue)	Food preservatives (e.g. benzoic acid, sorbic acid)
	Fragrances (cinnamic acid, balsam of Peru)
	Topical antibiotics (bacitracin, neomycin)
	Nettles, insect stings, caterpillar hairs, jellyfish

Associated Disorders

▶ There are several syndromes in which urticaria is a key component:
- *Muckle–Wells syndrome:* Urticaria, amyloidosis, and deafness, inherited in autosomal dominant manner.
- *Schnitzler syndrome:* Urticaria plus gammopathy.
- *Gleich syndrome:* Urticaria, angioedema and eosinophilia.
- *Wells' syndrome:* Eosinophilic cellulitis with flame figures; sometimes urticaria. Often related to arthropod assault.

10.3 Angioedema

▶ **Synonyms:** Angioneurotic edema, Quincke edema.
▶ **Definition:** Angioedema is the deep dermal and subcutaneous equivalent of urticaria, with increased vascular permeability and swelling.
▶ **Pathogenesis:** Common angioedema is caused by the same spectrum of factors as urticaria. Two common triggers are Hymenoptera stings and angiotensin converting enzyme (ACE) inhibitors. A rare form related to abnormalities in complement metabolism is discussed below. In addition, hereditary vibratory angioedema has been described, as well as rare cases of acquired vibratory angioedema.
▶ **Clinical features:** Angioedema can present in any site, but typically involves the face and neck. Many patients have massive facial swelling. Involvement of the tongue or of the neck can lead to airway obstruction. In addition, angioedema is far more likely to be accompanied by anaphylaxis than is urticaria. Thus angioedema is a potentially life-threatening situation. Many patients have accompanying urticaria, some do not. Pruritus is uncommon; some patients complain of burning.
▶ **Differential diagnosis:** Infections (cellulitis), trauma, superior vena cava syndrome, subcutaneous emphysema, Melkersson–Rosenthal syndrome.
▶ **Therapy:** Most patients are admitted because of the risk of airway obstruction and anaphylaxis. Treatment consists of antihistamines and usually i. v. corticosteroids with consideration for bronchodilators.

Hereditary Angioedema
► **Synonym:** Hereditary angioneurotic edema (HANE).
► **MIM code:** 106100.
► **Definition:** Defect in C1-esterase inhibitor, leading to unchecked complement activation and recurrent subcutaneous and mucosal swelling.
► **Pathogenesis:**
  • *Type I* (85%): reduced plasma C1-esterase levels (< 30% of normal).
  • *Type II* (10%): normal levels of functionally defective inhibitor.
  • *Type III* (5%): inhibitor inactivated by autoantibodies.
  • Excessive bradykinin release is the main cause of the angioedema.
► **Clinical features:** Recurrent swelling primarily in face and extremities. No urticaria. Nonpruritic. Rarely, transient or slight erythema before attack. Laryngeal edema can be life-threatening; gastrointestinal wall swelling is rare cause of acute abdomen.
► **Diagnostic approach:**
  ☒ *Note:* It is crucial to establish correct diagnosis in patient and family, because of the possibility of sudden death.
  • Measure C3, C4; C3 normal, C4 not identifiable; can use to monitor. Identify type of esterase defect in cooperation with immunology laboratory.
► **Differential diagnosis:**
  • Urticaria with angioedema, intolerance reactions (foods, drugs), physical angioedema (pressure, vibration).
  • Acquired angioedema with underlying hematologic disorder, usually monoclonal gammopathy (*Caldwell syndrome*) or systemic lupus erythematosus and in capillary leak syndrome.
  • Gleich syndrome (angioedema with urticaria and eosinophilia).
► **Therapy:**
  • *Acute attack*: C1-esterase inhibitor concentrate; if not available, 500–2000 mL fresh or fresh frozen plasma (p. 674).
  ☒ *Note:* Systemic corticosteroids, antihistamines, and norepinephrine have no effect.
  • *Prophylaxis:* Androgens (Danazol 200–600 mg daily); adjust based on clinical findings and inhibitor levels. C4 does not need to stabilize.

10.4 Food Allergies

► **Definition:** Immunologic reaction to foodstuff producing signs and symptoms of disease.
► **Clinical features:** Urticaria, anaphylaxis, allergic asthma, intestinal colic, nausea, vomiting, gas, diarrhea, vasculitis, arthralgias, hematogenous contact dermatitis, and oral allergy syndrome (OAS) may all be seen. In some cases atopic dermatitis can be provoked by foodstuffs; careful allergic testing and documentation is required.
► **Diagnostic approach:**
  • *History:*
    – Careful history; have patient keep detailed diary of what they eat.
    – Atopy—history of pollen allergies?
    – Cross-reaction between birch and hazelnut pollen with hazelnuts (filberts), walnuts, and fruits (apples, cherries, kiwi, peaches, and pears).
    – Cross-reaction between mugwort pollen and many spices and herbs (anis, basil, caraway, carrots, celery root, chamomile, chives, coriander, dill, fennel

seeds and leaves, legumes, lemon balm, lovage, paprika, pepper, peppermint, sage, soy, thyme, tumeric).
  – *Protein allergies:* Fish, shellfish (intolerance reactions to intrinsic histamine also possible), chicken eggs (white or yolk), milk (casein, lactalbumin, β-lactoglobulin); when gastrointestinal signs and symptoms present, always think of lactose intolerance.
  – Drug reactions, for example aspirin or penicillin.
• *Skin testing:*
  – Raw foodstuffs in scratch test; standardized allergen extracts (egg white, foodstuffs, spices, preservatives) in prick test, followed by intracutaneous test.
  – If the prick test reaction is as large as the histamine control, strong suggestion of sensitization.
  – If a hematogenous contact dermatitis or cross reaction is suspected in a patient where the history suggests allergic contact dermatitis, then patch testing.
• *IgE levels:* If the history strongly suggests a food allergy, then draw serum for IgE testing before skin testing. Always determine total serum IgE as well as specific IgE levels against suspected substances to be more precise. Basophil degranulation assay is another possibility in this group.
• *Provocation testing:*
  – Goal is to confirm a food reaction (allergic or toxic) following an elimination diet.
  – Foods should be tested in a placebo-controlled, double-blind setting. When testing children, the parents must also be blinded (proven critical in atopic dermatitis). Use results of history, skin testing, and IgE to determine which foods are tested.
  ⚠ *Caution:* Provocation testing should be done on in-patients in a facility where resuscitation is immediately available.
► **Differential diagnosis:**
• *Enzyme deficiencies:* Lactase (inherited, secondary), galactokinase, galactose-1-phosphate-uridyltransferase, phenylalanine 4-monooxygenase (*phenylketonuria*).
• *Vasoactive amines:*
  – *Histamine:* Dark fish meat (especially canned mackerel), sauerkraut, sausage, wine.
  – *Tyramine:* Cheese, yeast, herrings.
  – *Phenylethylamine:* Chocolate.
  – *Serotonin:* Bananas.
• *Pseudoallergic reactions:* Occur with both foodstuffs and additives; for example, tartrazine and naturally occurring salicylic acid may elicit reactions.
• *Reactions to impurities:* Foods contaminated with molds, bacteria, or chemicals from processing.
► **Therapy:**
• *Avoidance:* As far as possible.
• *Diet counseling:* Advice regarding hidden allergens, how to maintain balanced diet despite intolerance.
• *Diet manipulation:* In the case of pseudoallergy, elimination diet, followed by re-introduction of new food every 3 days.
• *Allergy emergency set:* Have patients with type I allergies carry an anaphylaxis kit containing an epinephrine autoinjection, solutions of antihistamines, and corticosteroids; issue an allergy pass.

- *Symptomatic therapy:*
  - Antihistamines (p. 618).
  - Cromolyn (p. 620) in patients with gastrointestinal signs and symptoms; poor absorption, only helps in 30% of cases.
  - Oral hyposensitization is only suggested in cases of confirmed type I allergy to milk or eggs. The response rate is lower than for pollen allergies. The dosage must be increased daily.
  - If there is a cross-reaction between foodstuffs and classic pollen allergies, hyposensitization against the pollens helps in up to 60% of patients.

10.5 *Other Allergic Diseases*

▶ **Overview:** In Germany, most dermatologists are trained in allergy, so they routinely do tests to identify airborne allergens causing allergic rhinitis and allergic conjunctivitis, and then offer hyposensitization in their offices. Some have more complex allergy practices dealing with food allergies and environmental diseases. Allergy testing may also help identify possible causes of drug reactions, as discussed in Chapter 11.

▶ **Hymenoptera stings:**
- About 5% of the population is allergic to bee, wasp, or hornet venom. Typically, after repeated stings patients develop a more severe reaction with marked local swelling or angioedema; many progress to anaphylaxis. The severity of the reaction is assessed by the history, as shown in Table 10.**5**.
- The diagnosis must be confirmed with skin testing (in a carefully controlled setting) and RAST. Hyposensitization is complex, as discussed below.
- ☐ *Note:* All patients with hypersensitivity to Hymenoptera venom should be given an emergency kit to carry at all times, containing epinephrine, antihistamines, and corticosteroids.

Table 10.5 · Classification of Hymenoptera toxin hypersensitivity

Grade	Signs and symptoms
0	Strong local reaction (> 10 cm, duration > 24 hours)
I	Generalized urticaria, pruritus, nausea
II	Grade I + angioedema, vomiting, diarrhea, dizziness, anxiety
III	Grade II + shortness of breath, stridor, dyspnea, dysarthria, hoarseness, confusion
IV	Grade III + hypotension, collapse, loss of consciousness, incontinence, cyanosis, cardiorespiratory arrest

10.6 *Hyposensitization*

▶ **Overview:** An antigen responsible for allergic rhinitis, allergic asthma, or Hymenoptera sensitivity is injected in increasing amounts with the goal of reducing the IgE-mediated hypersensitivity so that on subsequent exposures the patient remains symptom-free or reacts with less severe findings.

▶ **Mechanism of action:** The effectiveness and specify are well established. The mechanism of action remains unclear. Possibilities including blocking IgG antibodies, auto-anti-idiotype antibodies, an increase in specific suppressor T cells, and reduction of basophil function.

▶ **Indications and contraindications:**
  ◻ *Note:* The indications for hyposensitization are always based on history, skin testing, and RAST.
  • *Indications:*
    – Allergic asthma.
    – Allergic rhinitis.
    – Hymenoptera venom hypersensitivity.
    – *Atopic dermatitis:* Hyposensitization is only worthwhile if disease flares are clearly associated with one or a few seasonal allergens.
  • *Contraindications:*
    – *Absolute:* Use of β-blockers or ACE inhibitors, acute infections, severe chronic inflammatory diseases, chronic pulmonary disease, multiple sclerosis, pregnancy, immune defects.
    – *Relative:* Age <5 years, immunizations (leave 1–2 week window), malignancy, hyperthyroidism, cardiovascular disease, epilepsy, active tuberculosis, autoimmune diseases.

▶ **Hyposensitization against inhaled allergens:**
  • *Available agents:* A wide range of allergen extracts is available, in the from of aqueous solutions, semi-depot solutions, depot solutions, or allergoid solutions. The choice of the agent depends on the allergen spectrum.
  • The extracts are available in various concentrations with the proportions 1:10:100. Start with the weakest concentration and depending on tolerability, double the dosage every 7 days. Once 0.8–1.0 mL is reached, advance to the next concentration using 0.1–0.2 mL. The package instructions on increasing the dosage are only rough guidelines. Each hyposensitization program must be individually adjusted, depending on how the patient reacts to the injections.
  • The route of administration is subcutaneous. The physician must administer the injection. At each visit, document if the patient had a local or systemic reaction to the previous injection.
  ⚠ *Caution:* After each injection, the patient must wait 30 minutes because of the risks of severe anaphylactic reactions, especially with inadvertent intravascular injection.
  • Once the maximum dose is reached, it is then administered every 4–8 weeks.
  • Seasonal allergens can be given until just before the onset of the season and then continued as:
    – *Co-seasonal hyposensitization:* The maximum dose is reduced by two thirds and administered monthly. After the season, the dose is once again increased in weekly increments.
    – *Pre-seasonal hyposensitization:* No injections during the season; start from scratch again in the fall.
  • Total duration of treatment is usually 3 years.

▶ **Hyposensitization against Hymenoptera venom:** Once again, a wide range of products is available. Usually aqueous solution is used. Most patients are admitted to hospital for rush hyposensitization, which is then continued on an outpatient basis with depot products. The duration of treatment is 3–5 years. Specialized texts or local allergy centers should be consulted for exact details.

▶ **Anaphylactic reactions:** Hyposensitization can only be carried out in a clinic or practice where emergency resuscitation measures are available and where the physicians and office personnel receive routine training and testing in resuscitation. Treatment of anaphylaxis is discussed in detail (p. 673). The patient must be rapidly assessed and then treated according to Table 47.**1**.

► **Common errors:**
- Inaccurate or incomplete diagnosis.
- Incorrect assess of indications, usually failing to incorporate clinical features and treating based on prick testing or RAST results.
- Choosing the wrong extract.
- Mistakes in advancing dose.
- Terminating injections too soon.

11 Drug Reactions

11.1 Overview

▶ **Classification:** Drug reactions can be classified in many ways. One useful approach is to separate predictable reactions occurring in normal patients from unpredictable reactions occurring in susceptible patients, as proposed by Patterson and colleagues.

- *Predictable adverse reactions:*
  - Overdosage (wrong dosage or defect in drug metabolism).
  - Side effects (sleepiness from antihistamines).
  - Indirect effects (antibiotics change normal flora).
  - Drug interactions (alter metabolism of drugs; most commonly the cytochrome P-450 system).
- *Unpredictable adverse reactions:*
  - Intolerance (normal side effect occurs at low dose).
  - Allergic reaction (drug allergy or hypersensitivity; immunologic reaction to drug; requires previous exposure or cross-reaction).
  - Pseudoallergic reaction (nonimmunologic activation of mast cells).
  - Idiosyncratic reaction (unexplained reaction, not related to mechanism of action, without known or suspected immunologic mechanism).

◪ *Note:* Although we will concentrate on cutaneous drug reactions, remember that every organ system can be affected.

▶ **Epidemiology:** Many drug reactions start with skin findings. Thus, the skin can serve as an early warning for severe, potentially life-threatening reactions. At least 20% of patients hospitalized for 10 days or more develop some form of drug reaction.

- *Risk factors* for cutaneous drug reactions include:
  - *Patient factors:* age, sex, atopic predisposition, immune status.
  - *Underlying diseases.*
  - *Drug-related:* Dose, route of administration, number of drugs, drug interactions, drug metabolism.
  - *Genetic factors:* Pharmacogenetics is beyond our scope, but every individual has an almost unique array of enzymes that may influence how they react to medications.

◪ *Note:* The most common types of drug reactions are macular and maculopapular exanthems (40%), along with urticaria and angioedema (37%). Fixed drug eruption (6%) and erythema multiforme/toxic epidermal necrolysis (5%) are the only other frequently seen patterns; all others account for 0–3%, but may be clinically distinctive.

▶ **Pathogenesis:** In some instances, a drug reaction can be clearly assigned to an immunologic reaction type, although more often the mechanisms are not understood.

- *Type I:* Urticaria, angioedema, anaphylaxis.
- *Type II:* Thrombocytopenic purpura.
- *Type III:* Leukocytoclastic vasculitis, serum sickness.
- *Type IV:* Allergic contact dermatitis, some exanthems, photoallergic reactions.
- The mechanisms for the common maculopapular and erythema multiforme–like drug reactions are unknown, as is the reason why a fixed drug eruption recurs in exactly the same site.
- Pseudoallergic reactions (analgesics, contrast media, local anesthetics) are also common.

▶ **Clinical features:** There are two important rules:
- Almost every drug can cause almost every type of reaction. Clinically, one must learn which reactions are most likely to produce certain findings. The various drug reactions are covered below in detail.
- 80% of allergic and pseudoallergic drug reactions are caused by β-lactam antibiotics, aspirin, NSAIDs, and sulfonamides.

▶ **Diagnostic approach:**
- *History:*
  - The history is the most essential tool in diagnosing a drug reaction. Any exanthem in a hospitalized adult should be suspected of being a drug reaction. Obtain a complete list of all drugs; for in-patients, the chart offers complete documentation. For outpatients, even more effort is required. Ask about over-the-counter medications (laxatives, sleeping pills, herbal medications). Explore previous possible drug reactions and determine whether or not the current medications have been taken previously.
  - Determine the correct time course. If a patient is exposed to a medication for the first time, an allergic reaction cannot occur within the first 4–8 days. Re-exposure, cross-reactions, or pseudoallergic reactions all occur more rapidly, sometimes almost instantaneously (anaphylaxis).
  - *Ask about associated signs and symptoms*, such as fever, chills, diarrhea, or arthralgias.
  - *Does the patient have a known contact allergy to para-compounds?* This could explain a reaction to sulfonamides, oral hypoglycemic agents, thiazide diuretics, local anesthetics of the ester-caine type. Similarly, ethylene diamine sensitivity can explain sensitivity to theophylline and related products.
  - *Have other family members had unusual drug reactions (for example, drug induced-lupus erythematosus)?*
  - *How was the drug administered?* The likelihood of sensitization is topical > oral > intramuscular > intravenous. The best example is previous use of topical antihistamines sensitizing patient to oral agents.
  - *Does the patient have concurrent illnesses?* HIV/AIDS predisposes to sulfamethoxazole/trimethoprim reactions, while infectious mononucleosis is associated with a high incidence of reactions to ampicillin.
- **Allergy testing:** Patch, prick, scratch, and intracutaneous tests can all be used. In addition, oral exposition may be helpful but must be used carefully.
  - *Prick testing*: Useful when type I reaction has occurred, especially with agents of high molecular weight such as antisera, insulin, vaccines, and latex. Also helpful in evaluating IgE-mediated reactions to β-lactam antibiotics and sometimes other agents.
  - *Patch testing*: Patch testing is essential if allergic contact dermatitis is suspected, but may also be helpful if a drug has caused a dermatitic delayed reaction (type IV). Examples where patch testing has been helpful include chloramphenicol, diethyl barbiturate, ethylene diamine, gentamicin, mafenide, methimazole, neomycin, parabens, paraphenylenediamine, phenacetin, propylphenazone, thimerosal, and sulfamethoxazole/trimethoprim.
  - *Interpretation*: Such tests are read just like any other allergy test. The likelihood of reactions to the test solution or preservatives when employed intracutaneous tests is considerable. Anything other than a clearly positive reaction must be viewed skeptically.
  - *Photopatch testing*: If a photoallergic reaction is suspected (p. 45).
- *In-vitro diagnosis:* The possibilities for in-vitro diagnosis are limited, even though a rapid method of determining drug sensitivities is a great priority. One

explanation for the difficulties of skin or in-vitro testing is that many drug reactions are elicited by drug metabolites.

- Specific IgE levels can be measured for penicillin (major determinant), insulin, latex, gold, muscle relaxants, and sulfamethoxazole/trimethoprim. If positive, such tests are helpful, but a negative test does not exclude a reaction.
- Specific IgG and IgM antibodies may be useful for immune thrombocytopenia and purpura (type II).
- Coombs test is useful for drug-induced hemolysis, but rarely relevant in dermatologic disorders.
- Complement activation and immune complex assays may be helpful in evaluating vasculitis and serum sickness (type III).
- Lymphocyte transformation test has long been endorsed for determining drug sensitivities but is fraught with false-positive results and remains experimental.

- *Discontinuation:* Sometimes the diagnosis is made when the suspected agent is stopped and the skin disorder clears promptly. All drugs that are not essential should be stopped. Essential drugs should be replaced as far as possible with agents of a different chemical class. In some instances, one must treat the drug reaction (for example, urticaria with antihistamines) because the medication is required.
- *Provocation testing:* The patient can be challenged with the drug in question. This approach is potentially dangerous, and should be used only on in-patients and only by experienced physicians. Resuscitation facilities must be available for acute reactions, but the risk of severe chronic reactions is more difficult to estimate. A patient with erythema multiforme who is challenged could develop toxic epidermal necrolysis the next time—a potentially fatal disease with no effective therapy.

⚠ *Caution:* Never simply suggest that the patient try a pill!

▶ **Special cases:**
- *Penicillin:* This is a common allergen, but often still required in life-threatening situations. For these reasons, the ability to document penicillin allergy has been refined. Care is required, as small amounts of penicillin can elicit severe reactions and penicillin is a potent topical sensitizer. We employ the following stepwise scheme:
  - *IgE:* Specific IgE antibodies against the major allergenic determinants (penicilloyl G [benzylpenicillin], penicilloyl V [phenoxymethylpenicillin]) can be measured.
  - *Prick testing:* Use ampicillin, benzylpenicillin, benzyl penicilloic acid, cephalothin, methicillin, penicillin polylysine, as well as the penicillin taken by patient.
- *Local anesthetics:* There are two major groups of local "caine" anesthetics:
  - The *esters* include benzocaine and procaine; they cross react with *para*-substituted compounds and can lead to severe reactions.
  - The *amides*, including lidocaine, mepivacaine, and bupivacaine, are most widely used, and almost never cause allergic reactions.
  - More likely causes of allergic reactions are preservatives; single-dose vials are available without preservatives.
  - *Pseudoallergies* are more common. Systemic pharmacological effects of either the local anesthetic or epinephrine may be misinterpreted. Exceeding the maximum dose of the local anesthetic can result in cardiotoxicity. Hyperventilation and fainting (vasovagal syncope) are also often interpreted as allergies.

– *Procedure:* To exclude a rare type I reaction, the recommended test sequence is prick and then intracutaneous testing, followed by a subcutaneous therapeutic dose as an inpatient. Use of physiologic saline controls is required.
– If no reaction occurs, one can be assured that larger injections will not cause problems either.

- **Contrast media:** Patients who experience an anaphylactic reaction to contrast media have an increased risk of having a reaction on re-exposure. Less ionic solutions lower the risk somewhat. Most reactions are not allergic, so prick testing is usually negative. We still recommend it, to exclude the rare type I reactions. Then one can assume a pseudoallergy and suggest using alternative products that are less like to trigger reactions (although perhaps more expensive), and pretreatment with intravenous corticosteroids and antihistamines.

▶ **Therapy:** In most instances, discontinuation of the drug, topical antipruritic measures (polidocanol lotion), and systemic antihistamines suffice. The major area of concern is systemic corticosteroids, with recommendations ranging from "always use" to "never use." In our view, prompt administration early in suspected type I reactions is likely to help. Their use is discussed with some of the individual diseases below.

11.2 Common Reactions

Maculopapular Exanthem

▶ Most common reaction (Fig. 11.1); usual referral reads "rule out drug reaction." Main differential diagnostic consideration is viral exanthem or on occasion acute exanthem such as guttae psoriasis or pityriasis rosea.

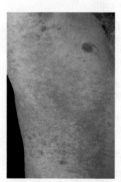

Fig. 11.**1** · Maculopapular reaction to ampicillin.

▶ **Drugs commonly responsible:** Ampicillin, amoxicillin, aminoglycosides, allopurinol, barbiturates, benzodiazepines, carbamazepine, co-trimoxazole, gold salts, penicillin, phenytoin, piroxicam.

▶ Patients with allergic contact dermatitis to a topical agent such as an antihistamine may react to the systemic administration of the agent with a widespread erythematous or urticaria-like eruption, known as *hematogenous contact dermatitis*. The extreme variant of this reaction is perhaps the *baboon syndrome* where patients have prominent flexural and genital erythema mimicking that of mandrils or baboons.

Urticaria (p. 169)

▶ **Drugs commonly responsible:** Penicillin and related antibiotics, aspirin, captopril, levamisole, NSAIDs, sulfonamides, insulin (Fig. 11.2), radiography contrast media.

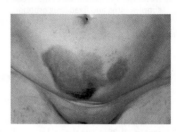

Fig. 11.**2** · Type I insulin allergy with hemorrhagic periphery.

Angioedema (p. 173)

▶ **Drugs commonly responsible:** ACE inhibitors.

Fixed Drug Eruption

▶ **Definition:** Cutaneous drug reaction that recurs at exactly the same site with repeated exposure to the agent.
▶ **Pathogenesis:** A mystery—totally unclear why the reaction remains so localized and recurs at same site.
  • *Drugs commonly responsible:* Ampicillin, aspirin, barbiturates, dapsone, metronidazole, NSAIDS, oral contraceptives, phenolphthalein, phenytoin, quinine, sulfonamides, tetracyclines.
▶ **Clinical features:** Typically red-brown patch or plaque; occasionally may be bullous (Fig. 11.3). Most common sites are genitalia, palms, and soles, as well as mucosa. Lesions typically 5–10 cm in diameter but can be larger; often multiple. Start as edematous papule or plaque; later becomes darker. Frequently resolves with postinflammatory hyperpigmentation. Very uncommon in children.
  ▣ *Note:* When confronted with hyperpigmented macule on genitalia, always think of fixed drug eruption.

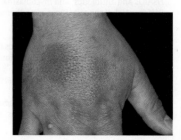

Fig. 11.**3** · Fixed drug reaction caused by barbiturates.

- Controversial variant is *diffuse bullous fixed drug eruption*, which is widespread; should only be diagnosed in patients with documented history of ordinary fixed drug eruption.
▶ **Diagnostic approach:** Patch testing within the site of the fixed drug eruption is helpful; it may be positive in 50% of cases.
▶ **Differential diagnosis:** Non-drug-related causes of similar lesions include fruits, tomatoes, UV light, additives and phytotoxins (shitake mushrooms).
◨ *Note:* The only two diseases that frequently come back in the same site are herpes simplex virus and fixed drug eruption.
▶ **Therapy:** Avoidance of triggering agent; topical corticosteroids may speed resolution.

11.3 Severe Skin Reactions

Erythema Multiforme and Erythema Multiforme-like Lesions

▶ Most erythema multiforme is caused by herpes simplex virus, especially if recurrent (p. 59, 281). The classical clinical findings are iris or target lesions, most often on the distal limbs. Lesions caused by mycoplasma or especially drugs are more often on the trunk and less like to have a target pattern. We prefer the term *erythema multiforme–like* for such lesions, which carry the risk of developing into severe skin reactions as discussed below.

Stevens–Johnson Syndrome (SJS)

▶ **Definition:** Combination of erythema multiforme with mucosal lesions as well as systemic signs and symptoms.
▶ **Epidemiology:** <2/1 000 000 yearly.
▶ **Clinical features:**
- Patients almost invariably have prodrome with fever, malaise, or arthralgias.
- Abrupt development of erythema multiforme.
- *Mucosal involvement* (Fig. 11.4 a):
  - *Mouth* (100%): Erosions, hemorrhage and crusts on lips, and erosions in mouth covered by necrotic white pseudomembrane.
  - *Eyes* (70–90%): Erosive conjunctivitis, can lead to scarring.
  - *Genitalia* (60–70%): Painful erosions.
- When mycoplasma is trigger, pulmonary involvement is possible (20%).
▶ **Histology:** Identical to erythema multiforme.
▶ **Diagnostic approach:** Clinical appearance, search for drugs (most common are NSAIDs and antibiotics) and mycoplasma.
▶ **Differential diagnosis:** Same as erythema multiforme; ocular lesions can be confused with cicatricial pemphigoid.
▶ **Therapy:**
- Short burst of systemic corticosteroids helpful in many cases but two problems:
  - Exclude or treat underlying infection, which could be worsened by immunosuppression.
  - Some studies suggest corticosteroids not helpful for toxic epidermal necrolysis (see below).
- Routine topical care: disinfectant mouth washes, antibiotic or corticosteroid eye drops (after ophthalmologic consultation).

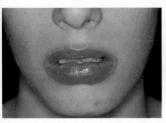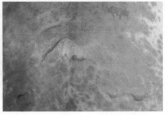

b

Fig. 11.4 · **a** Stevens–Johnson syndrome, labial lesions. **b** Toxic epidermal necrolysis.

Toxic Epidermal Necrolysis (TEN)

▶ **Synonym:** Lyell syndrome.
▶ **Definition:** Severe life-threatening disorder with generalized loss of epidermis and mucosa.
▶ **Epidemiology:** <2/1 000 000 yearly.
▶ **Pathogenesis:** The trigger is always drugs; there is a cytotoxic T-cell reaction with apoptosis of keratinocytes mediated by Fas-Fas ligand.
  • *Responsible drugs include:*
    – *Taken for short period of time:* Sulfamethoxazole/trimethoprim, sulfo-namides, aminopenicillins, quinolones, cephalosporins, corticosteroids (surprisingly).
    – *Taken for longer periods of time:* Carbamazepine, phenytoin, phenobarbital, valproic acid, lamotrigine, NSAIDs (especially oxicam types), allopurinol.
▶ **Classification:** The German Center for Documenting Severe Skin Reactions uses the following grouping: erythema multiforme, SJS (< 10% of body area involved), SJS–TEN overlap (10–30% involvement) and TEN (<30% involvement) (Table 11.1).

Table 11.1 · **Erythema multiforme and severe skin reactions**

Disease	Trigger	% Skin involved	Typical lesions	Location
Erythema multiforme	HSV	< 2	Target lesions	Distal limbs
SJS	Drugs ± HSV	< 10	Mucosal erosions, crusts	Mucosal surfaces
SJS–TEN overlaps	Drugs	10–30	Mucosal lesions, target-like lesions on trunk	Trunk, extremities
TEN	Drugs	> 30	Diffuse erythe-ma ± macules	Entire skin
SSSS	*Staphylococcus aureus* infection with exfoliation	Not defined; usually > 30	Diffuse skin loss	Entire skin

HSV = herpes simplex virus; SJS = Stevens–Johnson syndrome; SSSS = staphylococcal scalded skin syndrome; ten = toxic epidermal necrolysis.

► **Clinical features:**
- Prodrome depends on underlying disease and triggering drug.
- Sudden onset of either diffuse maculae (erythema multiforme–like drug reaction) or diffuse erythema without maculae. Then prompt progression towards widespread erythema and peeling of skin (Fig. 11.**4b**). Skin lies in sheets and folds on the bedding. Extensive mucosal erosions. Possible loss of hair and nails, as well as extensive postinflammatory hypopigmentation.
- Multiple systemic programs because of fluid and protein loss, difficulties in temperature regulation, fever, leukocytosis, and risk of secondary infections.
- Fatal in 10–30% of cases.

► **Histology:** Diffuse full-thickness epidermal necrosis with surprisingly little dermal change; stark contrast to staphylococcal scalded skin syndrome, which has only loss of stratum corneum.

► **Diagnostic approach:** Clinical picture, skin biopsy from erythematous non-eroded area. Granulocytopenia for more than 5 days is unfavorable sign.

► **Differential diagnosis:** Depending on severity, SJS and overlap syndromes; staphylococcal scalded skin syndrome has different histology and usually affects children; severe burn (history).

► **Therapy:** (p. 674).

  🔟 *Caution:* The outlook for TEN is grim and the therapy is controversial. Find out about local guidelines and follow them. The best example is corticosteroids, which are routinely used in some countries and totally contraindicated in others.

- The mainstay is excellent burn care, ideally in a burn center, with careful attention to electrolyte balance, topical disinfection, and prompt treatment of secondary infections.
- Systemic corticosteroids, if employed, should be used early to attempt to abort the immunologic reaction. Later in the course, they probably increase risk of infection and slow healing. Dosages in the range of 80–120 mg prednisolone daily have been suggested.
- Intravenous immunoglobulins are promising and should be employed in severe cases.
- Ophthalmologic monitoring is essential, as risk of scarring and blindness is significant.

11.4 Uncommon Reactions

► **Acral erythema:** Painful symmetrical erythema of the palms and soles, caused by a number of chemotherapy regimens. Appears days to weeks after treatment. More likely in drugs that are excreted in eccrine sweat with direct toxic effect. Self-limited and not a contraindication to further therapy.
- *Drugs commonly responsible:* 5-Fluorouracil, doxorubicin, cytarabine, methotrexate.

► **Acneiform lesions:** Papulopustular eruption, usually without comedones, different from acne because of sudden onset and unusual distribution.
- *Drugs commonly responsible:* Androgens (including danazol, body-building compounds), ACTH, cetuximab (EGFR inhibitor), corticosteroids, oral contraceptives (especially progesterone dominant), cyclosporine, halogenated compounds, lithium (p. 532).

► **Acute generalized exanthematous pustulosis:** Uncommon pustular eruption usually caused by drugs. Typically small nonfollicular pustules on erythematous background appear suddenly, sometimes associated with fever and neutrophilia. Onset usually abrupt, within 24 hours of drug exposure.

- *Drugs commonly responsible:* Penicillin, macrolide antibiotics.
- Patch testing is positive in up to 80% of cases.

► **Allergic contact dermatitis** (p. 196):

▣ *Note:* Don't forget that topical medications can cause allergies.

- *Drugs commonly responsible:* Antihistamines, benzocaine, neomycin, penicillin (so common as to limit topical use), sulfonamides.

► **Bullous reactions** (p. 230):

- *Drugs commonly responsible:* Vancomycin (IgA pemphigus), penicillamine (bullous pemphigoid, pemphigus foliaceus, pemphigus vulgaris).

► **Erythema nodosum** (p. 540):

- *Drugs commonly responsible:* Oral contraceptives, antibiotics, amiodarone, hypoglycemic agents, NSAIDs, sulfonamides.

► **Erythroderma** (p. 282):

- *Drugs commonly responsible:* Barbiturates, captopril, carbamazepine, cimetidine, NSAIDs, furosemide, sulfonamides, thiazides.

► **Hyperpigmentation** (p. 372):

- *Drugs commonly responsible:* ACTH, amiodarone, antimalarials, arsenic, chlorpromazine, estrogens, minocycline, phenytoin, phenothiazine, psoralens (with UV); chemotherapy agents (busulfan, 5-fluorouracil, cyclophosphamide).

► **Hypertrichosis** (p. 515):

- *Drugs commonly responsible:* Androgens, cyclosporine, minoxidil, phenytoin are most common; others include diazoxide, streptomycin, corticosteroids, penicillamine, psoralens.

► **Lichen planus-like eruptions** (p. 286): Many drug eruptions have a lichenoid histologic pattern but few clinically mimic lichen planus.

- *Drugs commonly responsible:* β-Blockers, gold salts, developing solutions for color film.

► **Lupus erythematosus** (p. 212):

- *Drugs commonly responsible:* Hydralazine, procainamide are most common; also isoniazid, minocycline and biologicals.

► **Photoallergic and phototoxic reactions:** There is considerable overlap between these two reactions and the lists of causative agents are often confusing (p. 297).

- *Photoallergic reaction:*
  - *Drugs commonly responsible:* Benzodiazepines, griseofulvin, nalidixic acid, NSAIDs, phenothiazines, sulfonamides, sulfonylureas, thiazides, triacetyldiphenylisatin (laxative).
- *Phototoxic reaction:*
  - *Drugs commonly responsible:* Amiodarone, furosemide, nalidixic acid, NSAIDs (especially piroxicam, carprofen, diclofenac), psoralens, phenothiazines, tetracyclines (especially doxycycline).

► **Psoriasiform eruption:**

- *Drugs commonly responsible:* ACE antagonists, β-blockers, antimalarials, gold, interferons, lithium, some oral contraceptives.

▣ *Note:* The clinical question is always if an underlying psoriasis was triggered, if a previously inapparent psoriasis was uncovered, or if the maculopapular eruption simply resembles psoriasis but has no biological connection. There are often medicolegal implications, so all statements should be worded carefully and documented. Look for evidence of other signs of psoriasis (nails, gluteal cleft, scalp, retroauricular region, joints) and take detailed personal and family history.

▶ **Purpura** (p. 245): May be divided into thrombocytopenic purpura and nonthrombocytopenic purpura.
- In *thrombocytopenic purpura*, antibodies may be formed against a complex of the medication and plasma proteins, but then be capable of attacking platelets (innocent bystander theory). Because the patient is thrombocytopenic, involvement of other organs may be seen, such as hematuria, hemoptysis, or gastrointestinal bleeding.
  - *Drugs commonly responsible:* Heparin, co-trimoxazole, gold salts, quinidine, quinine, sulfonamides. Heparin is so widely used that it is responsible for the bulk of clinical thrombocytopenia and thus purpura, with an incidence of around 5%. Type I heparin-induced thrombocytopenia (HIT) occurs with 1–2 days and is not serious, but type II HIT is life threatening with paradoxical thromboses. Use of low molecular weight heparin greatly reduces risk.
- In *nonthrombocytopenic purpura*, there are overlaps with progressive pigmented purpura (p. 247) and the entire picture is less clear. Excluding heparin, the same group of agents are implicated, with the addition of barbiturates, carbromal, allopurinol (Fig.11.**5**) meprobamate, and iodides.
▶ **Serum sickness:** The prototypical type III reaction, a hypersensitivity response to foreign proteins featuring fever, urticaria, arthralgias, edema, and lymphadenopathy. It is caused by deposition of circulating immune complexes in tissue. True serum sickness is rare today because most animal antisera have been replaced but a number of medications can cause a *serum sickness-like reaction.*
- *Drugs commonly responsible:* Penicillin; less often hydralazine, NSAIDS, *p*-aminosalicylic acid, sulfonamides, thiazides.
▶ **Vasculitis:** Drugs may be involved in leukocytoclastic vasculitis (p. 247), which also often presents as a purpura (see above).
- *Drugs commonly responsible:* ACE inhibitors, amiodarone, ampicillin, cimetidine, furosemide, NSAIDs, phenytoin, sulfonamides, thiouracil, and many more.
- In addition, some forms of ANCA-positive vasculitis are drug-related (p. 255).

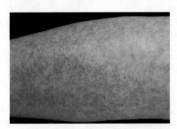

Fig. 11.**5** · Purpuric exanthem caused by allopurinol.

11.5 Drug Pseudoallergies

▶ **Synonyms:** Drug intolerance reaction, anaphylactoid drug reaction.
▶ **Definition:** Nonimmunologic reactions such as urticaria, asthma, and anaphylaxis caused by medications.
▶ **Pathogenesis:** The medications are multiple and not clearly understood. The common denominator is mast cell degranulation with release of histamine and other mediators (Table 11.**2**).

Table 11.2 · Medications causing histamine release

Group	Individual substances
Analgesics	Aspirin, codeine, morphine, papaverine
Antibiotics	Aminoglycosides, neomycin, polymyxin B, vancomycin
Antifungals	Ketoconazole, itraconazole, amphotericin B
Antihypertensives	Hydralazine, tolazoline
Anti-infectives	Pentamidine
Muscle relaxants	Alcuronium, decamethonium, pancuronium, succinylcholine, suxamethonium, tubocurarine
Narcotics	Opiates, thiopental
Contrast media	
Miscellaneous	ACTH, chloroquine, chlorpromazine, local anesthetics, phenyl-ethylamine, phenothiazine, reserpine, tyramine

▶ **Diagnostic approach:**
- Gradually increasing dosages are given; for example for aspirin, one proceeds with 1, 10, 50, 100, 250, 500 and finally 1000 mg. Most often 100–250 mg is required, but sometimes the 1 mg dose is sufficient to trigger an anaphylactoid reaction. Other medications are tested with analogous dosage schemes.
- ⚠ *Caution:* Severe acute and delayed reactions are possible, so testing is done on in-patients with resuscitation measures available.
- If a substance is tested and no reaction found, then it can be recommended. The allergy pass should indicate a pseudoallergy and ideally include recommendations for alternative medications.

▶ **Differential diagnosis:** Includes type I reactions, food intolerance reactions, and toxic reactions caused by overdosage.

12 Dermatitis

The terms *dermatitis* and *eczema* are among the most confusing in dermatology. Dermatitis means "inflammation of the skin," although some object to the term because it seems to omit the vital interplay between epidermis and dermis in cutaneous inflammation. Eczema comes from the Greek ekzein (= boiling) and is used by some to refer to an acute inflammation with vesicles and edema; others, however, are happy with the concept of chronic eczema. We have chosen only to use the term dermatitis, modify it with acute, subacute, or chronic, and regard eczema as a synonym. *Dermatosis* means "condition of the skin" and generally refers to noninflammatory disorders, although there is considerable overlap.

12.1 Atopic Dermatitis

Definitions

▶ **Atopy:** A familial predisposition to development of allergic asthma, conjunctivitis, rhinitis, and atopic dermatitis.
▶ **Atopic dermatitis:** In the best tradition of a circular definition, atopic dermatitis is the dermatitis that develops in individuals with atopy. It usually appears in infancy, is chronic and intensely pruritic with varying clinical patterns at different stages of life.

Epidemiology

Some 5–10% of the population of western Europe develop atopic dermatitis. The disease is familial, with apparent polygenic inheritance. A number of suspected gene loci have bene identified. A classic feature is that one family member may have allergic rhinitis and no skin findings, while another has only atopic dermatitis.

Pathogenesis

There appear to be two rather different ways to reach the same disease state:
▶ **Extrinsic atopic dermatitis syndrome (EADS):**
  • 80%.
  • Elevated total serum IgE.
  • Polyvalent type I sensitization (children against foods, adults against pollens and house dust mites).
  • CD4 cells dominate infiltrate.
▶ **Intrinsic atopic dermatitis syndrome (IADS):**
  • 20%.
  • No immunologic changes as in EADS.
  • CD8 cells dominate infiltrate.
▶ **Other features:**
  • Increased cholinergic reactions (white dermatographism, paradoxical sweat response to cholinergic agents).
  • Dry skin with distorted barrier function, perturbations in epidermal lipid composition (overlaps with ichthyosis vulgaris, p. 333).

Clinical Features

The clinical features of atopic dermatitis can be divided into the basic features and the facultative or associated features. There are many diagnostic scoring schemes for atopic dermatitis; if a patient has three major features and three minor features, they are likely to have the disorder.

▶ **Major features:**
- Pruritus.
- Typical dermatitis (face in children, flexures in adolescents, hands or nape in adults) (Figs. 12.**1**, 12.**2a–c**).
- Chronic or chronic, recurrent course (Fig. 12.**2 d**).
- Positive personal or family history for atopy.

▶ **Minor features:**
- *Cradle cap* as infant; yellow crusts on scalp.
- *Dry skin* with ichthyosis vulgaris, hyperlinear palms, keratosis pilaris.
- Thick, fine dry hair.
- Elevated serum IgE; IgE-mediated skin reactions.
- Predisposition to skin infections (*Staphylococcus aureus*, herpes simplex virus, human papilloma virus, molluscum contagiosum) because of selective reduced cellular immunity.
- Dermatitis on palms and soles (juvenile plantar dermatosis).
- Nipple dermatitis.
- Cheilitis (dry, inflamed lips, Fig. 12.**2e**).
- Lateral thinning of the eyebrows (Hertoghe sign).
- Double fold of lower lid (Dennie–Morgan fold or line).
- Periorbital hyperpigmentation, obvious facial paleness, or erythema.
- Pityriasis alba.
- White dermatographism.
- Increased pruritus with sweating.
- Diseases flares with emotional changes.
- Unable to tolerate wools or fat solvents.
- Food allergies.

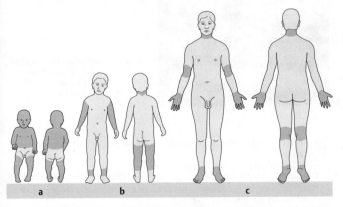

Fig. 12.**1** · **Distribution of lesions of atopic dermatitis over a lifetime. a** Infants. **b** children. **c** Adolescents and adults.

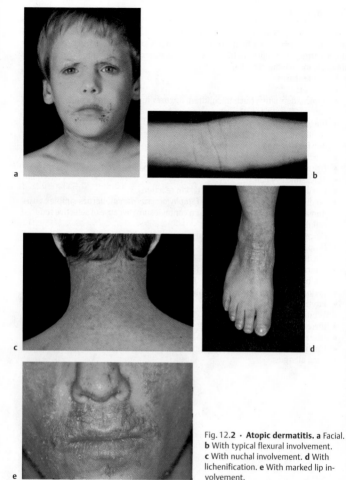

Fig. 12.**2** · **Atopic dermatitis. a** Facial.
b With typical flexural involvement.
c With nuchal involvement. **d** With
lichenification. **e** With marked lip involvement.

- Recurrent conjunctivitis, keratoconus, anterior and/or posterior subcapsular
  cataracts.
- Absent or reduced corneal or gag reflex.
► **Provocation factors:** Irritants, type I allergens, pseudoallergens (citrus fruits;
other foods or food additives), bacterial superantigens, hormones, increased
sweating, dry air, emotional stress.

Histology

▶ **Acute:** Parakeratosis, spongiosis, perivascular infiltrates.
▶ **Chronic:** Hyperkeratosis, acanthosis, sparse infiltrates.

Diagnostic Approach

▶ **Routine measures:.**
- Typical skin changes varying with age of patient.
- Family and allergy history.
- Serum IgE level, CBC (looking for elevated eosinophil count).
- White dermatographism, reduced gag reflex.
- Eye examination.

▶ **Special investigations:**
- Prick testing with common food and inhalant allergens.
- Allergen-specific IgE determinations.
- Atopy patch testing. Common aeroallergens are applied and interpret as in a routine patch test.

Differential Diagnosis

▶ The differential diagnostic considerations vary considerably over the lifetime of the patient and location of the findings. The classic pictures of facial, flexural, or nuchal dermatitis are extremely typical and can be diagnosed at a glance.

▶ In infants with scalp involvement, seborrheic dermatitis often is identical; often the diagnosis is made later in life as typical findings appear. Atopic dermatitis tends to appear after 6 months of age, whereas seborrheic dermatitis may be present earlier.

▶ Allergic contact dermatitis should be excluded; even though patients with atopic dermatitis are hard to sensitize, they are exposed to so many creams and ointments that sensitization is not uncommon.

▶ Adults may present with hand dermatitis (p. 200), eyelid dermatitis, or nuchal dermatitis.

Therapy

▣ *Note:* No disease is more complicated to treat than atopic dermatitis. It is absolutely essential to work with the patient (and the parents). Listen to their observations; make them a part of the treatment team. This is the easiest way to reduce the emotional aspects of the doctor–patient–parent relationship. For example, do not decide that a patient needs an ointment; instead ask the patient or parent "Do you do better with a cream or ointment—something that rubs in or something that stays a bit greasy?"

▶ **Topical:**
- Routine skin care with emollient creams or ointments; if tolerated, with urea as humectant; bath oils.
- *Topical anti-inflammatory agents:*
  - *Topical immunomodulators* (p. 599): Pimecrolimus (>6 months); tacrolimus 0.03 % >2 years, 0.1 % >15 years. Use b.i.d. until response, then taper; can combine with corticosteroids.
  - *Corticosteroids* (p. 596): Usually class I–II agents suffice; class III–IV reserved for flares, limited time period. In most instances once daily application is adequate; never more than b.i.d.

– *Tars:* Available as creams or mixed as ointments; perhaps for chronic lichenified lesions, such as hands; gels are designed for psoriasis and should not be used in atopic dermatitis.
– *Tannic acid creams or ointments* also useful on hands and feet.
– *Topical antiseptics,* used for baths and topical therapy; antiseptics (triclosan 1–3% cream) are preferable to antibiotics because of less sensitization.

► **Systemic:**
• *Antihistamines* for severe pruritus; in general, the sedating (older) agents work better; some evidence that cetirizine is anti-inflammatory.
• *Cyclosporine* (p. 628) for severe refractory disease.
• *Unsaturated fatty acids:* Efficacy unclear.
• *Antibiotics* for flares; cover for *Staphylococcus aureus,* which is usually involved.

► **Phototherapy:**
• Helpful in patients who report that they tolerate sunlight well.
• UVA1 is probably best for acute flares; selective UVB phototherapy (SUP) and 311 nm UVB best for chronic disease.

► Other measures:
• *Avoidance of triggers:* Wool clothes, fabric softeners often help, avoid work that requires frequent hand washing.
• If relevant type I allergens are identified, then avoidance: pollens, house dust mites.
• Elimination diet only if type I allergy is proven.
• Pseudoallergen-free diet if clinically suggested.
⚠ *Caution:* The routine use of restricted diets in infants with atopic dermatitis is to be discouraged.
• Psychologic counseling; job counseling.
• Training of parents and children at special centers or clinics.
• Vacation at high altitudes or sea level, especially if pollens appear to play role or disease is sunlight-responsive. House dust mites cannot live above 1500 m, perhaps explaining effectiveness of high altitude vacation.

12.2 Syndromes Associated with Atopic Dermatitis

There are a number of syndromes that are traditionally described as "associated with atopic dermatitis." When one examines the patients closely, they have a chronic dermatitis that may or may not be identical to atopic dermatitis.

Wiskott–Aldrich Syndrome

► **MIM code:** 301000. Gene locus Xp 11.23–11.22. Defect in *WAS* (Wiskott–Aldrich syndrome) gene.
► **Definition:** X-linked recessively inherited disease with triad of immune defects, thrombocytopenia, and atopic dermatitis.
► **Epidemiology:** Incidence of 4/1 000 000 men.
► **Pathogenesis:** WAS is involved in many signal transduction pathways. Major effects are on T-cell activation and actin polymerization (cell migration).
► **Clinical features:**
• *Immune defect*: Decreased humoral immunity against polysaccharides predisposes to recurrent infections with pneumococcus and other bacterial with polysaccharide cell walls; otitis media, pneumonia, meningitis, and sepsis. Later also herpes virus and *Pneumocystis carinii* infections.

- *Thrombocytopenia*: Purpura, prolonged bleeding time, bloody diarrhea. Mega-karyocytes in marrow normal.
- *Atopic dermatitis*: Onset in first year, more hemorrhagic than usual disorder; elevated IgE and IgA.
- Most patients die from infections or bleeding in the first 2 years; those who survive are at increased risk of malignancies, especially lymphomas.

▶ **Differential diagnosis:** Atopic dermatitis, other immune defects.
▶ **Therapy:** Intravenous immunoglobulin 0.2–0.6 g/kg every 4 weeks; bone marrow transplantation can be curative and also resolves skin problems.

Netherton Syndrome

▶ **MIM code:** 256500. Mutation in *SPINK5* gene, which encodes the serine protease inhibitor LEKT 1.
▶ **Clinical features:** Association of atopic dermatitis with keratinization disorders (ichthyosis linearis circumflexa; rarely other forms of ichthyosis) and bamboo hairs (p. 510).

12.3 Contact Dermatitis

▶ Contact dermatitis is divided into *allergic contact dermatitis* (ACD) and *irritant contact dermatitis* (ICD). These two processes are contrasted in Table 12.**1**. Although the theoretical differences are considerable, the two forms of contact dermatitis are usually grouped together because:
- Often both are present in the same individual.

Table 12.1 · Major differences between toxic and allergic reactions

Parameter	Toxic	Allergic
Dose-dependent	Yes	Usually not
Prior exposure required	No	Yes
Percentage exposed with reaction	High	Low
Adaptive immunity involved	No	Yes
Spread to nonexposed sites	No	Yes

- They can appear clinically quite similar.
- The two diagnoses are not mutually exclusive.

▶ **Pathogenesis:** In the sensitization phase of ACD, allergens are taken up by Langer-hans cells, processed and presented to T cells in the regional lymph node following migration. On re-exposure, the sensitized T cells are activated and trigger cutaneous inflammation at the site of exposure. The clinical reaction occurs 24–72 hours after antigen exposure. In ICD, cytokines are directly released by stimulated or damaged keratinocytes. Damage to the stratum corneum or epidermal lipids is intrinsic part of ICD, but also makes sensitization more likely.

▶ **Clinical features:** Acute contact dermatitis is pruritic, erythematous, and often vesicular. Subacute lesions may be crusted but still inflamed, while chronic contact dermatitis is dominated by lichenification, hyperkeratosis and rhagades with little sign of inflammation. Except for the distribution patterns, the two variants are identical.

▶ **Histology:** The microscopic pictures of ACD and ICD are identical. Acute disease will show spongiosis and a lymphocytic infiltrate perivascular infiltrate with dermal edema. More chronic lesions have signs of epidermal reaction including hyperkeratosis, parakeratosis, acanthosis and less infiltrate. ICD with toxic substances such as acids may show direct epidermal damage with necrotic keratinocytes, but this is the exception.

Allergic Contact Dermatitis

▶ **Definition:** Dermatitis resulting from type IV reaction following exposure to topical substances in sensitized individuals.

▶ **Epidemiology:** 2–5% of population are affected; much higher in some occupational groups.

▶ **Clinical features:**
- The hallmark of ACD is initial confinement to the area of skin that came into contact with an allergen (Fig. 12.3). This produces sharply localized, often irregular or unnatural patterns, which can suggest the correct diagnosis.
- If the allergen is absorbed or taken systemically, lesions may develop at sites that never came into contact with the trigger. The extreme version of this is *hematogenous contact dermatitis* when, for example, a patient sensitized to topical antihistamines takes the same medication systemically. Another variant of this is the *baboon syndrome*.

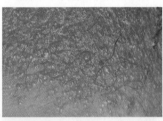
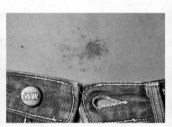
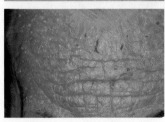

Fig. 12.3 · **Contact dermatitis. a** Acute allergic contact dermatitis with vesicles. **b** Allergic contact dermatitis to nickel in jeans button. **c** Subacute contact dermatitis with erythema and scales.

- The localization of ACD often gives clues as to the possible triggering agent (Table 12.2).
- The eyelids are very sensitive and often react to products simply transferred their by the hands, rather than being applied intentionally.
- Hand dermatitis is covered separately (p. 200).
- Some occupations have very high prevalence of ACD and often typical allergens, as shown in Table 12.3. Occupational skin diseases are also reviewed elsewhere (p. 565).

Table 12.2 · Common sources of allergens listed by body region

Region	Common allergen sources
Scalp	Cosmetics, hair ornaments
Forehead	Hat band, protective masks, airborne plant allergens, hair dyes
Eyelids	Cosmetics, ophthalmologic products, contact lens products, nail polish, airborne plant allergens
Ears	Hearing aids, glass frames, jewelry, ear drops
Oral mucosa	Dentures, other dental materials, chewing gum, toothpaste, foods
Face	Cosmetics, hair dyes, toiletries, shampoos, sun screens, protective masks, airborne plant allergens
Neck	Jewelry, cosmetics, clothing, hair dyes
Axilla	Deodorants and antiperspirants, other toiletries, clothing
Trunk	Clothing, metal zippers and buttons, cosmetics
Genitalia	Toiletries, condoms, spermicides, feminine hygiene products
Arms	Jewelry, cosmetics, clothing
Hands	Occupational exposure, gloves especially latex gloves, skin protective creams, cosmetics, toiletries, jewelry
Legs	Toiletries, cosmetics, stockings, other clothes
Legs in stasis dermatitis	Topical antibiotics, other topical medications
Feet	Shoe material (chromates, rubber, glues), antifungal agents, dyes in socks and stockings
Perianal region	Hemorrhoid medications, disinfectants, other toiletries

Table 12.3 · Common allergens in various occupations

Occupation	Allergens
Baker	Aromas and spices, lemon and almond oils, cinnamon, flour bleaches (ammonium persulphate), preservatives (benzoates), immediate-type allergy to proteins of eggs or flour
Office worker	Copy paper, printer and copy inks, glues, rubber
Electrician	Rubber and rubber-related products, metals, insulation material (colophony), resins (epoxy and formaldehyde)
Hairdresser	Permanents (glycerol monothioglycollate, ammonium thioglycollate), fragrances, dyes (para group, azo dyes), rubber, nickel (often present before entering profession)
Home maker	Foods, spices, rubber, soaps and cleansing supplies (fragrances, preservatives, turpentine) disinfectants, metals (chromates, nickel), cosmetics, immediate-type allergy to natural rubber latex
Gardener	Plant allergens (see text; think of airborne route), rubber, pesticides

Continued Table 12.3 ▶

Table 12.3 · **Continued**	
Occupation	Allergens
Health professional	Rubber, fragrances, disinfectants (formaldehyde, glutaraldehyde, mercury salts), medications, immediate type allergy to natural rubber latex
Farmer	Pesticides, conservatives in greases, airborne plant fragments, feed additives (often photosensitizers), rubber
Construction worker	Chromate and cobalt in cement, concrete hardeners, resins (epoxy and formaldehyde), insulation foam, rubber
Metal worker	Cutting oils, greases, soldering solutions, preservatives, fragrances, glues, rust preventatives, rubber, metals
Textile worker	Resins (formaldehyde), dyes, preservatives, stains, rubber

Table 12.4 · **Common allergens in topical medications**	
Category	Examples
Vehicle	Wool alcohols, cetyl alcohol
Preservative	Parabens, chloroacetamide, Euxyl K 400
Active ingredients	Antibiotics, local anesthetics, antihistamines, sun screens, corticosteroids, NSAIDs, older antifungal agents (not imidazoles)
Fragrances	Many

Tables 12.2–12.4 are based on material in Braun-Falco O, Plewig G, Wolff HH, Burgdorf WHC *Dermatology*, Springer Verlag, Berlin, 2000.

- An often overlooked cause of ACD is medication, especially over-the-counter products (Table 12.**4**).
- Rhus dermatitis is the most common cause of ACD in North America. Exposure to poison ivy, poison oak, or poison sumac typically causes a vesicular, often linear, pruritic eruption following outdoor exposure. Although the lesions look toxic, Rhus dermatitis is a true type IV allergy that develops only on repeated exposure to the plants.
  - There are very unusual clinical forms of Rhus dermatitis including eyelid involvement and perianal disease (using the leaves as outdoor toilet paper).
  - Patients with Rhus dermatitis may react to other plant products, such as some leather dyes, laundry marking ink in Asia, some varnishes, and the shell of cashew nuts (not the edible component).
- ▶ **Diagnostic approach:**
  - **History:**
    - A careful history and a bit of imagination are the keys to diagnosing contact dermatitis. Ask the patient about work and hobbies, and about what materials are likely to reach or be applied to the involved area.
    - Document the history carefully; some cases of contact dermatitis turn out to be work-related, and then documentation is crucial.
    - Onset of problem, occupation, course of disease on weekends or in vacation. Previous therapy. Exposure to common contact allergens such as chemicals, detergents, medications, cleansing products, rubber or latex gloves. Previous skin diseases.

◼ *Note:* Never forget the likelihood of contact dermatitis as a reaction to a medication (Table 12.**4**). Patients almost never think of this possibility, so you must.

- *Clinical features:* The location and pattern usually suggest the diagnosis of ACD. Always check for disease other than at sites of suspected contact.

- *Patch testing* (p. 43): The diagnosis is always confirmed with patch testing. The usual approach is to use an nationally accepted screening panel first, then specialized panels designed for a specific problem, such as for occupations (dentist), locations (hands), or special ingredients (fragrances or preservatives).

- *Testing with suspected product:* Patch testing with a suspected product is fraught with problems. False-positive reactions are common. Repeated open application test is better; product applied t.i.d. for 2 days to an antecubital fossa.

► **Differential diagnosis:**

- Main differential diagnostic consideration is ICD.

- ◼ *Note:* Both ACD and ICD can be present at same time, as patients with ICD dermatitis are inclined to develop ACD.

- *Erysipelas:* At first glance, can appear similar to well-defined erythematous area, but rapidly spreads, is not pruritic, and patient is sick.

- Atopic dermatitis and nummular dermatitis can be similar.

- ◼ *Note:* Clinical distinction is often difficult, so do patch testing when in doubt.

- *Tinea:* KOH examination.

- *Polymorphous light eruption:* Can be confusing when considering sunscreen allergy; otherwise, history clarifies.

► **Therapy:**

- Acute dermatitis of any sort is best treated with moist compresses and high-potency topical corticosteroid creams. In severe cases, a short burst of systemic corticosteroids, tapered over 7–10 days, is needed.

- More chronic cases can be treated with lower potency corticosteroids in an ointment base.

- Bath PUVA may be useful for severe hand and foot dermatitis.

- Oral cyclosporine is a last gasp measure for therapy-resistant chronic disease.

- The most important step is *avoidance.* Thus, the allergen or allergens must be exactly identified and the patient carefully counseled as to where the allergen and cross-reacting products can be encountered. Some allergens such as nickel or chromate are very difficult to avoid. In some instances, the patient must give up their occupation—an expensive and bureaucratic process.

Irritant Contact Dermatitis

► **Synonyms:** Toxic-irritant (contact) dermatitis.

► **Clinical features:** The clinical features are remarkably similar to allergic contact dermatitis. ICD never spreads beyond the area of contact, tends to be painful rather than pruritic, and, if the causative agent is strong enough, may form large blisters rather than tiny vesicles. ICD can either be very acute, such as when someone spills acid on their skin, or chronic, resulting from repeated exposures that individually would be harmless. In German, this type of irritant disease is known as *cumulative subtoxic dermatitis*—a most useful concept not easily translated into English. There are three special groups at risk: housewives, infants (diaper dermatitis), and healthcare workers.

- The prototype of ICD is hand dermatitis (see below).

► **Diagnostic approach:** The diagnosis is made on the basis of history of appropriate exposure. If clinical questions exist or if the ICD is work-related, the patch testing should be carried out to exclude ACD, which can accompany ICD and is more easily avoided.

▶ **Differential diagnosis:** As for allergic contact dermatitis.
▶ **Therapy:** The treatment is almost the same as for allergic contact dermatitis. Some tricks for hand dermatitis are discussed in the next section. More extensive blisters with skin loss may require antiseptics.

12.4 Other Forms of Dermatitis

Hand Dermatitis

Hand dermatitis is not a single disease, but it is such a great burden for patients and such a challenge for physicians that we discuss it separately.

▶ **Epidemiology:**
  • 1–4% of population affected; much higher among people with frequent exposure to moisture or hand washing.
  • 40% of hospital personnel have some degree of hand dermatitis.
  • Women are affected twice as often as men, showing the effect of domestic work.

▶ **Pathogenesis:**
  • Hand dermatitis is usually the summation of many factors. The hands are our interface with so many substances, whether it be at work or at home, that it is amazing they do not suffer more.
  • *Atopic dermatitis* is an important predisposing factor. Patients with atopy are more likely to develop hand dermatitis, as shown in long-term studies of individuals training to become barbers or hairdressers.
  • *Exogenous factors* include:
    – *Irritants:* Oils, paints, and solvents are typically implicated, but considering the population as a whole, water, soaps, and urine are even more important.
    – Repeated exposure is usually the determining factor.
    – Both allergic contact dermatitis and contact urticaria (common among cooks, caused by raw meats and vegetables) may play role.

▶ **Clinical features:**
  • Acute hand dermatitis is often vesicular, with tiny deep-seated lesions (Fig. 12.**4**); this form is also known as *dyshidrotic dermatitis* or *pompholyx*. Here the blisters are usually along the sides of the fingers and quite pruritic. We do not consider this process as a separate disease.
  • Severe blisters can lead to shedding of large pieces of the palmar skin.
  • Chronic hand dermatitis is usually hyperkeratotic with fissures, so that the hands are tender and easily hurt by motion or irritating fluids.

▶ **Diagnostic approach:**
  • The same detailed approach listed under contact dermatitis is required.
  • Do patch testing. Refer to special lists to test certain professions.

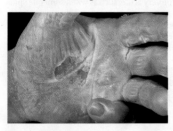

Fig. 12.**4** · Acute hand dermatitis with large blisters and desquamation of sheets.

Table 12.5 · Instructions for patients with hand dermatitis

Only wash your hands when they are dirty; use a mild synthetic detergent and lukewarm water. Dry hands carefully and then lubricate, using either the prescribed medication or hand care product. Also rinse and lubricate your hands after exposure to moisture or wet work.

In many instances you will need gloves. Choose plastic or vinyl gloves, not rubber gloves, as latex is a potent allergen. If possible, wear washable cotton gloves beneath the protective gloves. Try not to wear gloves for more than 20 minutes.

Avoid direct contact with soaps and detergents.

Avoid alcohol, gasoline, solvents, paint thinners and similar products; they are irritating and drying.

Avoid polishes, waxes, and household cleansers.

Wear gloves when you cut, peel, or press fruits or vegetables.

Wear gloves when you wash or treat your hair.

Do not wear a ring when washing your hands. Irritants accumulate beneath a ring. Ideally, you should not wear a ring until your dermatitis is entirely clear. If this is impossible, clean the ring each night with brush and soak it overnight in a mild ammonium solution.

Remember your hands have been injured—comparable to a broken bone. If all the triggering factors are removed, it will take 6 months for your hands to heal. You must follow these recommendations even after you start to feel better.

▶ **Differential diagnosis:**
- On physical examination, check the backs of the hands; their involvement suggests allergic contact dermatitis. Nail changes indicate chronic disease. Pustules point towards the psoriasis families.
- Foot involvement suggests ACD plays less of a role.
- Present of tinea on feet raises question of fungal id reaction (p. 106).
- Check for other features of atopic dermatitis.

▶ **Therapy:**
- ◘ *Note:* Remember the hands are constantly in contact with other body parts, clothing, and the rest of the environment. It is hard to keep medicine on the hands. Gloves are a two-edged sword; some patients benefit but others find the occlusion worsens their condition.
- Low- to mid-potency corticosteroids in emollient cream or ointment base are best. Most important time to apply is when there is some likelihood they will remain on the skin—such as when watching television!
- Patient counseling is crucial; we provide the instructions shown in Table 12.**5**.
- Use of protective creams may be helpful, especially in the work setting. Having the patient apply fluorescent-labeled protective cream and then examining the hands with a Wood's light can reveal how good a job they are doing of protecting their hands. The same check after a workplace exposure may show if the cream is staying on long enough to be beneficial. Different creams are available for wet and dry work.

Asteatotic Dermatitis

▶ **Synonyms:** Xerosis, dermatitis sicca.
▶ **Definition:** Dermatitis secondary to superficial cracks in epidermis as a result of dryness and reduced lipids.

Dermatitis

- ▶ **Epidemiology:** Common problem, more likely in elderly and those with atopic dermatitis or ichthyosis vulgaris.
- ▶ **Pathogenesis:** Exact lipid defects unclear, but older individuals has less of an epidermal lipid accumulation. Typical onset in early winter as central heating is started and room humidity drops. Also seen in compulsive shower takers or those who luxuriate in bubble baths. Acquired ichthyosis (p. 333) is probably a variation on this theme in some cases.
- ▶ **Clinical features:** Initially dry skin and pruritus. Sometimes erythematous cracks in skin (French: *eczema craquelé*). Later more diffuse inflammation.
- ▶ **Diagnostic approach:** Clinical diagnosis with typical history.
- ▶ **Differential diagnosis:** Atopic dermatitis, various forms of ichthyosis, especially acquired ichthyosis.
- ▶ **Therapy:** Avoidance of frequent baths or showers; use a synthetic detergent instead of soap; regular lubrication of skin, especially after bathing.

Nummular Dermatitis

- ▶ **Synonym:** Microbial dermatitis.
- ▶ **Definition:** Sharply circumscribed patches of dermatitis; nummular means "coin-shaped".
- ▶ **Epidemiology:** So poorly defined that no reliable numbers available; range in literature 0.1–10%.
- ▶ **Pathogenesis:** Probably reflects atopic dermatitis, xerosis, and on the legs stasis dermatitis coupled with hypercolonization by bacteria. More common in those with poor personal hygiene.
- ▶ **Clinical features:** 2–5cm plaques with erythema, papules, vesicles, and crusts (Fig. 12.**5**). Usually pruritic. Most often on extremities; legs in men, arms in women.
- ▶ **Histology:** Hyperkeratosis, acanthosis, focal spongiosis and perivascular infiltrates; corresponding to subacute to chronic dermatitis.
- ▶ **Diagnostic approach:**
  - Search for other signs of atopic dermatitis or dry skin.
  - Bacterial smear from recalcitrant lesions; also check for staphylococcal carriage in the throat, nares, or anogenital region.
  - Do patch testing; some are allergic or nickel, chromate, or other allergens.
- ▶ **Differential diagnosis:** Atopic dermatitis, psoriasis, tinea corporis, impetigo, petaloid seborrheic dermatitis.
- ▶ **Therapy:** Topical corticosteroids, perhaps combined with topical antibiotics or tar; if no response, try systemic antibiotics (penicillinase-resistant penicillins or cephalosporins); after healing, maintain lubrication.

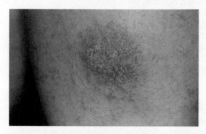

Fig. 12.**5** · Nummular dermatitis.

13 Collagen–Vascular Disorders

13.1 Classification and Overview

The collagen–vascular disorders (connective tissue disorders) are a complex group, without a unifying pathogenesis. All feature arthritis or arthralgias, and most have prominent skin involvement.

▶ **Lupus erythematosus**.
  • Chronic cutaneus lupus erythematosus.
  • Subacute cutaneous lupus erythematosus.
  • Systemic lupus erythematosus.
  • Drug-induced lupus erythematosus.
  • Antiphospholipid syndrome.
▶ **Dermatomyositis and polymyositis**.
▶ **Localized scleroderma**.
  • Morphea.
  • Linear scleroderma.
  • Disabling pansclerotic morphea.
▶ **Systemic sclerosis**.
▶ **Pseudoscleroderma**.
  • Eosinophilic fasciitis.
  • *Toxic forms:* Toxic oil syndrome, eosinophilia-myalgia syndrome, polyvinyl-chloride syndrome and others.
  • *Associated with other diseases:* graft-versus-host disease and porphyria cutanea tarda.
▶ **Mixed collagen–vascular disorders and other overlap syndromes**.
▶ **Other rheumatologic diseases**.
▶ **Raynaud syndrome**.

Many collagen–vascular disorders have some form of antinuclear antibodies (ANA), as shown in Table 13.**1**.

Table 13.1 · **Antinuclear antibodies with clinical relevance**

Antigen family	Specific antigen	Antinuclear antibody	Clinical association	Prevalence (%)
DNA	dsDNA	Anti-dsDNA IgG	SLE	45–90
			Sjögren syndrome	10
	ssDNA	Anti-ssDNA	SLE	50–95
Histone		Anti-histone		
	H1	Anti-H1	SLE	50–80
	H2A and H2B	Anti-H2A, anti-H2B	Drug-induced LE	90
Nucleosomes	Mono nucleosomes	Anti-nucleosome	Early marker for auto-immune disease	

Continued Table 13.1 ▶

Table 13.1 · **Continued**				
Antigen family	**Specific antigen**	**Antinuclear antibody**	**Clinical association**	**Prevalence (%)**
Low molecular weight RNP	U1 RNP/Sm	Anti-U1 RNP Anti-Sm	Overlap syndromes, SLE, systemic sclerosis, polymyositis, rheumatoid arthritis	90
	RNP-70	Anti-RNP-70	MCTD	
	RNP-A	Anti-RNP-A	SLE	
	Sm-B/B	Anti-Sm-B/B	Highly specific for SLE	20–30
	SS-A 60/Ro60	Anti-SSA60/ anti-Ro60	Sjögren syndrome SLE	70–80 20–60
	SS-A 52 / Ro52	Anti-SSA52/ anti-Ro52	Congenital heart block	95–100
	SS-B / La	Anti-SS-B, anti-La	Neonatal lupus Sjögren syndrome	75 40–90
Other	Jo-1(synthetase)	Anti-Jo-1	Polymyositis, idiopathic pulmonary fibrosis	30–40
	Scl-70 (topoisomerase)	Anti-Scl-70	Systemic sclerosis	30–40
	PM-Scl-100	Anti-PM-Scl-100	Systemic sclerosis, dermatomyositis, rheumatoid arthritis	
	Centromere protein B	Anti-centromere	CREST syndrome Primary biliary cirrhosis	40–80 10–30

13.2 Lupus Erythematosus (LE)

Overview

▶ **Definition:** A disease featuring autoimmune phenomena that may involve one or multiple organs, frequently has characteristic skin findings, and runs an acute or chronic course.

▶ **Classification:** The combination of history, clinical findings, and laboratory values can be used to classify LE as follows:
- *Chronic cutaneous LE*: Almost exclusively skin findings:
  - Discoid LE (DLE).
  - Lupus tumidus.
  - Lupus profundus.
- *Subacute cutaneous LE (SCLE)*: Predominantly skin findings, mild systemic involvement.
- *Systemic LE (SLE)*: Primarily systemic involvement.

Collagen–Vascular Disorders

▶ **Pathogenesis:**
- LE is a multifactorial disease with genetic and immunopathologic abnormalities. The release of nuclear antigens because of enhanced apoptosis (FAS-FAS-L) is a key factor.
- *Important predisposing factors:*
  - *Genetic predisposition:* HLA-B8, -DR2, -DR3, -DQwl, -DRB1; various polymorphisms—TNF-R gene, Fc-γ receptor, CD19 gene.
  - *Complement defects:* C1q, C1r, C1 s, C4, C2 (skin and renal disease).
  - *Exogenous factors:* UV radiation and medications.
  - *Individual factors:* Hormone status, altered immune status.
  - Transplacental transfer of maternal autoantibodies (anti-SSA, anti-SSB) can lead to neonatal LE.
▶ **Lupus band test:** This test identified the presence of immunoglobulins and complement at the dermoepidermal junction in both normal and lesional skin. Formerly used to classify LE, but now replaced by more sophisticated autoantibody determinations.

Chronic Cutaneous Lupus Erythematosus

▶ **Definition:** Chronic scarring erythematosquamous lesions primarily in sun-exposed skin. Some groups refer to all chronic cutaneous LE as discoid LE (DLE) but we prefer to reserve the term for a specific type of lesion, which may also be seen in SCLE or SLE.
▶ **Synonym:** Discoid lupus erythematosus.
▶ **Epidemiology:** More common in women (2–3:1); usually appears 15–60 years of age.
▶ **Clinical features:**
- Erythematous well-circumscribed persistent plaques with follicular hyperkeratoses, telangiectases; heal with scarring, peripheral hyperpigmentation and central hypopigmentation (Fig. 13.1). Sometimes tender or hyperesthetic.
- Sites of predilection include chronic sun-exposed areas: scalp, forehead, cheeks, ears, nose, upper lip, and chin. Usually limited number of lesions; occasionally disseminated.
- Common causing of scarring alopecia (p. 507), especially in blacks. About 1:250 black women in USA have LE alopecia.
- Small percentage of patients go on to develop SLE.
▶ **Histology:** The histologic findings exactly match the clinical: epidermal atrophy with vacuolar degeneration of basal cells, telangiectases, follicular plugs, lymphocytic infiltrate in dermis. Valuable clues are widened periodic acid–Schiff (PAS)-positive basement membrane and deposition of mucin.
▶ **Diagnostic approach:**
- Skin biopsy.
- *Direct immunofluorescence:* Deposits of IgG and C3 along the basement membrane in affected skin in up to 80%, but normal, nonexposed skin always negative.
- *Laboratory:* Negative or low-titer ANA; sometimes higher titer in disseminated.
- Exclude SLE.
▶ **Differential diagnosis:** Tinea faciei (KOH examination), granuloma faciale (brown color, no scarring), psoriasis (silvery scale), lupus vulgaris (diascopy), sarcoidosis (diascopy, no prominent follicles), rosacea (pustules, ears spared). In each case, histology is most helpful.
▶ *Therapy:*
- Sun avoidance and high-potency sunscreens (UVA, UVB).
- Short-term high-potency topical corticosteroids.

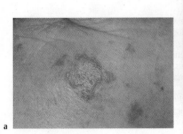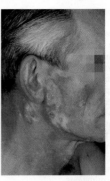

a b

Fig. 13.**1** · **Discoid lupus erythematosus. a** Early lesion. **b** Late lesion with scarring.

- Topical immunomodulators (pimecrolimus, tacrolimus) worth trying.
- Cryotherapy or intralesional corticosteroids for stubborn lesions.
- Systemic therapy for widespread, recalcitrant disease:
  - *Antimalarials:* Hydroxychloroquine 200–400 mg daily or chloroquine 250 mg daily; rarely need to go higher for skin findings alone; monitoring by ophthalmologist required every 6–12 months. With response, attempt to stop therapy.
  - Dapsone 50–100 mg daily.
  - Thalidomide 50–200 mg daily; special cases, contraception, watch for neuropathy.
  - Corticosteroids should generally be avoided; if disease is recalcitrant, then perhaps prednisolone 40 mg daily for 5 days a month.
  - ☑ *Note:* In general, cutaneous lesions are not an indication for systemic corticosteroids in LE.

Other Forms of Chronic Cutaneous Lupus Erythematosus

▶ **Lupus tumidus:**
  - *Clinical features:* Erythematous papules and nodules on face and upper trunk; very light-sensitive; histology shows rich amount of mucin and abundant dermal lymphocytes.
  - *Differential diagnosis:* Lupus tumidus is one of the common causes of benign lymphocytic infiltrates, along with lymphadenosis cutis benigna (borrelial infection), and arthropod bite and sting reactions.
  - *Therapy:* As for DLE; intralesional corticosteroids or antimalarials often useful.
▶ **Lupus profundus:**
  - *Synonym:* Lupus panniculitis.
  - *Definition:* LE with deep inflammation involving subcutaneous tissue.
  - *Clinical features:* Firm subcutaneous nodules on face, extremities or trunk; sometimes with overlying changes of DLE, but often with normal epidermis. Heal with sunken, cosmetically disturbing scars.
  - About $^1/_3$ of patients develop SLE.
  - *Differential diagnosis:* All forms of panniculitis; histology shows lobar panniculitis often rich in plasma cells.
  - *Therapy:* Dapsone most effective; also consider antimalarials.

► **Verrucous lupus erythematosus:** Hyperkeratotic plaques, especially on hands and feet; often mistaken for keratoacanthoma, hypertrophic lichen planus, or prurigo nodularis. Patients usually have other clues for LE elsewhere.
► **Chilblain lupus:** Blue-red plaques acral plaques that resemble pernio (p. 309) but are more permanent and patients do not give history of cold exposure; up to ¹/₃ develop SLE. Systemic therapy usually required.
► **Oral lupus erythematosus:** Typical lesions are palatal erythema or erosions; often overlooked. Rarely presenting feature. Try topical corticosteroids in gel or oral paste; otherwise intralesional corticosteroids or antimalarials.

Subacute Cutaneous Lupus Erythematosus

► **Definition:** Type of LE with widespread photosensitive skin disease, mild systemic involvement, characteristic autoantibody pattern, and good prognosis.
► **Epidemiology:** Women much more often affected (8:1).
► **Clinical features:**
  • Symmetrical widespread nonscarring erythematous patches and plaques with tendency to confluence (*psoriasiform*); usually light-exposed areas such as trunk and arms (Fig. 13.2 a). Sometimes *annular* or *target-like* (Fig. 13.2 b). Rarely erythema multiforme-like with blisters (*Rowell syndome*).
  • 60% fulfill ACR criteria for SLE; often arthralgias, rarely renal disease.

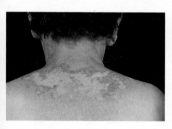 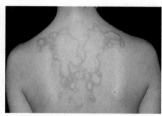

Fig. 13.2 · **a** Subacute cutaneous lupus erythematosus. **b** Annular form.

► **Histology:** Interface dermatitis with vacuolar degeneration and superficial dermal infiltrates; epidermal changes and deep infiltrates usually lacking.
► **Diagnostic approach:**
  • Skin biopsy.
  • Deposits of IgG and C3 along the basement membrane in lesional lesion in 50–60%; in normal skin in 10–20%.
  • *Laboratory*: 20–30% have low titer anti-dsDNA antibodies. Often positive for anti-SS-A and anti-SS-B (ANA-negative LE). Occasional complement defects.
► **Differential diagnosis:** The distinctions between discoid and subacute cutaneous LE are shown in Table 13.2. Other considerations include psoriasis, tinea corporis, annular erythemas, tinea versicolor, and rarely erythema multiforme.
► **Therapy:** Same as for discoid LE; emphasis on sun avoidance and sun screens. Antimalarials usually necessary, for either skin or arthritis. Also NSAIDs for joint pain.

Collagen–Vascular Disorders

Table 13.2 · Distinction between discoid and subacute cutaneous LE

Criteria	Discoid LE	Subacute cutaneous LE
Female:male ratio	3:2	8:1
Ethnicity	All	Favors whites
Location		
Head and neck	+	(-)
Trunk	(+)	+
Confluence of lesions	-	+
Follicular keratoses	+	-
Scarring	+	-
Photo-induced	++	++++
Histology		
Hyperkeratosis	+++	+
Epidermal atrophy	++	+
Superficial infiltrate	++	++
Deep infiltrate	++	-
Depots of IgG, C3 at BMZ		
Lesional skin	80%	50%
Normal skin	<10%	25%
ACR criteria	<10%	50–60%
Serology		
ANA	5–30%	80%
Anti SS-A, SS-B	<5%	70%

Neonatal Lupus Erythematosus

▶ **Pathogenesis:** Mothers with anti-SS-A and anti-SS-B transfer antibodies transplacentally. Anti-SS-A 52 cross-reacts with fetal cardiac conduction system antigens.
▶ **Clinical features:**
  • Mother may be normal (only serological evidence for LE), or have either discoid or subacute cutaneous lesions, or even Sjögren syndrome.
  • Infant has mild lesions of SCLE, often in annular pattern. Lesions are transient and heal without scarring over months. Major problem is congenital heart block, grade I–III, which occurs in 70%.
▶ **Histology:** Mild interface dermatitis with vacuolar change.
▶ **Diagnostic approach:**
  • *Laboratory:* Check anti-SS-A, anti-SS-B; rarely anti-U1 RNP positive.
  🔲 *Caution:* Check all infants with congenital heart block, and their mothers, for anti-SS-A and anti-SS-B.
▶ **Differential diagnosis:** Skin lesions confused with urticaria, annular erythema, and erythema multiforme; all uncommon in infants. Infantile LE starts later in life, has few cardiac manifestations and persistent skin lesions.

▶ **Therapy:** Skin lesions rarely require therapy. Heart block usually treated with plasmapheresis and dexamethasone (crosses placenta) if recognized during pregnancy; later with a pacemaker.

Systemic Lupus Erythematosus

▶ **MIM code:** 152700.
▶ **Epidemiology:** Annual incidence 25/100000; young women most frequently affected.
▶ **Clinical features:**
- *Cutaneous lesions:*
  - *Butterfly rash:* Classic lesion of SLE; mid-facial circumscribed erythema following sun exposure (Fig.13.**3a**); initially waxes and wanes; later permanent. 40–50% of patients have cutaneous disease at time of diagnosis.
  - Also may have diffuse erythema of scalp, ears, lips, upper trunk, forearms—sun-exposed areas—but also palmoplantar erythema. Some have transient exanthems, resembling drug eruption or erythema multiforme.
  - *Bullous lesions:* There are two distinct types of bullae:
  - Since LE has marked damage at the basement membrane zone (BMZ), the epidermis may separate. Common under the microscope, but some patients, especially with erythema multiforme lesions or sunburn, have bullae.
  - Some blacks often with LE nephritis have herpetiform blisters, mimicking dermatitis herpetiformis but on face, caused by antibodies to type VII collagen (as in epidermolysis bullosa acquisita). Very responsive to dapsone.
  - *Discoid lesions:* Many patients have hyperkeratotic scarring lesions.
  - Vasculitis may take many forms:
    - Typical leukocytoclastic vasculitis (p. 247).
    - Necrotic infarcted papules on digits, distal extremities; heal with white sunken scars.
    - Peripheral gangrene.
    - Subcutaneous nodules (nodular vasculitis).
    - Livedo racemosa (antiphospholipid syndrome, p. 258).
  - *Alopecia:* Common cause of scarring alopecia secondary to discoid lesions; also diffuse alopecia and association with alopecia areata.
  - *Nail fold changes:* Damaged cuticle with telangiectases (Fig. 13.**3b**). Similar changes in dermatomyositis, systemic sclerosis.
  - *Oral lesions:* Palatal erythema or erosions; less often elsewhere.
- *Systemic lesions:*
  - The American College of Rheumatology (ACR) criteria for the classification of SLE, formerly known as the American Rheumatologic Association (ARA) criteria (Table 13.**3**) illustrate how many organs are typically involved.
  - Most patients have arthritis; major life-threatening complications including renal and CNS disease; standard internal medicine textbooks should be consulted for details.
▶ **Diagnostic approach:**
- The ACR criteria were designed to identify patients in clinical studies; individuals with four or more criteria were accepted as having SLE. Although they were never intended as diagnostic criteria, they are widely so employed.
- A skin biopsy is useful for diagnosing LE, but not for separating the different types with certainty. Deposits of IgG and C3 along the basement membrane on normal, non–sun-exposed skin suggests SLE but is no longer an accepted criterion.

Table 13.3 · **ACR criteria for the classification of SLE**

Criterion	Definition
Malar rash	Fixed erythema over malar eminences (butterfly rash) sparing the nasolabial folds
Discoid rash	Lesions with follicular hyperkeratoses, erythema and scale; later atrophic scarring
Photosensitivity	Skin rash as reaction to sunlight
Oral ulcers	Oral or nasopharyngeal ulcerations, usually painless, observed by physician
Arthritis	Nonerosive arthritis involving two or more joints with tenderness, swelling, or effusion
Serositis	Pleuritis or pericarditis, appropriately documented
Renal disease	Persistent proteinuria $> 0.5\,g$ daily or cellular casts
Neurologic disease	Seizures or psychosis in the absence of any other explanation
Hematologic disorder	Hemolytic anemia with reticulocytosis, or leukopenia $< 4000/mm^3$ on 2 occasions, or lymphopenia $< 1500/mm^3$ on 2 occasions, or thrombocytopenia $< 100\,000/mm^3$ with no other explanation
Immunologic disorder	Anti-ds-DNA, or anti-SM, or anti-phospholipid antibodies (anticardiolipin, lupus anticoagulant, or false-positive syphilis test)
Antinuclear antibody	Positive ANA using immunofluorescence or equivalent assay at any point in course when patient not taking medications known to cause drug-induced lupus

▶ **Therapy:**
- *Cutaneous lesions:* Sunscreen avoidance and sun screens, topical corticosteroids or immune modulators; antimalarials.
- ⚠ *Caution:* With rare exceptions, cutaneous disease should not be taken as an indication for systemic therapy except for antimalarials.
- Table 13.**4** lists the major drugs recommended for SLE, with general indications.
- *Mild systemic diseases:* Arthritis, fever, headache, and other minor systemic complaints respond well to NSAIDs or antimalarials. If corticosteroids are used, the strategy must be to bring a flare under control and then eliminate or use as interval therapy.
- *Urticarial vasculitis:* Dapsone most effective.
- *Moderate systemic disease:* Serositis, pneumonitis, hematologic problems, vasculitis usually require corticosteroids (prednisolone 5–50 mg weekly, rapid taper or switch to interval therapy) and either azathioprine (100–150 mg daily) or methotrexate (7.5–20 mg weekly) for steroid sparing.
- *Severe systemic disease:* Renal, pulmonary, and CNS disease require aggressive therapy.
- High-dose corticosteroids (methylprednisolone pulse therapy 1000 mg daily for 3–5 days, then 1–2 mg/kg daily).
  - Cyclosporine 5 mg/kg daily, especially for membranous nephritis.
  - Mycophenolate mofetil (2 g daily), cyclophosphamide (50–100 mg daily or 500 mg every 4 weeks).

Table 13.4 · Major systemic medications for SLE

Drug	Indications	Comments
Antimalarials	Skin, arthritis, serositis	Eye exam every 6–12 months
NSAIDS	Arthritis, serositis, headache	Watch for GI bleeding, ↓ renal function
Corticosteroids		
Low-dose	Skin, arthritis, constitutional symptoms	Many complications
High-dose	Nephritis, CNS, vasculitis, hematologic problems	Use for control, then taper and add steroid-sparing agents
Azathioprine	Nephritis	Bone marrow, GI toxicity
Cyclophosphamide	Nephritis	Bone marrow toxicity, cystitis
Methotrexate	Arthritis	Hepatic disease
Mycophenolate mofetil	Nephritis	Leukopenia, GI distress
Cyclosporine	Nephritis	Hypertension, renal function

GI = gastrointestinal.

- *Experimental therapies:*
  - Intravenous immunoglobulins used for severe thrombocytopenia, other refractory life-threatening conditions.
  - Plasmapheresis for hyperviscosity syndrome, thrombotic thrombocytopenic purpura.
  - Anti-CD20, -CD40, and -TNF α antibodies.

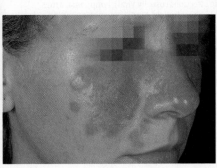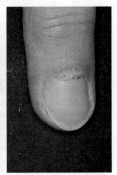

b

Fig. 13.**3** · **Systemic lupus erythematosus. a** Butterfly rash. **b** Nailfold telangiectases.

Drug-induced Lupus Erythematosus

▶ **Definition:** Clinical syndrome closely resembling LE, induced by various medications, features antihistone antibodies; usually resolves when drugs are stopped.
▶ **Pathogenesis:** The patients are usually slow acetylators who metabolize drugs slowly. Most of the triggering medications inhibit C4 and thus delay the breakdown of immune complexes. Normal individuals with HLA types associated with LE are at increased risk. Discrepancies between development of ANA and clinical findings of LE.
  • Responsible medications include:
    – *Biologicals:* IFA-α, IFN-γ, anti-TNF (ANAs common, LE rare).
    – *Antihypertensives:* Hydralazine, methyldopa.
    – *Antiarrhythmic agents:* Procainamide, quinidine.
    – *Others:* Minocycline, chlorpromazine, isoniazid.
▶ **Clinical features:** Similar to SLE, but usually less severe. Most often generalized systemic signs and symptoms; arthritis most common. Procainamide causes serositis and pulmonary disease; renal, CNS, and skin involvement uncommon.
▶ **Therapy:** Stop medication; manage as SLE but expect remission.
  ▶ *Note:* Monitor ANA baseline and every 6 months in patients on biologicals, minocycline for rheumatoid arthritis, hydralazine, or procainamide.

Antiphospholipid Syndrome

▶ **Synonyms:** Anticardiolipin syndrome, lupus anticoagulant syndrome.
▶ **MIM code:** 107320.
▶ **Definition:** Syndrome characterized by livedo racemosa, thromboembolic complications, abortion, and severe, otherwise unexplained headaches. Can be primary or secondary to a variety of diseases.
▶ **Epidemiology:** Most patients are young women.
▶ **Pathogenesis:**
  • Antiphospholipid antibodies (aPL) are commonly seen as normal variant in older individuals. Genetic predisposition (HLA-DR4, -DR7, -DRw53). Usual triggers include SLE, chronic infections (usually viral), lymphoma, drugs.
  • aPL appear to recognize phospholipid-binding proteins, not anionic phospholipids as initially thought.
  • Prominent target is β_2-glycoprotein I; after binding with aPL, it triggers activation of T cells, thrombocytes, and endothelial cells.
▶ **Clinical features:**
  • Arterial emboli, recurrent venous thromboses (CNS, lungs, legs) without other known risk factors in 30%.
  • Abortions, intrauterine death from placental insufficiency.
  • Valvular cardiac disease.
  • *Skin changes:* Livedo racemosa, Raynaud syndrome, persistent acral ulcerations, necrosis and gangrene.
  • *Sneddon syndrome:* Combination of livedo racemosa and CNS thrombotic events.
▶ **Diagnostic approach:**
  • The diagnosis of antiphospholipid syndrome is complex. Two major, not totally independent groups of antibodies can be identified:
    – Anticardiolipin antibodies (IgG), also responsible for false-positive VDRL titer (p. 143).
    – Lupus anticoagulant antibodies (IgG, IgM) against β_2-glycoprotein and phospholipid components of the prothrombin activator complex.

- The lupus anticoagulant inhibits the conversion of prothrombin to thrombin; it is found in 5–10% of LE patients (many without other findings of antiphospholipid syndrome).
  - ▶ *Note:* Although the lupus anticoagulant is associated with a prolonged partial thromboplastin time, it rarely causes bleeding but instead increases the risk of thromboembolism. The in-vivo defect in clot formation is misleading.
- Most patients have mild thrombocytopenia.
- *Skin biopsy:* May find a thrombus if lucky, but not a useful tool for routine work.
- *Diagnostic criteria* (Sapporo 1998):
  - History of abortion or thrombosis.
  - Presence of antiphospholipid antibodies or lupus anticoagulant.
► **Therapy:**
- Identification of either group of antibodies is not an indication for therapy.
- Treat underlying disease.
- Anticoagulation:
  - Prophylaxis with aspirin 325 mg.
  - After thrombosis, lifelong anticoagulation with coumarin.

13.3 Dermatomyositis and Polymyositis

Overview

► **Definition:** Uncommon group of diseases with loss of muscle strength secondary to autoimmune muscle damage.
- *Polymyositis:* No cutaneous involvement.
- *Dermatomyositis:* Both muscular and cutaneous abnormalities.
► **Epidemiology:** Incidence in children 3/million; in adults 0.5–1.0/100 000; women 1.5–2.0 times more often affected. In adults > 50 years of age, often paraneoplastic.
► **Pathogenesis:** Evidence for immune process is strong, including association with other autoimmune disorders and presence of circulating autoantibodies, both myositis-specific and overlapping. Suspected triggers include viral infections. In the case of polymyositis, the reaction appears primarily cellular with CD8+ cytotoxic T cells damaging muscles. In the case of dermatomyositis, humoral mechanisms appear more important, as complement activation leads to microangiopathy, with muscle necrosis secondary to impaired vascular supply. Invading cells are primarily CD4+. Mechanisms of paraneoplastic dermatomyositis unclear.
► **Classification:**
- *Polymyositis.*
- *Adult dermatomyositis:* Typical onset 40 years of age.
- *Juvenile dermatomyositis:* More acute onset with vasculitis (often leading to gastrointestinal hemorrhage), later calcification, lipodystrophy.
- *Paraneoplastic dermatomyositis:* Later onset, associated with those tumors common in older individuals (breast, head and neck carcinomas).
- *Amyopathic dermatomyositis:* Dermatomyositis with no evidence of muscle involvement over 6 months follow-up.

Clinical Features

► **Muscles:** Pain and then weakness in shoulder and hip girdle muscles. Typical problems include combing hair, getting out of chair, getting up from horizontal position, climbing stairs, or leaving a car. Difficulty swallowing and ptosis or strabismus can also occur. Early disease often associated with fever and malaise.

▶ **Skin:**
- Skin changes in 80–100% of cases; presenting sign in 25%.
- Periorbital and eyelid edema with violet tint to eyelids; known as *heliotrope lids* (sun-pointing lids); sometimes associated with reduced facial expression (Fig. 13.**4a**).
- Lichenoid papules over the finger joints and knuckles (*Gottron sign*, Fig. 13.**4b**).
- Erythematosus macules and plaques on forehead, chin, shoulders and upper arms (*shawl sign*) or anterior neck and upper chest (*V sign*).
- *Raynaud phenomenon:* Children frequently have distal sclerosis.
- Nail fold telangiectases and atrophy.
- Fissures and ulcers on tips of fingers and toes (*mechanic's hands*).

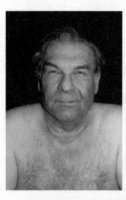
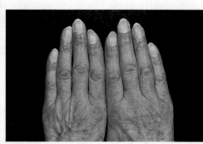

a

Fig. 13.**4** · **Dermatomyositis. a** Facial involvement with eyelid swelling. **b** Gottron papules.

▶ **Arthritis:** Most common at onset of disease; usually peripheral; 25% have morning stiffness.
▶ **Mucosa:** 10–20% have oral ulcers.
▶ **Calcinosis:** Distinctive feature of juvenile dermatomyositis; can be very extensive; soft tissue, vessel and muscle calcifications. Often most disturbing sequelae.
▶ **Lungs:** More common in patients with anti-Jo1; 20% have pulmonary fibrosis.
▶ **Gastrointestinal tract:** Children have vasculitis and frequent gastrointestinal ulcerations and hemorrhage. In adults, motility problems may occur.
▶ **Heart:** Asymptomatic EKG changes common; occasionally myocarditis or myopathy.
▶ **Histology:** The biopsy findings can best be remember as *almost LE*: vacuolar denegation, atrophy, perivascular inflammation, sometimes even a wisp of mucin.

Diagnostic Approach

▶ **Electromyogram (EMG):** Characteristic changes in affected muscles in 70%.
▶ **MRI:** Displays inflamed muscles; superior to sonarography or CT.
▶ **Muscle biopsy:** Most reliable diagnostic text; shows varying stages of necrosis and regeneration with inflammatory infiltrate. In polymyositis, CD8+ cells; in dermatomyositis, CD4+ cells, vasculitis, and perifascicular atrophy (almost diagnostic). Also helps exclude trichinosis.

🔏 *Caution:* Always biopsy muscle that EMG or MRI shows to be affected. Preserve muscle in solution provided by special muscle pathologist and keep under tension with muscle clamp. Otherwise, the procedure is worthless.

► **Laboratory:**
- Sed rate and C-reactive protein elevated in 50%.
- Creatine kinase (CK) is best marker; it is elevated at some point in disease. 24-hour urine creatine (*not creatinine—common error*) level > 200 mg is diagnostic. In children and pregnancy, more marked spontaneous variation. Other muscle enzymes can also be measured: AST, ALD, LDH.
- *Serology:*
  - *Myositis-specific antibodies(MSA):* Present in < 50%.
  - *Anti-Jo-1 (antisynthetase):* Present in 20%, correlates with lung disease and Raynaud phenomenon.
  - *Anti-SRP (signal recognition protein):* Acute disease, poor outlook.
  - *Anti-Mi2 (helicase):* Dermatomyositis, good outlook.
  - *Others:* Rheumatoid factor (10%), ANA (20%); no anti-DNA antibodies.
  - *Anti-PM-SCL (anti-PM1):* marker for polymyositis/systemic sclerosis overlap.
- *Skin biopsy:* Rarely diagnostic.
- *General evaluation:* Chest radiograph, EKG, echocardiogram pulmonary function.
- Search for underlying tumor in patients > 50 years of age or with suspicious history.

▣ *Note:* Do not overlook meticulous pelvic examination. Ovarian carcinoma is one of the more commonly associated tumors.

Differential Diagnosis

► **Other myopathies:** Inclusion body myositis (older, slow onset, 20% dysphagia, biopsy classic); muscular dystrophy (late-onset), neuromuscular atrophy (Charcot–Marie–Tooth disease), myasthenia gravis, thyrotoxic myopathy, Cushing disease, sarcoidosis, alcoholism.
► **Drugs:** Lipid-lowering agents, hydroxyurea, and NSAIDs (rarely) can produce dermatomyositis-like picture.
► **Overlap syndromes:** Polymyositis-systemic sclerosis, eosinophilic fasciitis, SLE. Childhood dermatomyositis often resembles systemic sclerosis, but is much more common.
► **Vasculitis:** May present with muscle weakness.
► **Polymyalgia rheumatica:** Older patients, slow onset, may be associated with temporal arteritis.
► **Trichinosis:** Can exactly mimic dermatomyositis with periorbital edema, nail fold hemorrhages and pain. More painful and usually has hypereosinophilia.

Therapy

► **Corticosteroids:**
- Start with 20 mg prednisolone b.i.d.; if needed, increase to 40 mg t.i.d. or use pulse therapy. In children with dermatomyositic vasculitis, t.i.d. regimens recommended to suppress disease rapidly.
- As soon as CK starts to drop, switch to single dose in morning and start tapering in 2 week intervals, checking clinical status and CK before each dose reduction.
- After several months, switch to alternate-day therapy for its adrenal-sparing role. Often long-term low-dose corticosteroids are needed, but a try at discontinuation is warranted.

▶ **Second-line agents:**
  • Methotrexate 5–15 mg p.o. or 15–50 mg i.v. weekly or azathioprine 1–3 mg/kg daily; either can be combined with corticosteroids.
  • Cyclophosphamide and cyclosporine are less effective.
▶ **Intravenous immunoglobulins:** 2 g/kg daily for 2 days; repeat every 4 weeks for 6–12 months; indicated for resistant cases, children with vasculitic component, and in those with steroid-induced diabetes mellitus.
▶ **Skin:** Antimalarials may help cutaneous lesions, as do topical corticosteroids. Sunscreens essential.
▶ **Other measures:** Bed rest during flares; physical therapy when stable; absolutely essential to avoid loss of function, especially for children, but if too strenuous, can trigger relapse. Watch for pneumonia—common complication.
▶ **Paraneoplastic disease:** Appropriate treatment of underlying malignancy; usually combined with or followed by corticosteroids, as recommended by oncologist.

13.4 Morphea

▶ **Overview:**
  • *Synonyms:* Localized scleroderma, circumscript scleroderma.
  • *Definition:* Cutaneous sclerosis without systemic involvement; several clinical variants.
  • *Epidemiology:* Uncommon disease; female: male 3:1; incidence around 3/100 000 yearly.
  • *Pathogenesis:* Poorly understood. Association with *Borrelia burgdorferi* not substantiated. Circulating autoantibodies support immune role.
▶ **Clinical features:**
  • *Classic morphea:*
    – Circumscribed sclerotic plaque with ivory center and red-violet periphery (*lilac ring*) (Fig. 13.**5a**). Starts as erythematous patch that slowly spreads. Rarely attached to underlying structures. Usually solitary; 5–20 cm.
    – *Course:* spontaneous or therapy-induced regression occurs.
    – Systemic findings uncommon; rarely malaise or Raynaud phenomenon.
  • *Variants:*
    – *Plaque form*: Larger solitary lesions.
    – *Atrophoderma of Pasini and Pierini:* Superficial erythematous variant of morphea, most common in young girls on trunk, resolves with atrophy and hyperpigmentation but no sclerosis. Clinically sharp vertical drop from normal skin into depressed lesion.
    – *Guttate*: Multiple small, often hypopigmented lesions.
    – *Nodular*: Keloid-like lesions, protuberant.
    – *Linear:* Lesion involving limb, usually leg, in children with bone loss and shortening of limb, as well as loss of function (Fig. 13.**5b**).
    – *Coup de sabre:* Lesion on forehead resembling scar from saber blow; may involve orbit and its content.
    – *Hemifacial atrophy (Parry–Romberg syndome):* Extreme form of linear morphea, distortion of one side of face with alopecia and abnormal pigmentation, sometimes with seizures or trigeminal neuralgia. Deeper involvement than coup de sabre. Some do not recognize it as morphea variant.
    – *Disabling pansclerotic morphea (generalized morphea):* Widespread morphea without systemic involvement. Muscle atrophy, loss of limb function, occasionally fatal.

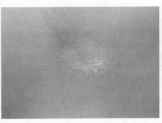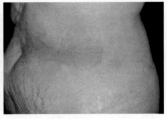

b

Fig. 13.**5** · **Morphea. a** Annular lesion. **b** Linear lesion.

– *Lichen sclerosus et atrophicus–like lesions:* Overlap, especially in nongenital lesions (see next section).
► **Histology:** Classic picture of thickened amorphous collagen with entrapment of adnexal structures and fat, occasionally eosinophilic infiltrate. Identical to systemic sclerosis.
► **Diagnostic approach:**
  • Skin biopsy can confirm diagnosis, but not distinguish between morphea and systemic sclerosis. Must rely on clinical findings.
  • ANA and anti-ss-DNA may also be found in linear and widespread morphea.
  • With widespread disease, evaluate joints and esophagus.
► **Differential diagnosis:**
  • Pseudoscleroderma, especially porphyria cutanea tarda and graft-versus-host disease.
  • Drug reaction (bleomycin-induced sclerosis).
► **Therapy:**
  • Solitary lesions with high-potency topical corticosteroids, also under occlusion or intralesional.
  • Bath PUVA or UVA1 (p. 606).
  • Sometimes large plaques respond to penicillin even though the proposed link between *Borrelia burgdorferi* and morphea has been dispelled. Proponents advise repeated courses of i. v. or i. m. penicillin.
  • For widespread or rapidly advancing disease, consider therapy usually reserved for systemic sclerosis.

13.5 Lichen Sclerosus

► **Synonyms:** Lichen sclerosus et atrophicus, lichen albus, white spot disease.
► **Definition:** Dermatosis that presents with either porcelain-white papules and plaques or atrophy and classic histological picture.
► **Epidemiology:** Women more often affected than men; two peaks—prepubertal and later in adult life—but onset at all ages possible.
► **Pathogenesis:** Not totally clear, but IgG antibodies against extracellular matrix protein 1 (EMP 1) identified in about 75% of patients.
► **Clinical features:**
  • *Cutaneous lesions:* Typically porcelain-white patches or plaques with an erythematous border. On trunk, very similar to morphea. Sometimes multiple smaller white papules are present (*confetti lesions, white spot disease*). Typically

on trunk, especially upper back, as well as flexures. Follicular hyperkeratoses or dilated follicles common; occasionally bullous or hemorrhagic. Asymptomatic.

- *Genital lesions in women:* White atrophic lesions involving vulva, labia minora, clitoris, and introitus (Fig. 13.**6a**). Involvement may spread to perianal region. Typically pruritic; often atrophic, may develop hemorrhage with trauma. Most common in older women (known to gynecologists as *kraurosis vulvae*), but also seen in prepubescent children. Latter sometimes resolves spontaneously, but may persist.

- ⚠ *Caution:* In young girls, lichen sclerosus with perianal involvement and hemorrhagic areas is frequently mistaken for child abuse.

- *Genital involvement in men*: Lichen sclerosus is a common cause of phimosis, usually not pruritic, and presents with easily damaged white atrophic patches (Fig. 13.**6b**). Often first identified on circumcision specimens; often resolves following procedure. Also known as balanitis xerotica obliterans.

- There is a slight risk of squamous cell carcinoma developing in genital lichen sclerosus, so patients should be monitored.

▶ **Histology:** Epidermal atrophy, follicular plugs, swollen edematous upper dermis with initial band-like infiltrate in upper–mid dermis. Sometimes subepidermal blister with hemorrhage. Older lesions closely resemble morphea. Possible distinction with elastin stain, as lichen sclerosus more likely to show damage.

▶ **Diagnostic approach:** Clinical examination, biopsy.

▶ **Differential diagnosis:** On trunk, morphea and vitiligo. Female genitalia: chronic dermatitis, vitiligo, erosive lichen planus, autoimmune bullous diseases. Male genitalia: balanitis in all its variants, idiopathic phimosis, erosive lichen planus.

▶ **Therapy:**

- *Trunk:* High-potency topical corticosteroids; also try selective UVB phototherapy (SUP) or bath PUVA.

- *Genitalia:* High-potency topical corticosteroids or intralesional corticosteroids (triamcinolone 10 mg/mL diluted 1:3 in lidocaine). Much more effective than topical estrogens or testosterone. Topical immunomodulators (tacrolimus or pimecrolimus).

- In young boys, topical corticosteroids can even reverse phimosis. If phimosis is persistent, then circumcision, perhaps with meatotomy.

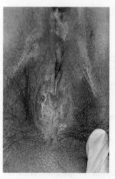 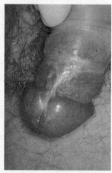

Fig. 13.**6** · **Lichen sclerosus. a** Extensive involvement of female genitalia. **b** Penile disease with phimosis.

a   b

13.6 Systemic Sclerosis

Overview

▶ **Synonyms:** Systemic scleroderma, progressive systemic sclerosis.
▶ **Definition:** Multiorgan disease with diffuse sclerosis of connective tissue favoring skin, lungs, gastrointestinal tract and kidneys.
▶ **Epidemiology:** Incidence 1–2/100 000 yearly; prevalence 20–75/100 000. Peaks between third and fifth decades; increases with age; female:male ratio 5:1, but men have worse prognosis; considerable geographic and ethnic variation.
▶ **Pathogenesis:**
  • Systemic sclerosis features small-vessel vasculopathy, fibrosis, immune activation.
  • Genetic predisposition (HLA-DR3, -DR5, -DRw6, -DRws52).
  • Current evidence favors vessel damage as the most likely primary event.
  • Autoreactive T cells appear, as in graft-versus-host disease; they may be transferred from fetus to mother during pregnancy (*microchimerism*).
  • Increased production of types I, III, and Iv collagen as well as fibronectin and proteoglycans with deposition in affected connective tissue.
▶ **Classification:** The German Dermatologic Research classification identifies three forms of systemic sclerosis with progressively worse prognosis:.
  • *Acral systemic sclerosis, type I:* Only involvement of hands and forearms.
  • *Acral systemic sclerosis, type II:* Starts on hands, but spreads to arms and trunk.
  • *Systemic sclerosis, type III:* Starts on trunk, usually severe facial involvement.
  • CREST syndrome can include types I or II. It features **c**alcinosis, **R**aynaud phenomenon, **e**sophageal disease, **s**clerodactyly, **t**elangiectases.

Clinical Features

▶ **Skin:**
  • *Hands:* Fingers initially puffy and edematous; later sclerodactyly (Fig. 13.**7a**), with loss of finger pads, tightening, reduced motion; painful fingertip ulcers (*rat bite ulcer*); loss of cuticle with telangiectases (*Heuck–Gottron sign*); peripheral calcinosis, often with ulceration of overlying skin and extrusion of calcified debris (*Thibierge–Weissenbach syndrome*).
  • *Face:* Microstomia with tightening of frenulum (Fig. 13.**7b**) (older denture wearers may have trouble inserting and removing dentures); reduced facial expression; prominent telangiectases.
  • Diffuse sclerosis of skin, sometimes restricts respiratory motion (Fig. 13.**7c**).
  • Raynaud phenomenon; often presenting sign.
  • Characteristic *confetti-like hypopigmentation:* focal hypopigmentation with follicular repigmentation; more dramatic in blacks; mistaken for vitiligo as skin often not yet sclerotic.
▶ **Histology:** Diffuse increase in collagen with loss of vessels and adnexal structures; perivascular infiltrates, sometimes eosinophils and plasma cells; identical to morphea.
▶ **Systemic findings:**
  • *Gastrointestinal tract:* Sclerosis of lingual frenulum reduces tongue motility; often sicca syndrome; swallowing problems; impaired esophageal motility; with more diffuse involvement, impaired transit and ileus.
  • *Lungs:* Problems both because skin restricts motion and pulmonary fibrosis interferes with oxygen diffusion.

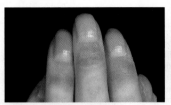
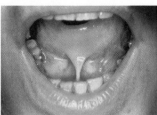
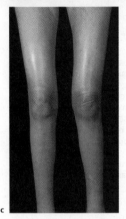

Fig. 13.**7** · **Systemic sclerosis. a** Arachnodactyly.
b Restriction of frenulum. **c** Diffuse skin thickening and tightness.

- *Kidneys:* Hypertension and progressive renal failure because of nephrosclerosis.
- *Heart:* Subtle and late, but can develop myocardial fibrosis and cor pulmonale. Pericardial effusions common, but usually asymptomatic.
- *Liver:* 15% have associated primary biliary cirrhosis and positive antimitochondrial antibodies.
- *Musculoskeletal:* Many present with arthralgias and muscle pain: later main problem is muscle atrophy. Overlap syndrome with polymyositis (anti-PM-Scl antibodies).
- *Bones:* Acro-osteolysis.
- *Teeth:* Widening of periodontal membrane (useful in radiologic diagnosis, but of little clinical significance).

Diagnostic Approach

- ▶ **Skin:** Check for cutaneous involvement and identify most urgent problems.
- ▶ **Lungs:** Chest radiograph, pulmonary diffusion studies, bronchoalveolar lavage (to assess inflammatory cells; prognostically useful).
- ▶ **Skeleton:** Radiologic documentation of osteolysis, calcification.
- ▶ **Gastrointestinal tract:** Esophageal manometry and functional scintigraphy.
- ▶ **Heart:** EKG, echocardiogram, cardiac catheterization if cor pulmonale is present.
- ▶ **Kidneys:** Renal function, urine status.

▶ **Laboratory:**
- Routine tests (CBC, liver function, sed rate, C-reactive protein).
- *Serology:*
  - More than 90% have positive ANA.
  - Anti-Scl-70 positive in 30–70%; usually with severe course.
  - Rarely (<5%) anti-RNA polymerase I–II; poor outlook.
  - Anti-centromere antibodies present in type I systemic sclerosis and CREST syndrome.
  - Anti-DM-Scl in overlap syndrome.
  - Rheumatoid factor positive in 30%.

Differential Diagnosis

▶ **Pseudoscleroderma:** see below.
▶ **Other collagen–vascular disorders:**
- Mixed collagen–vascular disorders.
- Overlap syndromes.
▶ **Graft-versus-host disease.**
▶ **Others:** Generalized morphea. Puffy hands can be confused with early stage of acrodermatitis chronica atrophicans.

Therapy

◻ *Note:* Types I and II can usually be treated conservatively, but type III requires immunosuppressive therapy. Each specific problem requires carefully adjusted therapy.
▶ **Raynaud phenomenon:** See below; same recommendations as for idiopathic disease.
▶ **Calcification:** Surgery sometimes required; low-dose coumarin may reduce inflammation.
▶ **Ulcers:** Occlusive dressings and skin equivalents are helpful for distal ulcers.
▶ **Sclerosis:** Neither penicillamine nor extracorporeal photophoresis has been proven definitely effective. For rapidly progressive disease, immunosuppression often tried.
- *Immunosuppressive agents:* Systemic corticosteroids (prednisolone 0.5 mg/kg daily), perhaps combined with azathioprine 1–2 mg/kg daily. Methotrexate 20–30 mg weekly, cyclosporine 3–5 mg/kg daily, or cyclophosphamide 2 mg/kg daily or as pulse therapy (500–800 mg once monthly) can be tried; none is overwhelmingly useful.
- *Aspirin:* Pain relief and inhibition of platelet function.
▶ **Internal organ involvement:**
- Angiotensin-converting enzyme (ACE) inhibitors are treatment of choice for renal hypertension.
- Proton pump inhibitors (omeprazole 20–40 mg daily) indicated for esophageal dysfunction.
- Pulmonary hypertension treated with i. v. prostacyclin; interstitial lung disease may respond best to cyclophosphamide.
▶ **Physical therapy:** Infrared light may help increase circulation by raising body temperature; physical therapy can help avoid contractures and retain function.

13.7 Pseudoscleroderma

Although the term "pseudoscleroderma" is not ideal, the concept is sound. There are a number of diseases that mimic morphea or systemic sclerosis, and in many instances appear to have similar causes. They are reviewed in Table 13.5.

Table 13.5 · Causes of pseudoscleroderma

Disease	Comments	See
Porphyria cutanea tarda	Sclerotic areas, usually on chest, coupled with skin fragility on hands and facial hirsutism	p. 312
Graft-versus-host disease	Chronic stage often features cutaneous sclerosis, usually depigmented	p. 227
Diabetes mellitus	Stiff hand syndrome, sclerodactyly in juveniles	p. 319
POEMS syndrome (Crow-Fukase syndrome)	**P**olyneuropathy, **o**rganomegaly, **e**ndocrinopathy, **m**onoclonal gammopathy (plasma cell dyscrasia), **s**kin changes (sclerosis, glomeruloid hemangiomas)	p. 322
Scleredema	Usually sclerosis of back; extensive mucin; associated with diabetes mellitus	p. 320
Scleromyxedema	Sclerosis associated with gammopathy	p. 320
Nephrogenic fibrosing dermopathy	Resembles scleromyxedema but found as complication of renal dialysis	p. 320
Phenylketonuria	Metabolic disturbance with mental retardation and hypopigmentation; usually detected and managed so sclerosis does not appear	p. 373
Stiff skin syndrome (congenital fascial dystrophy)	Fibrillin mutation leads to sclerodermoid changes, restriction of motion; neurological changes; hypertrichosis	
Carcinoid syndrome	Flushing more typical, but repeated vascular stimulation may lead to sclerosis	
Premature ageing syndromes	Both Werner syndrome and progeria may be confused with scleroderma initially	
Toxin exposure	*Eosinophilia–myalgia syndrome:* Ingestion of contaminated tryptophan led to pulmonary disease, hypereosinophilia, and cutaneous sclerosis *Toxic oil syndrome:* Ingestion of contaminated rapeseed oil caused similar picture	
Drugs	Bleomycin, administered locally or systemically, can cause sclerosis	

Eosinophilic Fasciitis

▶ **Synonym:** Shulman syndrome.
▶ **Definition:** Cutaneous induration, often acute onset, with joint contractions, eosinophilia and inflammatory infiltrate in fascia; no systemic involvement except joint contractures.
▶ **Epidemiology:** Uncommon; age peak 40 years.

► **Pathogenesis:** Unclear; sometimes follows excessive physical activity.
► **Clinical features:**
  • *Skin:* Symmetrical edematous, often painful induration, usually on distal limbs. Rarely associated with morphea.
  • *Musculoskeletal:* Arthralgias, myalgias; reduced range of motion and contractures usually affecting hands, occasionally elbows, shoulders, or other sites.
  • Patients may have malaise, fever, or other systemic complaints.
  • Sometimes associated with hematologic or lymphoproliferative disorders.
► **Histology:** Fascia markedly thickened; inflammatory infiltrate usually rich in eosinophils.
► **Diagnostic approach:**
  • Deep biopsy sampling the fascia; tissue should be preserved in muscle clamp to avoid artifacts.
  • *Laboratory:* Eosinophilia (90%), elevated sed rate (80%), hypergammaglobulinemia (80%), ANA (25%), rheumatoid factor (15%).
  • Borrelial serology to exclude Lyme disease.
► **Differential diagnosis:** Scleredema—not usually on limbs, scleromyxedema, eosinophilia-myalgia syndrome, generalized morphea.
► **Therapy:**
  • Often resolves spontaneously.
  • Prednisolone 60 mg daily; prompt improvement, rapid tapering; good outlook.
  • If poor response, bath PUVA or antimalarials.

13.8 Mixed Collagen–Vascular Disease

► **Synonym:** Sharp syndrome.
► **Definition:** Disease with features of SLE, systemic sclerosis and dermatomyositis, characteristic laboratory findings, and good prognosis.
► **Epidemiology:** Most patients are women; female: male ratio 4:1.
► **Pathogenesis:** Unknown.
► **Clinical features:**
  • Features of all three diseases, but nonetheless combine in a recognizable clinical pattern.
  • Raynaud phenomenon is obligatory; usual presenting sign.
  • Intermittent swelling of hands and feet with distal polymyositis.
  • Often lymphadenopathy.
  • Skin changes combine those of systemic LE with the confetti-like hypopigmentation of systemic sclerosis. Also diffuse nonscarring alopecia.
  • Wide variety of other signs and symptoms including serositis, fever, weight loss, pulmonary fibrosis, esophageal motility disturbances, trigeminal neuralgia. Renal disease uncommon.
► **Diagnostic approach:** Presence of high titer ANA; rarely anti-DNA antibodies; instead high titer anti-ENA (anti-U1-RNP) antibodies.
► **Differential diagnosis:** In addition to the obvious considerations of the three major collagen–vascular disorders, any one of which can appear dominant, one must consider other overlap syndromes such as polymyositis–systemic sclerosis. Usually the antibody pattern determines the answer.
► **Therapy:** Usually systemic corticosteroids are effective, although recurrence with tapering is common. Can be combined with azathioprine or other immunosuppressive agents. Milder cases respond well to antimalarials.

13.9 *Other Rheumatoid Diseases*

Rheumatic Fever

Streptococcus pyogenes causes several postinfectious immunologic disorders. Rheumatic fever is not associated with impetigo, but acute glomerulonephritis is. Rheumatic fever may be associated with erythema nodosum as well several distinctive cutaneous changes:

► *Erythema marginatum:* Perhaps 10% of patients develop unique rapidly moving, peripherally prominent patches and plaques; quickest of all the annular erythemas (p. 711).
► *Nodules:* Appear in first month of infection; usually along forearm (more distal than in rheumatoid arthritis); resolve spontaneously.

Rheumatoid Arthritis

► **MIM code:** 180300 (but usually not genetic).
► **Definition:** Most common of the autoimmune collagen–vascular disorders; primarily affects joints, with changes in synovial membranes and articular structures, leading to deformity and ankylosis.
► **Pathogenesis:** Viral triggers strongly suspected; possible gene locus at 6p21.3; HLA associations.
► **Clinical features:**
  • *Systemic findings:* multiple—should be reviewed in internal medicine texts.
  • *Skin findings:*
    – Rheumatoid nodules (see below).
    – Granulomatous dermatitis; often linear bands.
    – *Vasculitis:* many different forms possible but usually acral.
    – *Neuropathy:* paresthesias, pain, decreased sweating.
    – *Ulcerations:* sometimes caused by intimal proliferation (cut-onion pattern) without inflammation; also acral.
    – Pyoderma gangrenosum (p. 251).
► **Therapy:** Combination of anti-inflammatory and immunosuppressive therapy for underlying disease, coupled with specific dermatologic approaches.

Rheumatoid Nodule

► **Clinical features:** Common finding in rheumatoid arthritis; up to 2–3 cm nodules appear around elbows and on extensor surface of forearm; overlying skin usually unaffected, but lesions may drain.
► **Histology:** Classic palisading granuloma: macrophages surrounding area of necrobiotic collagen with fibrin. Similar picture in granuloma annulare (p. 292) but with mucin and in necrobiosis lipoidica but with plasma cells (p. 293).
► **Diagnostic approach:** Confirm serological diagnosis of rheumatoid arthritis. Excisional biopsy of small nodule if questions exists.
► **Differential diagnosis:** There are many lesions that appear similar:
  • *Subcutaneous granuloma annulare:* When a child has deep necrobiotic nodules, they do not have rheumatoid arthritis but just granuloma annulare. Also appears on hands in adults.
  ▣ **Note:** Consider the whole clinical picture; then there is no overlap between rheumatoid arthritis and granuloma annulare.
  • *Osteoarthritis: Heberden nodes* are cartilaginous and bony enlargements of the distal interphalangeal joints; when proximal, the same lesions are called *Bouchard nodes.* Both are much more common than rheumatoid nodules.

- *Gout:* Tophi are larger, more acral; uric acid answers question.
- Fibrous nodules and ulnar bands in acrodermatitis chronica atrophicans; no necrobiosis on biopsy; other clinical pattern.
- *Rheumatic fever:* 5% of patients may have nodules but they are transient and associated with acute disease; usually on forearms; on biopsy, not necrobiotic.
- *Syphilis:* Subcutaneous nodules can be seen in late syphilis; fibrosis and granulomatous inflammation with plasma cells.

▶ **Therapy:** Observe or consider excision; then risk of ulcers or sinus tracts.

Juvenile Rheumatoid Arthritis

▶ The systemic form (least common variant) of juvenile rheumatoid arthritis is known as *Still disease*. Patients are systemically ill with fever spikes coupled with a transient, pale pink, blanching nonpruritic rash. Also marked lymphadenopathy. May go on to have severe vasculitis, consumptive coagulopathy, and macrophage activation syndrome.

Sjögren Syndrome

▶ **MIM code:** 270150.
▶ **Definition:** Autoimmune disease with predilection for epithelial surfaces and exocrine glands.
▶ **Epidemiology:** More common in women; female:male ratio 9:1.
▶ **Pathogenesis:** Unknown; viral triggers suspected.
▶ **Classification:** Primary Sjögren syndrome vs. secondary Sjögren syndrome when associated with other defined collagen–vascular disorders (such as systemic sclerosis).
▶ **Clinical features:** Primarily affects the eyes and mouth; classic findings include dry eyes (reduced tears) and dry mouth (reduced saliva). The oral findings often lead to chronic burning or pain, difficulty swallowing, and caries. Also arthralgias and arthritis. Almost 50-fold increased incidence of B-cell lymphoma; usually MALT type.
  - Skin findings are uncommon:
    - Annular erythematous lesions common in Sjögren syndrome among East Asians.
    - Dry skin common but not diagnostically useful.
    - Variety of forms of vasculitis.
▶ **Diagnostic approach:** Primary Sjögren syndrome can be diagnosed when four of the following six points are present:
  - Dry eyes: symptoms.
  - Schirmer test.
  - Dry mouth: symptoms.
  - Reduced saliva production, abnormal sialogram or scintigraphy.
  - Abnormal salivary glands on labial biopsy.
  - Anti-SS-A/Ro or anti-SS-B/La antibodies.
▶ **Differential diagnosis:** Postradiation syndrome, HIV/AIDS, hepatitis C infection, lymphoma, sarcoidosis, graft-versus-host disease, and use of anticholinergic drugs should all be excluded, as well as associated collagen–vascular disorders.
▶ **Therapy:** Artifical tears and salvia; secretagogues; NSAIDs or antimalarials for arthritis; watch for oral candidiasis; management with internist, ophthalmologist, or oral medicine specialist.

13.10 Raynaud Syndrome

Overview

- **Definition:** Vascular spasms of digital arteries with distinct clinical patterns; often associated with autoimmune diseases.
- **Epidemiology:** Female:male ratio > 4:1.
- **Classification:**
  - *Raynaud phenomenon* is the classical clinical triad of ischemia (white), cyanosis (blue), and reactive hyperemia (red) occurring sequentially in a digit.
  - *Primary Raynaud syndrome (Raynaud disease)* is the presence of Raynaud phenomenon for more than 2 years without evidence of an underlying disease.
  - *Secondary Raynaud syndrome:* Same clinical findings, but associated with a variety of disorders:
    - *Collagen–vascular disorders* (especially systemic sclerosis or mixed collagen–vascular disorder, but any of the others is possible).
    - *Exogenous factors:* Vibration (jackhammer operator), repeated hammering (hypothenar hammer syndrome); injuries, postoperative; cold exposure; reflex sympathetic dystrophy (Sudeck atrophy).
    - Gammopathy with hyperviscosity syndrome; polycythemia vera, Waldenström macroglobulinemia.
    - Combination of vasculitis and hyperviscosity: paroxysmal nocturnal hemoglobinuria, cold agglutinin disease, cryoglobulinemia (p. 307), hot-cold hemolysin.
    - Obstructive arterial disease: arteriosclerosis, thromboangiitis obliterans (Buerger disease), thrombosis, thoracic outlet syndrome.
    - Neurological diseases with peripheral manifestations.
    - *Toxins:* Medications (amphetamines, β-blockers, clonidine, oral contraceptives, ergot derivatives—both in medications and in biological products, cytostatic agents (bleomycin, vinca alkaloids); heavy metals, vinyl chloride.
    - *Others:* Paraneoplastic, hypothyroidism.
- **Clinical features:**
  - Triad explained by pathophysiology:
    - *White:* Sudden vasospasm; cold numb fingers (*cadaver digit*).
    - *Blue:* Venous constriction persists even in face of arterial relaxation; cyanosis.
    - *Red:* Restored blood flow, pain, throbbing.
  - Features usually bilateral; typically start in only one digit. After years, may develop persistent finger swelling.
  - Cuticle thickens, proximal nail fold is thinned with telangiectases.
  - Occasionally involvement of toes, nose, or ears.
- **Diagnostic approach:**.
  - Careful history, confirming presence of white–blue–red triad and searching for triggering factors.
  - Clinical and laboratory evaluation to rule out the causes of secondary Raynaud syndrome, including sed rate, ANA, anti-DNA antibodies, anticardiolipin antibodies, β_2-glycoprotein, cold agglutinins, cryoglobulins, serum protein electrophoresis, blood viscosity test.
- **Therapy:** If an underlying disease is found, it should be treated. The Raynaud phenomenon is managed in the same way regardless of cause.

  Note: Patients with Raynaud phenomenon must not smoke.
  - Avoidance of cold: Warm gloves, hand warmers.

- Calcium channel blockers are treatment of choice; nifedipine 5 mg t.i.d.; if orthostatic hypotension is problem, try diltiazem 60–120 mg daily or verapamil 240–360 mg daily.
- Other vasodilators such as prazosin also useful, start with 1 mg daily; may increase slowly to as high as 6 mg daily.
- Calcitonin 100 IU i.v. daily for 10–14 days, or calcitonin nasal spray 100 IU 1–3× weekly.
- *Prostaglandins or prostacyclins:* All very expensive; given i.v. either continuously in hospital or daily for 6–8 hours over 5 days:
  – Alprostadil (PGI2).
  – Epoprostenol (prostacyclin).
  – Iloprost trometamol.
- *Topical nitroglycerine paste:* May help to avoid fingertip necrosis.
- *Supplemental measures:* Physical therapy, infrared light, windmilling (swinging hands like windmill to force blood to periphery).

13.11 Graft-Versus-Host Disease (GVHD)

▶ **Definition:** Disease following bone marrow transplantation or rarely blood transfusion where immunocompetent donor T cells recognize and attack host antigens.

Acute Graft-Versus-Host Disease

▶ **Epidemiology:** Occurs in 50% of bone marrow transplantation patients.

▶ **Pathogenesis:** The pathophysiology of GVHD is complex; through a variety of mechanisms donor T cells initiate processes damaging host tissue. GVHD is the greatest threat to the recipient. Even with highly improved matching techniques and many new avenues of immunosuppression, the problem persists. Prophylaxis measures include more refined tissue matching, treating graft material with anti-T-cell serum, specific monoclonal antibodies or mechanical measures to eliminate T cells, and modifying the immunosuppression regimens with immune modulators (cyclosporine, tacrolimus, pimecrolimus).

▶ **Clinical features:**
- Starts 1–5 weeks after procedure; occurs in 30–60% with a mortality of 10–15%.
- Most commonly affects gastrointestinal tract (diarrhea) and liver (elevated enzymes, decreased function, rarely failure).
- *Skin:*
  – Initially pruritus and tender skin; then macular exanthem favoring flexures, especially axilla.
  – Can progress to widespread skin loss.

▶ **Histology:** Sick epidermis, atrophy, vacuolar degeneration, apoptosis of keratinocytes; expression of HLA-DR on keratinocytes may precede morphologic changes.

▶ **Diagnostic approach:** Skin biopsy usually done, but diagnostic only in advanced disease. Early GVHD is very similar to drug reaction microscopically.

▶ **Differential diagnosis:** The usual clinical question is a drug reaction; many patients have received pre-transplant radiation or chemotherapy, further confusing the issue. When severe, resembles toxic epidermal necrolysis.

▶ **Therapy:** Mainstay is modifying immunosuppressive regimen, usually increasing corticosteroid dosage, or adding methotrexate.

Chronic Graft-Versus-Host Disease

▶ **Epidemiology:** Occurs in about 10% of patients; by definition >100 days after transplantation.

▶ **Clinical features:**
- *Skin:* Two basic patterns:
  - Sclerotic lesions, often with hypopigmentation; resembling morphea.
  - Lichenoid exanthem, similar to lichen planus, later more diffuse sclerosis and poikiloderma, with worse prognosis.
- *Systemic involvement:* includes liver, gastrointestinal tract, and also lungs with bronchiolitis obliterans.

▶ **Histology:** Either sclerosis or lichenoid infiltrate.

▶ **Diagnostic approach:** Usually clinically obvious because of past history.

▶ **Differential diagnosis:** Pseudoscleroderma (p. 222) or lichen planus and lichenoid drug reactions for the skin findings.

▶ **Therapy:** Immunosuppressive agents that disrupt activation of donor T cells are in wide use. Common choices include cyclosporine, corticosteroids, tacrolimus, mycophenolate mofetil, and T-cell depletion with monoclonal antibodies. Additional possibilities include bath PUVA for the sclerodermoid changes, thalidomide (initially 200–400 mg daily, then reduce to 100 mg daily), extracorporeal photophoresis, high-dose intravenous immunoglobulins, and anticytokine antibodies such as anti-TNFα.

14 *Autoimmune Bullous Diseases*

14.1 *Classification*

► **Loss of intraepidermal adhesion:**
► **Pemphigus vulgaris with subtypes:**
  • Classic.
  • Pemphigus vegetans (Neumann type, Hallopeau type).
► **Pemphigus foliaceus with subtypes:**
  • *Classic:*
    – Fogo selvagem (endemic variant).
    – Pemphigus erythematosus (Senear–Usher).
  • Paraneoplastic pemphigus.
  • Drug-induced pemphigus.
  • *IgA pemphigus:*
    – Subcorneal pustular dermatosis (Sneddon–Wilkinson).
    – Intraepidermal neutrophilic dermatosis.
► **Loss of subepidermal adhesion:**
  • *Pemphigoid:*
    – Bullous pemphigoid.
    – Pemphigoid gestationis.
    – Cicatricial pemphigoid.
    – Other variants.
  • *Linear IgA disease:*
    – Chronic bullous disease of childhood.
    – Adult form.
  • Epidermolysis bullosa acquisita.
  • Dermatitis herpetiformis.

14.2 *Pemphigus Group*

Pemphigus refers to a group of disorders with loss of intraepidermal adhesion because of autoantibodies directed against proteins of the *desmosomal complex* that hold keratinocytes together. The desmosome is a complex structure, with many of its components targets for autoantibodies.

Pemphigus Vulgaris (PV)
....

► **Definition:** Severe, potentially fatal disease with intraepidermal blister formation on skin and mucosa caused by autoantibodies against desmogleins.
► **Epidemiology:** Incidence 0.1–0.5/100 000 yearly, but higher in some ethnic groups. Most patients middle-aged.
► **Pathogenesis:**
  • Genetic predisposition: HLA-DRQ402, -DQ0505.
  • Patients develop antibodies against desmoglein 3 (Dsg3) and later desmoglein 1 (Dsg1) (see Fig. 1.6, p. 6). The bound antibodies activate proteases that damage the desmosome, leading to acantholysis.

- Serum antibody titer usually correlates with severity of disease and course.
  - Occasionally drugs cause pemphigus vulgaris and pemphigus foliaceus. Agents containing sulfhydryl groups (penicillamine, captopril, piroxicam) are more likely to cause pemphigus foliaceus; those without sulfhydryl groups tend to cause pemphigus vulgaris. The latter group includes β-blockers, cephalosporins, penicillin, and rifampicin.
  - ▶ *Note:* Drugs from either group can cause either type of pemphigus.
► **Clinical features:**
  - Sites of predilection include oral mucosa, scalp, face, mechanically stressed areas, nail fold, intertriginous areas (can present as intertrigo).
  - The blisters are not stable, as the epidermis falls apart; therefore, erosions and crusts common (Fig. 14.**1 a,b**).
  - Usually has three stages:
    - *Oral involvement:* In 70% of patients, PV starts in the mouth with painful erosions. Other mucosal surfaces can also be involved. Caused by anti-Dsg3 antibodies, as Dsg3 is the main desmoglein in mucosa.
    - Additional localized disease, often on scalp.
    - ▶ *Note:* Always check the scalp in patients with unexplained oral erosions.
    - Generalized disease because of development of antibodies against Dsg1 which is present in skin along with Dsg3. Painful, poorly healing crusted erosions and ulcers; blisters hard to find. Pruritus uncommon.
► **Histology:** When a fresh lesion is biopsied (small excision, not punch biopsy), acantholysis is seen (free-floating, rounded keratinocytes) with retention of basal layer keratinocytes (tombstone effect) and mild dermal perivascular infiltrates (Fig. 14.**1 c**).
► **Diagnostic approach:**
  - Clinical evaluation; check sites of predilection.
  - *Nikolsky sign:*
    - *True Nikolsky sign:* Gentle rubbing allows one to separate upper layer of epidermis from lower, producing blister or erosion—fairly specific for pemphigus.
    - *Pseudo-Nikolsky sign (Asboe–Hansen sign):* Pressure at edge of blister makes it spread—less specific, seen with many blisters.
  - *Histology:* Can be helpful, but often just erosions or nonspecific changes.
  - *Direct immunofluorescence:* Perilesional skin shows deposition of IgG (100%), C3 (80%) or IgA (<20%), as well C1q in early lesions. Antibodies surround the individual keratinocytes.
  - *Indirect immunofluorescence:* Using monkey esophagus, 90% of sera show positive reaction; titer can be used to monitor disease course.
  - *ELISA:* Can be used to identify anti-Dsg3 with mucosal disease or anti-Dsg1 or anti-Dsg3 with widespread disease.
  - Check for associated diseases, especially thymoma and myasthenia gravis.
► **Differential diagnosis:**
  - When the skin is involved, the question is usually which autoimmune bullous disease. On rare occasions, bullous impetigo, dyskeratotic acantholytic disorders (Darier disease, Hailey–Hailey disease, Grover disease) can cause problems.
  - When only the oral mucosa is involved, the following should be considered:
    - Denture intolerance reactions.
    - *Erosive candidiasis:* Not all oral candidiasis features white plaques (thrush); sometimes atrophy and erosions.
    - *Chronic recurrent aphthae:* Usually smaller lesions with erythematous border but sometimes large, persistent ulcers.

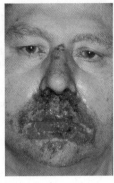
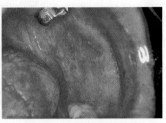
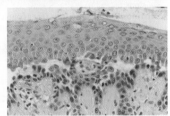

Fig. 14.1 · **Pemphigus vulgaris. a** With marked erosions. **b** With oral ulcerations. **c** Histology showing separation just above the basal layer.

– *Erythema multiforme:* Erosions on lips and mucosa associated with target lesions on skin.
– *Herpetic gingivostomatitis:* Usually in children.
– *Erosive lichen planus:* Look for signs of lichen planus elsewhere; if only in mouth, biopsy and direct immunofluorescence often needed.

▶ **Therapy:**
- Systemic corticosteroids are necessary for long periods of time. The main cause of morbidity and mortality today in patients with pemphigus vulgaris is corticosteroid side-effects. For this reason, corticosteroids are always combined with steroid-sparing agents.
- Patients should be screened for osteoporosis and latent tuberculosis before embarking on long-term corticosteroid therapy. Osteoporosis prophylaxis may be warranted.
- *Combination pulse therapy:* Treatment of choice. Every 3–4weeks, pulse of prednisolone 1.0g daily plus single dose of cyclophosphamide 7.5–15.0mg/kg; in interval cyclophosphamide 1–2 mg/kg daily.
- *Prednisolone-azathioprine therapy:*
  – Start with prednisolone 1.5–2.0mg/kg and azathioprine 2.5mg/kg.
  – Goal is to suppress blister formation within 1 week; if this is not achieved; double the prednisolone dose.
  – Once blister formation is suppressed, logarithmic tapering to maintenance dose of prednisolone 8mg daily and azathioprine 1.5mg/kg daily.
- *Alternative immunosuppressive agents:* Chlorambucil 0.1–0.2mg/kg daily; cyclosporine 5.0–7.5mg/kg daily; mycophenolate mofetil 2.0g daily.

- *Topical measures:* Local anesthetic gels in the mouth before meals may relieve pain and making eating less traumatic; antiseptics and anticandidal measures may also be useful.
- *Therapy-resistant course:* Drastic measures include high-dose intravenous immunoglobulins or column immune absorption of autoantibodies. The immunosuppressive therapy must be continued or a rebound invariably occurs.

Pemphigus Vegetans

▶ **Definition:** Unusual variant of PV with hyperkeratotic verruciform reaction (vegetans).
▶ **Clinical features:** Two forms:
- *Pemphigus vegetans Neumann type:* Originally typical PV, then development of white macerated plaques in involved areas.
- *Pemphigus vegetans Hallopeau type:* Also known as *pyodermite végétante*, limited to intertriginous areas, starts as pustules that evolve into vegetating lesions.

▶ **Histology:** Can be tricky; pseudoepitheliomatous hyperplasia and numerous eosinophils; acantholysis can be hard to find.
▶ **Diagnostic approach:** As for PV.
▶ **Differential diagnosis:** If mild and localized, can be confused with Hailey–Hailey disease.
▶ **Therapy:** See PV.

Pemphigus Foliaceus

▶ **Definition:** Form of pemphigus with superficial blisters caused by autoantibodies against Dsg1.
▶ **Epidemiology:** All age groups affected; not infrequently children.
▶ **Pathogenesis:**
- Autoantibodies against Dsg1, the main desmoglein in the upper epidermis; rarely antibody shift so that they later are formed against Dsg3 and patient develops PV.
- More often drug-induced than PV. Usual agents have sulfhydryl groups such as captopril, penicillamine, and piroxicam.
- May be caused by sunburn or as paraneoplastic sign.

▶ **Clinical features:**
- Sites of predilection include scalp, face, chest, and back (seborrheic areas) with diffuse scale and erosions (Fig. 14.2 a). Can progress to involve large areas (exfoliative erythroderma). Facial rash sometimes butterfly pattern. Oral mucosa usually spared (Dsg1 is scarcely expressed in oral epithelia).
- Individual lesions are slowly developing slack blisters that rupture easily, forming erosions and red-brown crusts.
- Several clinical variants discussed below.

▶ **Histology:** Blister forms in stratum corneum or stratum granulosum; acantholysis rarely seen; usually just a denuded epithelium and sparse dermal perivascular inflammation (Fig. 14.2 b).
▶ **Diagnostic approach:**
- Clinical appearance.
- Skin biopsy often not helpful.
- *Direct* and *indirect immunofluorescence* show superficial deposition of IgG.
- *ELISA* reveals IgG antibodies against Dgs1.

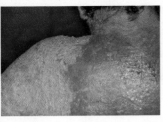 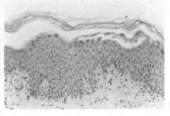

b

Fig. 14.**2** · **Pemphigus foliaceus. a** With diffuse, superficial erosions. **b** Histology showing subcorneal separation.

- *Medication history:* See PV. Agents with sulfhydryl groups most likely to cause pemphigus foliaceus; main actors are captopril, penicillamine, and piroxicam.
▶ **Differential diagnosis:** Frequently misdiagnosed, as blisters are so uncommon. Depending on clinical variant, possibilities include drug reaction, photodermatosis, seborrheic dermatitis, lupus erythematosus.
▶ **Therapy:** Same approach as PV but usually more responsive to therapy. Dapsone may be helpful.

Fogo Selvagem

▶ **Synonyms:** Brazilian pemphigus, South American pemphigus, wildfire pemphigus (fogo selvagem is Portuguese for wildfire).
▶ **Definition:** Endemic form of pemphigus foliaceus.
▶ **Epidemiology:** Found in areas where development is pushing back the jungle in Brazil; transfer of some infectious trigger suspected; common in families; patients usually < 30 years of age; women affected more often.
▶ **Clinical features:** Same as pemphigus foliaceus; burning is a typical feature, perhaps because of less adequate topical care; classic lesion is denuded burning erosion with roll of pushed-back upper epidermis at periphery. Can evolve into erythroderma. No oral involvement. Without therapy, 40% die within 2 years; others develop chronic disease persisting for decades.
▶ **Diagnostic approach:** Same as for pemphigus foliaceus.
▶ **Therapy:** Usually corticosteroids and steroid-sparing agent (azathioprine) suffice; otherwise, regimens as under PV.

Pemphigus Erythematosus

▶ **Synonym:** Senear–Usher syndrome.
▶ **Definition:** Uncommon variant of pemphigus foliaceus with additional features of lupus erythematosus.
▶ **Pathogenesis:** More likely to be triggered by sunlight or medications than other forms of pemphigus foliaceus.
▶ **Clinical features:** Older patients with erythema and crusting in butterfly distribution and seborrheic areas; often eroded.
▶ **Histology:** Superficial acantholysis and blister formation, sometimes vacuolar change in basal layer.
▶ **Diagnostic approach:**
- *Direct immunofluorescence:* Intercellular IgG, sometimes with C3; deposits of IgG, IgM, and C3 at BMZ in 50–70%. IgG and IgM can be found in normal skin.

- ANA positive in 80%; usually homogenous pattern; no specific autoantibodies for lupus erythematosus.
- Check drug history.
► **Therapy:**
- Usually responds to prednisolone 1–2 mg/kg tapered to low maintenance dose; can be combined with antimalarials.
- Meticulous sun avoidance and sunscreens.
- Dapsone also sometimes effective.
- If still not responsive, whole spectrum of agents discussed under PV can be used.

IgA Pemphigus

► **Definition:** Pustular acantholytic dermatosis with intercellular IgA deposition in epidermis.
► **Pathogenesis:** Unknown, but can be associated with gammopathy. Variety of different targets on keratinocyte; most common is desmocollin 1, but also Dsg1 and Dsg3.
► **Clinical features:** Two forms are identified:
- *Subcorneal pustular dermatosis (Sneddon–Wilkinson disease):* Lesions are broad annular erythematous patches with peripheral flaccid pustules and central crusting. Often serpiginous or arciform borders. Favor flexures and trunk; never mouth. Pruritic.
- *Intraepidermal neutrophilic dermatosis (Huff syndrome)* is clinically similar; *sunflower lesions* are considered typical—multiple pustules arranged like a flower.
  ▣ *Note:* There is disagreement whether an idiopathic form of Sneddon–Wilkinson disease with IgA antibodies exists. We feel the disease is IgA pemphigus and that if the antibodies are not found, once must search again in 6–12 months or seek consultation.
► **Histology:** Usually just a pustule is seen; the subcorneal lesions are flaccid, while the deeper ones are more likely to be intact. Acantholysis is often hard to find.
► **Diagnostic approach:** Diagnosis is made on basis of direct immunofluorescence showing only IgA directed against keratinocytes, either superficially or throughout epidermis.
► **Therapy:** Most cases are responsive to dapsone; if not, corticosteroids and immunosuppressive agents can be used, as for other forms of pemphigus.

Paraneoplastic Pemphigus

► **Definition:** Uncommon blistering disease with variety of clinical patterns and target antigens associated with underlying malignancy.
► **Pathogenesis:** Most often associated with lymphoma, leukemia, Castleman tumor, or thymoma; not with squamous cell carcinomas or adenocarcinomas. Presumably there are cross-reactions between tumor antigens and desmosomal antigens such as all the plakins, desmogleins, and even bullous pemphigoid antigen. The anti-Dsg antibodies seem pathogenetically most important; cell-mediated immunity also plays a role.
► **Clinical features:**
- The most constant feature is severe, persistent painful stomatitis extending from the lips into the pharynx, larynx, and esophagus. Conjunctival involvement may lead to blindness.
- The cutaneous changes are polymorphic, ranging from erythematous macules to lichenoid papules to blisters and erosions.

▣ *Note:* If a patient is sick and has lesions resembling erythema multiforme, lichen planus, and a blistering disease, be highly suspicious of paraneoplastic pemphigus.

- Some patients develop bronchiolitis obliterans, which is usually fatal.

▶ **Histology:** The histologic pattern is as variable as the clinical, so it rarely helps in diagnosis.

▶ **Diagnostic approach:** If indirect immunofluorescence is positive on rat bladder epithelium, this strongly suggests paraneoplastic pemphigus, but such a test is negative in 25% of cases. The combination of IgG antibodies against plakins and desmogleins confirms the diagnosis. In about $1/3$ of patients, the underlying tumor is diagnosed after the mucocutaneous disease; "tumor-free" patients deserve a thorough tumor search.

▶ **Differential diagnosis:** Erythema multiforme, lichen planus, PV, cicatricial pemphigoid, chemotherapy-induced stomatitis, persistent herpes simplex infections.

▶ **Therapy:**
- Treating the underlying tumor comes first. The prognosis correlates with the response.
- There is no consensus on what immunosuppressive regimen to employ, especially in those patients required chemotherapy. Recent reports of good success with anti-CD20 antibodies (rituximab).

14.3 *Pemphigoid Group*

Bullous Pemphigoid (BP)

▶ **Definition:** Subepidermal blistering disease caused by autoantibodies to components of the hemidesmosomes in the basement membrane zone (BMZ).

▶ **Epidemiology:** Most common autoimmune bullous disease; incidence around 1/100 000 yearly. Favors elderly, and incidence clearly much higher in older age groups; one estimate 300× more likely at 90 years of age than at 60 years of age. Men more frequently affected (male:female ratio 2:1).

▶ **Pathogenesis:**
- Figure 1.7 (p. 8) shows the components of the basement membrane zone including the hemidesmosome and extracellular proteins, which anchor the epidermis to the dermis. Structural or genetic defects in components of the hemidesmosome, which serves to anchor the epidermis to the dermis, cause epidermolysis bullosa (p. 351); autoantibodies cause BP or other related diseases.
- Autoantibodies are directed against two hemidesmosomal proteins:
  - BP 230 or BP antigen 1 (BPAG1), a 230 kD component of the inner plaque of the hemidesmosome.
  - BP 180 or BP antigen 2 (BPAG2), a 180 kD transmembrane glycoprotein also known as type XVII collagen.
- BP 180 is likely to be more involved in the initial immune response, since it is transmembrane.
- The binding of autoantibodies leads to complement activation, attraction of eosinophils, release of proteases, and separation between the epidermis and dermis.
- Less common causes include drugs (benzodiazepine, furosemide, penicillin, sulfasalazine), sunlight, and ionizing radiation.

► **Clinical features:**

- Before blisters develop, pruritus, dermatitic, and urticarial lesions may be present. The blisters tend to develop in these areas.
- ◪ *Note:* Always keep BP in mind when confronted with an elderly patient with persistent "urticaria."
- Since the entire epidermis is the blister roof, the blisters are very stable. They are tense, often have a fluid level, and can reach 10 cm in diameter (Fig. 14.**3a,b**).
- Oral mucosal involvement in <20%; rarely presenting sign.

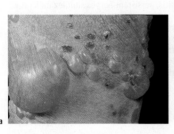
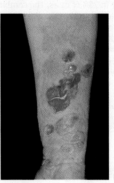

Fig. 14.**3** · **Bullous pemphigoid. a** With large blisters and hemorrhagic crusts. **b** With blisters, erosions, and crusts.

- *Several clinical variants:*
  - *Dyshidrotic BP:* Occasionally starts as acute vesicular dermatitis on palms and soles.
  - *Localized BP:* Limited to one area; typical for disease induced by ionizing radiation, but also occurs spontaneously.
  - *Erythrodermic BP:* Presents as erythroderma, with no previous blisters.
  - *Herpetiform (vesicular) BP:* Clinically mimics dermatitis herpetiformis.
  - *Prurigo nodularis–like BP:* Pruritic lesions with rapid progression into prurigo nodularis; few blisters.
  - *Pemphigoid vegetans:* Vegetating intertriginous lesions; analogous to pemphigus vegetans.
  - *Lichen planus pemphigoides:* Combination of BP and lichen planus (p. 286).

► **Histology:** In the prebullous lesions, the presence of unexpected eosinophils is a good clue. Later subepidermal blister formation. Two forms: a cell-rich form that contains many eosinophils and neutrophils and a cell-poor form with a sparse infiltrate. The lamina lucida remains on the roof of the blister; the lamina densa, on the floor.

► **Diagnostic approach:**

- *Laboratory:* Elevated sed rate, eosinophilia, increased IgE in 60%.
- *Direct immunofluorescence:* Best taken from erythematous area at periphery, not blister itself; band of IgG and C3 along BMZ.
- *Indirect immunofluorescence:* Using NaCl split skin, the autoantibodies usually attach to just the roof of the blister, but can appear on the dermal side or in both locations.

- ELISA identifies antibodies against both BP 230 and BP 180 in 60–80% of patients. Those directed specifically against the NC16 epitope of BP 180 correlate best with disease course.

▶ **Differential diagnosis:** Epidermolysis bullosa acquisita (see below), linear IgA disease (see below), generalized bullous fixed drug reaction, other bullous drug reactions, erythema multiforme, bullous systemic lupus erythematosus.

▶ **Therapy:**
- Mainstay is systemic corticosteroids:
  - Prednisolone 1 mg/kg daily.
  - As soon as control is reached, tapering to maintenance dose of 8 mg daily.
  - Try to taper to alternate-day dosage for adrenal-sparing effect.
- Most widely used steroid-sparing agent is azathioprine; mycophenolate mofetil also appears promising.
- Methotrexate 15–20 mg weekly is also effective; it can be combined with high-potency topical corticosteroids during the 4–6 weeks of induction.
- Some patients do well on high-potency topical corticosteroids; worth a try with localized disease or systemic problems (especially diabetes mellitus).
- Large open blisters and erosions may require topical antiseptics.

Cicatricial Pemphigoid

▶ **Synonyms:** Benign mucous membrane pemphigoid, benign mucosal pemphigoid.
▶ **Definition:** Chronic subepidermal blistering disease favoring mucous membranes, especially mouth and eyes.
▶ **Epidemiology:** Most patients > 65 years of age; women more often affected.
▶ **Pathogenesis:** Poorly understood; several different target antigens—BP 180, BP 230, laminin 5, α6β4 integrin.
  ◘ *Note:* Topical ophthalmologic medications can also cause disease; usually unilateral and resolves when medication is stopped.
▶ **Clinical features:**
- *Conjunctiva:* Affected in 75% of cases; when sole site—*ocular pemphigoid.* Starts unilaterally, within 2 years usually bilateral. Adhesions, ectropion, corneal damage (Fig. 14.4).
  ⚠ *Caution:* The name "benign" is a misnomer—25% of patients lose their vision.
- *Oral mucosa:* Also affected in 75% of cases; vesicles, blisters, erosions, scarring. *Desquamative gingivitis* occurs. Much less painful than PV.
- Esophagus and larynx can also develop strictures, requiring surgery.
- *Genitalia:* In women, narrowing of vaginal orifice; in men, adhesions between glans and foreskin.

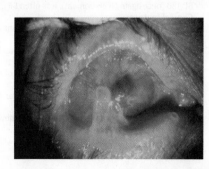

Fig. 14.**4** · Cicatricial pemphigoid with ocular involvement. (Image courtesy of Uwe Pleyer MD Berlin, Germany)

- *Skin:* Only involved in 25 % of cases; usually generalized disease similar to BP. Localized form is known as *Brunsting–Perry disease* with persistent plaques on which recurrent blisters develop.
▶ **Histology:** Subepidermal blister, usually cell-poor.
▶ **Diagnostic approach:**
  - *Direct immunofluorescence:* IgG (60 %) and C3 (40 %) along BMZ in lesional skin, also occasionally IgM and IgA; in normal skin, about 30 % IgG.
  - *Indirect immunofluorescence:* When NaCl split skin is used, IgG reactivity can be seen on either side of the split, or in both locations, depending on target antigen.
  - *Identify target antigens:*
    – BP 180 is most common; patients have mucosal and skin disease.
    – α3 subunit of laminin 5 (formerly known as epiligrin); patients have mucosal and skin disease.
    – α6β4-integrin; these patients have only ocular disease.
▶ **Differential diagnosis:** Bullous pemphigoid, epidermolysis bullosa acquisita, erosive lichen planus, paraneoplastic pemphigus, Stevens–Johnson syndrome.
▶ **Therapy:**
  - Ocular disease: topical or systemic corticosteroids; consultation with ophthalmologist.
  - Mucosal disease: try topical corticosteroids first.
  - *Widespread or resistance disease:*
    – Prednisolone 1–2 mg/kg plus azathioprine 2 mg/kg or prednisolone-cyclophosphamide pulse therapy (p. 231).
    – High-dose intravenous immunoglobulins or immune absorption, maintaining immunosuppression to avoid rebound.
  - Persistent localized lesions: excision and grafting (donor dominance).

Pemphigoid Gestationis

▶ **Synonym:** Herpes gestationis.
▶ **Definition:** Form of BP occurring during pregnancy.
▶ **Epidemiology:**
  - Occurs in 1:10 000–40 000 pregnancies; if same father, high likelihood of recurrence in subsequent pregnancies.
  - No maternal risk; no increase in birth defects, but complications of pregnancy in 15–30 % with 8 % fetal death rate.
▶ **Pathogenesis:** Mothers often HLA-B8, -DR3, or -DR4; father often HLA-DR2. Possible that mothers are sensitized against placental antigens. Target antigens are BP 180 (once again NC16 domain), less often BP 230.
▶ **Clinical features:**
  - Sites of predilection include the protuberant abdomen and extremities; mucosal involvement < 20 %.
  - Grouped stable blisters with pruritus develop in second or third trimester and persist until delivery. Rarely appear postpartum. Resolve within 3 months. Occasionally recur with menses or ingestion of oral contraceptives. Tends to be worse in next pregnancy.
  - ◪ *Note:* If pemphigoid gestationis persists after delivery, a hydatidiform mole or choriocarcinoma must be excluded.
  - The autoantibodies cross the placenta; the newborn can have blisters for a few weeks.
▶ **Histology:** Subepidermal blister, usually with cell-rich pattern.

▶ **Diagnostic approach:**
- *Direct immunofluorescence:* Band of C3 along BMZ; occasionally IgG; all the others uncommon.
- *Indirect immunofluorescence:* The IgG antibodies cannot always be demonstrated directly, but their strong complement-fixing properties allow identification (herpes gestationis factor). On NaCl split skin, the IgG attaches to the blister roof.
- **Laboratory:** Often hypereosinophilia.

▶ **Differential diagnosis:** Papular eruption of pregnancy and other disorders of pregnancy (p. 570).

▶ **Therapy:**
- Topical corticosteroids first; then systemic prednisolone 20–40 mg daily, which should be continued through delivery.
- ⚠ *Caution:* The newborn is at risk of adrenal suppression and must be checked carefully.
- In severe cases, high-dose intravenous immunoglobulins, immune absorption, or cyclosporine.
- Persistence after delivery may be indication for luteinizing hormone-releasing hormone (administered by gynecologist).

Epidermolysis Bullosa Acquisita (EBA)

▶ **Definition:** Subepidermal blistering disease with predilection for areas subject to mechanical forces.

▶ **Epidemiology:** Uncommon disorder, seen in adults in 4th–5th decades; not to be confused with epidermolysis bullosa (p. 351).

▶ **Pathogenesis:** Autoantibodies directed against type VII collagen, a component of the lamina densa.

▶ **Clinical features:** Several different forms:
- *Acral mechanobullous form* closely resembles porphyria cutanea tarda; fragile skin and blisters on backs of hands healing with milia and scarring; nail dystrophy. Foot involvement is clue to EBA.
- *Inflammatory form* is very similar to BP with stable blisters; less often resembles cicatricial pemphigoid or dermatitis herpetiformis; heals with scarring; sometime scarring alopecia. About 50% of patients have mucosal involvement.
- *Associated diseases:* Occasionally seen with inflammatory bowel disease, lupus erythematosus, or rheumatoid arthritis.

▶ **Diagnostic approach:**
- *Direct immunofluorescence:* Deposition of IgG (rarely IgA) in BMZ.
- *Indirect immunofluorescence:* IgG with ability to bind complement found in 50%. Using NaCl split skin, IgG binds to base of blister.
- *ELISA* identifies antibodies against type VII collagen.

▶ **Differential diagnosis:** Before the ability to identify antibodies to type VII collagen, EBA was lost either as BP with negative immunofluorescence or as porphyria cutanea tarda with negative urine studies. Bullous lupus erythematosus also has antibodies to type VII collagen but is clinically quite different (p. 209).

▶ **Therapy:**
- Corticosteroids only effective for the inflammatory form, but not as effective as in pemphigoid. With localized disease, try topical corticosteroids first.
- Prednisolone 60–80 mg daily, combined with azathioprine 1–2 mg/kg daily, cyclosporine 3–5 mg/kg daily or cyclophosphamide 50 mg daily; steroid component tapered as soon as improvement seen.
- Plasmapheresis can help to spare systemic medications.

- Other alternatives include dapsone 100–150 mg daily, colchicine 0.5–1.5 mg daily, high-dose intravenous immunoglobulins.

14.4 Subepidermal IgA-mediated Disorders

Linear IgA Disease of Adults (LAD)

▶ **Definition:** Subepidermal blistering disease caused by deposits of IgA along BMZ.
▶ **Epidemiology:** Uncommon disease; female: male ratio 2:1.
▶ **Pathogenesis:**
  - Multiple target antigens have been identified; issue still unclear. Some stain lamina lucida; others attach to type VII collagen in lamina densa.
  - Several drugs cause LAD; most common is vancomycin but also penicillin, sulfamethoxazole/trimethoprim, vigabatrin.
▶ **Clinical features:** LAD may be identical to dermatitis herpetiformis but without gastrointestinal involvement, or resemble BP or even cicatricial pemphigoid with ocular involvement. Over 50% have mucosal involvement; sometimes limited to these tissues. In adults, chronic disease. Histology corresponds to clinical pattern.
▶ **Diagnostic approach:**
  - IgA antibodies by definition present best seen with direct immunofluorescence.
  - Additional tests should include eye examination and jejunal biopsy to exclude celiac disease (see below).
▶ **Therapy:** Corticosteroids work best for lamina lucida type; dapsone often helpful for lamina densa type.

Linear IgA Disease of Childhood

▶ **Synonym:** Formerly known as chronic bullous disease of childhood.
▶ **Definition:** Most common subepidermal blistering disorder in childhood.
▶ **Epidemiology:** Usually occurs before 5 years of age and resolves spontaneously.
▶ **Pathogenesis:** Most common target antigen is LAD1, a proteolytic fragment of BP 180.
▶ **Clinical features:** Large tense blisters, almost always arranged in rosette fashion with predilection for abdomen, groin, axillae, and face (Fig. 14.5). Also urticarial plaques with peripheral blisters. Mucosal disease very common; as high as 90% in some series. Gastrointestinal disease extremely rare.

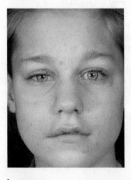

Fig. 14.5 · Linear IgA disease of childhood with periorbital involvement.

▶ **Histology:** Subepidermal blister; usually with inflammatory infiltrate.

▶ **Diagnostic approach:** Obligatory presence of IgA deposits along BMZ identified by direct immunofluorescence in 100% and indirect immunofluorescence (when trying to avoid skin biopsy in child) in 40–70%.

▶ **Differential diagnosis:**

- Bullous pemphigoid also occurs in childhood; usually even earlier. It is clinically identical except for a lower incidence of mucosal involvement and can only be identified with immunofluorescence studies. Treatment is the same.
- Dermatitis herpetiformis only occurs in small children who are heterozygous for predisposing HLA genes.

▶ **Therapy:** Both dapsone (0.5–2.0 mg/kg) and sulfapyridine may be useful. If not, systemic corticosteroids.

14.5 *Dermatitis Herpetiformis*

▶ **Definition:** Pruritic vesicular disease caused by IgA autoantibodies directed against epidermal transglutaminase and presenting with granular pattern in papillary dermis.

▶ **Epidemiology:** Men are affected twice as often women. Disease of young adults.

▶ **Pathogenesis:**

- Dermatitis herpetiformis and gluten-sensitive enteropathy are closely related. They are the result of an abnormal immune response to gluten antigens. Gluten is the main adhesive substance of many grains. The most important sensitizing protein is gliadin, which is the substrate for tissue transglutaminase. Autoantibodies against tissue transglutaminase also cross-react with the similar epidermal transglutaminase, producing dermatitis herpetiformis. The antibodies in dermatitis herpetiformis patients have more affinity for epidermal transglutaminase than do those in patients with gluten-sensitive enteropathy.
- There is a strong HLA association, as 90% of patients are HLA-DQ2 (A1*0501 and B1*02). The other 10% are HLA-DQ8 (A1*03, B1*03). Other genetic factors are involved.
- Rare patients with enteropathy have skin involvement; few patients with skin findings have symptomatic bowel disease, but most have an abnormal bowel biopsy.
- Patients in both groups are at increased risk for B-cell lymphoma of the MALT type.

▶ **Clinical features:**

- Sites of predilection include the knees and elbows (*Cottini type* when limited to these areas), as well as buttocks and upper trunk. Facial involvement rare.
- Hallmark is intensely pruritic or burning tiny vesicles, which are usually scratched away by the time the patient presents (Fig. 14.**6**).
- In undisturbed lesions, there may be a rim of peripheral vesicles arranged in herpetiform fashion. Less often there are larger blisters.
- Occasional signs and symptoms of enteropathy with malabsorption, voluminous loose stools, and weight loss.
- Occasional association with other autoimmune diseases such as diabetes mellitus, pernicious anemia, thyroid disease, and vitiligo.
- Patients often are not able to tolerate iodine and flare with exposures, such as when eating seafood. Iodine challenge or iodine patch test are old diagnostic measures.
- Spontaneous remissions may occur, but disease often lifelong.

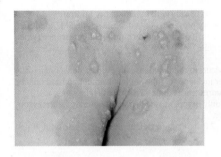

Fig. 14.**6** · Dermatitis herpetiformis.

▶ **Histology:** Neutrophilic microabscesses in the papillary dermis are the hallmark. Often admixed with eosinophils. Edema leads to subepidermal blister formation.

▶ **Diagnostic approach:**
  - Skin biopsy; often hard to obtain fresh lesion.
  - *Direct immunofluorescence:* Granular deposits of IgA in dermal papillae; sometimes granular-linear along BMZ. Present in >95% of patients, also in normal skin (buttocks); persist long after therapy is started.
  - *Indirect immunofluorescence:* IgA antibodies against smooth muscle endomysium (source of tissue transglutaminase) present in 80%.
  - *ELISA* identifies IgA antibodies against tissue transglutaminase in at least 80%; antigliadin antibodies also present, but less specific.
  - *Jejunal biopsy:* flattening of villi (85%) with intraepithelial lymphocytes in 100%.

▶ **Differential diagnosis:** Dermatitis herpetiformis is probably incorrectly invoked as a differential diagnostic consideration more than any other skin disease as it is suspected in anyone with pruritus where there is no obvious cause. Scabies, BP before the development of blisters, and the prurigo group are the main issues.

▶ **Therapy:**
  - The mainstay of therapy is a gluten-free diet (Table 14.**1**), which also protects against gastrointestinal lymphoma. The diet is hard to follow and only takes effect after months, but is essential.

Table 14.1 · **Gluten-free diet**

Forbidden	Allowed
Wheat, rye, barley, oats, spelt	Potatoes, rice, corn, millet, buckwheat, chestnut meal, quinoa, amaranth
Grain products: grits, cream of wheat, wheat germ, oatmeals, and others	Gluten-free binders, potato starch, corn starch, rice flour, soy flour
Commercial breads, cakes, cookies, crackers, pasta	Gluten-free bread and cookies, rice cakes
Malt, coffee substitutes, beer	
Careful with sausage, processed meats or fish, spices, cheeses (gluten binders), cheese substitutes, soups, sauces, puddings	Look for products with gluten-free marking Check www.gluten.net

- Dapsone is amazingly effective; hours to days after the first dose, the pruritus disappears. Usually a low dose of 25–50 mg suffices; for details on usage.

14.6 Overview of Diagnostic Approach

Table 14.2 · Diagnostic criteria for autoimmune bullous diseases

Clinical features	Histology	Direct immuno-fluorescence	Indirect im-munofluores-cence	Target antigens
Pemphigus vulgaris (PV)/pemphigus foliaceus (PF)				
Blisters, erosions on mucosa (PV) and skin (PV,PF)	Suprabasal acantholysis	Intercellular IgG and C3	Intercellular IgG (monkey esophagus)	Dsg3 (PV)[a] Dsg3 (PV,PF)[a]
Paraneoplastic pemphigus				
Hemorrhagic sto-matitis, polymor-phic exanthems	Suprabasal acantholysis with inter-face der-matitis	Intercellular IgG and C3; also IgG and C3 at BMZ	Intercellular IgG (rat bladder)	Plakins Dsg1/Dsg3[a] 170 kD antigen
IgA pemphigus				
Fragile blisters, pustules with ero-sions, crusts	Subcorneal or intra-epidermal neutrophilic abscesses	Intercellular IgA and C3	Intercellular IgA (monkey esophagus) in 50%	Desmocollin 1 Dsg1/Dsg 3[a]
Bullous pemphigoid				
Pruritus, urticarial plaques, large stable blisters	Subepider-mal blister with eosinophils	Linear IgG (IgA) and C3 at BMZ	IgG on epider-mal side of split skin	BP 180[a] BP 230
Pemphigoid gestationis				
Pruritus, urticarial plaques, large stable blisters in pregnancy	Subepider-mal blister with eosinophils	Linear IgG < C3 at BMZ	IgG on epider-mal side of split skin	BP 180[a]

Continued Table 14.2 ▶

Autoimmune Bullous Diseases

Table 14.2 · Continued

Clinical features	Histology	Direct immuno-fluorescence	Indirect im-munofluorescence	Target antigens
Cicatricial pemphigoid				
Oral and ocular blisters, erosions and scars; 25% skin lesions	Subepidermal blister, later atrophy and scarring.	Linear IgG ± IgA ± C3 at BMZ	IgG ± IgA on both sides of split skin	BP180[a] Laminin 5 A6β4 integrin
Linear IgA disease				
Grouped tense blisters, mucosal involvement common	Subepidermal blister with neutrophils	Linear IgA (and C3) at BMZ	IgG on epidermal (sometimes dermal) side of split skin	LAD-1 BP 180[a] BP 230
Epidermolysis bullosa acquisita				
Inflammatory (BP-like) and atrophic (porphyria cutanea tarda-like) variants; mechanobullous; frequent mucosal disease	Subepidermal blister; often with neutrophilic infiltrate	Linear IgG and C3 at BMZ; rarely linear IgA and C3 at BMZ	IgG (or IgA) and C3 on dermal side of split skin	Type VII collagen
Dermatitis herpetiformis				
Pruritic grouped vesicles, usually excoriated	Subepidermal blister, papillary neutrophilic microabscesses	Granular IgA in papillae	IgA directed against endomysium (monkey esophagus)	Transglutaminase[a] Gliadin[a]

BMZ = basement membrane zone; Dsg = desmoglein.
[a] commercially available test systems

15 Purpura and Vasculitis

15.1 Overview

Purpura is the result of red blood cells leaking through vessel walls into the dermis. It can be caused by hematologic abnormalities, increased venous pressure, or vessel damage—*vasculitis*. The causes of vasculitis are multiple, as there are a variety of triggers and several pathological mechanisms. The classification of vasculitis is controversial but we will simply consider those forms primarily seen in the skin as "cutaneous vasculitis" and those with primary systemic findings as "systemic vasculitis."

15.2 Purpura

Classification

▶ **Definition:** Spontaneous small areas of bleeding into the skin. The lesions of purpura consist of *petechiae*, tiny pinpoint areas of bleeding, as well as *ecchymoses*, which are larger (Fig. 15.**1**).

▶ **Purpura secondary to coagulopathies:**
- *Changes in platelet number and function:*
  - *Thrombocytopenia:* Idiopathic thrombocytopenic purpura (ITP) is caused by autoantibodies directed against platelets. Secondary causes include radiation, medications, bone marrow diseases with reduced production, splenomegaly and Kasabach–Merritt syndrome (with increased destruction).
  - *Thrombocythemia:* Too many platelets may also cause purpura; many cases are pre-leukemic.
  - *Platelet dysfunction:* Wiskott–Aldrich syndrome (p. 194) is a good dermatological example.
- *Abnormalities in the coagulation factors:* Disseminated intravascular coagulation (DIC), including purpura fulminans (p. 81).

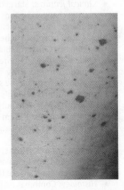

Fig. 15.**1** · Purpura with vasculitis.

► **Purpura secondary to vascular disorders:**
- Vasculitis (palpable purpura).
- Vasculitis with purpura and arthralgias in cryoglobulinemia and cryofibrino-genemia.
- Vascular malformations: hereditary hemorrhagic telangiectasia (Osler–Weber–Rendu disease).
- Increased intravascular pressure: stasis purpura.
- Toxic vessel damage (septic purpura, drug-induced purpura).

► **Purpura secondary to collagen-vascular disorders:**
- Senile purpura (limited to severely actinically damaged skin of arms and face).
- Steroid purpura.
- Several genodermatoses: Pseudoxanthoma elasticum, Marfan syndrome, and Ehlers–Danlos syndrome.

Idiopathic Purpura

☐ *Note:* The idiopathic purpuras are also known as the progressive pigmented purpuras or the purpuric oddities. Their etiology is unclear; some favor a localized form of increased intravascular pressure or other causes of a leaky vessel; others consider them a forme fruste of a lymphocytic vasculitis. The disorders discussed below have frequent overlaps.

► **Progressive pigmented purpuric dermatosis:**
- *Synonym:* Schamberg disease.
- *Epidemiology:* Men are more often affected.
- *Clinical features:*
  - Chronic course.
  - Circumscribed several-centimeter patches, usually on shins, with tiny punctate red-brown hemorrhages at the periphery, often compared to sprinkled cayenne pepper; foci tend to become confluent centrally.
  - Lesions are entirely asymptomatic, but may rarely spread to involve entire limb or even trunk.
- *Histology:* Lymphocytic perivascular infiltrate and hemorrhage.

► **Eczematoid purpura:**
- *Synonyms:* Doucas–Kapetanakis syndrome.
- *Epidemiology:* Men more often affected.
- *Clinical features:* Starts on legs but likely to spread. Foci of purpura with dermatitic changes. Lesions pruritic.
- *Histology:* Purpura, but also scale and spongiosis.

► **Pigmented purpuric lichenoid dermatitis:**
- *Synonyms:* Gougerot–Blum syndrome.
- *Epidemiology:* Men more often affected.
- *Clinical features:* Early lesions similar to Schamberg disease, but lichenoid papules develop on the shins.

► **Purpura anularis telangiectodes:**
- *Synonyms:* Majocchi purpura.
- *Clinical features:* 1–3 cm patches, not limited to the legs, containing both purpuric macules and telangiectases. Chronic course.

► **Lichen aureus:**
- *Clinical features:* Often sharply localized over or near a perforating vein, characteristic gold-brown color, more often seen in younger patients and away from the lower legs than are the other forms. Asymptomatic.
- *Histology:* Combination of purpura and lichenoid infiltrate.

▶ **Differential diagnosis:** Vasculitis, drug-induced purpura, as well as the different forms of pigmented purpura. Overlaps occur; not mutually exclusive. Always exclude chronic venous insufficiency.

▶ **Therapy:** Topical corticosteroids can suppress the occasional itching, but there is no truly effective approach. Most patients require nothing but reassurance.

15.3 Cutaneous Vasculitis

Leukocytoclastic Vasculitis

▶ **Synonyms:** Hypersensitivity angiitis, allergic vasculitis, "palpable purpura".
▶ **Definition:** Inflammation of dermal venules with immune complex deposition and fibrinoid necrosis.
▶ **Epidemiology:** Favors children and young adults; in older patients often drug reaction or reflection of systemic vasculitis.
▶ **Pathogenesis:** The many possible triggers are shown in Table 15.1. Usually immune complexes are formed, then deposited in the venules, where they activate complement and establish an inflammatory reaction that damages the vessel wall.

Table 15.1 · Leukocytoclastic vasculitis: associated diseases and diagnostic procedures

Associated diseases	Diagnostic procedures
Infections: streptococci, tuberculosis, hepatitis B and C	Throat culture, antistreptolysin, chest radiograph, hepatitis serology
Lupus erythematosus, Sjögren syndrome	Antinuclear antibodies, autoantibodies
Rheumatoid arthritis	Rheumatoid factor
Cryoglobulinemia	Cryoglobulins
Gammopathy	Serum protein electrophoresis
Complement defects	CH50, C3, C4
Serum sickness	History: vaccines, anti-thymocyte globulin, streptokinase, immunoglobulins
Systemic vasculitis (Wegener granulomatosis, polyarteritis nodosa)	Look for extracutaneous manifestations.
Drugs	ACE inhibitors, NSAIDs, phenytoin, sulfonamides, thiouracil and many more

▶ **Clinical features:**
- The hallmark of leukocytoclastic vasculitis is purpura. More advanced lesions are often palpable. Other lesions may be urticarial, pustular, or necrotic (Fig. 15.**2a,b**).
- Sites of predilection include the lower legs (100%), arms (15%), mucosa (15%), external ears (10%), and conjunctiva (5%).
- The most common clinical findings are purpura (99%), papules (40%), ulcerations (30%), pustules (20%), urticaria (10%), subcutaneous nodules (10%), and livedo racemosa (<5%).

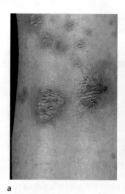 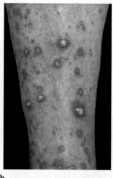

Fig. 15.**2** · **Leukocy-toclastic vasculitis.**
a With necrosis.
b With pustules.

a   b

- **Specific variants:**
  - *Henoch–Schönlein purpura:* Appears primarily in children, purpura associated with gastrointestinal distress and arthralgias; IgA immune complexes in kidneys and skin.
  - *Acute hemorrhagic edema:* Target-like purpura in infant and small children.
- ▶ **Histology:** Necrotic vessel wall with fibrin, nuclear dust (leukocytoclasia), and exocytosis of erythrocytes.
- ▶ **Diagnostic approach:** A biopsy is essential for the diagnosis. Direct immuno-fluorescence studies are often done but rarely affect diagnosis (IgA for Henoch–Schönlein purpura).
- ▶ **Differential diagnosis:** Septic vasculitis (gonorrhea, meningococcemia, candidiasis, many others); livedo vasculitis.
- ⓘ *Caution:* Leukocytoclastic vasculitis is common in Wegener granulomatosis and polyarteritis nodosa; a positive biopsy does not exclude systemic vasculitis.
- ▶ **Therapy:**
  - If acute insult, treat the trigger.
  - Often no therapy is needed; bed rest and compression stockings help.
  - Corticosteroids: prednisolone 60 mg for 3–5 days.
  - If recurrent, dapsone 0.5–2.0 mg/kg daily or colchicine 0.5–1.0 mg daily.

Urticarial Vasculitis

- ▶ **Definition:** Leukocytoclastic vasculitis with urticarial lesions persisting more than 24 hours, systemic signs and symptoms, and often hypocomplementemia.
- ▶ **Epidemiology:** Uncommon.
- ▶ **Pathogenesis:** Can be primary or associated with systemic lupus erythematosus, Sjögren syndrome, cryoglobulinemia, or Wegener granulomatosis.
- ▶ **Clinical features:**
  - The urticarial lesions persist more than 24 hours and resolve, leaving behind hemosiderin, causing red-brown maculae.
  - ▷ *Note:* Even though many patients have hives persisting more than 24 hours, few have urticarial vasculitis with signs and symptoms.
  - Systemic lesions include arthritis, nephritis, and abdominal distress.
  - Pulmonary involvement can be fatal.

▶ **Histology:** Typical hive with edema but also with leukocytoclastic vasculitis. A perivascular lymphocytic infiltrate is not sufficient for the diagnosis.
▶ **Diagnostic approach:** Assuming biopsy is positive:
  ● *Laboratory:*
    – Sed rate, C-reactive protein, serum protein electrophoresis.
    – ANA, autoantibodies (anti-SS-A/Ro; anti-SS-B/LA).
    – Assess complement levels: CH50, C3, C4.
  ● Further evaluation based on signs and symptoms, but can include chest radiograph, pulmonary function testing, renal evaluation.
▶ **Therapy:** Difficult; try antihistamines, NSAIDs, dapsone and antimalarials; if not responsive or with systemic involvement, corticosteroids and perhaps additional immunosuppressive agents.

15.4 *Variants of Cutaneous Vasculitis*

There disorders show leukocytoclastic vasculitis or a variant thereof in their early lesions, although the later well-developed lesions have other clinical and histological features.

Sweet Syndrome

▶ **Definition:** Acute illness with fever, leukocytosis, and erythematous succulent cutaneous plaques.
▶ **Epidemiology:** Female:male ratio 3.5:1, more common in spring and fall.
▶ **Pathogenesis:** In most cases, the cause of Sweet syndrome is unclear but viral or bacterial triggers have long been suspected. Other cases are associated with an underlying malignancies or are drug reactions, particularly to granulocyte colony-stimulating factor (G-CSF). The most common associated malignances are hematologic, usually acute myelogenous leukemia, although solid tumors are also occasionally found. Finally, Sweet syndrome may appear in association with inflammatory disease such as inflammatory bowel disease, rheumatoid arthritis, or even lupus erythematosus.
▶ **Clinical features:**
  ● Prodrome and arthralgias most common in patients with idiopathic Sweet syndrome. Not all patients have fever and leukocytosis.
  ● Succulent plaques, as large as 10–15 cm, with irregular border (*rocky island pattern*); sometimes *illusion of vesiculation*—look vesicular but are solid when pressed; plaques may be dotted with pustules. Leg lesions may resemble panniculitis.
  ● Oral lesions seen in 20%; more common in drug-related: aphthae, erosions.
  ● Uncommon forms include chronic neutrophilic plaques and acute lesions confined to hands.
▶ **Histology:** Distinctive band of subepidermal edema with band-like infiltrate rich in neutrophils. Vasculitis in 30%. Early lesions dominated by lymphocytes. Later nuclear dust and ingestion of neutrophils by macrophages (*bean bag cells*). In some instances, leukemic cells identified in infiltrate.
▶ **Diagnostic approach:** Clinical features, histology; search for underlying tumor, infection, inflammatory disorder or drug exposure.
▶ **Differential diagnosis:** While the juicy plaques are distinctive, other possibilities include leukemic infiltrates, pyoderma gangrenosum, erythema elevatum et diutinum (more chronic), granuloma faciale (more chronic), leukocytoclastic vasculitis, erythema nodosum, and true abscesses.

► **Therapy:**
- Prednisolone 60 mg daily tapered over 2–3 weeks.
- If recurrent, consider methotrexate, clofazimine, or thalidomide.

Erythema Elevatum et Diutinum

► **Synonym:** Extracellular cholesterosis.
► **Definition:** Chronic cutaneous vasculitis with formation of fibrotic plaques.
► **Epidemiology:** Uncommon.
► **Pathogenesis:** Suspicion that streptococci are trigger for chronic immune complex reaction. Occurs in HIV/AIDS but unclear if result of immunosuppression or other factors.
► **Clinical features:** Symmetrical, slowly-developing red-brown papules and nodules favoring backs of hands, over the digital joints and knees and elbows. Rarely more widespread. Usually asymptomatic. Association with IgA monoclonal gammopathy or even multiple myeloma.
► **Histology:** Leukocytoclastic vasculitis with thickening of vessel walls; later fibrosis, granulomatous inflammation, occasional cholesterol deposits.
► **Diagnostic approach:** Skin biopsy; serum protein electrophoresis.
► **Differential diagnosis:** Sweet syndrome far more acute; granuloma faciale looks similar but has a different distribution; early lesions indistinguishable from more usual leukocytoclastic vasculitis.
► **Therapy:**
- Limited disease; intralesional or high-potency topical corticosteroids.
- More widespread or resistant disease: dapsone 0.5–2.0 mg/kg daily.
- Systemic corticosteroids usually disappointing; nicotinamide and tetracycline may help.

Granuloma Faciale

► **Definition:** Chronic form of leukocytoclastic vasculitis causing red-brown facial plaques.
► **Epidemiology:** Uncommon.
► **Pathogenesis:** Unknown, perhaps similar to erythema elevatum et diutinum.
► **Clinical features:** Usually solitary or limited number of red-brown plaques limited to face, typically cheeks, chin, forehead or ears. Occasionally multiple or scattered lesions. Lesions are soft, poorly circumscribed, and asymptomatic, but a cosmetic problem.
► **Histology:** Name is misnomer, as lesion is not a granuloma. Perivascular infiltrate of neutrophils and eosinophils; initially leukocytoclastic vasculitis. Characteristic Grenz zone between normal epidermis and infiltrate. Old name of "eosinophilic granuloma" should be avoided because of confusion with Langerhans cell histiocytosis.
► **Diagnostic approach:** Skin biopsy.
► **Differential diagnosis:** Lupus tumidus, mast cell tumor, xanthogranuloma, sarcoidosis, lymphoma, leukemic infiltrate.
► **Therapy:** Intralesional corticosteroids, laser destruction, cryotherapy. Dapsone 0.5–2.0 mg/kg daily sometimes induces prompt remission.

Pyoderma Gangrenosum

▶ **Definition:** Neutrophilic dermatosis, noninfectious, with rapid tissue destruction.
▶ **Epidemiology:** Uncommon.
▶ **Pathogenesis:** Mechanism still unknown; abnormal neutrophil trafficking and immunologic dysfunction are the best guesses. Association with inflammatory bowel disease, rheumatoid arthritis, and monoclonal gammopathy (usually IgA) is clear; less often associated with lymphomas and leukemias.
▶ **Clinical features:**
  • Ulcer with prominent undermined border and boggy necrotic base (Fig, 15.**3**). Grows rapidly. May start as pustule. Can become extremely large and extend to fat, fascia, or even muscle.
  • Heals with cribriform (sieve-like) scars.
  • Displays *pathergy*: skin trauma (needle stick, insect bite, biopsy) can trigger lesions.
  • Facial pyoderma gangrenosum tends to be more superficial and less destructive.
  • Other variants include peristomal pyoderma gangrenosum and postoperative cutaneous gangrene (*Cullen syndrome*). Important to document in case of future surgeries.
▶ **Histology:** Massive destruction; at periphery neutrophils about vessels, but classic leukocytoclastic vasculitis is rare.
▶ **Diagnostic approach:** Diagnosis of exclusion—culture for bacterial, viral (herpesviruses in immunosuppressed) and deep fungal agents; suspect artifact; skin biopsy also only helps for exclusion; direct immunofluorescence identifies immune deposits but of uncertain utility.
▶ **Differential diagnosis:** Many infections, pemphigus vegetans, brown recluse spider bite, artifact, other forms of vasculitis, calciphylaxis, cryofibrinogenemia, coumarin, heparin necrosis.
▶ **Therapy:**
  • Treat associated disease.
  • Topical therapy usually inadequate; exception is intralesional corticosteroids in early lesions.
  • Systemic corticosteroids are mainstay: prednisolone 1–2 mg/kg daily tapered as healing occurs. The use of systemic corticosteroids makes it even more mandatory to exclude underlying infections.
  • Cyclosporine (and presumably also tacrolimus and pimecrolimus) is amazingly effective, suggesting that T cells play a role in the primary pathogenesis. Usual dose 5–10 mg/kg daily, reduced to half as healing starts but continued for several months.
  • Inhibitors of TNFα are also dramatically effective, even though no role for this cytokine had been expected in pyoderma gangrenosum.

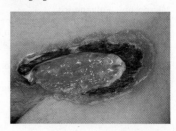

Fig. 15.**3** · Pyoderma gangrenosum.

Other Forms of Cutaneous Vasculitis

► Nodular vasculitis is a form of panniculitis, in some instances caused by *Mycobacterium tuberculosis*, when it is known as *erythema induratum*.
► All of the collagen–vascular diseases can feature vasculitis, but it is very rare for any of them to present with leukocytoclastic vasculitis. A possible exception is childhood dermatomyositis where vasculitis can be the overriding problem.

15.5 Systemic Vasculitis

The current standard Chapel Hill classification is based on the size of vessels most often involved. It fails to do justice to cutaneous vasculitis, but is very useful for understanding larger vessel disease. We have simply divided systemic or medium-sized and large vessel vasculitis into ANCA-associated and non-ANCA diseases.

ANCA-positive Vasculitis

ANCA stands for **a**nti**n**eutrophil **c**ytoplasmic **a**ntibody. ANCA are almost always of pathogenic significance; they are IgG antibodies directed against lysosomal antigens of neutrophils and macrophages. There are two major types:
► **cANCA:** directed against proteinase 3 and most common in Wegener granulomatosis.
► **pANCA:** directed against myeloperoxidase and most common microscopic polyangiitis but also seen in connective tissue vasculitis of various sorts with a wide variety of target antigens (Table 15.**2**).

Table 15.2 · **Associations with ANCA**

Type of vasculitis	cANCA	pANCA
Microscopic polyangiitis	10	60
Wegener granulomatosis	50–90	< 5
Churg-Strauss syndrome	20	20
Henoch-Schönlein purpura	–	< 5
Polyarteritis nodosa	< 5	< 5
Connective tissue diseases	–	20–50

Based on Table 16.9, p. 532 in Fritsch P, *Dermatologie, Venerologie,* 2nd ed, Springer Verlag, Berlin, 2004.

Microscopic Polyangiitis
► **Synonyms:** Pauci-immune vasculitis, microscopic panarteritis.
► **Definition:** Necrotizing vasculitis with few immune deposits, always involving smallest blood vessels but capable of affecting medium-sized vessels and with tropism for kidneys and lungs.
► **Epidemiology:** Much more common than polyarteritis nodosa; perhaps 2–5/100 000 yearly.
► **Pathogenesis:** Unknown; no relation to hepatitis B.

▶ **Clinical features:**
- *General findings:* Fever, weight loss.
- *Skin:* Leukocytoclastic vasculitis (30–40%).
- *Kidneys:* Pauci-immune necrotizing glomerulonephritis with casts (70%).
- *Lungs:* Pulmonary vasculitis with alveolar hemorrhage and hemoptysis (10–15%).

▶ **Diagnostic approach:**
- Skin biopsy doesn't help distinguish from cutaneous leukocytoclastic vasculitis.
- Check kidneys and lungs.
- 60% positive for pANCA.

▶ **Differential diagnosis:**
- *Leukocytoclastic vasculitis:* Confined to skin, no glomerulonephritis.
- *Wegener granulomatosis:* More severe upper airway problems, granulomatous inflammation, cANCA.

▶ **Therapy:** Prednisone and cyclophosphamide, as in polyarteritis nodosa (see below).

Wegener Granulomatosis

▶ **Definition:** Systemic vasculitis with aseptic granulomatous inflammation, primarily involving upper and lower respiratory tract, as well as kidneys.

▶ **Epidemiology:** Incidence 0.3/100000 yearly; USA study: prevalence of 1/25000.

▶ **Pathogenesis:** Unknown; infections have long been suspected as trigger.

▶ **Clinical features:**
- *1st stage:* General signs and symptoms such as fever, malaise coupled with upper airway problems (rhinitis, sinusitis).
- *2nd stage:* Lower airway problems: cough, dyspnea, hemoptysis, pleurisy.
- *3rd stage:* Generalized involvement including skin.
- *Frequency of organ involvement:* Lungs (95%), upper airway (90%), kidneys (85%), joints (70%), eyes (60%), ears (60%), skin (45%), nerves (20%), heart (10%).
- *Skin:* Polymorphic picture including leukocytoclastic vasculitis, urticarial vasculitis, necrotizing pyodermas (mini-pyoderma gangrenosum), panniculitis.

▶ **Histology:** Triad of necrotizing leukocytoclastic vasculitis, necrosis, and granuloma formation. The granulomas can be in the vessel walls or adjacent; they can be palisading (thus microscopically mistaken for granuloma annulare) or rich in giant cells. The necrosis is irregular and often described as "geographic."

▶ **Diagnostic approach:**
- *Tissue diagnosis:* Usually airway or renal biopsy; sometimes skin biopsy helps.
- Investigate upper airways, lungs, and kidneys.
- cANCA positive in 50% during early phases, >90% when generalized.

▶ **Differential diagnosis:**
- *Pulmonary disease:* microscopic polyangiitis, infections.
- *Kidneys:* other causes of glomerulonephritis.
- Destructive upper airway disease: NK/T-cell lymphoma (nasal type), formerly known as lethal midline granuloma.

▶ **Therapy:**
- Before immunosuppressive therapy, the 1 year survival for generalized Wegener granulomatosis was <20%. Now >90% response rates, although many patients are left with organ defects.
- *Fauci regimen:* Prednisone 1 mg/kg daily and cyclophosphamide 2 mg/kg daily. If not responsive, either agent can be increased. Once response occurs, taper predinsone with goal of stopping. Cyclophosphamide is continued for at least 1 year at the standard dose before being slowly tapered.

- Many other immunosuppressive regimens under investigation, such as cyclo-phosphamide induction followed by methotrexate; consult literature.
- Recurrences or localized disease can often be treated with co-trimoxazole; mechanism of action is unclear but enhances speculation about infectious trigger.

Churg–Strauss Syndrome

▶ **Synonym:** Allergic granulomatosis and angiitis.
▶ **Definition:** Systemic vasculitis favoring small vessels with triad of asthma, granulomatous vasculitis of lungs and skin, and eosinophilia of tissues and blood.
▶ **Epidemiology:** Extremely rare; 0.3/100000 yearly; perhaps association with atopy.
▶ **Pathogenesis:** Unknown; speculation about role of leukotriene antagonists in triggering this disorder.
▶ **Clinical features:**
- *Asthma* is present in over 80% and often the presenting symptom, present for years before other features develop.
- Pulmonary infiltrates and vasculitis come later. Nasal and sinus disease is not destructive.
- Transient pulmonary eosinophilic infiltrates occur; resembles Löffler syndrome.
- Multiple other organs involved: mononeuritis multiplex (60%), kidneys (50%), heart (40%), gastrointestinal tract (40%).
- *Skin:* Involved in 70%: purpura, nodules, and urticarial vasculitis.
- *Localized Churg–Strauss granulomas:* Sometimes disease process limited to skin, most often in association with rheumatoid arthritis but also infections, lymphoma, and idiopathic.
▶ **Histology:** Striking palisading granulomas with marked necrosis, both associated with vessels and at a distance, highlighted by marked eosinophilia, nuclear dust ,and giant cells.
▶ **Diagnostic approach:**
- Tissue diagnosis: skin or lung biopsy.
- Investigate lungs and other organs on the basis of signs and symptoms.
- *Laboratory:* Elevated sed rate, hypereosinophilia, elevated IgE, cryoglobulins, immune complexes.
- Both cANCA and p ANCA can be positive; estimated 20% for each.
▶ **Differential diagnosis:**
- *Microscopic polyangiitis:* Pulmonary hemorrhage, no asthma or eosinophilia.
- *Wegener granulomatosis:* Histological overlaps but different pattern of airway involvement.
- *Allergic aspergillosis:* Identify fungus in lungs, positive skin test.
- *Löffler syndrome:* Search for worms, other triggers.
- *Eosinophilic pneumonia:* Impaired pulmonary function, no vasculitis.
▶ **Therapy:**
- Very steroid responsive: initially use prednisolone 1 mg/kg daily.
- Reserve immunosuppressive agents (cyclophosphamide, mycophenolate mofetil, cyclosporine) for treatment failures or life-threatening disease.
- Both IFN-α and intravenous immunoglobulins have shown promise.

Drug-induced ANCA Vasculitis

Many drugs induce the production of ANCA but only a few produce a clinical vasculitis, often with renal disease. Examples include:

► Hematopoietic growth factors (G-CSF, GM-CSF), especially when used in patients with chronic benign neutropenia whose counts then go up as they develop vasculitis. Same factors may cause Sweet syndrome and pyoderma gangrenosum.
► Asthmatic patients receiving leukotriene inhibitors appear at risk of developing Churg–Strauss syndrome.
► Vaccination-induced vasculitis has been described with hepatitis B and influenza immunizations; it remains puzzling, but the risk is not a justification for withholding these vaccines from patients with vasculitis or collagen–vascular disorders.

Polyarteritis Nodosa

► **Synonyms:** Panarteritis nodosa, Kussmaul–Maier disease.
► **Definition:** Necrotizing segmental vasculitis involving small and medium-sized arteries with infarctions.
► **Epidemiology:** Rare; incidence 0.5/100 000 yearly; most commonly affects middle-aged men.
► **Pathogenesis:** Association with hepatitis B; also with HIV/AIDS. Involvement in segmental and favors areas where branching occurs. Small aneurysms frequently develop. Thromboses lead to infracts and vessel-wall obliteration.
► **Clinical features:**
  • *General symptoms:* fever, weight loss, arthralgias.
  • *Skin:* Frequently involved; livedo racemosa, digital gangrene, subcutaneous nodules, ulcers, leukocytoclastic vasculitis.
  • *Cutaneous polyarteritis nodosa:* Disease limited to skin for long periods of time; nodules and ulcers, usually on legs.
  • *Gastrointestinal tract:* "Intestinal angina"—postprandial abdominal pain because of inadequate blood supply; drastic problems include ischemic bowel perforation and mesenteric artery thrombosis or rupture.
  • *Peripheral neuropathy:* Vasculitic neuropathy in up to 80%; involves larger peripheral nerves (mononeuritis multiplex) with sensory and in some instances motor problems.
  • *Kidney:* Almost 100% involvement, but usually subclinical except for hypertension.
  • *Heart:* Can lead to myocardial infarction or congestive heart failure.
  • *CNS:* Risk of strokes, as well as hypertensive changes.
► **Histology:** Segmental involvement makes it hard to find lesions. Initial inflammatory infiltrate is neutrophilic, later replaced by mononuclear cells with intimal proliferation, finally granulomas and fibrosis.
► **Diagnostic approach:**
  • *Histologic confirmation:* Usually skin or muscle biopsy from affected area; blind biopsies, such as testicular biopsy, have low yield.
  • *Imaging:* Angiography can reveal microaneurysms in gastrointestinal or renal arteries.
  • *Laboratory findings:*
    – Few changes considering severity of disease: elevated sed rate, anemia, thrombocytosis, microscopic hematuria.
    – Check for HBsAg positivity.
    – ANCA positive in <5%.

► **Differential diagnosis:**
- *Microscopic polyangiitis:* Glomerulonephritis, alveolar hemorrhage, pANCA).
- *Other forms of vasculitis:* Kawasaki (children, acute picture), Wegener (head and neck, lungs, cANCA), leukocytoclastic vasculitis (little systemic involvement), lupus erythematosus (other skin findings, ANA, autoantibodies).

► **Therapy:**
- Systemic corticosteroids: prednisolone 1 mg/kg daily; can start with pulse therapy 1.0 g daily for 3 days.
- If unresponsive or with major organ involvement, add cyclophosphamide (2 mg/kg daily) or other immunosuppressive agents.
- If patient is HBsAg positive, then start therapy with prednisone and plasma exchanges, followed by IFN and lamivudine—consult hepatology.

Mucocutaneous Lymph Node Syndrome

► **Synonym:** Kawasaki disease.
► **Definition:** Systemic vasculitis in children with acute onset and involvement of coronary arteries.
► **Epidemiology:** 80% of patients < 5 years of age, male:female ratio 1.7:1; incidence 100/100000 yearly in Japan but < 10/100000 in Germany.
► **Pathogenesis:** Infectious agent or superantigen suspected but not proven.
► **Clinical features:** Six main findings present in > 95% (except for cervical lymphadenopathy):
- Unexplained high temperature.
- Bilateral conjunctivitis.
- Oral involvement with pharyngeal erythema and strawberry tongue.
- Maculopapular or urticarial exanthem.
- Acral edema, palmoplantar erythema and then characteristic desquamation of fingertips after 10–14 days.
- Cervical lymphadenopathy (50%).
- *Coronary artery disease:* The real problem is coronary artery inflammation with the formation of aneurysms, occurs in around 20% of untreated patients in week 2–3.

► **Histology:** Nonspecific changes; not diagnostically helpful.
► **Diagnostic approach:**
- Diagnosis certain when five of six features present, or four plus coronary artery disease.
- ⚠ *Caution:* In older children, cardinal signs and symptoms are often missing so life-threatening cardiac disease may be overlooked (*incomplete Kawasaki disease*). Be suspicious.

► **Differential diagnosis:** Scarlet fever, toxic shock syndrome, viral exanthems, Stevens–Johnson syndrome, drug reactions.
► **Therapy:** High-dose intravenous immunoglobulins (single dose 2 mg/kg over 8 hours) plus aspirin 30–40 mg/kg daily until defervescence, then 3–5 mg/kg daily for 2 months. If aneurysms are present, consult with cardiology regarding further anticoagulation and management.

Behçet Syndrome

► **Definition:** Systemic vasculitis with recurrent aphthae, genital ulcerations, and involvement of many other organs.
► **Epidemiology:** Common disease in Middle East and East Asia (*Silk Road disease*); prevalence 1/1000 in Japan; 1/500000 in North America.

▶ **Pathogenesis:** Complex; in Japan strong association with HLA-B51; heat shock proteins (especially HSP60) may be involved in stimulating γδ + T-cell response in susceptible individuals; infectious triggers (streptococci, herpes simplex) also long suspected.

▶ **Clinical features:**
- *Main features:*
  - Recurrent oral aphthae (p. 494), at least 3× in 12 months (100%).
  - Indolent genital ulcers (90%).
  - Chronic recurrent uveitis (50%).
- *Other features:*
  - *Skin:* Erythema nodosum (80%), recurrent thrombophlebitis, pathergy (pustular response at site of trauma).
  - *Large vessel vasculitis:* Pulmonary artery aneurysms (arterial-bronchial fistula formation), aortic aneurysms.
  - *Arthritis and arthralgias:* Favor hands, wrists, ankles, knees.
  - Gastrointestinal ulcers, distal ileum and cecum.
  - *CNS:* Stroke, aseptic meningitis.
  - Kidney disease and peripheral neuropathy rare.
- *MAGIC syndrome:* Overlap between Behçet syndrome and relapsing polychondritis.

▶ **Histology:** Three categories:
- Early lesions show leukocytoclastic infiltrates similar to Sweet syndrome or sometimes leukocytoclastic vasculitis with fibrinoid change.
- Later lesions with lymphocytic or granulomatous inflammation.
- *Aphthae:* Intense neutrophilic infiltrate with necrosis.

▶ **Diagnostic approach:**
- Diagnosis likely with two of the three main symptoms and two additional symptoms.
- No specific laboratory tests; screen for organ involvement.
- *Pathergy test:* Inject 0.1 mL of physiologic NaCl with fine needle on forearm; read after 24–48 hours. Pustule or papule suggests diagnosis; histology shows neutrophilic infiltrate or vasculitis.

▶ **Differential diagnosis:** Long list because of multisystem involvement:
- *Other forms of vasculitis:* None typically have aphthae.
- *Other ocular–oral–genital syndromes:* Erythema multiforme, cicatricial pemphigoid, Reiter syndrome (reactive arthritis), erosive lichen planus.
- *Crohn disease:* Often with aphthae, and bowel changes similar.
- Cyclic neutropenia.
- ◨ *Note:* Do not diagnose Behçet syndrome on the basis of severe aphthae alone.

▶ **Therapy:**
- *Oral and genital lesions:* Topical or intralesional corticosteroids.
- Cyclosporine most effective for uveitis; azathioprine also effective.
- *Other systemic therapy:*
  - Colchicine 0.5–1.5 mg daily.
  - Dapsone 0.5–2.0 mg/kg daily.
  - Corticosteroids ± immunosuppressive agents.
- Each of many systemic complications requires specialized therapy, often in consultation.

15.6 Livedo

▶ **Definition:** Net-like blue-red erythema.
▶ **Pathogenesis:** Livedo results from reduced arteriolar flow and accumulation of deoxygenated blood in venules. There are two forms (Fig. 15.**4**):
  • *Livedo reticularis:* Functional or physiologic, transient; result of vasoconstriction.
  • *Livedo racemosa:* Pathologic, permanent; result of vascular occlusion or malformation.
▶ **Clinical features:**
  • Livedo reticularis more common on legs; if arms or trunk involved, think of livedo racemosa.
  • Livedo reticularis is common:
    – *Transient:* Results from exposure to cold or other triggers; also known as *cutis marmorata.*
    – *Permanent:* Mechanisms poorly understood.
  • Livedo racemosa is persistent, progressive; associated with variety of underlying diseases; always requires investigation (Table 15.**3**).
▶ **Histology:**
  • *Livedo reticularis:* Normal skin.
  • *Livedo racemosa:* Fibrin in vessel wall, thrombi in small vessels, extravasation of erythrocytes.
  ◻ *Note:* The pathological findings are in the arterioles, which are in "normal" skin, not in the blue areas; the choice of biopsy site is extremely important.
▶ **Therapy:**
  • *Livedo reticularis:* None required, or warming.
  • *Livedo racemosa:* Treat associated disease.

Table 15.3 · Diseases associated with livedo racemosa

Inflow impaired (arterial)	Outflow impaired (venous)	Hyperviscosity
Arteriosclerosis	Leukocytoclastic vasculitis	Cryoglobulinemia
Cholesterol emboli	Thrombi	Thrombocytosis
Sneddon syndrome[a]	Emboli	Macroglobulinemia
Arteritis: polyarteritis nodosa, connective tissue disease, thromboangiitis obliterans		Cold agglutinin disease
		Anti-phospholipid syndrome

[a] Subtimal hyperplasia leads to livedo racemosa and a variety of CNS findings (seizures, stroke, hemiparesis, visual loss, speech disturbances).

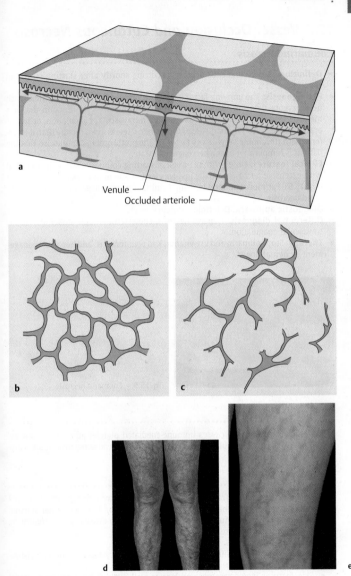

Fig. 15.**4** · **Livedo. a** Anatomic basis of livedo reticularis. **b** Livedo reticularis—regular closed circles. **c** Livedo racemosa—irregular broken arcs. **d** Livedo reticularis. **e** Livedo racemosa.

15.7 Vessel Occlusion and Cutaneous Necrosis

Coumarin Necrosis

▶ **Definition:** Acute cutaneous necrosis occurring shortly after starting coumarin therapy.

▶ **Pathogenesis:** The unifying factor is reduced protein C levels; either those with heterozygous defect or secondary to disorders such as liver dysfunction, diabetes mellitus, postoperative status, disseminated intravascular coagulation, or use of oral contraceptives. Coumarin drops the protein C levels more rapidly than it interferes with the counter-regulatory factors of the prothrombin complex, so that the patient is temporarily in a hypercoagulable state.

▶ **Clinical features:** Onset within 1 week of starting coumarin. Vascular occlusion with extensive necrosis; usually involves fatty tissue of buttocks, breasts, thighs (Fig. 15.5). Far more common in women. Initially hemorrhage, then blisters, then rapid necrosis.

▶ **Diagnostic approach:** Determine protein C levels.

▶ **Differential diagnosis:** Heparin necrosis, cholesterol emboli, disseminated intravascular coagulation.

▶ **Therapy:** Stop coumarin and use vitamin K to counteract it; add heparin; management by hematologist.

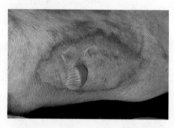

Fig. 15.5 · Coumarin necrosis.

Heparin Necrosis

▶ Extremely rare; heparin causes immune-mediated platelet adherence, clotting, and necrosis. Low molecular weight heparin can thus cause necrosis at sites distant from injection.

Cholesterol Emboli

▶ **Pathogenesis:** Emboli from cholesterol plaques; may develop following endovascular surgery (mechanically dislodged), trauma or 3–8 weeks after starting anticoagulant therapy. Often history of coronary artery disease, aortic aneurysm, or cerebrovascular disease.

▶ **Clinical features:**
• Renal involvement is life-threatening; cholesterol crystals can often be visualized in retinal vessels.
• Skin features livedo racemosa on legs as well as "blue toe syndrome." Pedal pulses usually intact. Necrosis develops promptly. Up to 90% have skin involvement.

▶ **Histology:** Cholesterol crystals or clefts can be seen in vessels.
▶ **Diagnostic approach:** History, clinical examination, biopsy.
▶ **Differential diagnosis:** Exclude other forms of occlusive vascular disease, such as vasculitis, other emboli, thrombi, hyperviscosity syndrome.
▶ **Therapy:** No satisfactory therapy exists.

Fat Emboli

▶ **Pathogenesis:** Small pieces of fat get into circulation either from bone marrow (fractured femur, polytrauma) or fat (trauma, liposuction).
▶ **Clinical features:** Multiple petechiae, favoring axillae and conjunctivae. Variety of systemic signs and symptoms such as fever, confusion, cardiovascular problems.
▶ **Histology:** Cutaneous vessels occluded by particles of fat, along with hemorrhage.
▶ **Therapy:** Heparin, fluids, sometimes systemic corticosteroids.

Calciphylaxis

▶ **Pathogenesis:** Rare effect usually occurring in patients with chronic renal disease, secondary hyperparathyroidism, and elevated calcium and phosphate levels. Media of deep dermal and cutaneous vessels become calcified and then occluded.
▶ **Clinical features:** Livedo changes with extensive necrosis. Other organs such as coronary vessels, lungs, or fatty tissue may also show calcium deposition.
▶ **Histology:** Calcium salt deposits in vessel walls.
▶ **Therapy:** No standard therapeutic approach. Fatality rate $> 50\%$, usually with sepsis. Attempt to lower calcium levels, anticoagulated with heparin; hyperbaric oxygen has shown some promise.

Nicolau Syndrome

▶ Cutaneous necrosis following intramuscular injection. Either medication is injected into an artery or its local irritant effects causes arteriospasm. Livedo reaction with pain, hemorrhage, bullae, and then necrosis. Onset minutes to hours after injection. No good therapy other than standard wound care. Medication can be re-administered at later date without problems.

Extravasation of Chemotherapeutic Agents

▶ Clinically identical to Nicolau syndrome and more common because of widespread use of locally toxic chemotherapy agents such as doxorubicin and daunorubicin. Either medication is administered outside the vein, or vessel leakage occurs. Intense pain, rapid blanching, livedo pattern, and then necrosis. In some instances antidotes are recommended, but in most cases only good wound care is available. Occasionally recall reactions occur; when same medication is administered properly at a different site, the formerly damaged site may flare up.

16 Papulosquamous Disorders

16.1 Psoriasis

Overview

▶ **MIM code:** 177900.
▶ **Definition:** A chronic recurrent dermatosis characterized by a T cell-mediated inflammatory reaction and subsequent epidermal hyperproliferation.
▶ **Epidemiology:**
  • 1–3% of individuals in Western Europe and USA affected.
  • Incidence varies between different ethnic groups and geographic locations.
  • Female:male ratio is 1:1.
▶ **Pathogenesis:**
  • *Genetics:* Polygenic inheritance with variable penetrance. Two types can be identified:
    – *Type I psoriasis:* Onset < 40 years of age, with positive family history and association with HLA-Cw6, -B13, -B57, -DR7.
    – *Type II psoriasis:* Onset > 40 years, sporadic, no HLA associations.
  • The sequence of events is unclear. The initial reaction is possibly an intrinsic defect of keratinocytes with increased cytokine production which leads to expansion of CD45RO+ T cells with resultant production of type 1 cytokines. Sequelae include epidermal proliferation, migration of neutrophils into the epidermis, proliferation of vessels in papillary dermis.
  • Known triggers include streptococcal infections, medications (angiotensin converting enzyme [ACE] antagonists, β-blockers, antimalarials, gold, interferons, lithium, some oral contraceptives), alcoholism, stress, nonspecific skin injury.
  • *Köbner phenomenon:*
    – Minor skin damage or injury can lead to the development of psoriasis in the lesion (isomorphic response).
    – Systemic factors must play a role as the Köbner phenomenon can occur anywhere on skin, but is far more likely to develop during a time when psoriasis is on the upsurge than when it is stable or resolving.
    ▷ *Note:* Köbner phenomenon is not restricted psoriasis; it may occur with lichen planus, vitiligo, and many other diseases..
▶ **Classification:**
  • *Psoriasis vulgaris:*
    – Chronic stable, plaque-type psoriasis.
    – Guttate psoriasis.
    – Inverse psoriasis.
  • *Psoriatic erythroderma.*
  • *Pustular psoriasis.*
    – Palmoplantar pustular psoriasis (Barber–Königsbeck).
    – Acrodermatitis continua suppurativa (Hallopeau).
    – Generalized pustular psoriasis (von Zumbusch).
    – Annular pustular psoriasis.
    – Impetigo herpetiformis (pustular psoriasis in pregnancy).
  • *Drug-induced psoriasis and psoriasiform drug reactions.*
  • *Psoriatic nail disease.*
  • *Psoriatic arthritis.*

Clinical Features

▶ **Sites of predilection:** Include scalp, retroauricular area, knees, elbows, sacrum, nails (Fig. 16.**1**).

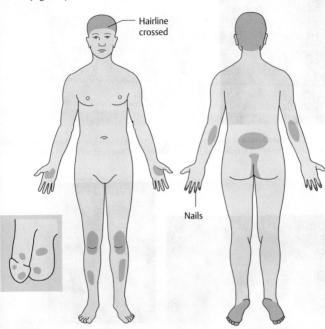

Hairline crossed

Nails

Fig. 16.**1** · Sites of predilection for plague-type psoriasis.

▶ **Lesion morphology:** Sharply bordered erythematous patches and plaques with silvery scale (Fig. 16.**2**).
▶ **Psoriasis vulgaris:**
 • *Chronic plaque-type psoriasis:*
  – Small papules evolve through confluence into large irregular, well-circumscribed plaques, 3–20 cm.
  – *Silvery scale* is extremely typical.
  – Sites of predilection include knees, elbows, sacrum, scalp, retroauricular area (Fig. 16.**3 a**).
  – Untreated, the plaques can remain stable for months or years.
  – May be less distinct in dark skin (Fig. 16.**3 b**).
 • *Guttate psoriasis:*
  – Appears as exanthem over 2–3 weeks; starting with small macules and papules that evolve into 1–2 cm plaques with silvery scale (Fig. 16.**3 c**).
  – Favor the trunk, less often extremities or face.

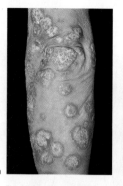
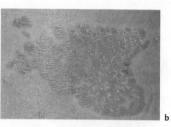

Fig. 16.**2** · **Psoriasis. a** Sharply bordered erythematous plaques with silvery scale—typical of psoriasis. **b** Similar lesions after the scales have been removed with keratolytics.

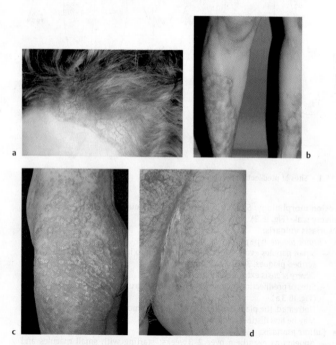

Fig. 16.**3** · **Psoriasis. a** Psoriasis of scalp; note sharp delineation between diseased and normal skin. **b** Psoriasis in dark skin. **c** Guttate psoriasis with transition to psoriatic erythroderma. **d** Inverse psoriasis without scale but with fissures.

- Most patients are children or young adults, usually after a streptococcal pharyngitis; sometimes following treatment or tonsillectomy, the psoriasis resolves completely and never returns.
- Differential diagnosis includes pityriasis lichenoides et varioliformis acuta, pityriasis rosea.

- *Intertriginous psoriasis* (Fig. 16.**3 d**):
  - Involves axillae and groin; often misdiagnosed.
  - Differential diagnosis includes candidiasis and other forms of intertrigo.
  - Macerated and fissured; thick plaques and silvery scale usually missing.
  - Requires less aggressive therapy.
- *Inverse psoriasis:*
  - Overlaps with intertriginous; describes form where involvement is flexural and classical sites such as knees and elbows are spared.

► **Psoriatic erythroderma:**
- Involves the entire integument: can develop suddenly out of a guttate psoriasis, or from a long-standing psoriasis following too aggressive therapy or abrupt discontinuation of medications.
- When confronted with possible psoriatic erythroderma, always think about pityriasis rubra pilaris (p. 278). In erythrodermic form, very hard to separate. Other forms of erythroderma also must be considered (p. 282).

► **Pustular psoriasis:**
- *Palmoplantar pustular psoriasis (Barber–Königsbeck):*
  - Numerous pustules on palms and soles (Fig. 16.**4 a**).
  - Always check for psoriasis elsewhere and in history.
  - Diagnosis confusing—two entities cause trouble:
  - *Palmoplantar pustulosis:* Similar clinically without evidence for psoriasis. Often blamed on foci of infection (pustular bacterid of Andrews) but little proof. Patients tend to be women who smoke; lacks HLA association to psoriasis. Female:male ratio 4:1; average age 30–50 years. We regard this entity as different from psoriasis.
  - *Dyshidrotic dermatitis* (p. 200): Initial lesions are clear vesicles; a form of hand dermatitis; may evolve into pustules.
- *Acrodermatitis continua suppurativa (Hallopeau):* Pustules limited to one or a few fingertips including nail bed. Nail loss not uncommon. Once again relationship to psoriasis controversial, but we view this as localized psoriasis.

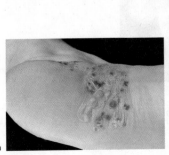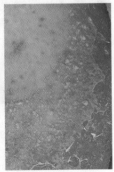

Fig. 16.**4** · **Psoriasis. a** Psoriasis with palmoplantar pustulosis. **b** Annular pustular psoriasis.

- *Generalized pustular psoriasis (von Zumbusch):* Patients with widespread psoriasis and on the verge of erythroderma develop diffuse pustules and are critically ill with fever, chills, and malaise.
- *Annular pustular psoriasis:*
  - 5–30 cm dusky erythematous lesions with peripheral rim of pustules and a collarette scale pointing toward the center (Fig. 16.**4b**).
  - Often associated with psoriasis vulgaris; in other instances, an intermediate stop on the way to erythroderma.
  - Differential diagnosis includes the figurate erythemas (p. 285).
- *Impetigo herpetiformis (pustular psoriasis in pregnancy):* Rare febrile disease of 3rd trimester with annular pustular psoriasis; abnormal calcium metabolism endangers fetus; likely to recur with subsequent pregnancies or oral contraceptives.

▶ **Histology:** Many distinctive features: acanthosis with parakeratosis, lack of stratum granulosum, elongation of rete ridges, dilated tortuous vessels in papillary dermis, dermal lymphocytic infiltrate, exocytosis of neutrophils into epidermis producing spongiform pustules (*Kogoj*), or subcorneal microabscesses (*Munro*).

▶ **Drug-induced psoriasis and psoriasiform drug reactions:**
- Medications are common triggers for psoriasis.
- The following groups can cause problems:
  - β-Blockers: mechanism well-understood; block the β_2 adrenergic receptors of keratinocytes, elevating cAMP, which increases cell proliferation. If a psoriatic patient needs a β-blocker, try to use a more cardiac-selective β_1 adrenergic blocker.
  - ACE inhibitors; use angiotensin II antagonists instead.
  - Chloroquine (although risk seems somewhat overrated, as American troops in Viet Nam all took chloroquine and there was not an epidemic of psoriasis).
  - Immunomodulators (various interferons, imiquimod).
  - Lithium salts.

▶ **Psoriatic nail disease:** Valuable diagnostic clues (Fig. 16.**5**):
- *Dorsal nail matrix:* Pitting of nail plate.
- *Ventral nail matrix:* Onycholysis, oil spots (greasy dark stain; preonycholysis), distal subungual debris, red spots on lunula.

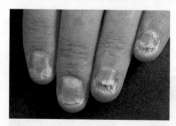

Fig. 16.5 · **Psoriasis.** Psoriatic nail changes.

Diagnosis and Differential Diagnosis

▶ **Diagnostic approach:**
- The diagnosis of psoriasis can usually be made clinically with ease; the problem is therapy.

■ *Note:* If you suspect the diagnosis of psoriasis, always check the gluteal cleft, scalp, and nails for typical changes.

▶ **Difficulties in diagnosis:**
- Treated lesions (loss of scale or redness).
- Early or eruptive lesions (no scale has developed, smaller lesions).

▶ **Skin biopsy:** Not as helpful as it sounds, because classic lesions are rarely biopsied, and clinically difficult lesions often puzzle microscopists.

▶ **Psoriasis Area and Severity Index** (PASI): An widely used system to assess the severity of psoriasis. It is extremely useful in following individual patients and in clinical studies.
- The body is divided into four segments: head (H), trunk (T), upper extremities (U), and lower extremities (L), which are weighted based on percentage of body surface area: H = 0.1, T = 0.3, U = 0.2, L = 0.4.
- The area involved (A) is then assessed for each segment: 0 = none, 1 = < 10%, 2 = 10–30%, 3 = 30–50%, 4 = 50–70%, 5 = 70–90%, 6 = 90–100%.
- To assess severity (S), a four-point scale is used: 0 = no symptoms, 1 = sight symptoms, 2 = moderate symptoms, 3 = marked symptoms, 4 = very marked symptoms. The points erythema (E), infiltration (I), and desquamation (D) are assessed.
- The regional scores are calculated and then summed as follows:
- $PASI = 0.1 (E_H + I_H + D_H) A_H + 0.3 (E_T + I_T + D_T) A_T.$
- $+ 0.2 (E_U + I_U + D_U) A_U + 0.1 (E_L + I_L + D_L) A_L.$
- A sample PASI calculation with maximum involvement and severity in shown in Table 16.**1**. The score can range from 0 to 72, moving in 0.1 increments.

Table 16.1 · Sample PASI calculation

Region	Surface area	Erythema	Infiltration	Desquamation	Area of involvement	Regional score
Head	0.1	4	4	4	6	7.2
Trunk	0.3	4	4	4	6	21.6
Arms	0.2	4	4	4	6	14.4
Legs	0.4	4	4	4	6	28.8
PASI						72

▶ **Differential diagnosis:**
- Considerations include tinea, contact dermatitis, nummular dermatitis. Secondary syphilis can be psoriasiform clinically; it is always so under the microscope. Acute cases resemble pityriasis lichenoides et varioliformis acuta and pityriasis rosea.
- The distinction between psoriasis and seborrheic dermatitis can be extremely difficult. In HIV/AIDS, the two appear to overlap with Reiter syndrome.
- Pityriasis rubra pilaris is another diagnostic challenge; if palms and soles are prominently involved, if there are areas of sparing, or if things just don't fit with psoriasis, always think of pityriasis rubra pilaris.
- Always take a drug history; many drug reactions are psoriasiform, and in some instances lead to true psoriasis in susceptible hosts.

Basic Aspects of Therapy

▶ An overview of the many topical and systemic measures available for psoriasis and how we tend to employ them is shown in Table 16.**2**.

Table 16.2 · Treatment of psoriasis

Type of psoriasis	Therapy	Comments
Psoriasis vulgaris	Anthralin Vitamin D analogues Retinoids (topical, systemic) UVB 311 nm narrow band PUVA	For more severe disease: Biologicals Cyclosporine Fumaric acid Methotrexate
Psoriatic erythroderma	Biologicals Cyclosporine A Methotrexate	Low doses can be combined; treat "gently"
Pustular psoriasis	Retinoids (systemic) Cyclosporine A Methotrexate	Every case is a special case! Stop smoking!
Drug-induced psoriasis	Stop medication; find suit- able alternatives	If needed, treat as above with standard measures.
Psoriatic arthritis	NSAIDs Methotrexate Cyclosporine	Biologicals (TNF-α antago- nists)

▶ The choice of which mediation to use must always be based on the age, sex, social setting, and ability of the patient to apply topical medications or travel for light therapy, as well as on contradictions.

▣ *Note:* The social and psychological implications of psoriasis are almost impossible to overemphasize. Always be aware of how much the patients are disturbed by their disease, and seek help and support where available.

▶ It is important to adjust the treatment of psoriasis to fit the changing physical findings. Experience is the best teacher in this respect, but Table 16.**3** provides a few suggestions.

Table 16.3 · Psoriasis: therapeutic implications of clinico-pathologic findings

Clinical finding	Pathologic correlate	Therapy
Scales	Hyperkeratosis Parakeratosis	Keratolytics Emollients
Thickness	Acanthosis (psoriasiform hyperplasia)	Anthralin Topical corticosteroids Vitamin D analogues Phototherapy
Erythema	Dilated vessels Lymphocytic infiltrates	Topical corticosteroids Cyclosporine Fumaric acid Biologicals
Pustules	Collections of neutrophils in epidermis	Retinoids Methotrexate

Topical Therapy

► **Salicylic acid:**
  - 2–5% salicylic acid is a useful keratolytic to remove scales. It facilitates all other topical measures. Concentrations up to 20% may be used on the palms and soles.
  - ⚠ *Caution:* Salicylic acid can be irritating and then induce new lesions (Köbner phenomenon). It should not be used over wide areas in children because of the risk of systemic resorption and side effects (salicylism and nephrotoxicity).
► **Anthralin:** The keystone for most topical regimens. It requires a well-trained, compliant patient and is easier to use in in-patients than outpatients. It can easily be combined with phototherapy (Ingram regimen).
► **Vitamin D analogues:** Most widely available are calcipotriol and tacalcitol; they are most useful for small areas of moderate psoriasis. Roughly as effective as mid-potency corticosteroid, with fewer side effects. Combination products containing both vitamin D analogues and corticosteroids are available, but costs limit their use on widespread disease; also, they can potentially effect calcium metabolism.
► **Retinoids:** Tazarotene is effective in moderate psoriasis, with few irritating effects. The other more widely available retinoids are less well suited for psoriasis.
► **Corticosteroids:** Useful for small areas, on scalp and in inverse psoriasis; simple for patient to use; available in many forms (creams, ointments, lotions); can be combined with occlusion.
  - ⚠ *Caution:* Long-term widespread use of potent topical corticosteroids can lead to adrenal suppression and cushingoid effects. The most important side effect is cutaneous atrophy (p. 596). When discontinued, there is often a rebound effect. On the scalp, steroid side effects simply don't occur, so high-potency products should be used.
► **UVB 311 narrow band light (TL01):** Relatively long wavelength UVB has good penetration and has both anti-inflammatory (induces apoptosis of immune cells) and antiproliferative effects. The more carcinogenic shorter wavelength UVB is avoided. Suitable for all forms of psoriasis except pustular psoriasis.
► **Balneophototherapy:** Combination of selective ultraviolet phototherapy (SUP) (305–325 nm) with prior bath in 5–10% table salt or solution simulating ocean water. Based on climatotherapy regimens at Dead Sea and other health spas. Because the Dead Sea is 400 meters below sea level, UVB is increasingly absorbed, so the radiant light is dominated by UVA.
► **PUVA (psoralens and UVA) (p. 607):**
  - PUVA is well-established for severe forms of psoriasis.
  - In young patients, be aware of increased lifetime risk for skin cancers and increased photodamage.
  - Systemic PUVA has been to a great extent replaced in Germany by bath PUVA, which is simpler to use and just as effective. Both widespread and pustular psoriasis respond well.

Systemic Therapy

▶ *Note:* Systemic therapy is very attractive to patients. Just try smearing your body with any cream or ointment 2–3 times a daily for a weekend and you will appreciate what psoriatic patients go through for a lifetime. It is little wonder they invariably ask about and prefer systemic therapy. Fortunately many options are available.
► **Fumaric acid:**
  - Fumaric acid esters are helpful in all forms of psoriasis and have been successfully used for moderate to severe disease. They can be tried for therapy-re-

sistant forms, such as severe scalp psoriasis, pustular psoriasis, inverse psoriasis and even psoriatic arthritis.
- The standard product in Germany is Fumaderm — a combination of fumaric acid esters, available as Fumaderm Initial and Fumaderm. The main component is dimethyl fumarate, with either 30 mg or 120 mg in the respective forms.
- The exact details for administering fumaric acid esters as Fumaderm are outlined in Chapter 42 (p. 634).
- The clinical response is slow and first comes as the dosage is slowly increased. Although almost all patients have a drop in lymphocyte count, they do not have an increased susceptibility to infections.

🔃 Always warn the patient that a response may take as long as two months. Such a warning avoids much disappointment and explaining later on.
- Its advantages are effectiveness and a lack of cumulative toxicity. The disadvantages are flushing and gastrointestinal side effects, which can be reduced with the following therapy plan.

🔃 If gastrointestinal problems appear when the dosage is increased, go back to the previously tolerated dosage until all problems resolve, then attempt once again to increase dosage.

► **Methotrexate** (p. 629):
- Methotrexate is the most widely used disease-modifying agent for both psoriasis and psoriatic arthritis. Dermatologists initially used methotrexate for psoriasis in dosages high enough to completely control disease (24–45 mg/ weekly) and encountered many side effects. Rheumatologists started with much lower dosages (7.5–15 mg / weekly with a maximum of 25 mg /weekly) and noticed that both joints and skin improved.
- The usual form of administration is the Weinstein regimen, designed to adjust timing of methotrexate dose to decreased keratinocyte cell cycle time in psoriasis and at the same time reduce toxicity. The drug is given in three divided dosages at 12-hour intervals once a week; in other words, perhaps 5 mg Saturday evening, 5 mg Sunday morning, and 5 mg Sunday evening.
- Today most experienced dermatologists in USA view methotrexate as the most effective form of systemic therapy. Nonetheless, it is clearly more toxic than fumaric acid esters. The organ of most concern is the liver, but hepatotoxicity has dropped markedly since lower dosages became standard. Methotrexate is bound to serum proteins; when other medications bind in a competitive manner, higher free concentrations of methotrexate may result with subsequent bone marrow toxicity.

► **Retinoids** (p. 622):
- The most effective retinoid for psoriasis is acitretin.
- Retinoids suppress epidermal proliferation, leading to a reduction in thickness of psoriatic lesions and therefore increasing the effectiveness of other measures, especially phototherapy. Therefore, retinoids are most often used in combination.
- Retinoids have a wide variety of side effects including elevation of serum cholesterol and triglycerides, triggering of pancreatitis, and musculoskeletal problems, as well as inevitable skin and mucosal dryness.
- They are potent teratogens and cannot be used in women capable of childbearing without undue precaution.
- Photosensitization is a common side effect, but may also explain partially the efficacy of such combination therapy. In any event, it must be closely monitored.

► **Cyclosporine** (p. 628):
- Cyclosporine is highly effective for psoriasis and capable of perhaps inducing the most rapid response of any of the systemic agents. Often improvement is seen in a manner of a few days.

- The dramatic effectiveness of cyclosporine was the first hard clue pointing to the central role of T cells in psoriasis and triggering the many investigative efforts that made possible the host of biological agents that are now available.
- The long-term side effects of cyclosporine are too great to make it a routine drug for psoriasis.

▶ **Biologicals:** These are therapeutic molecules that are specifically targeted in order to imitate or inhibit naturally occurring proteins. The main categories currently used are antibodies and fusion proteins, which either antagonize mediators with a central pro-inflammatory role or interfere with the interactions between T cells and endothelial cells or antigen-presenting cells (APC). Table 16.5 summarizes the biologicals available in Europe for the treatment of psoriasis. The fascinating scientific background, targeting, efficacy, and relative paucity of side

Table 16.4 · Biological agents for psoriasis and psoriatic arthritis

Indications	Dose	75% PASI ↓	Joint response	Side effects
Alefacept				
Moderate to severe psoriasis	7.5 mg i.m. weekly	35% after 14 weeks	55%	↘CD4+ T cells Autoantibodies (2%)
Efalizumab				
Moderate to severe psoriasis	1 mg/kg subq. weekly	36% after 12 weeks	None	Guttate flares during initial treatment; risk of rebound when treatment stopped
Etanercept				
Psoriatic arthritis, rheumatoid arthritis	25–50 mg subq. 2× weekly	35% after 12 weeks	60–70%	Delayed hypersensitivity reaction at injection site Anti ds-DNA antibodies Infections (long-term therapy)
Infliximab				
Psoriatic arthritis, rheumatoid arthritis, Crohn disease, others	5 mg/kg i.v. at weeks 0, 2, and 6	>80% after 10 weeks	~70%	Infusion reactions Autoantibodies (10%) Infections (tuberculosis) Anaphylaxis (<0.1%)

effects are unfortunately balanced by a cost so high as to threaten the best of reimbursement plans.

- *Modifiers of T-cell response:*
  - *Alefacept:* A fusion protein combining LFA-3 (CD58) and the constant region (Fc) of human IgG antibody. The LFA-3 component binds to CD2 on T cells and blocks a costimulatory molecule required for interaction with APC. The antipsoriatic effect comes from the reduction in the number of CD45 RO-memory T cells. The Fc fragment attracts natural killer (NK) cells, which cause apoptosis of these T cells. Since CD2 is highly up-regulated in activated T cells, this important component of the psoriatic pathway is to a large extent eliminated.

    The usual regimen involves a single 7.5 mg i.m. injection once weekly for 12 weeks. Effects can be seen as early as after two injections, but usually peak 6–8 weeks after therapy is concluded. About 40% of patients achieve a PASI reduction of 75%. A rebound flare is not seen. Lymphocyte counts should be monitored.
  - *Efalizumab:* A humanized monoclonal anti-CD11a antibody that blocks the interaction of CD11a (LFA-1) with a variety of molecules. It inhibits both interaction between T cells and APC, as well as the attachment of T cells to endothelium via ICAM-1.

    The usual dosage is 1 mg/kg subq. once weekly for continuous use. The PASI can be expected to drop by about 50% in most patients after 3 months. In these responders the response will continue to improve over time and side effects are remarkably low, even with long-term treatment.

    May be associated with *flares* (papular eruption in previously uninvolved sites), which may sometimes resolve with continuing treatment and in other instances get progressively worse. In the latter case, *rebound* may occur (PASI >125% as compared with status at onset), requiring cyclosporine or TNF antagonists for control.
- *TNF antagonists:* TNF α is the key pro-inflammatory cytokine in psoriasis stimulating keratinocytes and causing T-cell activation. It is produced early in psoriatic inflammation and then induces further pro-inflammatory mediators. Elevated TNFα levels are found in skin lesions, in joint fluid, and systemically in psoriatic patients. Its central role in inflammation has made TNFα an attractive target for blocking inflammation. Two biologicals that inhibit it were first proven effective in rheumatoid arthritis and then employed for both joint and skin manifestations of psoriasis. Both biologicals occasionally induce antibodies to ds-DNA and in rare instances cause a systemic lupus erythematosus-like reaction.
  - *Etanercept:* A fusion protein containing the soluble TNFα receptor protein (p75) and the Fc component of IgG. It binds to circulating TNF and blocks its function. The usual regimen is 25–50 mg subq. 2× weekly for 12 weeks or longer. The joint involvement improves in almost 75% of patients, while the PASI score can be expected to drop by 50%. Injection site reactions can occur, but otherwise well tolerated.
  - *Infliximab:* A chimeric antibody linking a murine anti-TNF monoclonal antibody to human Fc component of IgG. It too blocks TNFα and additionally induces apoptosis in cells with membrane-bound TNF. The usual regimen is 5 mg/kg i.v. in physiologic saline administered at weeks 0, 2, and 6. It can be repeated as required when the skin or joint condition worsens. Within 3 weeks, a mean 50% improvement in PASI can be seen. After 10 weeks, 80% of patients have an improvement of 75% in PASI. Well tolerated.

▶ *Note:* All patients should be checked before therapy for latent or active tuberculosis, for example with skin testing and chest radiograph. Local guidelines for
the diagnosis and monitoring of tuberculosis should be followed. Activation of
tuberculosis may be a problem with both etanercept and infliximab.

16.2 Psoriatic Arthritis

▶ **Epidemiology:**
- 3–5% of psoriatic patients have joint involvement; male:female ratio 1:1.
- ▶ *Note:* The real problem is the 15% of adults with *arthritis sine psoriasis*—that is,
  they have psoriatic arthritis but no skin findings, or skin findings so subtle that a
  rheumatologist overlooks them.

▶ **Clinical features:**
- Three main types of psoriatic arthritis:
  - Mono- or oligoarthritis with muscular or tendon attachment pain (enthesi-
    tis) similar to reactive arthritis (30–50%).
  - Symmetric polyarthritis resembling rheumatoid arthritis (30–50%)
    (Fig. 16.**6**).
  - Axial disease resembling ankylosing spondylitis (< 10%).
- Clinical examination should search for all three types of disease, looking for
  swollen or painful joints. Definite identification of joint fluid is a crucial diag-
  nostic skill. It is unusual to have psoriatic arthritis in a digit with an entirely normal nail.

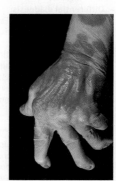

Fig. 16.**6** · Psoriatic arthritis with marked deformities.

▶ **Diagnostic approach:**
- Our scheme for evaluating the hands and feet in patients with psoriatic arthritis
  is shown in Table 16.**5**.
- Develop a standardized radiographic evaluation scheme: both hands and feet in
  two planes, as well as sacrum to assess sacroiliac joints; if clinical and radiographic findings do not agree, then scintigraphy or symptom-directed MRI; repeat in 2 years or with new joint disease.
- *Laboratory evaluation:* ANA, autoantibodies, rheumatoid factor, uric acid; for
  seronegative arthritis without skin changes, check for HLA-B13, -BW57, -B27.

Table 16.5 · Joint evaluation

Digit	Hands								Feet							
	Nails		DIP		PIP		MCP		Nails		DIP		PIP		MCP	
	L	R	L	R	L	R	L	R	L	R	L	R	L	R	L	R
I																
II																
III																
IV																
V																

▶ *Note:* Important clues to diagnose of psoriatic arthritis include:
  – Skin or nail changes of psoriasis.
  – Positive family history of psoriasis.
  – Mono- or oligoarticular involvement at onset.
  – Sausage finger(s): multiple joints on same digit involved, with marked swelling.

▶ **Differential diagnosis:**
  • *Rheumatoid arthritis:* Female:male ratio 3:1, symmetrical involvement of small distal joints, + rheumatoid factor, ↑ sedimentation rate, distinctive radiographic appearance.
  • *Gout:* Female:male ratio 1:7, usually involves single joint (great toe), ↑ serum uric acid, crystals in joint fluid.
  • *Osteoarthritis:* Female:male ratio 10:1, characteristic combination of small joints of hands and feet with larger joints, such as knees, hips, sacrum, and cervical spine, no inflammation, no joint fluid, Heberden nodes, characteristic radiographic picture.

▶ **Therapy:**
  • Mainstay is NSAIDs; COX2 inhibitors are probably best forgotten, although they initially seemed promising.
  • If patients do not experience prompt control with NSAIDs, then consider should be given to disease-modifying agents such as methotrexate. Sulfasalazine has no effect on skin disease or axial skeletal disease, but is a second choice for distal joint disease.
  • The next step is usually TNFα blockers, which first proved their worth in rheumatoid arthritis. Response rates in the neighborhood of 50% are expected, with improvement seen in a matter of weeks.
  • Agents employed for severe psoriasis are also useful, including cyclosporine and retinoids.
  • Physical therapy should be incorporated into the treatment plan at an early point, in order to maximize retention of function. Surgery may be required for severe pain or loss of function. The fear of infection when operating through or near psoriatic plaques is almost certainly overrated, but is a common point of interaction between dermatologists, rheumatologists, and orthopedic surgeons.

16.3 Reiter Syndrome

▶ **Definition:** A form of reactive arthritis often with psoriasiform skin changes, which may be associated with urethritis or conjunctivitis depending on the triggering agent.

▶ **Pathogenesis:** Genetic factors are important, as up to 75% of white patients are HLA-B27 positive; much lower in other ethnic groups; HLA-BW22 or -BW42 may also be involved. Molecular mimicry or bacterial superantigens appear to be involved, as signs and symptoms often develop 1–4 weeks after an infection. Several different clinical settings can be observed:

- *Postdysentery Reiter syndrome*: Causative agents include *Shigella flexneri* (serotype 1b and 2a), *Salmonella typhimurium*, *Yersinia enterocolitica* (serotypes 3 and 9), *Campylobacter jejuni*. Clinical changes begin within weeks of a gastrointestinal infection, which may or may not be symptomatic. Male:female ratio is 1:1.
- *Posturethritis Reiter syndrome* (p. 150): Causative agent *Chlamydia trachomatis* (serotypes D–K). Signs and symptoms start 1–3 weeks after sexual contact, often with a new partner. Men far more often affected.
- *HIV-associated Reiter syndrome:* In advanced HIV infection, appearance of overlapping features of severe psoriatic arthritis and Reiter syndrome.

▶ **Clinical features:**
- *Cardinal features:*
  - *Circinate balanitis*: Annular erosive lesions on glans, often polycyclic with white periphery.
  - *Keratoderma blennorrhagicum*: Pustular and hyperkeratotic lesions on palms and soles, similar to pustular psoriasis. Previously mistakenly associated with gonorrhea.
  - *Other features of psoriasis:* Nail changes, involvement of scalp, knees, elbows.
  - *Oral lesions* (much more common than in psoriasis): Erythema and even ulcerations.
  - *Arthritis:* Asymmetric, favors lower extremities; rheumatoid factor negative. Known as reactive arthritis or seronegative spondyloarthropathy. 10% have ankylosing spondylitis.
- Patients may be ill with fever, chills, and malaise. They may have lumbar or sacral pain. Other features include urethritis or cervicitis (only when *Chlamydia trachomatis* is involved), dysentery (with other triggers), and conjunctivitis or iritis. The conjunctivitis is more common with *Chlamydia trachomatis* triggers and is bilateral. The iritis comes later and is usually unilateral. About 1–2% develop aortitis with aortic valve regurgitation and heart block; usually occurs in those with long-standing arthritis. Reactive (serum amyloid A protein, SAA) amyloidosis and an IgA nephropathy are rarely seen.
- Course usually self-limited, with resolution within 12 months. About 15% relapse; another 15% develop chronic disease.

▶ **Diagnostic approach:**
- The presence of two cardinal symptoms and one other feature should strongly suggest the diagnosis.
- Leukocyte count, sedimentation rate, C-reactive protein all elevated.
- Determination of HLA type may be useful.
- EKG, eye examination, and appropriate joint imaging (including MRI) after rheumatologic evaluation.
- If septic arthritis is suspected, then tap joint and culture fluid.
- Search for causative organisms depending on clinical presentation (dysentery versus urethritis) and exclude HIV infection.

► **Differential diagnosis:**
- *Skin:* Primarily psoriasis, on scalp seborrheic dermatitis.
- *Joints:* Psoriatic arthritis, rheumatoid arthritis, ankylosing spondylitis, septic arthritis.

► **Therapy:**
- If an infection is identified, then treat. Often doxycycline 100 mg b.i.d. is used, even empirically.
- NSAIDS are standard for arthritis; if more severe, systemic corticosteroids (prednisolone 60–100 mg daily until improvement, then taper over 2–4 weeks).
- For chronic arthritis consider methotrexate (15–25 mg weekly) or TNF antagonists (see psoriasis treatment, p. 269). Methotrexate should be used with care in HIV.
- For skin disease, standard psoriasis therapy; if severe, consider acitretin.

16.4 Seborrheic Dermatitis

► **Definition:** Erythematous scaly eruption, usually in areas rich in sebaceous glands.

► **Epidemiology:** Very common; occurs in most infants and in many elderly patients.

► **Pathogenesis:** Two main factors are presence of generous amount of epidermal lipids and colonization, at least transiently by *Malassezia* species (lipophilic, usually nonpathogenic yeasts). Immune response also plays a role; tends to be far more severe in HIV/AIDS. In our view seborrheic dermatitis overlaps with psoriasis and may well be a minimal form of this disorder.

► **Clinical features:**
- Erythematous red-yellow, poorly circumscribed patches with fine scale; only mildly pruritic (Fig. 16.**7**).
- Common sites: scalp (dandruff), eyebrows, perinasal areas, ears, retroauricular area; less often anterior chest; annular or petaloid form most common on neck.

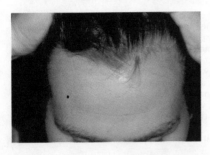

Fig. 16.**7** · Seborrheic dermatitis.

► **Diagnostic approach:** Clinical diagnosis. If severe and acute, think of HIV/AIDS.

► **Differential diagnosis:**
- *Psoriasis:* Lesions better circumscribed, thicker scale (definite overlap).
- *Allergic contact dermatitis:* more pruritic, less chronic. If in doubt, patch testing.
- *Truncal lesions:* Tinea corporis, pityriasis versicolor–do KOH examination.
- Look for atopic stigmata; scalp dermatitis in infants can be atopic, seborrheic, or a combination thereof.

▶ **Therapy:**
- *Medicated shampoos:* Antimycotic forms (ketoconazole or ciclopiroxolamine), zinc pyrithione, selenium sulfide or tar; alternate with regular shampoo. Frequent shampooing helps.
- For cutaneous lesions, either imidazole creams or lithium succinate cream. If refractory, low-potency corticosteroid cream for 2–3 days or topical immuno-modulatory agent (pimecrolimus or tacrolimus).
- Rare patients may benefit from UV light, tar, or low-potency anthralin preparations.

16.5 Pityriasis Amiantacea

▶ **Definition:** Not a disease, but a very uncommon reaction pattern on the scalp, seen with seborrheic dermatitis, psoriasis, contact dermatitis, or atopic dermatitis.
▶ **Pathogenesis:** Reasons for disordered keratinization not understood.
▶ **Clinical features:** Massive white adherent scales on scalp (Fig. 16.**8**); sometimes arranged like roof tiles. The scales are firmly adherent to hairs; bundles of hair frequently accompany them as they are removed.

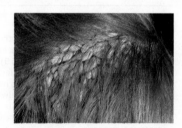

Fig. 16.**8** · Pityriasis amiantacea with thick scales and severe dermatitis.

▶ **Diagnostic approach:** Clinical diagnosis.
▶ **Differential diagnosis:** In children exclude tinea capitis—KOH examination. Look for signs of seborrheic dermatitis, psoriasis, or atopic dermatitis.
▶ **Therapy:**
- The first step is to remove the scales. Apply a 5–10% salicylic acid in a washable base or mixed with a potent corticosteroid cream overnight under shower cap occlusion. In the morning, shampoo using a salicylic acid or tar shampoo. Then apply a corticosteroid lotion. Repeat the process each night until improvement is seen; then cut back on both the frequency and strength of the corticosteroids.
- If an underlying disease can be identified, adjust the treatment to that diagnosis (i.e. tars for psoriasis, less helpful for atopic dermatitis).
- In many instances, the patients are amazingly passive about what must be a distressing condition and do not treat their scalps aggressively. Sometimes a brief stay in the hospital or daycare clinic is useful to insure that they are actually treating themselves.

16.6 *Pityriasis Rubra Pilaris*

▶ **Definition:** Group of uncommon chronic erythematosquamous disorders with palmoplantar hyperkeratosis, follicular papules, and often erythroderma.
▶ **Pathogenesis:** Unknown; increased epidermal turnover but not as severe as in psoriasis. Some suspect infectious origin.
▶ **Classification:** The Griffiths classification is shown in Table 16.**6**.

Table 16.6 · **Classification of pityriasis rubra pilaris**

Form	E	PPK	FK	Spontaneous healing	Recurrences
Classic					
Adult	+	+	+	+	+
Juvenile	+	+	+	(+)	+
Atypical					
Adult	(+)	(+)	(+)	?	?
Juvenile	(+)	(+)	(+)	?	?
Circumscript	–	–	+	+	–

E = erythroderma; FK = follicular keratosis; PPK = palmoplantar keratoderma.

▶ **Clinical features:** Areas of diffuse erythema with fine scale and often weeping; follicular hyperkeratoses, often prominent on backs of fingers; salmon color; often areas of sparing (*nappes claires*, Fig. 16.**9**). Scalp, face, and palmoplantar involvement common; often site of first manifestations. Often provoked by light.
   ◼ *Note:* Pityriasis rubra pilaris is often mistaken for months as psoriasis. If a case of psoriasis just doesn't look right, always think of pityriasis rubra pilaris.
▶ **Histology:** Difficult histologic diagnosis; may have parakeratosis at shoulders of follicles or alternating hyper- and parakeratosis. Neutrophils not prominent, in contrast to psoriasis.
▶ **Diagnostic approach:** Almost entirely a clinical diagnosis; skin biopsy for possible aid. Follicular areas and nappes claires are best clues.

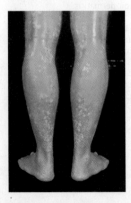

Fig. 16.**9** · Pityriasis rubra pilaris with areas of sparing (nappes claires).

▶ **Differential diagnosis:** Biggest problem is psoriasis; prominent facial involvement or follicular lesions speak against it. Early scalp involvement often mistaken for atopic dermatitis or seborrheic dermatitis. Early diffuse lesions confused with lichen planus, pityriasis lichenoides et varioliformis acuta.

▶ **Therapy:**
- Very difficult to treat; responds poorly to many psoriasis regimens such as PUVA, methotrexate, or anthralin.
- With acute flares, systemic corticosteroids may be useful (prednisolone 60–100 mg tapered rapidly). Introduce retinoids at same time; usually acitretin although some prefer isotretinoin; must use either dosages than in acne.
- Recently we have seen good responses to infliximab.

16.7 Pityriasis Rosea

▶ **Definition:** Acute self-limited erythematosquamous exanthem with classical clinical pattern.

▶ **Epidemiology:** Most patients young adults; male:female ratio 1:1. More common spring and fall; tends to occur in mini-epidemics.

▶ **Pathogenesis:** Viral etiology long suspected, but no single virus convincingly implicated.

▶ **Clinical features:**
- Initial lesion is often large 2–6 cm annular patch with collarette scale (*herald patch*, Fig. 16.**10a**); usually on trunk.
- After 1–2 weeks, typical exanthem with 1–3 cm patches with fine scale (Fig. 16.**10b**), often arranged along skin folds creating *Christmas tree pattern* on back. Typically not found on face or distal extremities. Easily irritated, producing dermatitic appearance.

b

Fig. 16.**10** · **Pityriasis rosea. a** Typical herald patch. **b** Multiple inflamed patches.

- Pruritus rare, unless treated with drying agents.
- Typically resolves spontaneously over 6–12 weeks.
- In blacks, facial and acral involvement common; known as *inverse pityriasis rosea*. More chronic, often pruritic, heals with hypopigmentation.

▶ **Histology:** Microscopic picture not diagnostic; helpful only for differential diagnostic considerations.

▶ **Diagnostic approach:** Almost exclusively a clinical diagnosis; KOH examination and syphilis serology.

▶ **Differential diagnosis:** Herald patch often mistaken for tinea corporis.
  ▣ *Note:* If patient gives history of tinea corporis spreading rapidly under therapy, suspect pityriasis rosea.
  • Diffuse exanthem suggests secondary syphilis, subacute cutaneous lupus erythematosus, guttate psoriasis, pityriasis lichenoides et varioliformis acuta.
▶ **Therapy:**
  • The most important step is to lubricate the skin and avoid drying therapies (frequent washing, antibacterial soaps, lotions, alcohol-based products).
  • On occasion, topical corticosteroids may be used briefly; low to midpotency in emollient base b.i.d.
  • Topical antipruritic agents and systemic antihistamines are rarely needed for the pruritus.

16.8 Small-Patch Parapsoriasis

▶ **Synonyms:** Chronic digitate dermatitis, parapsoriasis *en petites plaques*.
▶ **Definition:** Chronic superficial scaly dermatosis with distinctive clinical pattern and controversial relationship to large-patch parapsoriasis and mycosis fungoides.
▶ **Epidemiology:** Most common in adults >50 but seen in all ages; male:female ratio 5:1.
▶ **Pathogenesis:** Unknown; some consider it related to T-cell lymphoma.
▶ **Clinical features:**
  • Sites of predilection include trunk, upper arms, thighs.
  • Oval poorly circumscribed macules with fine (pityriasiform) scale, often following skin lines. Wrinkled appearance but not truly atrophic. Usually yellow-brown, not red.
  • Lesions are chronic; may be present for decades.
▶ **Histology:** Banal dermatitis with slight spongiosis and mild parakeratosis. Marked interface change suggests large-patch parapsoriasis.
▶ **Diagnostic approach:**
  • Clinical picture, chronicity, and lack of evidence of mycosis fungoides on biopsy.
  • Molecular biology not answer; over 50% have circulating monoclonal T-cell population, but such a clone is rarely found in the skin. Significance unclear.
▶ **Differential diagnosis:**
  • Main question is mycosis fungoides; we believe useful to separate, as so few patients with small-patch parapsoriasis advance to mycosis fungoides.
  • Other possibilities include pityriasis lichenoides chronica, psoriasis, lichenified dermatitis of all type, tinea corporis.
▶ **Therapy:**
  • Usually asymptomatic and no treatment required.
  • Phototherapy is most useful; bath PUVA or narrow-band 311 nm irradiation work best.
  • Topical midpotency corticosteroids can be used for pruritic or inflamed lesions; also emollients containing urea.

16.9 Erythema Multiforme

- **Definition:** Acute self-limited inflammatory reaction with typical target or iris lesions.
- **Epidemiology:** Affects young adults (20–40 years of age) with male dominance.
- **Pathogenesis:** The vast bulk of recurrent cases are triggered by herpes simplex virus (HSV) infections. Immune complexes containing HSV DNA can be found in the lesions. Other triggers include mycoplasma and only rarely drugs.
- **Clinical features (Fig. 16.11a):**
  - The classic lesion is a target lesion (Fig. 16.**11b**) found on the distal extremities. The rings come from:
    - Central dark hemorrhagic zone, which becomes blue-violet.
    - Intermediate white area.
    - Peripheral erythematous ring.

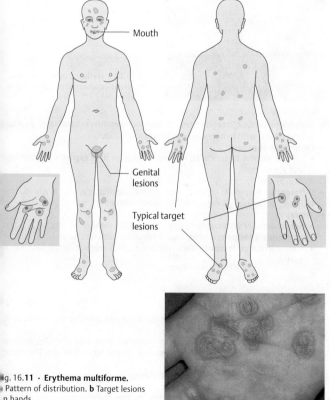

Mouth

Genital lesions

Typical target lesions

a

Fig. 16.**11** · **Erythema multiforme.**
a Pattern of distribution. **b** Target lesions on hands.

b

Papulosquamous Disorders

- ► Typically 1–3 cm in diameter; rarely clinically bullous or urticarial. Heals spontaneously over weeks, sometimes with residual hyperpigmentation.
- ► The presence of a prodrome is often emphasized, but the prodrome is caused by the HSV, mycoplasma, or underlying disease requiring drug therapy. While erythema multiforme can involve the mucosa, in most cases lip involvement is HSV, not erythema multiforme.
- ► The assessment of erythema multiforme is usually straightforward when HSV is the trigger. In the case of other causes, the picture is complicated by a series of other more severe skin findings:
  - *Erythema multiforme-like drug eruption:* Lesions are usually on the trunk, not forming excellent target lesions (Fig. 16.12) and far more likely to progress to Stevens–Johnson syndrome and toxic epidermal necrolysis (p. 184).

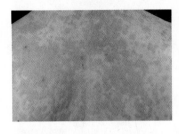

Fig. 16.**12** · Erythema multiforme-like drug eruption which is truncal and lacks target lesions.

- ► **Histology:** Necrotic keratinocytes, vacuolar degeneration in basal layer, papillary dermal edema with lymphocytic perivascular infiltrates.
- ► **Diagnostic approach:**
  - Clinical pattern, history of HSV (often missing) or drug exposure, related signs and symptoms.
  - Skin biopsy.
- ► **Differential diagnosis:** Erythema multiforme-like drug eruption, erythema multiforme-like lupus erythematosus (Rowell syndrome).
- ► **Therapy:**
  - Short course of systemic corticosteroids (prednisolone 60–80 mg for 3–5 days) dramatically shortens course. Topical corticosteroids less helpful.
  - If recurrent, suppressive therapy with antiherpetic medications (p. 615) is most useful.

16.10 Erythroderma

- ► **Definition:** Abnormal redness (erythema) of the skin covering wide areas or the entire skin surface.
- ► **Epidemiology:** Reliable information on incidence is not available. Men are more frequently affected, and mean age of onset is around 50 years of age. Three main causes (Fig. 16.13):
  - Exacerbation of underlying dermatitis (atopic dermatitis, psoriasis, pemphigus foliaceus).
  - *Drug reactions:* Most common drugs include barbiturates, captopril, carbamazepine, cimetidine, NSAIDs, furosemide, sulfonamides, thiazides.
  - Malignancies, including lymphomas and paraneoplastic reactions.

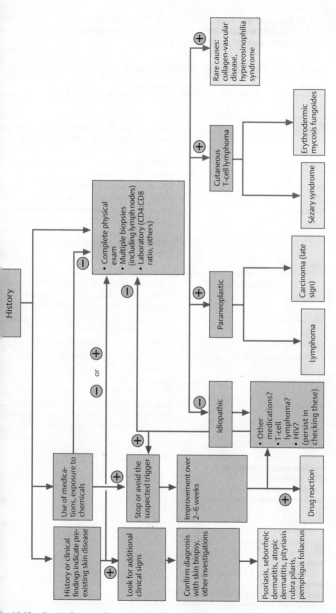

Fig. 16.**13** · Practical approach to patients with erythroderma

- In one large series, the most common causes were dermatitis (24%), psoriasis (20%), drug reactions (19%), cutaneous T-cell lymphoma (8%). Table 16.7 shows possible causes of erythroderma in adults.

Table 16.7 · **Possible causes of erythroderma**

Disease	Comments
Common	
Psoriasis	Usually pre-existing disease, especially pustular; flares likely with discontinuation of corticosteroids or methotrexate
Atopic dermatitis	Intensely pruritic, usually multiple atopic stigmata
Drug reactions	Usually start as morbilliform reaction; can be purpuric; resolves when drug is stopped
Idiopathic	More common in elderly people. Detailed clinical and histological studies reveal no cause; re-examine periodically to exclude cutaneous T-cell lymphoma (also called red man syndrome)
Less common	
Cutaneous T-cell lymphoma	Both Sézary syndrome and erythrodermic mycosis fungoides possible; massive lymphadenopathy; circulating atypical lymphocytes
Pityriasis rubra pilaris	Often starts on hands, scalp; islands of sparing and follicular involvement
Contact dermatitis	Distant spread; history usually clear
Chronic actinic dermatitis	Usually starts on face and neck, intensely pruritic
Paraneoplastic	Usually occurs late in course of solid-organ malignancies; not really a clue to diagnosis
Bullous diseases	Pemphigus foliaceus especially likely to evolve into erythroderma; occurs less often in bullous pemphigoid and paraneoplastic pemphigus
Rare	
Hypereosinophilia syndrome	
Ofuji syndrome	
Crusted scabies	
Severe collagen-vascular disorders	
Lichen planus	
Dermatophyte infections	
Erythroderma in children	
Ichthyoses	
Immunodeficiency syndromes	
Atopic dermatitis	
Staphylococcal scalded skin syndrome	

▣ *Note:* Even after extensive evaluation, the cause of erythroderma remains unclear in about $^1/_3$ of patients.

▶ **Pathogenesis:**
- Erythroderma demonstrates the "systemic signs of cutaneous disease".
- Erythroderma is major medical problem; patients suffer from impaired temperature control (too much skin blood flow) with chills, as well as protein loss (scales) and water loss.
- Problems include edema (ankle, facial), tachycardia, both hyperthermia (increased blood flow) and hypothermia (evaporative cooling). They may develop a enteropathy because of the protein loss. 20% have hepatomegaly.
- Lymphadenopathy is the most common extracutaneous finding and does not always indicate cutaneous T-cell lymphoma. *Dermatopathic lymphadenopathy* as a response to severe cutaneous disease is a well-established clinicopathologic entity.

▶ **Histology:** Microscopic examination is essential, but not always capable of providing the answer. Severe psoriasis may appear similar to severe atopic dermatitis or a drug reaction. Sézary syndrome and mycosis fungoides can, however, usually be identified.

▶ **Diagnostic approach:** The most information is obtained form a detailed history, examination of old records or biopsies, and search for subtle clues to underlying disease.

▶ **Therapy:**
- Initially, good supportive care, fluid management, and attention to secondary infections are essential.
- Systemic corticosteroids are sometimes used empirically with an initial dose of 1–3 mg/kg daily of prednisolone tapered rapidly to 0.5 mg/kg daily.
- Cyclosporine 4–5 mg/kg daily for 3 months as a last resort.
- Topical treatment should be bland.
- Once the erythroderma is resolving, primary treatment for the underlying disease can be started.

16.11 Figurate Erythemas

▶ **Definition:** The figurate erythemas are a group of totally unrelated disorders, having in common only the tendency to form annular or polycyclic lesions (p. 711).

▣ *Note:* The most common figurate diseases are urticaria, tinea, and erythema migrans. Always think of them first.

▶ **Classification:** The figurate erythemas are typically divided into superficial and deep, based clinically on tendency to have scale or not. Some authors regard perivascular cuffing as suggestive of figurate erythema and then histologically divide based on involvement of superficial vascular plexus alone or both the superficial and deep plexuses. These distinctions are not clinically helpful.

- *Erythema annular centrifugum* is the classic figurate erythema. It presents as slowly expanding erythematous rings often with collarette scale. Roughly the same factors that trigger urticaria are implicated in erythema annulare centrifugum. It is usually asymptomatic, but cosmetically disturbing. Most important is search for underlying cause.
- *Erythema gyratum repens* moves more rapidly than erythema annulare centrifugum, has a *woodgrain* pattern and is almost always a sign of underlying malignancy (p. 486).
- *Erythema marginatum* is associated with rheumatic fever (p. 224).

- *Necrolytic migratory erythema*: Marker for glucagonoma; acral and orificial erosions plus figurate erythema (p. 486).
- *Granuloma annulare:* Ring-shaped but rarely polycyclic and extremely slowly expanding (p. 292).
- *Subacute cutaneous lupus erythematosus* is often annular and can evolve into complex patterns (p. 207); *lupus tumidus* is the classic example of a deep figurate erythema.
- *Sjögren syndrome* in Japanese patients often has associated annular erythema.
- Carrier females of x-linked recessive chronic granulomatous disease have an *arcuate erythema*—subtle and very rare.
- Some cases of hereditary angioedema are annular.
- *Acral erythema:* Recurrent eruption in summertime in patients lacking the M component of lactate dehydrogenase.

16.12 Lichenoid Dermatitis

The term lichenoid is confusing; clinically it suggests a disease resembling lichen planus (flat-topped papules, violaceous color) but histologically it refers to a bandlike infiltrate of lymphocytes at the dermoepidermal junction.

Lichen Planus

▶ **Definition:** Common inflammatory disease featuring pruritus, distinctive violaceous flat-topped papules and often oral erosions.

▶ **Epidemiology:** Appears at all ages, but most common between 30–60 years of age.

▶ **Pathogenesis:**
- Infiltrate of Th1 cells and cytotoxic cells → IFN-γ and TNF → expression of HLA-DR8+ adhesion molecules on keratinocytes → basal cell layer damage → reactive hyperkeratosis (model of T-cell-mediated epidermal damage).
- In some countries, especially Italy, association between lichen planus and hepatitis viruses (usually hepatitis C). IFN therapy for hepatitis can trigger lichen planus.
- Eruptions resembling lichen planus are frequently induced by medications (a long list, including pain medications, antibiotics, antiepileptics, chloroquine, quinidine, ACE inhibitors, antituberculosis agents, and hypoglycemic agents and chemicals) and chemicals (most often color film processing materials).

▶ **Clinical features:**
- *Classic skin finings:*
  - Classic lesions are glistening *violaceous flat-topped papules* (Fig. 16.**14 a**), usually 2–10 mm in diameter. Fine lacy white markings on top of papules known as *Wickham striae*. Scratching and trauma induce new lesions: Köbner phenomenon. In exanthematous form, sudden development of widespread disease.
  - Pruritus usually present and sometimes intense.
  - Sites of predilection include inner aspects of wrists, ankles, anterior shins, buttocks.
- *Many cutaneous variants:*
  - *Hypertrophic lichen planus*: Verrucous persistent plaques, especially shins and ankles; painful when on soles.

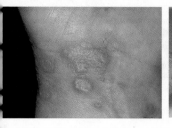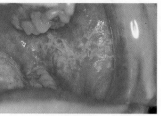

b

Fig. 16.**14** · **Lichen planus. a** Violaceous flat-topped papules. **b** Lacy network on oral mucosa.

- *Lichen planopilaris:* Hyperkeratotic follicular papules, usually on scalp (*Graham–Little syndrome*); infiltrate confined to follicular epithelium; can lead to scarring alopecia (p. 506) and one of precursors of pseudopelade.
- *Linear lichen planus:* Linear grouping of lichen planus papules that cannot be explained by Köbner phenomenon; usually on legs of children.
- *Erosive lichen planus:* Most common on oral mucosa, less often genital mucosa or soles; painful, often chronic erythematous erosions.
- ▣ *Note:* The chronic irritation can lead to development of squamous cell carcinoma, so erosive lichen planus must be monitored closely.
- *Bullous lichen planus:* Sometimes ordinary lesions become bullous because of intensity of dermoepidermal junction damage.
- *Lichen planus pemphigoides:* Combination of lichen planus and bullous pemphigoid (p. 236); separation from bullous lichen planus has been controversial, but now better established. Also triggered by drugs such as captopril, PUVA, and cinnarizine.
- *Atrophic lichen planus:* Atrophic, often hyperpigmented areas, sometimes with violaceous rim.
- *Mucosal findings:*
  - Large lacy white network on buccal mucosa, less often on tongue, lips or labial mucosa (Fig. 16.**14 b**). Painful erosions also present, often on hard palate.
  - Similar reticulate pattern with erosions can be seen on genital mucosa.
- 80–90% clear within 2 years; isolated mucosal disease more likely to be chronic.

▶ **Histology:** Acanthotic epidermis with prominent stratum granulosum and saw tooth pattern of rete ridges; band-like dermal lymphocytic infiltrate that damages basal layer. In drug-induced lichen planus, histologic changes often less pronounced.

▶ **Diagnostic approach:** Clinical features, histology, drug history; depending on local pattern, hepatitis screening.

▶ **Differential diagnosis:**
- *Classic lesions:* Lichenoid drug eruptions, lichen nitidus, secondary syphilis, pityriasis lichenoides et varioliformis acuta, early pityriasis rubra pilaris.
- *Hyperkeratotic lesions:* Lichen simplex chronicus, prurigo nodularis, warts.
- *Linear lesions:* Lichen striatus, linear epidermal nevus, linear psoriasis.
- *Lichen planopilaris:* Early lesions → keratosis pilaris, other follicular keratoses, Darier disease, early pityriasis rubra pilaris. Advanced lesions → lupus erythematosus; other forms of scarring alopecia.
- *Erosive lichen planus:* Oral lesions → lupus erythematosus, autoimmune bullous diseases. Soles → secondary syphilis.

► **Therapy:**
- In most instances, high-potency topical corticosteroids, perhaps under occlusion are most effective. For erosive lichen planus, either corticosteroid solutions or intralesional injections; hypertrophic lesions may also do better with intralesional corticosteroids.
- Systemic corticosteroids is needed for widespread or rapidly spreading disease. Usually 60 mg daily, tapered over 6–8 weeks.
- **⚠ Caution:** Risk of rebound flare is considerable; it is wise to taper slowly, if medically tolerable.
- Other choices include acitretin, antimalarials, and even cyclosporine as a last resort.
- Bath and cream PUVA are promising alternatives; effective and with much less risk of triggering flare than ordinary PUVA.

Lichen Nitidus

► **Definition:** Uncommon dermatosis featuring tiny white papules; considered by some as lichen planus variant.
► **Epidemiology:** Either more common or more easily noticed in blacks.
► **Clinical features:**
- Multiple pinhead-sized glistening white papules, favoring forearms, abdomen, penis, buttocks. May be accompanied by typical lesions of lichen planus.
- Mucosal lesions less common; tiny yellow papules, less often lacy network as in lichen planus.
- Pruritus uncommon.
► **Histology:** Small granulomatous infiltrate just beneath the epidermis, involving only 2–3 rete ridges; very early lesions may have minuscule band-like infiltrate.
► **Diagnostic approach:** Clinical examination, biopsy.
► **Differential diagnosis:** Lichen planus, sarcoidosis, disseminated granuloma annulare, eruptive xanthomas, plane warts.
► **Therapy:** Nothing standard, spontaneous healing occurs; if symptomatic, try topical corticosteroids.

Pityriasis Lichenoides et Varioliformis Acuta

► **Synonyms:** PLEVA, pityriasis lichenoides acuta, Mucha–Habermann disease.
► **Definition:** Acute dermitis with hemorrhagic crusted papules.
► **Epidemiology:** Most patients are children or young adults.
► **Pathogenesis:** Cause unknown, but viral triggers long suspected.
► **Clinical features:** Sudden appearance of red-brown 0.5–3.0 cm papules that rapidly develop hemorrhagic crusts. Sometimes necrotic, ulcerated, and heal with scars. Rarely associated with systemic signs and symptoms.
► **Histology:** Prototype of lymphocytic vasculitis with dense wedge-shaped lichenoid infiltrate and vascular damage in upper dermis.
► **Diagnostic approach:** Clinical examination, biopsy.
► **Differential diagnosis:** Severe varicella, leukocytoclastic vasculitis, secondary syphilis, drug reaction. Some patients with lymphomatoid papulosis (p. 478) clinically have this disorder, but reveal highly atypical CD30 + lymphocytes on biopsy.
► **Therapy:** Often resolves spontaneously. Systemic antibiotics (erythromycin or tetracycline) frequently tried. If symptomatic, consider systemic corticosteroids or PUVA. Exquisitely sensitive to methotrexate but rarely indicated in young patients.

Pityriasis Lichenoides Chronica

▶ **Synonyms:** Parapsoriasis guttata, Juliusberg disease.
▶ **Definition:** Chronic lichenoid dermatitis with persistent scale.
▶ **Pathogenesis:** In some instances, evolves out of PLEVA, but also occurs spontaneously.
▶ **Clinical features:** Flat brown papules, usually on trunk, covered with a sheet of large adherent scale that can be peeled off in one piece; fancifully compared to communion wafers in some countries (Fig. 16.**15**). Lesions symmetrical, often following skin lines. Asymptomatic, but lasts for years or decades.
▶ **Histology:** Hyperkeratotic scale with parakeratosis, modest lichenoid infiltrate.
▶ **Diagnostic approach:** Clinical examination, biopsy.
▶ **Differential diagnosis:** Lichen planus, small-patch parapsoriasis, PLEVA, secondary syphilis, nummular dermatitis.
▶ **Therapy:** Extremely difficult; light is best—either PUVA or SUP. Oral antibiotics can also be tried, but less helpful than with PLEVA. Methotrexate not as effective as in PLEVA and not warranted because of chronic course.

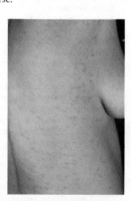

Fig. 16.**15** · Pityriasis lichenoides chronica.

Other Lichenoid Disorders

▶ **Lichen sclerosus** (p. 217): Often has a band-like infiltrate but rarely papules. Closely related to morphea and not to other lichenoid disorders.
▶ **Lichen aureus**: Is a form of pigmented purpura (p. 246) but may have a lichenoid infiltrate.
▶ **Lichen Striatus**.
   • **Definition:** Grouped usually linear lichenoid papules most common in children.
   • **Pathogenesis:** Unknown, most likely inflammatory response in area limited by mosaicism (p. 350).
   • **Clinical Features:** Initially non-distinct erythematous papules whose linear arrangement soon becomes apparent. Typically as linear band down leg. Usually self-limited with spontaneous regression.
   • **Histology:** Subacute dermatitis with scattered dyskeratotic cells in epidermis and dermal lymphocytic infiltrate without lichenoid pattern.
   • **Differential Diagnosis:** Linear lichen planus, perhaps early cases of ILVEN.
   • **Therapy:** No good therapy; if pruritic, try topical corticosteroids or calcineurin inhibitors.

17 *Granulomatous and Necrobiotic Disorders*

17.1 *Granulomatous Disorders*

A granuloma is a small nodular aggregate of macrophages, often admixed with inflammatory cells and giant cells. This chronic inflammatory response in the skin is most often elicited by infections and foreign bodies. In this section, we consider two idiopathic granulomatous disorders.

Sarcoidosis

▶ **Synonym:** Boeck disease.
▶ **Definition:** Multisystem granulomatous disease that favors the lungs, lymph nodes, and skin.
▶ **Epidemiology:** Prevalence in Western Europe 20–30/100 000, but tremendous regional and racial variation. For example, in southeastern USA more common among blacks. Male:female ratio 1:1; onset typically < 40 years of age.
▶ **Pathogenesis:**
  • Etiology unclear. An infectious cause has long been suspected, but no agent has been unequivocally identified.
  • The T-cell response is diminished while at the same time B-cell and antibody response is stimulated. Such a constellation is common in infections.
▶ **Clinical features:**
  • *Systemic findings:* Any organ can be involved, but most commonly affected are the hilar lymph nodes, lungs, joints, and skin. Refer to internal medicine textbook for details.
  • *Cutaneous findings:*
    – *Erythema nodosum:* Usually associated with fever, arthralgias; appears in 10% of patients and is good prognostic sign (p. 540). *Löfgren syndrome:* erythema nodosum, hilar lymphadenopathy, arthritis.
    – *Lupus pernio*: Red-violet chronic infiltrate on tip of nose; looks as if it should be cold-related (true pernio) but is not; often associated with chronic pulmonary involvement and digital bone cysts (*Jüngling syndrome*).
    – *Nodular sarcoidosis:* Red-brown plaques and nodules, often symmetrical, favor the thighs; associated with hilar lymphadenopathy and splenomegaly (Fig. 17.**1a**).
    – *Maculopapular sarcoidosis:* Transient red-brown papules, appear early in disease and may reappear, heralding disease flares. Favor trunk, but may appear on face and extremities. Can be annular (Fig. 17.**1b**), especially in blacks.
    – *Scar sarcoidosis:* Nodular changes in scars may be early sign of sarcoidosis. Sometimes subtle trauma, such as venipunctures is sufficient trigger.
▶ **Histology:** Small well-circumscribed dermal granulomas with few accompanying lymphocytes (naked granulomas) and variety of giant cells.
  ⚠ Caution: The presence of a foreign body in a cutaneous granuloma does not exclude sarcoidosis, as patients with sarcoidosis are more likely to react to such materials.
▶ **Diagnostic approach:**
  • Clinical examination, biopsy; skin is often easiest place to document sarcoidal granuloma histologically.

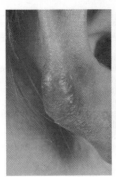 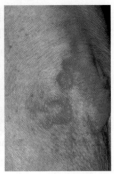

Fig. 17.**1** · **Sarcoidosis.**
a Nodular infiltrate.
b Annular lesion.

a   b

- Chest and hand radiographs.
- Serum calcium level (granulomas produce 1,25-dihydroxycholecalciferol) and serum angiotensin-converting enzyme (ACE) level may both be elevated, as are urine hydroxyproline and calcium levels.
- Document increased antibodies and reduced cellular immune response.
- Ophthalmologic consultation.

▶ **Differential diagnosis:**
- *Lupous pernio:* Pernio, granulomatous rosacea, lupus vulgaris.
- *Nodular sarcoidosis:* Lymphoma, leukemic infiltrates, lupus tumidus, lymphadenosis cutis benigna.
- *Maculopapular sarcoidosis:* Disseminated granuloma annulare, lichen planus, lichen nitidus, secondary syphilis.

▶ **Therapy:**
- Treatment based on general condition of patient.
- Topical corticosteroids usually helpful for cutaneous lesions; if not, consider PUVA for maculopapular disease.
- Allopurinol has been successful in some cases of skin involvement; can also be combined with pentoxifylline.
- Both systemic corticosteroids and methotrexate may be employed, but usually for systemic problems, not skin changes alone.

Melkersson–Rosenthal Syndrome

▶ **Definition:** Rare combination of granulomatous cheilitis, facial nerve paralysis (*Bell palsy*), and fissured tongue.
▶ **Pathogenesis:** Unknown.
▶ **Clinical features:**
- *Granulomatous cheilitis:* Initially spontaneous swelling of lips (usually upper) with resolution but frequent recurrences; over time, permanent swelling and distortion (*tapir lip*). Other sites rarely involved.
- ▷ *Note:* Granulomatous cheilitis may also appear as isolated disease, or in association with sarcoidosis or Crohn disease.
- *Facial nerve paralysis:* Either isolated attack or persistent disease.
- *Fissured tongue:* Present long before other findings, but connection totally mysterious.

- *Other findings:* Patients may have lymphadenopathy (mistaken for sarcoidosis) migraine headaches, visual disturbances, hearing problems.
▶ **Histology:** Initially edema and perivascular infiltrate, later small granulomas often difficult to find.
▶ **Diagnostic approach:** Clinical examination, biopsy.
▶ **Differential diagnosis:** Angioedema, recurrent herpes simplex, recurrent erysipelas, *Ascher syndrome* (double lip, blepharochalasis, and thyroid problems), hemangioma, lymphedema, amyloidosis.
▶ **Therapy:**
- Intralesional corticosteroids (triamcinolone 10 mg/mL dilated 1:3 with lidocaine) are best approach; painful but effective.
- Excision and plastic repair, if disease is stable.
- Clofazimine 100 mg daily or q.o.d. for 6–12 months or dapsone 50–100 mg daily for same time period.

17.2 Necrobiotic Disorders

Necrobiosis is a very bad term—poorly defined and linguistically impossible. It literally means "condition of living and dying," but describes a peculiar histological change in the dermis with basophilia, mucin deposition, swelling, and distortion of collagen fibers.

Granuloma Annulare

▶ **Definition:** Dermatosis usually with small grouped papules or subcutaneous nodules that show necrobiosis on biopsy.
▶ **Epidemiology:** Typically affects children and young adults; more common in those with atopy.
▶ **Pathogenesis:** Unknown.
▶ **Clinical features:**
- Classic lesion is ring on dorsum of hand or foot consisting of many small papules 1–3 mm in diameter (Fig. 17.2). Often with a distinction pale blue-red color. Entire lesion up to 5 cm. Also appear on distal extremities. Asymptomatic and usually resolves spontaneously without scarring (75% disappear over 2 years).
- *Variants:*
  – *Giant granuloma annulare:* Lesions up to 20 cm.

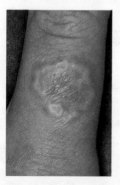

Fig. 17.**2** · Granuloma annulare.

- *Disseminated granuloma annulare:* Young adults, favors wrists and ankles, but also trunk; many tiny papules without annular pattern, often hyperpigmented and generally persistent. In older adults, associated with diabetes mellitus.
- *Subcutaneous granuloma annulare:* Deep nodules, usually on palms and soles, or near joints; *pseudo-rheumatoid nodules.*
- *Light-induced granuloma annulare.*
- *Perforating granuloma annulare:* Discharge of damaged collagen through epidermis with crust and scars.

▶ **Histology:** Foci of basophilic collagen surrounding by macrophages (*palisading macrophages*); sometimes with mucin.

▶ **Diagnostic approach:** Clinical examination usually suffices; biopsy if questions exist. Rule out diabetes mellitus in older patients.

▶ **Differential diagnosis:**
- Abundant opportunities for mistakes:
  - The classic lesions in small children usually misdiagnosed as tinea corporis because they are annular, even though no scale or inflammation is seen.
  - The subcutaneous nodules are designated rheumatoid nodules and the patient worked up for rheumatoid arthritis; if no other signs and symptoms, subcutaneous granuloma annulare is the answer.
- *Disseminated disease:* Planar warts, eruptive xanthomas, steatocystoma multiplex, eruptive vellus hair cysts, sarcoidosis, lichen planus (should itch), drug reactions.

▶ **Therapy:**
- Since spontaneous resolution is the rule, usually no therapy is required.
- Lesions often disappear following biopsy or other minor trauma.
- Topical corticosteroids under occlusion or intralesional.
- For disseminated disease, bath PUVA or short burst of systemic corticosteroids. Isolated reports of good responses to fumaric acid for 6 weeks.

Necrobiosis Lipoidica

▶ **Definition:** Chronic atrophic dermatosis usually on shins with distinctive yellow telangiectatic appearance, often associated with diabetes mellitus.

▶ **Epidemiology:** Female:male ratio 2:1; usually middle-aged women. 60–70% of patients have diabetes mellitus but only 0.3% of patients with diabetes mellitus have necrobiosis lipoidica.

▶ **Pathogenesis:** Primary event appears to be vasculopathy, followed by damage to collagen and granulomatous response.

▶ **Clinical features:**
- Asymptomatic oval dark red patches and plaques, almost always on shins. Slowly spread, coalesce, and develop diagnostic yellow color with numerous telangiectases (Fig. 17.**3**). Borders remain irregular, sharply defined, and dark red.
- Biggest problem is ulceration, which develops in 25% and is very difficult to heal.
- Other sites of involvement include thigh, distal extremities, trunk, and even scalp (with scarring alopecia).
- Disseminated necrobiosis lipoidica, also known as granulomatosis disciformis chronica and progressiva may rarely occur.

▶ **Diagnostic approach:** Clinical examination; biopsy sites often heal poorly. Exclude diabetes mellitus.

▶ **Differential diagnosis:** Typical lesion on shins unique and diagnostic; perhaps confused with statis dermatitis and dermatosclerosis, but latter is far more diffuse. Disseminated disease overlaps with granuloma annulare and actinic granuloma.

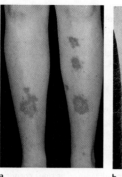
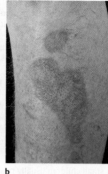

Fig. 17.**3** · **Necrobiosis lipoidica. a** General appearance. **b** A close-up view shows the distinctive yellow color.

► **Therapy:**
- Despite atrophy, best approach is topical corticosteroids under occlusion or intralesional corticosteroids.
- If lesions are identified early, anti-inflammatory therapy with dapsone or colchicine may help.
- Cream PUVA also effective in early phase.
- Compression stockings and pentoxifylline may be useful.
- If ulcerated, consider excision and coverage with mesh graft.
- ▣ *Note:* Control of diabetes mellitus is essential, but does not influence necrobiosis lipoidica.

Other Conditions with Necrobiosis

- Rheumatoid nodules (p. 224), usually in patients with obvious rheumatoid arthritis; thus not a diagnostic clue.
- *Actinic granuloma:* Also known as elastolytic granuloma or O'Brien granuloma. May be granuloma annulare in sun-damaged skin. Large bizarre atrophic patches with prominent red-brown border. Typically sites include arms, face, and nape. Biopsy shows necrobiosis, solar elastosis, and ingestion of elastin by giant cells. Treatment same as granuloma annulare.
- *Necrobiotic xanthogranuloma:* Rare condition with yellow patches and plaques; almost always periorbital findings (initially mistaken for xanthelasma) but also involves face or trunk (Fig. 17.**4**). Biopsy shows necrobiosis, foam-laden macrophages, and lymphoid clusters. Associated with monoclonal gammopathy. No effective treatment.

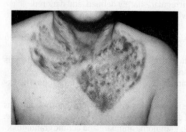

Fig. 17.**4** · Necrobiotic xanthogranuloma (Image courtesy of Prof. N. Hass MD, Berlin, Germany)

18 Dermatoses Caused by Physical and Chemical Agents

18.1 Photodermatoses

Overview

▶ **Definition:** Skin diseases caused or exacerbated by exposure to light.
▶ Almost all cutaneous light reactions are caused by UV radiation of wavelength 280–400 nm. Shorter wavelengths are filtered out by the atmosphere; longer wavelengths only rarely play a role. The electromagnetic spectrum is shown in Table 18.**1**.

Table 18.1 · Electromagnetic spectrum	
Region	**Wave length (nm)**
Gamma	0.0001–0.14
X-ray	0.0005–20
Ultraviolet	
	UVC
40–280	
	UVB
280–320	
	UVA
320–400	
	UVA2
320–340	
	UVA1
340–400	
Visible light	400–800
Infrared	800–10^5
Radio waves	10^5–10^{15}

▶ **Minimal erythema dose:** The amount of light required to produce a barely visible erythema (p. 49); it depends on the wavelength, skin type, and amount of previous light exposure. UVB is about 1000× as rich in energy as UVA; in other words, about 1000× as much UVA exposure is required to produce the same erythema.
▶ **Depth of penetration:** Depends on wavelength; the longer wavelengths penetrate deeper. Thus UVA reaches deeper into the dermis than UVB, while lasers designed to selectively reach and interact with dermal vessels or pigment are all in the visible light spectrum or longer.
▶ **Physiological light protection:** The skin has many intrinsic mechanisms to protect against light damage:
   • Epidermal acanthosis and hyperkeratosis. Reaches maximum after 2–3 weeks.
   ◪ *Note:* For a long time the major role of the stratum corneum in light protection was overlooked or underestimated.

- Increased melanin synthesis and transfer of melanosomes to keratinocytes.
- Natural free radical or activated oxygen scavengers (glutathione, catalase, vitamin C, vitamin E, melatonin, others).
- DNA repair mechanisms, most important is nucleoside excision repair to remove thymine dimers and photo adducts.
► **Other important physiologic processes** in the skin include:
- Synthesis of vitamin D and *cis–trans* isomerization of urocanic acid.
- *Immunosuppressive effects:* Inhibition of Langerhans cells and release of suppressive cytokines that can have systemic effects.

Sunburn

► **Definition:** Acute sun damage to skin, caused primarily by UVB.
► **Clinical features:** Known to everyone; painful, sharply demarcated erythema limited to areas of sun exposure (Fig. 18.1); if severe, blister formation; later, peeling.
🔳 *Caution:* A widespread blistering sunburn is comparable to a second-degree burn and requires similar treatment.
► **Histology:** Apoptotic keratinocytes (sunburn cells), widened vessels, marked edema, lymphocytic infiltrate.
► **Differential diagnosis:** Always consider a phototoxic drug reaction as a possible contributing factor to bad sunburn.
► **Therapy:**
- Immediate use of NSAIDs may help.
🔳 *Caution:* Paradoxically, NSAIDs can also cause phototoxic reactions.
- If sunburn is severe, then fluid replacement may become important. Otherwise, simply lubricate the skin and await natural healing.
🔳 *Note:* Both topical and systemic corticosteroids are overrated in sunburn. The popular topical anesthetics and antihistamines sold over the counter in the USA and Europe are likely causes of allergic contact dermatitis.

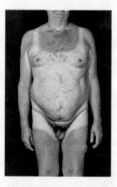

Fig. 18.**1** · Sunburn.

Phototoxic and Photoallergic Reactions

▶ **Definition:** The combination of light and certain topical or systemic agents can lead to an enhanced reaction.

▶ **Epidemiology:** Phototoxic reactions are far more common than photoallergic reactions. Some substances, such as psoralens, cause a phototoxic reaction in almost everyone exposed to them and the appropriate wavelength of light.

▶ **Pathogenesis:** In contrast to the discussion of allergic versus toxic contact dermatitis, the situation with photodermatoses is less clear. It can be difficult to decide if a reaction is toxic or allergic, and some medications cause both.

- A *phototoxic reaction* is an exaggerated sunburn; the photosensitizers make the skin make sensitive to light, often by causing the production of free oxygen radicals. A phototoxic reaction can occur the first time the patient uses the medication or product. The likelihood of reaction is dose-related (Figs. 18.**2**, 18.**3**).
- Causes of phototoxic reactions include:
  - *Tars* and their derivatives such as acridine or anthracene.
  - *Dyes:* Bengal red, eosin, fluorescin, methylene blue, riboflavin, acridine, thiopyronine.
  - *Medications:* Amiodarone, furosemide, NSAIDs (especially piroxicam, carprofen, diclofenac), psoralens, phenothiazines, tetracyclines (especially doxycycline).
  - *Furocoumarins* in a wide variety of plants and grasses; also source of psoralens; plants include giant hogweed (most notorious in Europe), celery, parsley, turnip, citrus fruits (including bergamot), St. John's wort.
  - Exposure to plant sap or juice plus sun exposure leads to streaking bullous dermatosis, known as *phytophotodermatitis* (*dermatitis pratensis* or meadow grass dermatitis). Individuals exposed to giant hogweed may have large blisters mistaken for burns.
  - *Berloque dermatitis* is caused by using perfumes or after shave lotions containing bergamot oil; typical picture is streaked hyperpigmented rash on side of neck where perfume is often applied. Acute reaction often overlooked; only pigmentary changes noted.
- In contrast, a *photoallergic reaction* requires previous exposure, the development of sensitization and then a repeated exposure with the right combination of sensitizer and light exposure. Sometimes a different wavelength of light is required for the sensitization and then the re-elicitation of the dermatitis, which can have a variable morphology ranging from exanthem to urticaria.
- Typical causes of photoallergic reactions include:
  - *Medications:* Benzodiazepines, nalidixic acid, NSAIDs, phenothiazines, sulfonamides, sulfonylureas, thiazides, triacetyldiphenylisatin (laxative).
  - *Antimicrobial agents*, such as halogenated salicylanilides formerly added to deodorant soaps.
  - *Bleaches and blankophores* in laundry soaps.
  - *Sunscreens* (*para*-amino benzoic acid, benzophenone).
  - *Cyclamates* (artifical sweeteners).

▶ **Clinical features:** Clinical features and localization are distinctive.

▶ **Diagnostic approach:** Clinical examination and history usually suffices for phototoxic dermatitis. For photoallergic dermatitis, photopatch testing useful (p. 45).

▶ **Differential diagnosis:**
- *Phototoxic dermatitis:* Sunburn, other toxic (non-photo) reactions.
- *Photoallergic dermatitis:* Allergic contact dermatitis via aeroallergens.

▶ **Therapy:** Same as for allergic and toxic contact dermatitis (p. 199).

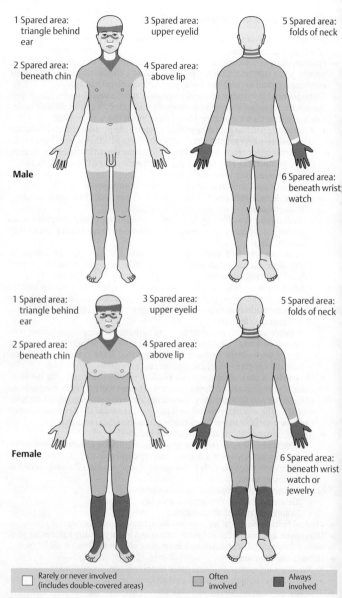

Fig. 18.2 · Typical localization of photoallergic and phototoxic reactions.

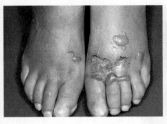 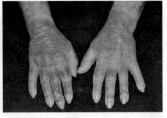

b

Fig. 18.3 · **a** Phototoxic dermatitis. **b** Photoallergic dermatitis.

Chronic Actinic Dermatitis

▶ **Synonyms:** Persistent light reaction, actinic reticuloid (when histology shows atypical lymphocytes).
▶ **Definition:** Persistent photoallergic dermatitis following sensitization but without further antigen exposure.
▶ **Pathogenesis:** Poorly understood; presumably photohaptens induce autoimmune response including persistent lymphocytic infiltrates.
▶ **Clinical features:** Pruritic chronic dermatitis in light-exposed areas, most common on nape. Lichenified skin with multiple excoriations and erosions.
▶ **Histology:** Acanthosis, dermal fibrosis, lymphocytic infiltrates which in some instances may show marked atypia (actinic reticuloid). Progression to lymphoma most uncommon.
▶ **Diagnostic approach:** Clinical examination, biopsy. Photo provocation (UVA, UVB, and visible light) as well as photopatch testing.
▶ **Differential diagnosis:** Atopic dermatitis, mycosis fungoides, Sézary syndrome.
▶ **Therapy:** Azathioprine 50 mg daily or 3× weekly can be almost miraculous; PUVA hardening also helpful. In severe cases, cyclosporine.

Polymorphous Light Eruption

▶ **Definition:** Idiopathic eruption caused by UV exposure; appears in hours to days with morphology varying considerably between patients.
▶ **Epidemiology:** Far and away the most common photodermatosis, with an estimated prevalence of 10–20%. Usually starts in adolescents or young adults.
▶ **Pathogenesis:** Unknown; perhaps autoimmune response to damaged keratinocytes.
▶ **Clinical features:** Wide spectrum of clinical patterns ranging from papulovesicular exanthem (most common) to plaques, erythema multiforme–like lesions, hemorrhagic or purpuric changes (Fig. 18.4). The eruption is usually most prominent following the first UVA exposure in the spring—thus often a feature of a winter trip to sunny climes. Appears hours to days after exposure, lasts for several days and resolves spontaneously without scarring. Some degree of hardening over the summer and recurrences each year are to be expected.
☒ *Note:* The lesions in any one patient are relatively uniform and remain so over the life of the disease. The term polymorphous refers to the *different patterns in different patients.*
▶ **Histology:** Dermal edema, lymphocytic perivascular infiltrates and minimal epidermal damage; no mucin (in contrast to lupus erythematosus).

Dermatoses Caused by Physical and Chemical Agents

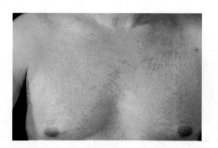

Fig. 18.**4** · Polymorphous light eruption.

▶ **Diagnostic approach:** Clinical examination; provocation testing is useful; 60–100 J/cm² UVA to individual site of predilection can reproduce lesions.

▶ **Therapy:**
- Avoidance of sunlight via sunscreens and protective clothing; gradual increases in light exposure rather than intensive exposure on first day.
- Use of antioxidant for 1 week before exposure; then on vacation combination of antioxidant and sunscreen (for example Eucerin Phase 1 and Phase 2 gel-cream containing α-glucosyl rutin as antioxidant).
- Hardening with UVB or PUVA before exposure.
- If lesions develop, topical corticosteroids and oral antihistamines.
- Severe, persistent disease: consider azathioprine 50–100 mg daily to 3× weekly for 3 months.

Mallorca Acne

▶ **Synonym:** Acne aestivalis.
▶ **Definition:** Acneiform eruption developing following excessive sun exposure.
▶ **Epidemiology:** First described in European tourists going to Mallorca in mid-winter; more common in women 20–40 years of age.
▶ **Pathogenesis:** Unclear, but likely variant of polymorphous light eruption. Most patients without history of acne vulgaris, but develop follicular lesions with sun exposure. Roles of sweating and topical agents such as emollients or sunscreens long disputed.
▶ **Clinical features:** Monomorphic small skin-colored follicular papules with tiny red rim; usually on shoulders, mid–upper back, or upper arms. Generally pruritic. Face spared; no comedones or pustules. Changes persist for days to weeks; little hardening, so unlucky patients are affected from spring to fall.
▶ **Histology:** Follicular plugging with inflammatory reaction.
▶ **Diagnostic approach:** Clinical examination; search for acne elsewhere; exclude photoallergic reaction; later try to reproduce lesions with photo provocation.
▶ **Differential diagnosis:** Acne vulgaris is common and Mallorca acne uncommon. Sun-aggravated acne vulgaris with comedones and pustules is not Mallorca acne.
▶ **Therapy:** Sun avoidance; clothing better than sunscreens; gels preferred over creams because of confusion over role of topical occlusion. Topical corticosteroids for pruritus. Same hardening approaches as tried for polymorphous light eruption may help here.

Actinic Prurigo

▶ **Definition:** Common form of photosensitivity among natives of North and South America, with distinctive clinical pattern.

▶ **Epidemiology:** Rare and sporadic in Europe; usually associated with atopic dermatitis. Among Native Americans, prevalence rates can be as high as 20–30%, varying with tribe.

▶ **Pathogenesis:** Unknown, but distinct HLA-DR4 associations.

▶ **Clinical features:** Starts in childhood or adolescence as overlap between atopic dermatitis and photosensitivity. More common in women. Pruritic dermatitic lesions that evolve into prurigo papules and lichenified plaques. Some patients have vesicular hydroa vacciniforme–like lesions on nose and ears. Lesions begin in spring or summer months and recurrences are the rule. Among Native Americans, associated with cheilitis and conjunctivitis with pterygium formation.

▶ **Histology:** Varies with stage of lesion and is not diagnostic: lymphocytic infiltrates and spongiosis dominate.

▶ **Diagnostic approach:** Clinical examination, detailed history; look for associated atopy; perhaps photo provocation.

▶ **Differential diagnosis:** Polymorphous light eruption, light-sensitive atopic dermatitis, and in adults chronic actinic dermatitis.

▶ **Therapy:** Avoidance and sun protection; easier to achieve among European patients than Native Americans. Topical corticosteroids; pulses of systemic corticosteroids for severe flares.

Hydroa Vacciniforme

▶ **Definition:** Rare photodermatosis in children with blisters and scars formerly felt to resemble the morphology of smallpox.

▶ **Pathogenesis:** Unknown, but Epstein–Barr virus (EBV) may play a role.

▶ **Clinical features:** Blue-red erythema that develops into blisters with serous or hemorrhagic contents (Fig. 18.**5**). Almost always involves face, occasionally hands. Heals with hypopigmented scars.

▶ **Histology:** Similar to polymorphous light eruption.

▶ **Diagnostic approach:** Clinical examination, biopsy. exclude porphyrias via blood, urine and stool examinations; search for herpes simplex virus and EBV.

▶ **Differential diagnosis:** Erythropoietic porphyria and erythropoietic protoporphyria can be similar; initially severe herpes simplex virus infection often sus-

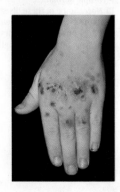

Fig. 18.**5** · Hydroa vacciniforme.

pected. A form of panniculitic T-cell lymphoma has been described in Japan and Mexico that clinically resembles hydroa vacciniforme.

▶ **Therapy:** Mainstay is light avoidance and maximum sunscreen protection. UVB or PUVA hardening is difficult but worth trying. Neither β-carotene nor antimalarials proven effective. For flares, zinc oxide shake lotions or topical corticosteroids.

Pellagra

▶ **Definition:** Deficiency in nicotinic acid, part of the vitamin B complex.

▶ **Epidemiology:** Common worldwide dietary defect, often association with other deficiencies such as kwashiorkor. In the early 1900s, very common in rural southeastern USA; Goldberger won Nobel Prize for identifying vitamin deficiency.

▶ **Pathogenesis:** In addition to inadequate dietary vitamins and malabsorption, nicotinic acid deficiency can result from interference by various medications such as isoniazid and phenytoin.

▶ **Clinical features:** The classic features are the 4 Ds: diarrhea, dementia, dermatitis, and death. Patients have photosensitivity and develop hyperpigmented scaly patches; the lesions on the V of the neck as known as *Casal necklace*; other typical sites include cheeks, backs of hands and backs of feet in those working outdoors barefoot.

▶ **Therapy:** Adequate diet and nicotinic acid replacement.

Light-sensitive Dermatoses

There are many dermatoses that can worsen with light exposure, including the following:
▶ Lupus erythematosus.
▶ Dermatomyositis.
▶ Rosacea.
▶ Recurrent herpes simplex virus infections.
▶ Erythema multiforme (via connection with herpes simplex).
▶ Lichen planus.
▶ Darier disease.
▶ Disseminated superficial actinic porokeratosis.
▶ Pityriasis rubra pilaris.
▶ Allergic contact dermatitis; for example, allergy to chromium salts in cement workers.
▶ Atopic dermatitis.
◨ *Note:* Some of these diseases are routinely treated with light, such as atopic dermatitis. Most patients will improve with UVA1 or selective UVB phototherapy (SUP), but some will worsen. Therefore, always ask about previous improvement or worsening with sunlight exposure before starting phototherapy.

18.2 Light-induced Aging and Photocarcinogenesis

Skin and Light

Modest sun exposure has healthy effects, including stimulation of vitamin D synthesis and a positive influence on the psyche. All that is needed for healthy living is 10–15 minutes a day. In the past 50 years there have been dramatic changes in lifestyle, such as vacations in sunny climates in the winter, population shifts toward sunnier climates (in the USA), more outdoor living, and greater emphasis on tanning especially with artifical light sources (tanning studios). All these factors have contributed to overwhelm the skin's intrinsic defense and regeneration mechanisms, leading to an increase in photoaging and carcinogenesis. The loss of atmospheric ozone has also contributed by allowing more UVB light to reach the Earth's surface, but this contribution is far less than that of lifestyle changes.

Molecular Biology

UV irradiation is a potent and complete carcinogen. Absorption of UVB by DNA leads to formation of thymine dimers. Incorrect or inadequate repair leads to carcinogenesis by producing stable mutations in critical growth control genes. UVA leads more to breaks in DNA and DNA–protein complexes. In addition, the irradiation reduces Langerhans cells and causes cutaneous immunosuppression.

Chronic Effects of Light on the Skin

▶ **Aging:** One must distinguish between intrinsic aging and extrinsic or photoaging. Intrinsic aging is best seen on the buttocks; there is epidermal atrophy, a loss in dermal connective tissue, and other relatively minor changes. A dramatic comparison is that the buttock skin of a 60-year-old is about as "aged" as the facial skin of a 20-year-old.

▶ **Photoaging:** There are many stigmata of chronic light exposure. The degree of photoaging is proportional to the total UV exposure; the skin never forgets a ray of sunlight. Many different names have been applied to photoaged skin:
  - *Sailor's skin* or *farmer's skin:* Two names applied to the overall appearance.
  - *Solar elastosis:* The most common change skin microscopically is basophilic staining of the dermis, reflecting an increase in abnormal elastic fibers. Occasionally focal intense elastosis presents as a yellow nodule or plaque. The following terms all refer to various manifestations of elastosis:
    - *Cutis rhomboidalis nuchae:* Multiple deep furrows as seen on the nape.
    - *Favre–Racouchot disease:* Cysts and comedones especially in periorbital location.
    - *Lemon skin:* Pale yellow color and thickened skin.
  - Focal areas of hypopigmentation: *idiopathic guttate hypomelanosis*, most common on arms and less often legs.
  - *Solar lentigines (actinic lentigenes):* Irregular hyperpigmented macules with increased basal layer melanin; most common on face and backs of hands. Flat seborrheic keratoses. Unlike freckles (ephilides), not reversible as exposure is decreased.
  - *Poikiloderma:* Combination of hyper- and hypopigmentation, telangiectases, and atrophy.

▶ **Carcinogenesis:** Skin cancers are the most common human malignancies. For the three main types, there are varying degrees of evidence for solar carcinogenesis.

Many other co-factors are involved, such as exposure to other forms of ionizing radiation, heat, trauma and chemical carcinogens, certain scars (such as those associated with tuberculosis and osteomyelitis), immunosuppression, and selected pre-existing dermatoses such as mucosal lichen planus or lichen sclerosus. The main tumor types are all covered later in more detail.

- **Squamous cell carcinoma (p. 417):** The most common cutaneous tumor is actinic keratosis, which is microscopically a squamous cell carcinoma in situ. There are atypical keratinocytes with individual cell keratinization and mitoses. Almost every white individual with even modest sun exposure develops some actinic keratoses. Long-term regular exposure seems to be the risky behavior. The rate of conversion to squamous cell carcinoma is low and not exactly defined; one rule of thumb is that 1% convert each year, but this seems high to us.
- **Basal cell carcinoma (p. 433):** In most instances this is a malignant tumor of hair follicle origin. Most tumors occur in sun-exposed skin, but are rare on the back of the hands (high sun exposure) and also occur on nonexposed skin. Patients with nevoid basal cell carcinoma syndrome have a mutation in the *PTCH* gene and numerous basal cell carcinomas; the same mutation is seen in sporadic basal cell carcinoma.
- **Malignant melanoma (p. 396):** Has been increasing dramatically in incidence; the rate in Australia is now 40–50/100 000 year and in Western Europe 10–15/100 000. Sun exposure appears to be a major factor; studies in the USA have shown that incidence increases with decreasing latitude (living further south) and, for the same latitude, increases with increasing altitude. Exposure during childhood, and occasional excessive exposure (weekends or vacations), appears more dangerous than long-term chronic exposure; the latest studies in Western Europe and USA show that the most excessive overexposure occurs in teenage and young adult life.

18.3 Photosensitive Genodermatoses

All these disorders present with varying degrees of photosensitivity in infancy or childhood. In each instance the differential diagnostic considerations include most of the other disorders, depending on the associated findings such as premature aging or mental retardation. In photosensitivity in infants, erythropoietic porphyria and other forms should be excluded; at birth, neonatal lupus erythematosus must also be considered.

Xeroderma Pigmentosum
· ·

- ▶ **MIM code:** 278700; gene locus 9q22.3–31 and at least three other loci.
- ▶ **Definition:** Defect in DNA excision repair mechanism with autosomal recessive inheritance, leading to marked photosensitivity and multiple cutaneous malignancies.
- ▶ **Epidemiology:** Prevalence of 1–3/million.
- ▶ **Pathogenesis:** Divided into 10 different complementation groups, each representing a different defect in part of the complex DNA excision repair mechanism. When fibroblasts from patients in two different complementation groups are fused, they have normal repair capabilities.
- ▶ **Clinical features:**
  - Clinical variations depending on the complementation group.
  - Predominant feature is extreme photosensitivity with sunburn as infant with minimal exposure.

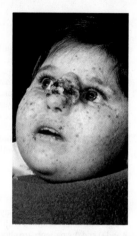

Fig. 18.**6** · Xeroderma pigmentosum: child with destructive basal cell carcinoma and marked actinic damage.

- Soon multiple actinic lentigines of varying size and color develop, along with areas of hypopigmentation, telangiectases, and atrophy, leading to poikiloderma at an early age (Fig. 18.**6**).
- *Multiple skin tumors:* Most common are basal cell carcinoma, squamous cell carcinoma, and malignant melanoma. Incidence of basal cell carcinoma estimated at 1000× normal. Almost every patient has a malignant melanoma by 20 years of age.
- Internal malignancies are also increased by 10–20-fold, including oral squamous cell carcinomas, CNS tumors, and almost every other organ.
- *Associated disorders:*
  - *DeSanctis–Cacchione syndrome:* Several complementation groups have associated neurological disorders including mental retardation and motor defects.
  - Overlaps with Cockayne syndrome (see below) and trichothiodystrophy (p. 512).
  - *Pigmented xerodermoid:* Also known as xeroderma pigmentosum variant, adults with later onset of photosensitivity, similar clinical picture, but no established repair defect.

▸ **Histology:** Nothing in tumors offers clue to xeroderma pigmentosum except early age of patients.

▸ **Diagnostic approach:** Clinical examination; repair defect can be identified in fibroblasts and complementation group typing performed; both highly specialized.

▸ **Therapy:**
- Absolute light avoidance; development of nocturnal habits; careful use of sunscreens is not enough.
- High-dose retinoids reduce incidence of tumors but have considerable side effects.
- Topical bacterial endonuclease (T4) shows promise to improve cutaneous repair mechanisms.
- Regular monitoring and prompt removal of tumors at less advanced stage.

Cockayne Syndrome

► **MIM code:** 216400.
► **Definition:** Rare disorder with photosensitivity and growth defects, inherited in autosomal recessive manner.
► **Pathogenesis:** Two responsible genes (*CKN1* and *CKN2*). Also overlaps with several xeroderma pigmentosum groups (B, D, G).
► **Clinical features:** Patients present with photosensitivity, growth retardation, premature aging, optic atrophy, and deafness. Profound retardation. Develop characteristic bird-like facies. Those with xeroderma pigmentosum–Cockayne syndrome overlap have more photosensitivity and freckling but do not develop tumors as do ordinary xeroderma pigmentosum patients.
► **Diagnostic approach:** Genetic diagnostic methods are only way to sort out complex picture.
► **Therapy:** Nothing effective; death at early age.

Trichothiodystrophy

Some patients with trichothiodystrophy (p. 512) have photosensitivity. In one form the genetic defect is linked with xeroderma pigmentosum complementation group B and D and the patients are photosensitive, but do not develop cutaneous malignancies at an early age.

Bloom Syndrome

► **MIM code:** 210900: gene locus 15q26.1.
► **Definition:** Rare genodermatosis with triad of photosensitivity, facial telangiectases, and dwarfism.
► **Pathogenesis:** Defect in *BLM* gene, encoding a DNA helicase known as RecQL3 3
► **Clinical features:** Patients present with low birth weight as well as both telangiectases and photosensitivity in infancy. Also have café-au-lait macules. No increase in cutaneous malignancies, but high lifetime risk of systemic malignancies especially leukemias and lymphomas.
► **Diagnostic approach:** Clinical suspicion, genetic studies; exclude porphyria.
► **Therapy:** Sun protection; monitoring for internal malignancies.

Rothmund–Thomsen Syndrome

► **MIM code:** 268400; gene locus 8q24.3.
► **Definition:** Combination of early onset of poikiloderma associated with cataracts, photosensitivity, dwarfism, and hypogonadism.
► **Pathogenesis:** Most patients have defect in DNA helicase RecQL4. Unclear if different genetic defects lead to different clinical patterns.
► **Clinical features:** Rothmund first described patients with poikiloderma and cataracts, while Thomsen's patients had no cataracts. This controversy still continues. Patients present with photosensitivity and poikiloderma; about half have juvenile cataracts. Later develop hyperkeratotic lesions over flexors. Adults have increased risk of squamous cell carcinoma. Facies features a saddle nose with prominent forehead and chin. Growth retardation, hypogonadism, and multiple epithelial defects (hair, nails, teeth). High risk of osteosarcoma.
► **Diagnostic approach:** Clinical suspicion, genetic studies.
► **Therapy:** Sunscreens, cataract surgery, baseline bone surveys and then monitoring for osteosarcoma.

Hartnup Syndrome

► **MIM code:** 234500; gene locus 11q13.
► **Definition:** Disturbance in intestinal absorption and renal reabsorption of neutral amino acids; autosomal recessive inheritance.
► **Pathogenesis:** The most striking problem is low levels of tryptophan, leading to reduced levels of nicotinic acid.
► **Clinical features:**
  • Photosensitivity, usually appearing in childhood. May sometimes mimic hydroa vacciniforme. Red-brown hyperpigmentation with scaling develops.
  • Neurological findings include ataxia and other cerebellar problems.
► **Diagnostic approach:** Prenatal screening performed in some countries; for example Massachusetts where incidence is 1/15000 births (the Hartnups were a Massachusetts family). Otherwise, measure urine amino acid levels or indol bodies.
► **Therapy:** Nicotinic acid replacement dramatically improves the skin and usually helps the neurological signs and symptoms. Usual dose 50–100 mg daily. Sunscreens.

18.4 Diseases Caused by Cryoproteins

Cryoproteins are proteins with special physicochemical properties, whose structures or binding capacities change with temperature. In the human system, the relevant cryoproteins are those that are not aggregated at body temperature but aggregate when modest degrees of cooling take place, usually in acral sites. They can be found in a variety of disorders and lead to a number of dermatologic signs and symptoms.

Cryoglobulinemia

► **Definition:** Presence of circulating immunoglobulin complexes that precipitate when incubated at $<4°C$.
► **Pathogenesis:**
  • There are three types of cryoglobulins, as shown in Table 18.**2**.
  • Types II and III are known as mixed cryoglobulinemias; when no underlying disease is present, the term essential mixed cryoglobulinemia may be employed. Over 80% are associated with hepatitis C infection; the main difference between types II and III is a higher incidence of renal disease in the former.

Table 18.2 · Cryoglobulins

Type	Composition	Associated disease	Clinical features
I	Monoclonal IgG or IgM	Myeloma, Waldenström macroglobulinemia, lymphoma	Thrombosis, livedo, Raynaud syndrome, ulcers
II	Monoclonal IgM (rheumatid factor) plus polyclonal IgG	Same B-cell disorders as for type I, Sjögren syndrome, rheumatoid arthritis, hepatitis C	Chronic immune complex vasculitis, skin and kidneys
III	Polyclonal Ig	Connective tissue disease, primary biliary cirrhosis, hepatitis C	Chronic immune complex vasculitis, skin and kidneys

▶ **Clinical features:** The unifying clinical feature is acral skin changes in response to cold exposure, sometimes as subtle as entering an air-conditioned building.
  ● In type I disease, thrombosis, hyperviscosity, Raynaud phenomenon, necrotic lesions and CNS lesions dominate.
  ● In types II and III disease, the classic finding is leukocytoclastic vasculitis with superficial ulcerations, favoring the region about the ankles. Raynaud phenomenon, cold urticaria, purpura, arthralgias, polyneuritis, and glomerulonephritis (up to 50%) are seen.
▶ **Diagnostic approach:** The blood must be transported to the laboratory at 37°; there it is cooled to < 4°C; then cryocrit is determined and then the proteins selectively analyzed. Reactive hypocomplementemia. Other laboratory testing is designed to exclude various underlying diseases.
▶ **Differential diagnosis:** Other forms of vasculitis; other cryoprotein disorders.
▶ **Therapy:**
  ● Avoid cold, especially sudden shifts in temperature.
  ● When hepatitis C is involved, then treatment with interferon (pegylated IFN α2b) and ribavirin is most important.
  ● If underlying disease is indicated, then appropriate follow-up and therapy.
  ● For progressive disease, methotrexate or cyclophosphamide plus systemic corticosteroids, perhaps combined with plasma exchange.

Cryofibrinogenemia

Patients have fibrinogen that aggregates at lower temperatures, creating a complex of fibrin, fibronectin and fibrinogen. They develop a combination signs and symptoms based on thrombi and coagulation defects. Skin findings include Raynaud phenomenon, acrocyanosis, urticaria, and purpura. Diagnosis is based on identifying the abnormal cryofibrinogen. Treatment includes streptokinase or urokinase for acute thrombosis, as well as plasma exchange to reduce risk.

Cold Agglutinin Disease

▶ **Definition:** Disease caused by erythrocyte aggregation following exposure to cold.
▶ **Pathogenesis:** Cold agglutinins are antibodies that agglutinate erythrocytes more efficiently at temperatures below body temperature. They are usually IgM antibodies directed against erythrocyte polysaccharides. Caused by proliferation of B cells; sometimes they appear transiently following mycoplasma, EBV, or *Treponema pallidum* infection. When chronic, often associated with low-grade B cell lymphoma. Following cold exposure, there is intravascular coagulation (vessel occlusion) and hemolysis (hemolytic anemia). Key factor is how active antibodies are at 30°C.
▶ **Clinical features:** Typical cutaneous features include acrocyanosis following cold exposure, accompanied by paresthesias and rarely necrosis. May also present as cold urticaria or livedo racemosa. Also episodes of hemolytic anemia following cold exposure; if severe and persistent, hepatosplenomegaly.
▶ **Diagnostic approach:**
  ● Blood clots at room temperature; must be kept at body temperature until serum is separated.
  ● Sedimentation rate increased at room temperature, normal at body temperature.
  ● Measure cold agglutinins and determine target antigen (anti-I suggests infection; anti-i suggests EBV or lymphoma).

Differential diagnosis: Other cryoprotein disorders. Raynaud phenomenon has three phases; cold agglutinin response faster and much more dramatic. Also exclude anticardiolipin, lupus erythematosus, systemic sclerosis.

Therapy: Nothing very good for chronic form; avoid cold. In severe chronic forms, immunosuppressive therapy with chlorambucil or cyclophosphamide, perhaps combined with plasmapheresis. Corticosteroids ineffective. Watch for hemochromatosis.

8.5 Disease Caused by Cold

Pernio
....

Synonym: Chilblain.

Definition: Localized erythema caused by exposure to damp cold.

Pathogenesis: Trigger is modest cold (freezing temperatures not required) coupled with moisture; usually toes involved, but also perniones of thighs in riders.

Clinical features: Blue-purple papules and nodules, slowly developing; usually on toes, can also involve shins, thighs, fingers; more common in women who are overweight and not physically active.

Histology: Papillary dermal edema and lymphocytic perivascular infiltrates.

Diagnostic approach: Exclude hyperviscosity syndrome, other myeloproliferative disorders.

Differential diagnosis: Lupus erythematosus (chilblain lupus), sarcoidosis (lupus pernio). In both instances, permanent and not cold-related.

Therapy: Protection from cold; if severe and chronic, topical calcium channel blockers (usually nifedipine) may help.

19 Metabolic Diseases

19.1 Porphyrias

▶ **Definition:** Porphyrias are the result of enzymatic defects in heme synthesis (heme or its ferric chelate is the active site in hemoglobin).
▶ **Classification** (summarized in Table 19.1):
- *Based on most severely affected organ:*
  - Erythropoietic porphyrias.
  - Hepatic porphyrias.
- *Based on clinical features:*
  - Acute porphyrias that can present with life-threatening crises and neurological signs and symptoms (acute intermittent porphyria, porphyria variegata, hereditary coproporphyria).
  - Chronic, non-life-threatening porphyrias (all the erythropoietic porphyrias and porphyria cutanea tarda).

Table 19.1 · Important features of the porphyrias

Enzyme	Disease	Main site of involvement	Excess production of:	Skin findings	Inheritance
PBG deaminase	Acute intermittent porphyria	Liver	PBG, ALA	–	AD
Uroporphyrinogen-III-co-synthetase	Congenital erythropoietic porphyria	RBC	Uroporphyrin I, coproporphyrin II	+++	AR
Uroporphyrinogen decarboxylase	Acquired type I PCT	Liver	Uroporphyrin	+ →	Acquired
	Hereditary type II PCT Hepatoerythropoietic porphyria	(also RBC)	(Protoporphyrin in RBC in hepatoerythropoietic porphyria)	+++	AD AR
Coproporphyrinogen oxidase	Hereditary coproporphyria Homozygous coproporphyria	Liver	Coproporphyrin III PBG, ALA	– +	AD Homozygous AD
Protoporphyrinogen oxidase	Porphyria variegata	Liver	Protoporphyrin, coproporphyrin, PBG, ALA	+	AD
Ferrochelatase	Erythropoietic protoporphyria	RBC	Protoporphyrin	++	AD

AD = autosomal dominant; ALA = aminolevulinic acid; AR = autosomal recessive; PBG = porphobilinogen; PCT = porphyria cutanea tarda

Congenital Erythropoietic Porphyria

- ► **Synonyms:** Günther disease, erythropoietic uroporphyria.
- ► **MIM code:** 263700.
- ► **Definition:** Rare defect in heme synthesis caused by point mutations in uro-porphyrinogen-III co-synthetase gene; autosomal recessive inheritance.
- ► **Clinical features:** Extreme photosensitivity; marked mutilation of sun-exposed skin; massive porphyrinuria (dark-red urine); fluorescent teeth; onset of problems in infancy.
- ► **Diagnostic approach:** Markedly elevated uroporphyrin I, coproporphyrin I in urine, feces, RBC, and plasma; stable fluorescence of RBC.
- ► **Differential diagnosis:** Other childhood photosensitivity disorders.
- ► **Therapy:** Light avoidance or extreme photoprotection (clothing better than sun-screens); bone marrow transplantation successful in some cases.

Erythropoietic Protoporphyria

- ► **MIM code:** 177000.
- ► **Definition:** Defect in ferrochelatase; autosomal dominant inheritance.
- ► **Pathogenesis:** Ferrochelatase mutation on one paternal allele (*cis*) and low ex-pression of ferrochelatase polymorphism on the allele (*trans*).
- ► **Clinical features:**
  - Onset of photosensitivity in first year of life; either sunburn or urticarial lesions can appear, sometimes followed by purpura.
  - Evolves into persistent acral or nasal lichenoid papules, pitted scars and thick-ening (Fig. 19.1).
  - In 5–10% of cases, rapid hepatic fibrosis with liver failure and need for trans-plantation.
- ► **Diagnostic approach:** Elevated protoporphyrin levels in RBC, which show tran-sient fluorescence.
- ► **Differential diagnosis:** Other childhood photosensitivity disorders, hyalinosis cutis et mucosae, p. 354.
- ► **Therapy:**
  - Light avoidance or extreme photoprotection (clothing better than sunscreens).
  - Systemic β-carotene is effective; dosage of 75–100 mg daily (adjusted for sea-son and weight of patient); takes several weeks to be effective (skin must get a bit orange); start in February, discontinue in November.

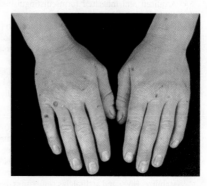

Fig. 19.1 · Erythropoietic proto-porphyria.

Porphyria Cutanea Tarda (PCT)

▶ **MIM codes:** 176100; 176090.

▶ **Definition:** Defect in uroporphyrinogen decarboxylase that can be either acquired or inherited, causing hepatic and cutaneous findings.

▶ **Classification:**

- *Acquired PCT (type I) (MIM code 176090):* Caused by liver damage (estrogens, alcohol, viral hepatitis, hexachlorobenzene [insecticide], drug-induced hepatic dysfunction, hemochromatosis).
- *Autosomal dominant PCT (type II) (MIM code 176100):* Provoked by same factors
- *Hepatoerythropoietic porphyria:* Autosomal recessive defect in uroporphyrinogen decarboxylase gene.

▶ **Clinical features:**

- Skin changes in sun-exposed areas, especially backs of hands and face. Patients are photosensitive, but rarely enough to be a complaint.
- Increased skin fragility; minor trauma leads to erosions, blisters, and crusts (Fig. 19.**2**); usually first finding noticed by patient. Later hyperpigmentation blisters, and milia. Hypertrichosis on cheeks and temples. Marked solar elastosis.
- Rarely, patients develop sclerotic plaques (pseudoscleroderma, p. 222).
- In homozygotes, clinical picture is that of congenital erythropoietic porphyria.

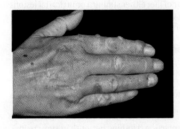

Fig. 19.**2** · Porphyria cutanea tarda with blisters and crusts in light-exposed areas.

▶ **Diagnostic approach:**

- Total porphyrins and uroporphyrins raised in urine; coproporphyrins raised in stool; porphobilinogen (PBG) and δ-aminolevulinic acid (ALA) normal.
- Acquired and inherited forms distinguished by enzyme essay or mutation analysis.
- Exclude other causes of hepatic dysfunction (liver function, hepatitis serology CBC, Hgb, Hct, ferritin (iron overload common).
- Careful history of medications and occupational or hobby exposure to potential hepatotoxins.

▶ **Differential diagnosis:** Limited differential diagnostic considerations when classic picture present; some forms of epidermolysis bullosa acquisita look similar, as does drug-induced pseudoporphyria (usually furosemide) in renal dialysis patients.

▶ **Therapy:**

- Avoid hepatotoxic agents.
- If hepatitis C is documented, treat it with interferon and ribavirin.
- Chloroquine 125 mg 2 × weekly. Chloroquine makes the uroporphyrin crystals in the liver more soluble so they can be excreted. One must start treatment slowly, ideally on an inpatient basis, and increase dosage slightly as urine values stabilize. Fever and arthralgias sometimes develop during induction.

☑ *Caution:* Chloroquine is also one of the drugs that can trigger PCT. The dosage for PCT is only 250 mg weekly, in contrast to 250–500 mg daily for anti-inflammatory action (as in collagen–vascular diseases).

• *Bloodletting:* Remove 500 mL every 2 weeks, monitoring Hgb, iron, and ferritin. Decrease frequency of bleeding when clinical improvement has occurred and Hgb is at low normal level.

cute Intermittent Porphyria

MIM code: 176000.
Definition: Defect caused by reduced activity of porphobilinogen deaminase; autosomal dominant inheritance.
Clinical features:
• No cutaneous findings.
• Patients experience acute life-threatening attacks, usually triggered by medications (barbiturates, estrogens, psychotherapeutic agents).
• *Findings include:*
    – *Gastrointestinal:* bowel cramps, constipation, diarrhea, ileus, vomiting.
    – *Cardiovascular:* tachycardia, hypertension (rarely hypotension).
    – *Neurological:* paresis, psychosis, sensory disturbances, seizures.
    – *Others:* anemia, dark urine, decreased urine output.
☑ *Note:* When any of these findings are present and not clearly explained, think of acute intermittent porphyria. Remember that porphyria variegata and hereditary coproporphyria can present in the same way.
Diagnostic approach: Reduced porphobilinogen deaminase activity; during acute attack, increased amounts of porphobilinogen, aminolevulinic acid, uroporphyrin, and coproporphyrin in urine.
Differential diagnosis: The trick is thinking of acute intermittent porphyria when confronted with a critically ill patient. Lead poisoning can produce a similar laboratory picture, but is easily excluded by lead levels.
Therapy:
• Treatment should be multidisciplinary.
• Stop all possible triggering medications.
• Pain control with opiates (preferably pethidine).
• Antiemetics (promazine, chlorpromazine).
• Infusion of heme arginate 3 mg/kg in 100 mL saline over 20 minutes; daily for 4 days (Heme arginate is not available in the USA, but other heme products can be used.).
• Watch fluids carefully.
Prophylaxis:
• Instruct patient and family doctor on medications that can trigger attacks.
• *Safe list:*
    – *Analgesics:* Aspirin, indomethacin.
    – *Sleep:* Chloral hydrate, phenothiazine, lorazepam.
    – *Coughing:* Codeine, dihydrocodeine.
    – *Local anesthetics:* Amethocaine, bupivacaine, procaine.
    – *General anesthetics:* Nitrous oxide, atropine, cyclopropane, suxamethonium, tubocurarine.

orphyria Variegata

MIM code: 176200.
Definition: Defect in protoporphyrinogen oxidase, autosomal dominant inheritance; variegata means "variable" or "changing".

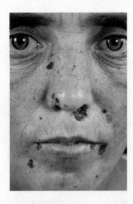

Fig. 19.**3** · Porphyria variegata caused by estrogens

► **Epidemiology:** Very common in Scandinavia and in whites in South Africa (ma⸤ssive⸥ founder effect from single immigrant with disease).
► **Clinical features:** Combination of skin changes of porphyria cutanea tarda a⸤nd⸥ acute disturbances of acute intermittent porphyria; either can domina⸤te⸥ (Fig. 19.**3**).
► **Diagnostic approach:** Increased uroporphyrin and coproporphyrin in urine; ⸤in⸥ contrast to PCT the precursor substances are also increased. Protoporphyrin a⸤nd⸥ coproporphyrin in stool.
► **Therapy:** Photoprotection usually suffices for skin; antimalarials or bleedi⸤ng⸥ rarely needed. Acute attacks and prophylaxis as for acute intermittent porphyri⸤a.⸥

Hereditary Coproporphyria

► **MIM code:** 121300.
► **Definition:** Defect in hepatic coproporphyrinogen oxidase, autosomal domina⸤nt⸥ inheritance.
► **Clinical features:** Same as porphyria variegata.
► **Diagnostic approach:** Increased levels of coproporphyrin in urine and stool; no⸤r⸥mal RBC porphyrin level.
► **Therapy:** Same as porphyria variegata.

19.2 Disorders of Lipid Metabolism

► **Definition:** Complex group of disorders of cholesterol and triglyceride metab⸤o⸥lism, with abnormal or increased plasma lipoproteins.
► **Clinical features:** The cutaneous consequence of elevated plasma lipoprote⸤in⸥ levels is the uptake of lipids by macrophages following leakage through vesse⸤ls,⸥ leading to the formation of xanthomas and xanthelasma. The difference types ⸤of⸥ xanthoma include:
  • *Plane xanthoma:* Irregular yellow-tan macules and flat-topped papules.
  • *Tuberous xanthoma:* Larger red-brown or yellow nodules on pressure points⸤,⸥ elbows, knees, hands, feet.
  • *Tendon xanthoma:* Large subcutaneous nodules over Achilles' or digital tendo⸤ns.⸥
  • *Eruptive xanthoma:* Numerous small yellow papules, often with red border, th⸤at⸥ appear suddenly.

- *Palmar xanthoma:* Yellow streaks (*striae*) or papules in the palmar creases.
- *Xanthelasma:* Most common xanthoma; yellow flat-topped papules and plaques on lids, especially upper lid; no clear association with lipid abnormalities.

Diagnostic approach: The role of the dermatologist is to identify a lesion as a xanthoma. Then the patient must evaluated first for abnormalities of cholesterol and triglyceride metabolism and treated according the latest guidelines.

Note: There is no point in trying to guess the underlying defect based on the skin findings.

Normolipemic Xanthomas

In some instances, xanthomas are identified clinically but the serum cholesterol ands triglyceride levels are normal. Possibilities include xanthomas composed of plant sterols (sitosterolemia, cerebrotendinous xanthomatosis), apolipoprotein defects, xanthomatous forms of Langerhans cell histiocytosis or xanthogranulomas, storage disorders, foreign bodies (some tissue fillers look xanthomatous under the microscope), and even trauma.

There are several rare but distinctive forms of normolipemic xanthomas:

Diffuse normolipemic plane xanthoma: Large yellow-tan patches and plaques favoring trunk, flexures, neck, eyelids; associated with gammopathy.

Necrobiotic xanthogranuloma: Yellow nodules and plaques, favor periorbital region; associated with gammopathy (p. 294).

Xanthoma disseminatum: Diffuse yellow-orange papules involving axilla, groin, neck, and eyelids; mucosal surfaces also affected; pituitary involvement with diabetes insipidus occurs, but disease is entirely distinct from Hand–Schüller–Christian disease.

Verruciform xanthoma: Verruciform papule with foam cells in tips of elongated dermal papilla. Most common on lips and genitalia following trauma, but also occurs in resolving severe dermatoses and in the lesions of CHILD syndrome (p. 414).

Diagnostic approach: Clinical examination, biopsy, normal cholesterol and triglyceride levels.

Therapy: Normolipemic xanthomas do not respond to diet and medical management as do true xanthomas. Localized lesions can be ablated or excised; there is no satisfactory treatment for widespread disease.

19.3 Disorders of Amino Acid Metabolism

Some disorders of amino acid metabolism with skin findings are listed in Table 19.2.

Table 19.2 · Skin findings in disorders of amino acid metabolism

Disease	MIM code	Pathogenesis	Skin findings
Phenylketonuria (p. 373)	261600	Phenylalanine hydroxylase deficiency	Pale skin and hair, photosensitivity, rarely sclerosis.
Hartnup syndrome (p. 307)	234500	Resorption disturbance for neutral amino acids	Pellagra-like signs and symptoms.
Alkaptonuria (p. 381)	203500	Homogentisic acid dioxygenase deficiency	Darkening of nasal, auricular cartilage

Continued Table 19.2 ▶

Table 19.2 · Continued			
Disease	**MIM code**	**Pathogenesis**	**Skin findings**
Homocystinuria	236200	Cystathionine synthetase deficiency	Livedo reticularis, atrophic scars, facial erythema, Marfanoid facies thin hair
Richner–Hanhart syndrome (p. 347)	276600	Tyrosine aminotransferase deficiency	Palmoplantar keratoses

19.4 Disorders of Mineral Metabolism

Hemochromatosis

▶ **Definition:** Disorder due to deposition of hemosiderin causing tissue damage.
▶ **Epidemiology:** The most common genetic disease, as about 10% of individuals have one abnormal *HFE* gene and in Europe about 1:300 are homozygous for the defect.
▶ **Pathogenesis:** Patients with two abnormal *HFE* genes are at risk of developing iron overload. HFE controls the intestinal absorption of iron. The most common mutation is C282Y; other mutations are less damaging. Only about 25% of homozygotes develop clinical findings. Men develop problems far more often (M 10:1) and earlier than women, because of the protective efforts of menstruation. Secondary hemochromatosis occurs following repeated transfusions for a variety of hematological diseases. Juvenile hemochromatosis is caused by mutations in a different gene and is very rare but much more aggressive.
▶ **Clinical features:**
• The major problems result from iron deposition in the liver (cirrhosis, liver cancer, more problems with PCT), pancreas (diabetes mellitus, *bronze diabetes*), heart (conduction disturbances, congestive heart failure), joints (arthritis), and gonads (loss of libido, secondary sexual characteristics).
• The skin becomes bronzed but the increased pigment is melanin, not iron; patients with vitiligo and hemochromatosis have no bronzing in their white spots.
▶ **Diagnostic approach:** Serum transferrin saturation and then serum ferritin levels, followed by genetic testing and perhaps liver biopsy.
▶ **Therapy:** Therapeutic withdrawal of blood.

Acrodermatitis Enteropathica

▶ **MIM code:** 201100.
▶ **Definition:** Defect in intestinal zinc transport gene *SLC39A4* with distinctive cutaneous findings; autosomal recessive inheritance. Acquired zinc deficiency produces the same clinical picture.
▶ **Pathogenesis:** SLC39A4 is primarily expressed in the duodenum and jejunum and functions as a zinc-specific intestinal transport protein. Both homozygous and heterozygous mutations lead to abnormal zinc metabolism. The body normally stores 4 g of zinc; the average daily requirement is 10–15 mg. Table 19.**3** provides more details.

Table 19.3 · Zinc deficiency and related parameters

Zinc status	Plasma zinc level	Hair growth rate	Hair zinc levels
Normal	Normal	Normal	Normal
Mild deficiency	Normal	Normal	↓
Severe deficiency	↓	↓	Normal/ ↑

- **Clinical features:**
  - Acral, well-circumscribed, erythematous weeping plaques; most prominent around mouth, nares, anogenital region. When not moist, such as on the hands, can be psoriasiform. Also telogen effluvium loss of eyebrows and eyelashes.
  - Frequent secondary infections, usually with *Candida albicans*.
  - Diarrhea, photophobia, loss of smell.
  - Most common causes of acquired zinc deficiency are inflammatory bowel diseases; today, all parenteral nutrition includes adequate zinc.
- **Diagnostic approach:** Serum for determination of zinc level must be obtained using zinc-free needles and collecting system; marked diurnal variation, so always draw in a.m. Values vary from laboratory to laboratory, so always use same service; in our hospital 10–20 µmol/l is normal.
- **Differential diagnosis:** Most patients initially misdiagnosed as severe candidiasis.
- **Therapy:** Oral zinc replacement therapy produces miraculous results: improvement within days and soon total clearing.

Menkes Syndrome

- **Synonym:** Kinky hair syndrome.
- **MIM code:** 309400.
- Rare defect in copper transport protein inherited in x-linked recessive manner. Patients have sparse, brittle, twisted scalp hair (pili torti and trichorrhexis nodosa), profound mental retardation, and elastic fiber defects, primarily in arteries. Death occurs in infancy.

19.5 Endocrine Disorders

Pituitary Gland

- **Prolactinoma** is caused by a pituitary adenoma composed of lactotrophs secreting excessive amounts of prolactin. The main side effects are delayed puberty in either sex, galactorrhea–amenorrhea in women, and decreased libido in men. Some drugs (including haloperidol, trifluoperazine, metoclopramide) also cause elevated prolactin levels, as does hypothyroidism and other tumors in or near the pituitary gland. Treatment consists of bromocriptine or cabergoline as well as neurosurgery.
- **Acromegaly** (MIM code 102200) results from oversecretion of growth hormone by pituitary tumors, in adolescents or adults resulting in excessive bone growth of the face, hands and face with coarsening of facial features, and a host of medical problems. Dermatologic findings include thickening of the skin, seborrhea, hyperhidrosis, hypertrichosis, and acanthosis nigricans (p. 485).

▶ **Cushing disease** is the result of hyperadrenocorticism caused by excessive pituitary secretion of ACTH, usually because of a pituitary adenoma.

Thyroid Gland

▶ **Hyperthyroidism:**
- Warm moist skin, telogen effluvium with increased number of dystrophic hairs, onycholysis, increased incidence of alopecia areata and vitiligo.
- In the case of immunogenic hyperthyroidism (Graves disease) associated proliferation of fibroblasts, T cells and then mucin:
  - *Pretibial myxedema:* Red-yellow plaques over shins, often with orange peel texture.
  - *Acropathy:* Swollen fingers.
  - *Orbital deposits* cause exophthalmos.
▶ **Hypothyroidism:**.
- *Generalized myxedema:* Widespread puffy, doughy skin; usually cool and dry; hair loss (primarily occipital and frontal).
- More prominent edema infraorbital and on backs of hands (Fig. 19.**4**).
- Yellow skin tones because reduced conversion from carotene to retinal.

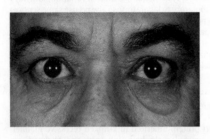

Fig. 19.**4** · Hypothyroidism: yellow skin tones and lid edema.

Parathyroid Gland

▶ **Hyperparathyroidism:** Skin findings most common with renal disease and secondary hyperparathyroidism including pruritus, calcinosis, and sometimes *calciphylaxis* (intravascular calcification causes lightening strike—like livid erythema with subsequent necrosis). Treatment consists of excision of all parathyroid glands, with one placed in an accessible subcutaneous location.
▶ **Hypoparathyroidism:** Associated with T-cell defects because of close origins of parathyroid glands and thymus; seen in mucocutaneous candidiasis, Di George syndrome; most common following thyroid surgery with accidental removal of parathyroids. Clinical findings: tetany, dry skin, and hair.

Adrenal Glands and Gonads

▶ **Cushing syndrome:** Endogenous or exogenous excess amount of corticosteroids leads to steroid acne, hirsutism, hyperpigmentation, striae, telangiectases, hypertrichosis and purpura (weakened vessels).
  ◨ *Note:* Cushing **disease** is a neurosurgical problem, as the hyperadrenocorticism results from a pituitary tumor in most cases; Cushing **syndrome** is the result of hyperadrenocorticism from any other cause.

Addison disease: Diffuse bronze hyperpigmentation, even darker with light exposure, darkened scars, reduced sebum flow.

Androgens: Secreted by adrenal glands and gonads; terminal hair follicles and sebaceous glands are major target organs for testosterone and its conversion product 5-hydrotestosterone. Clinical findings include androgenetic alopecia, hirsutism, acne. In women with atypical acne, consider Stein–Leventhal syndrome.

Adrenogenital syndrome: Includes a variety of syndromes in which defective production of cortisol leads to elevated ACTH levels, which trigger the overproduction of intermediary hormones by the adrenal with potential virilization and sometimes precocious puberty. The most common defect is 21-hydroxylase deficiency, inherited in an autosomal recessive manner. Some patients may have late-onset disease, presenting with therapy-resistant acne.

Pheochromocytoma: Rare adrenal tumor (85% of cases); may also arise in parasympathetic ganglia (paraganglioma). Most are benign and often bilateral; about 15–20% are malignant. Associated with neurofibromatosis 1, von Hippel–Lindau syndrome, and MEN2 syndrome. Oversecretion of catecholamines, usually epinephrine and norepinephrine. Main symptom is hypertension, but occasionally cause pale skin. Often mistakenly included in approach to flushing (p. 707), but usually erroneously. Diagnosis based on increased urine or serum catecholamines.

Pancreas: Diabetes Mellitus

50–70% of patients with diabetes mellitus have cutaneous changes, which can be divided into four groups:

Skin infections: *Candida albicans* is the most common pathogen, causing perlèche, vulvitis, balanitis, paronychia, common bacterial infections include staphylococcal and streptococcal pyodermas, and erythrasma. Less common but more serious are mucormycosis, clostridial gangrene, and malignant otitis externa (*Pseudomonas aeruginosa*).

Markers of diabetes mellitus:

- *Necrobiosis lipoidica* (p. 293): Over 50% of patients with necrobiosis lipoidica have or develop diabetes mellitus, but less than 0.1% of diabetics have this skin change (female:male 3:1).
- *Disseminated granuloma annulare* (p. 292) is likely to be marker, but not highly predictive.
- *Acanthosis nigricans* (p. 485), lipodystrophy (p. 538) signs of insulin resistance.
- *Glucagonoma syndrome* (*necrolytic migratory erythema*), hyperlipidemia, PCT reflect underlying metabolic problems.
- *Bullous disease of diabetes:* Controversial disease; most have either bullous pemphigoid or epidermolysis bullosa acquisita; some suggest associated with retinal disease.
- *Prurigo:* Diabetes mellitus may lead to renal failure and then a vicious cycle of pruritus leading to nodular skin lesions (prurigo) and perhaps other perforating dermatoses (p. 330).
- Scleredema (see below).
- Hemochromatosis or *bronze diabetes* (see above).

Complications of diabetes:

- *Macroangiopathy:* Cutaneous atrophy, especially on soles, dry skin, hypothermia, nail dystrophy, hair loss.
- *Microangiopathy:* Perhaps *Binkley spots:* tiny brown macules on shins.
- *Diabetic stiff skin syndrome.*
- *Neuropathy:* Hyperhidrosis, malum perforans.

▶ **Complications of diabetic therapy:**
- Oral hypoglycemic agents: allergic reactions, photosensitivity.
- *Insulin:* Allergic reactions (5–10%), lipoatrophy, lipohypertrophy.

Neuroendocrine Tumors

▶ The scope of neuroendocrine tumors is beyond this book. Patients have tumors of the pancreas, intestine, thyroid gland, and many other sites secreting hormones such as insulin, glucagon, gastrin, histamine, serotonin, and calcitonin (medullary or C-cell of thyroid). Several points are of dermatologic interest.

▶ Patients with multiple endocrine neoplasia (MEN) have a variety of cutaneous findings, including multiple mucosal neuromas, angiofibromas, connective tissue nevi, and lichen amyloidosus (p. 324).

▶ Pancreatic glucagonomas are often associated with necrolytic migratory erythema (p. 486).

▶ Carcinoid tumors may cause flushing when they release serotonin or bradykinin. About 70% of patients have flushing, often associated with warmth or sweating and sometimes evolving into cyanosis. Diagnosed on elevated serum serotonin levels or elevated urine 5-hydroxy indolacetic acid (5-HIAA) levels.

19.6 Mucinoses

▶ **Definition:** Deposition of mucopolysaccharides (ground substance) in dermis. Unifying factor is histological identification of mucin, either with H&E stain as thready basophilic material or with alcian blue or Hale stain for more specific confirmation.

▶ There are a number of disorders with mucin deposits, including:
- **Thyroid-associated mucinoses:** Pretibial myxedema and generalized myxedema (p. 318).
- **Lichen myxedematosus and scleromyxedema:**
  - Lichen myxedematous presents with multiple small papules or urticarial lesions. When the papules are disseminated, likely to progress to sclerotic changes (scleromyxedema); latter sometimes presenting problem.
  - Unifying feature is thickening of the skin with mucinous infiltrate. Lichen myxedematosus: pruritic firm 5 mm white papules, closely grouped; usually on extremities. Scleromyxedema often has mask-like facies, tightened digits and diffuse sclerosis.
- Almost always associated with monoclonal gammopathy (IgG with γ light chains); also in HIV/AIDS.
- Therapy very unsatisfactory. Plasmapheresis, extracorporeal photophoresis, bath PUVA, and systemic retinoids worth trying.

▶ **Nephrogenic fibrosing dermopathy** (p. 222): Resembles scleromyxedema but associated with renal dialysis.

▶ **Scleredema adultorum:**
- Patients develop thickened, tightened skin on nape and upper back (Fig. 19.5); when arms are pushed backward, skin of back forms into folds. Typically follows infections, such as streptococci, measles, influenza, HIV; usually regresses.
- Also associated with diabetes mellitus; little likelihood of regression.
- Prompt treatment of initial infection. Penicillin G 1 million IU daily for 14 days sometimes tried empirically. Both systemic corticosteroids and penicillamine controversial. Physical therapy to retain motility.

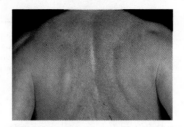

Fig. 19.5 · Scleredema adultorum.

▶ **Reticulated erythematous mucinosis:** REM syndrome, sometimes considered form of cutaneous lupus erythematosus with reticulated erythematous plaques on midback and chest. Responds to antimalarials.

☑ *Note:* The most common cause of mucin identified histologically is lupus erythematosus. Always exclude this diagnosis.

▶ **Focal cutaneous mucinosis:** Isolated papules or nodules containing mucin, with no obvious cause. Excision if disturbing.

19.7 Cutaneous Signs of Monoclonal Gammopathy

▶ **Cutaneous plasmacytoma:** Terminology confusing, as in some European countries multiple myeloma is known as plasmacytoma; in others, plasmacytoma is a type of B-cell lymphoma unrelated to multiple myeloma. Cutaneous involvement by multiple myeloma is very rare. Plasma cell infiltrates more likely to be reactive; always do light-chain clonality studies. One typical clinical setting is in the pseudo-recurrence following a curetted or otherwise ablated basal cell carcinoma or squamous cell carcinoma, in which a red-brown nodule develops and causes clinical alarm but is found to be a reactive polyclonal plasma cell infiltrate.

▶ **Increased tumor and infection rate:** Presumably because of immunosuppression; a variety of infections as well as squamous cell carcinoma, basal cell carcinoma, malignant melanoma, and Kaposi sarcoma are more common.

▶ **Cutaneous deposits:** Amyloidosis, scleromyxedema, scleredema, POEMS syndrome, diffuse normolipemic plane xanthoma, necrobiotic xanthogranuloma, xanthoma disseminatum, IgM papules.

▶ **Neutrophilic dermatoses:** Pyoderma gangrenosum, Sweet syndrome especially when atypical, IgA pemphigus (Sneddon–Wilkinson variant), erythema elevatum et diutinum, leukocytoclastic vasculitis.

▶ **Urticarial dermatoses:** Angioedema with C-1 esterase deficiency; Schnitzler syndrome (urticaria plus IgM gammopathy).

▶ **Autoimmune disorders:** Epidermolysis bullosa acquisita, paraneoplastic pemphigus, IgA pemphigus, atypical scleroderma, Sjögren syndrome.

▶ **Side effects of immunoglobulins:** Hyperviscosity syndrome, cryoglobulinemia (type I), Waldenström macroglobulinemia, Waldenström purpura, Raynaud phenomenon, follicular hyperkeratoses and spikes (crystalloid immunoglobulins).

▶ **Acquired cutis laxa:** Rare disease but can accompany gammopathy.

POEMS Syndrome

▶ POEMS is an acronym for **p**olyneuropathy, **o**rganomegaly, **e**ndocrine disorders, **m**onoclonal gammopathy, **s**kin disease.
▶ Diffuse sclerosis with hyperpigmentation.
▶ Glomeruloid hemangiomas, perhaps caused by elevated VEGF levels.

19.8 Gout

▶ **Definition:** Hyperuricemia associated with crystal-induced arthritis, tophi and in some instances renal stones.
▶ **Pathogenesis:** Over 99% of cases associated with decreased renal excretion of uric acid. Rarely, overproduction of uric acid (*Lesch–Nyhan syndrome* with self-mutilation). Secondary elevation in leukemia, polycythemia, hemolytic anemia, tumor chemotherapy; also caused by diuretics, chronic renal disease, and ketoacidosis (diabetes mellitus, fasting).
▶ **Clinical features:** Acute arthritis with exquisite pain, swelling; most often involves great toe (*podagra*) (60%), less often other digits (10%), feet (10%), or other joints. Renal stones a risk. Cutaneous findings include uric acid deposits (*tophi*) most often on ears or periarticular; in later case, differential diagnostic considerations include rheumatoid nodule.
▶ **Therapy:** Acute flares treated with NSAID or colchicine; prophylaxis with diet, probenecid or allopurinol.

19.9 Amyloidosis

Introduction

▶ **Definition:** A condition where amyloid, a β-pleated stable protein, is deposited in tissues.
▶ **Diagnostic approach:**
 • Amyloid can only be diagnosed with certainty with a biopsy. The following stains can be used:
  – *Congo red:* When examined in polarized light, amyloid is doubly refractive and apple green.
  – *Thioflavine S:* Yellow fluorescence.
  – *Acridine orange:* Red fluorescence.
 • Immunohistochemical studies with antibodies can also be used to further identify the type of amyloid.
 • *Biopsy sites:* Most useful sites for primary amyloidosis include:
  – Rectal mucosa (85%).
  – Transverse carpal ligament (almost 100%).
 ▣ *Note:* If patient presents with bilateral carpel tunnel syndrome, always think amyloid.
  – Subcutaneous fat tissue (biopsy or aspirate; <50%).
  – Bone marrow (circa 40%, but only for primary amyloidosis).
  – Other sites may include skin, oral mucosa, muscle, sural nerve, liver, gastrointestinal wall, heart (depending on type of involvement).

Overview

The unifying theme of amyloid is β-pleated protein sheets combined with glyco-protein components. Most typical is amyloid A protein, which is related to the serum amyloid A (SAA) protein and in turn to C-reactive protein. Table 19.4 lists some of the different types of amyloid and Table 19.5 summarizes the different types of amyloidosis, some of which are discussed below.

Table 19.4 · Types of amyloid

Type	Abbreviation	Clinical designation	Precursor protein
Immune amyloid	AL	Primary amyloidosis	Light chain immuno-globulins (λ > ϰ)
Classic amyloid	AA	Secondary amyloid (leprosy, rheumatoid arthritis, inflammatory bowel disease, familial Mediterranean fever, many more)	Apolipoprotein with properties of acute phase protein (SAA)
Endocrine amyloid	AE	APUD tumors (thyroid C cells, islet cells, others)	Prohormone
Familial amyloid	AF	Usually associated with polyneuropathy	Prealbumin variant
	AF	Nonneuropathic form (renal disease)	SAA
Senile amyloid	AS	Cerebral or cardiac forms	Variety of precursor proteins; related to prion disease and Down syndrome
Hemodialysis amyloid	AH	Side effects of long-term hemodialysis; carpel tunnel syndrome and cystic bone lesions	B2 microglobulin
Cutaneous amyloid	AK	Localized skin involvement	Keratins

Table 19.5 · Cutaneous amyloidosis

Type	Characteristics
Primary cutaneous amyloidosis	
Lichen amyloidosus	Papules on shins
Macular amyloidosis	Intra-scapular hyperpigmentation and papules
Nodular amyloidosis	Yellow nodules with central atrophy; can be primary or secondary to AL amyloid

Continued Table 19.5 ▶

Table 19.5 · Continued	
Type	Characteristics
Secondary cutaneous amyloidosis	
With epithelial tumors	Basal cell carcinoma, seborrheic keratosis, actinic keratosis
With actinic elastosis	
With excessive light exposure or PUVA therapy	
Cutaneous signs of systemic amyloidosis	
AL type	Hemorrhage and deposits about vessels; rarely nodular deposits
AA type	Hemorrhage and deposits around vessels
Amyloid elastosis	Rare, progressive fatal variant

Lichen Amyloidosus

▶ **Epidemiology:** Most common form of cutaneous amyloidosis; more common in Asians.
▶ **Pathogenesis:** Patients have severe pruritus, whatever the cause. Excessive scratching and rubbing damages keratinocytes; keratin drops into dermis and is somehow processed into amyloid.
▶ **Clinical features:** Pruritic, closely grouped firm glistening papules; often with fine scale; pink to red-brown; almost always on shin (Fig. 19.**6**).
   ☐ *Note:* Amyloid deposits in AL and AA amyloid never itch.
▶ **Histology:** Dermal papillae dilated and filled with subtle deposits of amyloid K. Incontinence of pigment, acanthosis confirm previous manipulation.
▶ **Diagnostic approach:** Clinical examination, biopsy. No extensive immunologic workup needed.
▶ **Differential diagnosis:** Lichen planus, lichen simplex chronicus.
▶ **Therapy:** No good solution; antipruritic measures (such as topical corticosteroids, perhaps under occlusion), PUVA, or even systemic retinoids.

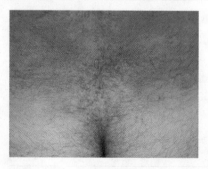

Fig. 19.**6** · Lichen amyloidosus.

Macular Amyloidosis

- ► **Synonyms:** Interscapular amyloidosis, bath brush amyloidosis.
- ► **Epidemiology:** Uncommon; seen more often in Asians and darker-skinned individuals; usually affects adults.
- ► **Pathogenesis:** Once again self-induced in patients with marked pruritus; often associated with notalgia paresthetica. Some patients use a back scratcher or bath brush to alleviate itching on their back.
- ► **Clinical features:** Modest pruritus, disseminated often confluent small tan macules; poorly circumscribed. Typically interscapular but can occur at other sites. Overlaps with lichen amyloidosis.
- ► **Histology:** Very subtle deposits of amyloid A in dermal papillae; easily missed.
  - ▣ *Note:* In pure cutaneous amyloidosis with amyloid K, there are no perivascular deposits.
- ► **Diagnostic approach:** Clinical examination, biopsy.
- ► **Differential diagnosis:** Postinflammatory hyperpigmentation, atopic dermatitis, other forms of dermatitis, lichen simplex chronicus, fixed drug reaction.
- ► **Therapy:** As for lichen amyloidosus; capsaicin solution once daily for long period of time has helped some.

Nodular Amyloidosis

- ► **Synonyms:** Amyloidosis cutis nodularis atrophicans, plaque-like amyloidosis.
- ► **Pathogenesis:** Association with AL; some patients have isolated cutaneous disease, other share evidence of systemic involvement.
- ► **Clinical features:** Red-brown nodules and plaques, often with central thinning so that underlying fat is seen with yellow shimmer; often on scalp.
- ► **Histology:** Massive deposits of amyloid L, diffusely filling dermis, also involves vessels and sweat glands.
- ► **Diagnostic approach:** Clinical examination, biopsy. Exclude systemic involvement with gammopathy.
- ► **Differential diagnosis:** Nevus lipomatosus, lipoma, cysts, lymphoma; histologically, all forms of amorphous deposits, such as gout and nodular elastosis.
- ► **Therapy:** Excision.

Secondary Cutaneous Amyloidosis

Secondary deposits of amyloid K in the skin are almost always an incidental finding in histology reports. The presence of secondary amyloid has no clinical significance. The most common setting is in tumors such as basal cell carcinoma, seborrheic keratosis, and actinic keratosis. Any lichenified dermatitis may also show deposits, as can skin damaged by light or PUVA.

Primary Systemic Amyloidosis

- ► **Synonym:** Immunocyte-derived amyloidosis.
- ► **Definition:** Amyloidosis caused by a monoclonal gammopathy with deposition of AL in many organs.
- ► **Pathogenesis:** Uncommon disorder; associated with variety of monoclonal B-cell proliferations including multiple myeloma, Waldenström macroglobulinemia, plasma cell dyscrasia with Bence Jones proteins, heavy chain disease, and B-cell lymphomas. In some instances, no underlying disease is found and the cause provisionally designated as "idiopathic" but the disease eventually evolves into a gammopathy.

► **Clinical features:**
- A wide variety of organs can be involved, so the signs and symptoms are highly variable. Most commonly involved organs include kidneys, heart, peripheral nervous system, tongue, gastrointestinal tract.
- Skin findings include:
  - Spontaneous purpura, often facial with many colorful names such as "pinch purpura" or "postproctoscopic purpura." The message is that minor trauma damages vessel walls infiltrated by amyloid and leads to unexpected purpura.
  - Tiny amyloid deposits, often periorbital or intertriginous, and often with subtle purpura.
  - Nodular amyloidosis (see above).
  - Macroglossia.
  - Peripheral neuropathy can indirectly lead to malum perforans; involvement of carpel ligament to carpel tunnel syndrome.

► **Histology:** Deposits of amyloid found in small blood vessels in dermis or subcutaneous fat. If skin lesions are present, yield is high. Best site for blind biopsy is rectal mucosa or subcutaneous fat.

► **Diagnostic approach:** Clinical examination, biopsy; once amyloid has been confirmed, then extensive search for underlying disease.

► **Differential diagnosis:**
- All the different causes of purpura.
- *Papules:* Xanthoma, xanthelasma, lipoid proteinosis, lichen myxedematosus.
- *Nodules:* Cysts, lipomas, nevus lipomatosus, lymphoma, and others.

► **Therapy:** Skin disease requires no therapy; B-cell proliferations treated by hematology-oncology, with secondary signs and symptoms managed in multidisciplinary fashion.

Secondary Systemic Amyloidosis

► **Synonyms:** Reactive amyloidosis, wear-and-tear amyloidosis.

► **Pathogenesis:** Deposition of AA amyloid secondary either to chronic inflammatory diseases (tuberculosis, leprosy, inflammatory bowel disease, rheumatoid arthritis) or to variety of malignant tumors. Familial Mediterranean fever features an abnormality in SAA and invariably progresses to AA deposits.

► **Clinical features:**
- Depend heavily on underlying disease; most likely organs are kidney, liver, spleen adrenal glands, and gastrointestinal tract. Main problem is progressive renal failure.
- Cutaneous findings uncommon: purpura or rarely deposits.

► **Histology:** Same as with AL amyloid; blind skin biopsies once again unlikely to be useful.

► **Therapy:** Treat underlying disease; possibility of regression if control is achieved.

19.10 Smoking and the Skin

Overview

The detrimental effects of smoking are well known. In Germany about 25% of the population smokes, with an disturbing increase in young smokers, especially young women. About 25% of deaths are blamed on smoking, although some estimates are much higher. The main problems are carcinoma of the lung and cardiovascular disease. There is no other risk factor with such clearly proven adverse effects on human health.

Cutaneous Manifestations

▶ **Premature aging:** Smokers' skin is often excessively wrinkled, has a yellow-orange tint. Although excessive sun exposure is a greater risk factor, the two effects are cumulative. Favre–Racouchot disease is especially common in smokers.

▶ **Yellow fingers:** Direct discoloration of the finger tips and nails from smoke.

▶ **Impaired wound healing:** Combination of impaired collagen synthesis, reduced oxygen supply because of excessive carbon monoxide and decreased circulation (nicotine-induced vasoconstriction, hyperviscosity).

Diseases Associated with Smoking

▶ **Well established:**
  • Palmoplantar pustulosis.
  • Psoriasis, especially pustular psoriasis.
  • Acne inversa.
  • Squamous cell carcinoma of the lips and oral mucosa.
  • Condylomata acuminata (and carcinoma of cervix).

▶ **Possible associations:**
  • Atopic dermatitis; also passive exposure from smoking parents.
  • Malignant melanoma (smokers have worse prognosis).
  • Lupus erythematosus (also worse response to antimalarials).

▶ **Other dangers:** Smokers should not be prescribed inflammable topical agents, such as those in alcohol base.

▶ **Possible positive effects:** There are rare diseases that seem to improve with smoking—Behçet syndrome and Crohn disease. We mention them only for completeness, and do not encourage patients with either of these disorders to start smoking.

20 Pruritus and Prurigo

20.1 Pruritus

Overview

▶ **Definition:** *Pruritus or itching* is an unpleasant cutaneous sensation that makes the individual scratch.
▶ **Pathogenesis:** Pruritus is a physiologic protective mechanism, stimulating the host to scratch away stinging insects or scabies mites. It is thus similar to other protective mechanisms against heat, cold, or pain. Numerous mediators, including histamine, cytokines, opiates and others, can induce pruritus. Itch impulses are transmitted by slow-firing unmyelinated C fibers. The receptors have not been completely identified, but probably consist of a group of structures that cross-modulate each other. Minimal stimulation of single fibers can cause itching, tickling, or tingling; more aggressive stimulation of bundles of fibers by rubbing or scratching temporarily inhibits the unpleasant stimuli.
▶ **Clinical features:** Pruritus may be localized or generalized. It tends to be worse at night when the patient is less distracted. Patients with pruritus may have either normal skin or excoriations, as well as signs of an underlying skin disease.

Diagnostic Approach

◼ **Note:** The challenge is to determine whether the patient has a pruritic skin disease that has not been identified or whether an underlying systemic disease is causing their symptoms (Table 20.1).
▶ **History:** Severity of pruritus, interferes with sleep.

Table 20.1 · Causes of pruritus

Category	Examples
Metabolic and endocrine diseases	Diabetes mellitus, hyperthyroidism, hypothyroidism, chronic renal disease, uremia, carcinoid syndrome
Malignancy	Hodgkin disease (most common), other lymphomas and solid tumors
Hematologic diseases	Polycythemia vera, monoclonal gammopathy, mastocytosis, hypereosinophilia syndrome
Hepatic disease	Primary biliary cirrhosis, hepatitis, cholestasis (pregnancy, drug-induced), biliary obstruction
Infections and infestations	Scabies, pediculosis, onchocerciasis, arthropod assault reactions, any systemic worm infestation
Psychogenic factors	Acute—reaction to stress, anxiety, depression Chronic—delusions of parasitosis
Skin diseases	Allergic contact dermatitis, atopic dermatitis, bullous pemphigoid, dermatitis herpetiformis, dermatophyte infections, fiberglass dermatitis, pediculosis, polymorphous light eruption, scabies, urticaria, xerosis

▶ **Physical examination:** Excoriations, xerosis, scabies, pediculosis, dermographism, lymphadenopathy.

▣ *Note:* Scabies can present with virtually no cutaneous findings, especially in meticulous patients (*scabies of the cleanly*).

▶ **Laboratory:** Sedimentation rate, CBC, liver function tests, glucose, serum IgE, hepatitis serology, stool for ova and parasites.

▶ **Imaging:** Chest radiograph.

▶ **Additional studies:** Based on the history, additional studies might include thyroid function tests, α-fetoprotein, carcinoembryonic antigen (CEA), ferritin, creatinine, creatinine clearance, blood urea nitrogen (BUN), serum protein electrophoresis, serotonin levels, urine electrophoresis.

Therapy

▶ Treat the underlying disease, if one has been identified.
▶ Antihistamines, tranquilizers, opiate antagonists.
▶ Topical capsaicin.
▶ Optimal skin care (lubricants).
▶ **UVB irradiation:**
  • **Uremic pruritus:** UVB irradiation, charcoal tablets, lidocaine i.v., cholestyramine, ondansetron, naloxone i.v, plasmapheresis, subtotal parathyroidectomy.
  • *Cholestatic pruritus:* UVB irradiation, cholestyramine, plasmapheresis.

20.2 Prurigo

Overview

The combination of pruritus and associated skin lesions, produced by scratching, is known as prurigo. The cause of prurigo is unknown. It is unclear why in some clinical settings pruritus leads to excoriations, and in others to the development of dome-shaped papules. Many different unrelated diseases are lumped together under the rubric of prurigo; we will discuss only a few common examples. All can be treated in the same way with systemic antihistamines, topical anesthetics (polidocanol), or distractors (menthol), and in some instances with topical corticosteroids.

Prurigo Simplex Acuta

Acute reaction usually in children, induced by arthropod bites or stings, also known as *strophulus.* Typical prurigo seropapule (tiny papule with marked edema producing a vesicle at top) develops; intensely pruritic. Self-limited; treat with antihistamines.

Prurigo Simplex Subacuta

The least well-defined member of a fuzzy group. We view this as synonymous with *"pruritogenic excoriation."* Patients present with papules, excoriations, and the history that the pruritus is greatly relived when the papules are excoriated and damaged. When only the face is involved, the term *acne urticata* is applied. Probably many different causes of pruritus, which meet in a common pathway in susceptible individuals. Chronic problem; extremely difficult to treat. Try antihistamines, anesthetics, topical corticosteroids; some patients respond to phototherapy or minor tranquilizers.

Prurigo Nodularis

▶ **Clinical features:** Patients develop red-brown hyperkeratotic nodules several centimeters across, typically on the extremities. Formerly felt to be almost pathognomic of uremia, but also seen in atopic dermatitis and without obvious cause. More common in women. Complain of pruritus.

▶ **Histology:** Prototype of pseudoepitheliomatous hyperplasia, with marked acanthosis and hyperkeratosis. In some instances, hypertrophied cutaneous nerves, but unclear if causative or reactive.

▶ **Diagnostic approach:** Look for other signs of atopic dermatitis; exclude renal disease and other systemic causes of pruritus if clinically plausible.

▶ **Differential diagnosis:** Difficult to separate from verrucous lichen planus; look for signs of disease elsewhere.

▶ **Therapy:** Most effective are high-potency corticosteroids under occlusion or intralesional corticosteroids, coupled with systemic antihistamines.

Lichen Simplex Chronicus

▶ **Clinical features:** One or several lichenified patches, almost always on nape or dorsal aspect of hands or feet. Facial involvement uncommon. Patient manipulates just this localized area, in contrast to prurigo nodularis where broad areas are attacked. Rarely complain of pruritus. When examined closely, often consists of central plaque surround by multiple small papules and rim of postinflammatory hyperpigmentation. Also more common in atopic dermatitis.

   ◩ *Note:* Often the patient will manipulate the area during the short course of an office visit.

▶ **Histology:** Epidermal reaction as in prurigo nodularis but less severe.

▶ **Diagnostic approach:** Look for other signs of atopic dermatitis.

▶ **Differential diagnosis:** Usually diagnosis is obvious, but patient is unwilling to accept. Occasionally confused with tinea or lichen amyloidosus; overlaps with prurigo nodularis.

▶ **Therapy:** Same as prurigo nodularis; see above.

Perforating Disease of Renal Dialysis

▶ **Synonyms:** Perforating folliculitis, hyperkeratosis follicularis et parafollicularis in cutem penetrans (Kyrle disease).

▶ **Definition:** Pruritic papules usually in patients with diabetes mellitus, renal failure, and dialysis, although all three components are not always present.

▶ **Pathogenesis:** Although this disorder is common in dialysis patients, it is nonetheless surrounded by both linguistic and scientific confusion. Kyrle disease is illogical; he described epidermal keratoses penetrating into the dermis. Perforating folliculitis is an oxymoron, as all folliculitis shows some degree of follicle wall damage by definition. These patients have pruritus induced by their renal disease (or occasionally by other factors), and react with a follicular type of prurigo nodularis.

▶ **Clinical features:** Intense pruritus; numerous 3–6 mm hyperkeratotic nodules, usually clearly in a follicle, are seen on the shins, forearms, and sometimes elsewhere on the body. Areas with no follicles, such as palms, soles, and mucosa are spared.

▶ **Histology:** Highly confusing; varying combinations of follicular plugging, follicle wall damage, reactive epidermal changes, excoriations, chronic inflammation.

▶ **Diagnostic approach:** Clinical examination and history.

▶ **Differential diagnosis:** The perforating dermatoses are considered under elastosis perforans serpiginosa (p. 359). The true differential diagnostic considerations are lichen simplex chronicus and prurigo nodularis; we view the three entities as part of a spectrum.

▶ **Therapy:**
- Maximize management of renal disease; investigate dialysis system with nephrologists, as some feel types of filters and dialysates plays a role; UV light effective for renal pruritus; also try topical antipruritic agents.
- In more severe cases, charcoal tablets (12–16 daily), lidocaine i.v., cholestyramine, ondansetron, naloxone i.v, plasmapheresis, subtotal parathyroidectomy.

Prurigo Pigmentosa

▶ **Definition:** Uncommon pruritic disorder that heals with distinctive hyperpigmentation.

▶ **Epidemiology:** Originally described in Japanese, but seen occasionally in all races; more common in women.

▶ **Clinical features:** Intensely pruritic inflammatory papules usually favoring breasts and anterior chest; often arranged in reticular pattern. Heal with striking postinflammatory hyperpigmentation.

▶ **Histology:** Dense subepidermal lymphohistiocytic infiltrate with pronounced epidermotropism and numerous necrotic keratinocytes.

▶ **Therapy:** Symptomatic care, topical corticosteroids or anesthetics (polidocanol).

Other Types of Prurigo

Many other diseases are designated as prurigo. All are pruritic are some point in their course, but not otherwise related. Table 20.2 summarizes this mixed group.

Table 20.2 · Other types of prurigo

Disease	Comments
Actinic prurigo	Uncommon form of photosensitivity combining dermatitis, cheilitis and prurigo; most common in Native Americans
Prurigo aestivalis (Hutchinson prurigo)	Polymorphous light eruption in childhood
Besnier prurigo	Atopic dermatitis with prurigo nodularis
Prurigo diabetic	Diabetes mellitus with prurigo nodularis
Prurigo dermatographica (Marcussen prurigo)	Prurigo following pressure urticaria
Prurigo gestationis	Old term for pruritic disease in pregnancy; probably represents flare of atopic dermatitis in pregnancy, but unclear
Prurigo hepatica	Prurigo secondary to liver disease
Prurigo melanotica (Pierini–Borda)	Prurigo plus postinflammatory hyperpigmentation, usually in dark-skinned individuals
Prurigo uremica	Prurigo in renal failure; formerly very common diagnosis

21 *Genodermatoses*

Although this chapter is devoted to genodermatoses, many acquired disorders are also considered when they seem to fit into the general clinical picture. For example, acquired forms of porokeratosis are considered along with the less common inherited ones.

21.1 *MIM Code*

What is the MIM Code?

Victor A. McKusick, one of the giants of clinical human genetics, started using a numerical code when he began compiling his books entitled *Mendelian Inheritance in Man*. The books evolved into a website, OMIM (*Online Mendelian Inheritance in Man*), which today serves as the standard for clinical genetics and the most convenient way to acquire updated information on all genetic disorders.

The MIM code is given throughout this book whenever it is relevant. The first digit identifies the pattern of diagnosis: 1 = autosomal dominant inheritance; 2 = autosomal recessive inheritance; 3 = X-linked inheritance.

How to Use OMIM

1 Simply enter ONIM in Google or any search engine and you will land on OMIM—or enter www.ncbi.nlm.nih.gov/OMIM.
2 Search OMIM.
3 Enter the MIM code, or a key word or two if you are looking for a syndrome or set of findings.
4 You will see a list of disease descriptions likely to be relevant to your query; chose whichever ones seem most useful.
5 Now you can read an update about the disease, the gene, find extensive references, or be linked to Medline.

21.2 *The Ichthyoses*

Overview

The primary ichthyoses are a heterogenous group of inherited disorders featuring excessive scale. The alternate term *disorder of keratinization* is less offensive to patients who do not enjoy being told they resemble fish (ichthyosis is Greek for "fishlike condition"). Secondary or acquired ichthyosis describes similar scaly conditions appearing later in life.

The "brick and mortar" model of the epidermis helps one understand the genetic basis of the primary ichthyoses. The stratum corneum is made up of keratins and lipids. Mutations in keratins usually have autosomal dominant inheritance and can be viewed as "defective bricks." Mutations in the enzymes needed to produce and metabolize lipids are usually autosomal recessive, and represent "defective mortar."

Classification

▶ **Primary ichthyoses:**
  • *Common:*
    – Ichthyosis vulgaris (see below).
    – X-linked recessive ichthyosis.
  • *Rare:*
    – Congenital autosomal recessive ichthyoses:
    – Nonbullous congenital ichthyosiform erythroderma.
    – Lamellar ichthyosis.
    – Autosomal dominant lamellar ichthyosis.
    – Ichthyoses with epidermolytic hyperkeratosis:
    – Bullous congenital ichthyosiform erythroderma (Brocq).
    – Ichthyosis hystrix (Curth–Macklin).
    – Ichthyosis bullosa (Siemens).
    – Harlequin fetus.
    – Syndromes with ichthyosis:
    – Ichthyosis linearis circumflexa (Netherton syndrome).
    – X-linked dominant chondrodysplasia punctata (Conradi–Hünermann–Happle syndrome).
    – Refsum syndrome.
    – Sjögren–Larsson syndrome.
▶ **Secondary or acquired ichthyoses:**
  • Paraneoplastic marker for lymphoma and internal malignancies.
  🛑 *Caution:* Whenever ichthyosis appears in adult life for the first time, exclude an underlying malignancy.
  • *Infections:* Leprosy, tuberculosis, syphilis.
  • *Vitamin deficiency:* Vitamin A, vitamin B6, and nicotinic acid deficiency (pellagra, p. 302).
  • *Medications:* nicotinic acid (most common), triparanol, butyrophenone.
  ◼ *Note:* Any drug that alters lipids is potentially capable of inducing an ichthyosis-like condition.
  • **Miscellaneous:** Sarcoidosis, hypothyroidism, Down syndrome, long-term renal dialysis, severe xerosis in the elderly.

Ichthyosis Vulgaris

▶ **MIM code:** 146700.
▶ **Definition:** Most common form of ichthyosis and also the mildest.
▶ **Epidemiology:** Prevalence of 1:250.
▶ **Pathogenesis:** Abnormal formation of keratohyalin granules and delayed destruction of desmosomes because of defective or absent production of profilaggrin and filaggrin, producing a *retention hyperkeratosis*.
▶ **Clinical features:**
  • Usually starts in first year of life (months 3–12; not at birth), progressive until puberty, then usually improvement. Better in summer.
  • Clinically overlaps with xerosis, sometimes making definitive diagnosis difficult.
  • White fine scales of varying intensity on extensor surfaces (especially shins), trunk and lateral aspects of face. Flexures always spared (Fig. 21.1). No mucosal involvement.
  • Exaggerated palmoplantar markings (ichthyosis hand or foot).
  • Callus-like lesions on knees and elbows.

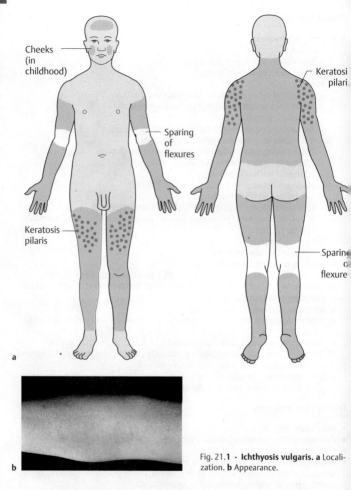

Cheeks
(in
childhood)

Keratosis
pilaris

Sparing
of
flexures

Keratosis
pilaris

Keratosis
pilaris

Sparing
of
flexures

a

b

Fig. 21.1 · **Ichthyosis vulgaris. a** Localization. **b** Appearance.

- Follicular hyperkeratoses on shoulders (keratosis pilaris); sometimes also involves buttocks, thighs and upper arms.
  ▢ *Note:* When confronted with extensive keratosis pilaris, always think of ichthyosis vulgaris.
- *Associated disorder:* Atopic dermatitis (50%).
► **Histology:** Mild hyperkeratosis with an absent granular layer; normal dermis.
► **Diagnostic approach:** Clinical examination; biopsy may be helpful, but often equivocal. Best clues are family history, early onset, spared flexures, and hyperlinear palms.

▶ **Differential diagnosis:** Other forms of ichthyosis, acquired ichthyosis, extreme xerosis (particular problem in blacks).
▶ **Therapy:** Topical urea compounds most useful; watch concentration (irritating if too high) and chose a well-tolerated vehicle; alternatives include lactic acid and salicylic acid or combinations thereof. Lubrication of skin after bathing most crucial; defatting soaps should be avoided.
> ▶ *Note:* Topical corticosteroids absolutely useless—just a very expensive cream!

X-linked Recessive Ichthyosis

▶ **Synonym:** Steroid sulfatase deficiency.
▶ **MIM code:** 308100.
▶ **Definition:** Ichthyosis seen only in men as a result of steroid sulfatase deficiency.
▶ **Epidemiology:** Prevalence of 1:6000 among men.
▶ **Pathogenesis:** Mutation in steroid sulfatase gene *STS* at Xp22.32 means that the mortar (cholesterol sulfate) cannot be broken down, so once again a *retention hyperkeratosis* develops.
▶ **Clinical features:**
- *Ichthyosis* (100%):
    - Starts in first 6 months, progressive until puberty, then stable; improves in summer.
    - Large brown polygonal scales divided by wide splits (Fig. 21.2).

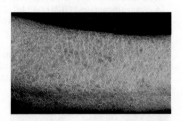

Fig. 21.2 · X-linked recessive ichthyosis: coarse brown scales.

- In younger patients, prominent involvement of scalp, ears, and neck (*dirty neck*).
    - On trunk and extremities, typically localized severally involved areas.
- *Ocular involvement* (100%):
    - Asymptomatic corneal opacities.
    - May also be found in carrier females.
- *Complications of pregnancy* (30–40%):
    - Deficiency of placental steroid sulfatase leads to low levels of estrogens.
    - Often delayed onset of labor or inadequate contractions.
- *Hypogonadism* (25%):
    - Reduced androgen synthesis leads to hypergonadotropic hypogonadism.
    - Testes often undescended with increased risk of testicular carcinoma.
▶ **Histology:** Hyperkeratosis, normal to thickened granular layer.
▶ **Diagnostic approach:**
- Clinical examination (dirty neck), history of abnormal delivery or affected uncles; elevated plasma cholesterol sulfate level or lipoprotein electrophoresis showing increasing motility of β- and pre-β-lipoproteins.
- Also arrange for ophthalmologic and urologic consultation; consider testosterone replacement.

▶ **Differential diagnosis:** In contrast to ichthyosis vulgaris, no hyperlinear palms, no keratosis pilaris, flexural involvement and larger, darker scales.

▶ **Therapy:** Same as ichthyosis vulgaris; also worth trying 10% cholesterol ointments topically, especially in infants who do not tolerate urea or lactic acid.

Collodion Baby

A number of forms of ichthyosis present at birth with infant encased in a tight membrane of adherent keratinocytes, which has been compared to parchment or collodion. Kollodes is the Greek word for glutinous or glue-like. The membrane is then shed, leaving either normal skin (*lamellar exfoliation of newborn*) or, more often, one of the forms of nonbullous congenital ichthyosiform erythroderma or lamellar ichthyosis. Both disorders are heterogenous and also show overlaps. Our listing and description is deliberately simplified; when confronted with a case, consult OMIM or a specialized text.

Nonbullous Congenital Ichthyosiform Erythroderma

▶ **MIM code:** 242100.

▶ **Definition:** Rare severe ichthyosis presenting at birth.

▶ **Pathogenesis:** One of the first examples of proven genetic heterogeneity, as several different mutations cause the same clinical syndrome. All three involve lipid metabolism and have autosomal recessive inheritance:

- Tranglutaminase-1 (*TGM1*) at 14q11.2; also involved in lamellar ichthyosis.
- Two lipoxygenases at 17p13.1 (*ALOX12B* and *ALOXE3*).

▶ **Clinical features:**

- Frequently born as collodion baby.
- Fine white scales and erythroderma (usually severe but variable). Also ectropion and scarring alopecia (Fig. 21.3).
- Nail dystrophy, hypotrichosis, short stature, cardiac malformations.

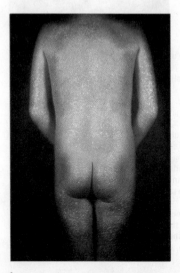

Fig. 21.3 · Nonbullous congenital ichthyosiform erythroderma.

▶ **Histology:** Hyperkeratosis with focal parakeratosis, hypergranulosis and acanthosis; keratinocyte membranes periodic acid–Schiff (PAS) positive.

▶ **Therapy:** Systemic retinoids may be helpful, but long-term use problematic; otherwise, as for ichthyosis vulgaris.

Chanarin–Dorfman syndrome

▶ MIM code 275630; *CG158* gene at 3p21; similar to nonbullous congenital ichthyosiform erythroderma but with lipid inclusions in epidermal cells, cataracts, deafness, and often mental retardation.

Autosomal Recessive Lamellar Ichthyosis

▶ **MIM code:** 242300.

▶ **Definition:** Severe uncommon (1:100000) ichthyosis.

▶ **Pathogenesis:** Several genes identified; most common is transglutaminase-1 (*TGM1*) at 14q11.2, but several other loci known. Unique problem in that one mutation can produce two clinical patterns: fine scale and erythroderma or thick scales and prominent ectropion.

▶ **Clinical features:**

• Frequently born as collodion baby.

• Thick dark scales, marked facial involvement, often ectropion, sometimes persistent erythroderma, temperature intolerance (sweat ducts clogged or defective) (Fig. 21.**4**).

▶ **Histology:** The transglutaminase-1 can be stained in frozen sections of skin; if absent, suggests diagnosis.

▶ **Diagnostic approach:** Very confusing; both autosomal dominant lamellar ichthyosis and lamellar ichthyosis/nonbullous congenital ichthyosiform erythroderma overlap. Both are much more rare than lamellar ichthyosis.

▶ **Therapy:** Patients often require systemic retinoids; otherwise, same treatment as ichthyosis vulgaris.

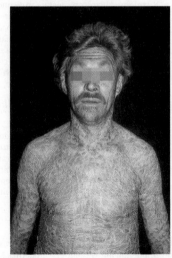

Fig. 21.**4** · Autosomal recessive lamellar ichthyosis.

Autosomal Dominant Lamellar Ichthyosis

▶ **MIM code:** 146750.
▶ Rare form of ichthyosis; autosomal dominant inheritance with gene undetermined. Can mimic either lamellar ichthyosis or less often nonbullous congenital ichthyosiform erythroderma. *TGM1* not involved. Treatment difficult but identical to other forms of lamellar ichthyosis.

Ichthyoses with Epidermolytic Hyperkeratosis

▶ Epidermolytic hyperkeratosis is a specific histologic finding with clumped keratohyaline granules and vacuolization of stratum spinosum and granulosum. It is found in several types of ichthyoses, as well as in palmoplantar keratoderma (Vörner type), epidermal nevi, sporadic papules (epidermolytic acanthoma), and as a chance focal finding in normal skin.

Bullous Congenital Ichthyosiform Erythroderma (Brocq)

▶ **Synonym:** Epidermolytic hyperkeratosis.
▶ **MIM code:** 113800.
▶ **Definition:** Uncommon (1:100000) severe generalized disorder with blisters and hyperkeratotic lesions.
▶ **Pathogenesis:** Mutations in keratin 1 and 10 genes; this keratin pair is expressed above the basal layer. Structural mutation with autosomal dominant inheritance about 50% of cases familial and 50% new mutations.
▶ **Clinical features:**
  • At birth, widespread blisters and erosions; child looks as if burned.
  • During infancy, flaccid blisters at sites of pressure or friction.
  • Then development of distinctive dirty, spiny, hyperkeratotic lesions, often scattered on an erythematosus background; most often in flexures.
  • Palmoplantar keratoderma common, especially with keratin 1 mutation.
▶ **Histology:** Microscopic picture so distinctive that skin biopsies were used for prenatal diagnosis; intracellular vacuolization in stratum spinosum and granulosum clumped keratohyaline granules, compact hyperkeratosis.
▶ **Diagnostic approach:** Clinical examination, biopsy.
▶ **Differential diagnosis:** At birth, confused with epidermolysis bullosa and staphylococcal scalded skin syndrome. Later, clinically distinctive.
▶ **Therapy:** Systemic retinoids help with keratoses but may increase tendency to blister; watch for infections; otherwise, same as ichthyosis vulgaris.

Ichthyosis Hystrix (Curth–Macklin)

▶ **MIM code:** 146590.
▶ Rare ichthyosis showing autosomal dominant inheritance with characteristic spines (hystrix means porcupine, referring to spikes or spines), palmoplantar keratoderma, and epidermolytic hyperkeratosis. One family had keratin 1 mutation but probably heterogenous. Peculiar binucleated keratinocytes. Treatment with systemic retinoids. There are other even rarer forms of ichthyosis and epidermal nevus with a hystrix appearance and with varying histologic pictures.

Ichthyosis Bullosa (Siemens)

▶ **MIM code:** 146800.
▶ Mild form of congenital ichthyosis resembling congenital ichthyosiform erythroderma but without erythroderma. Mutation in keratin 2e gene, which is ex-

pressed even higher in epidermis. Patients described in German as "molting," as frequently sheets of skin are shed in irregular pattern. Histology shows epidermolytic hyperkeratosis. Treatment same as bullous congenital ichthyosiform erythroderma.

Harlequin Fetus

▶ **Synonym:** Ichthyosis congenita gravis.
▶ **MIM code:** 242500.
▶ Rare devastating disorder, barely compatible with life. Children born with extremely thick scales separated by erythematous fissures, fancifully compared to a harlequin's costume. Massive ectropion, eclabium; respiratory problems from construction by scales. Exact defect in keratin not known. Few survivors, with lifelong systemic retinoids.

Syndromes with Ichthyosis

Netherton Syndrome
▶ **Synonym:** Ichthyosis linearis circumflexa, Comèl–Netherton syndrome.
▶ **MIM code:** 256500.
▶ **Definition:** Distinctive syndrome with ichthyosiform skin changes, trichorrhexis invaginata, and atopic dermatitis.
▶ **Pathogenesis:** Mutation in *SPINK5* gene at 5q32, which codes for serine protease inhibitor; autosomal recessive inheritance.
▶ **Clinical features:**
  • Skin changes include:
    – Generalized erythroderma, especially severe on face; about 20% of childhood erythroderma are Netherton syndrome.
    – Circinate slightly raised erythematous bands on trunk (*ichthyosis linearis circumflexa*) with distinctive *double-edged scale*.
    – Complicated by overlapping features of atopic dermatitis including flexural and facial dermatitis; more difficult to treat than ordinary atopic dermatitis.
  • Hair shaft shows trichorrhexis invaginata (bamboo hairs) (p. 510).
  • Increased frequency of food allergies, urticaria, and infections.
  • Sometimes failure to thrive, rarely mental retardation.
▶ **Diagnostic approach:** Clinical examination, examination of hairs; often elevated IgE levels. Occasionally aminoaciduria.
▶ **Therapy:** Difficult to manage; keratolytics for ichthyotic lesions; in testing of topical tacrolimus, only patients to absorb significant amounts were those with Netherton syndrome who experienced considerable toxicity. Sometimes systemic retinoids help.

Conradi–Hünermann–Happle Syndrome
▶ **Synonym:** X-linked chondrodysplasia punctata.
▶ **MIM code:** 302960.
▶ **Definition:** Rare complex of cutaneous, ocular, and bony disorders.
▶ **Pathogenesis:** Mutation in *EBP* gene, a sterol isomerase located at Xp11.22–11.23. Lethal in males; presents in mosaic pattern in female infants.
▶ **Clinical features:**
  • Skin at birth shows ichthyosiform erythroderma; later hyperkeratotic areas as well as pigmentary changes following Blaschko lines. Also scarring alopecia and unruly hair.
  • Radiograph of epiphyses shows stippling (chondrodysplasia punctata); resolves with time, so not reliable for diagnosis later in life.
  • Scoliosis, nasal hypoplasia, cataracts.

► **Diagnostic approach:** Clinical examination, radiography, genetic analysis.
► **Differential diagnosis:** Several other disorders diagnosed as chondrodysplasia punctata, with different patterns of inheritance and varying degrees of skeletal change. Consult OMIM or geneticist.
► **Therapy:** Interdisciplinary management; skin tends to be major problem only early in life.

Sjögren–Larsson Syndrome
► **MIM code:** 272200.
► Rare ichthyosis; autosomal recessive inheritance with defect in *FALDH* at 17p11.2 coding for fatty aldehyde dehydrogenase. Common only in northern Sweden. Fine scaling of neck and abdomen, coupled with ophthalmologic and CNS abnormalities, as well as mental retardation.

Refsum Syndrome
► **MIM code:** 266500.
► Rare ichthyosis; autosomal recessive inheritance, with defect in *PAHX* at 10pter-p11.2 coding for a phytanic acid hydroxylase. Fine white scale resembling ichthyosis vulgaris but coupled with peripheral and cranial nerve dysfunction and cardiomyopathy. Increased plasma phytanic acid.

CHILD Nevus or Syndrome
► Peculiar type of ichthyosiform epidermal nevus (p. 414), often listed with ichthyosis.

21.3 Other Keratinization Disorders

Follicular Keratoses
....

Just as the stratum corneum sheds scales, the hair follicle epithelium must shed its outermost keratotic material. Normally the combination of lipid secretion and hair growth cleanses the follicle, but sometimes a plug of keratin is retained. After a follicle has been plugged, it may become gaping or patulous, producing *follicular atrophoderma*. A comedo in acne sounds similar, but it is an intrafollicular plug without an elevated component.
Conditions with plugged follicles include:
► **Keratosis pilaris:**
  • Most common; seen in almost everyone at some time in life.
  • Plugs accompanied by mild follicular erythema.
  • Usually over triceps area, but may also involve shoulders, buttocks, and thighs.
  • Associated with atopic dermatitis, ichthyosis vulgaris, and vitamin A deficiency.
  • Treatment consists of soaking, aggressive scrubbing, and using keratolytic lotions (such as urea or lactic acid lotions). Although topical retinoids sound as if they should work, they are surprisingly ineffective.
► **Keratosis pilaris atrophicans:** Also known as ulerythema ophryogenes, features plugged follicles on cheeks and eyebrows, leading to alopecia and follicular atrophoderma.
► **Keratosis spinulosa:** Also known as lichen spinulosus, consists of localized grouped white plugs usually on trunk of children.
► **Keratosis follicularis spinulosa decalvans:** MIM code 308800; uncommon disorder with X-linked recessive inheritance; features follicular keratoses on exposed areas along with scarring alopecia, palmoplantar keratoderma, photophobia, corneal dystrophy, and often atopic dermatitis.

► **Other disorders:** Both Darier disease (see below) and pityriasis rubra pilaris (p. 278) can start with follicular keratosis.

Darier Disease
....

► **MIM code:** 124200.

► **Definition:** Common genodermatosis with primarily follicular keratoses, distinctive histology, and autosomal dominant inheritance.

► **Epidemiology:** One of the most common genodermatoses; prevalence 1 : 30 000; little interference with fertility, so larger pedigrees common.

► **Pathogenesis:** Darier disease provided one of the first surprises in the search for genes causing dermatoses. The defect is in a calcium-channel regulating gene *ATP-2A2* at 12q24.1 which codes for SERCA2, an ATPase isoform. The disturbance in calcium homeostasis is thought to interfere with desmosome stability.

► **Clinical features:**

• Onset of skin disease usually around puberty. Multiple tiny (2–4 mm) rough brown papules; most common in seborrheic areas (midchest, face, retroauricular) (Fig. 21.5). Sometimes provoked by light.

• Also abnormal digital hieroglyphics, tiny palmoplantar pits, and longitudinal white or red nail stripes.

• Occasionally painful palmoplantar keratoderma with bullae.

• Cobblestone papules seen on palate, but also on pharyngeal, genital, and rectal mucosa.

• *Acrokeratosis verruciformis Hopf:* Flat papules on the sides and backs of hands; genetic studies have shown same mutation, indicating that this is simply one manifestation of Darier disease and not a separate entity, although it often appears without other stigmata.

• Increased likelihood of generalized infections with herpes and vaccinia viruses.

► **Histology:** Distinctive combination of acantholysis and individual cell keratinization, producing *corps ronds* (cells with peculiar keratin inclusions) and *grains* (parakeratotic material).

► **Diagnostic approach:** Clinical examination, biopsy; family history often positive.

► **Differential diagnosis:** Well-developed cases distinctive; early lesions confused with other follicular keratoses. Same histologic picture can be seen in Grover disease (see below) as well as epidermal nevi and acquired acanthomas, so clinicopathologic correlation required.

► **Therapy:** Acitretin 25–50 mg daily is probably the best treatment; should be used until disease under control and then stopped because of side effects. Tendency to secondary infections; some patients improve dramatically with antibiotics. Drastic approach is excision of severely affected area, such as soles, with skin grafting; donor dominance persists for months to years. Topical retinoids and keratolytics disappointing at best.

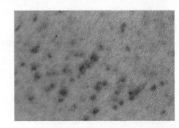

Fig. 21.**5** · Darier disease: keratotic brown papules.

Hailey–Hailey Disease

▶ **Synonym:** Familial benign chronic pemphigus.
▶ **MIM code:** 169600.
▶ **Definition:** Genodermatosis with frequent weeping dermatitis flexural patches; autosomal dominant inheritance.
▶ **Pathogenesis:** Mutation in *ATP2C1*, another calcium pump gene, at 3q21-q24; analogous to pathophysiology of Darier disease.
▶ **Clinical features:** Intertriginous areas are involved. Highly typical superficial erosions with fissures and splits; described as resembling "dusty road drying out after a rainstorm" (Fig. 21.**6**). Often foul-smelling. Occasionally nail streaks. Also predisposed to herpes and vaccinia infections, but less so than Darier disease.

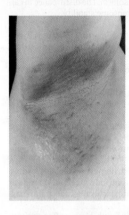

Fig. 21.**6** · Hailey–Hailey disease.

▶ **Histology:** Prominent acantholysis with little dyskeratosis ("collapsing brick wall") and frequent inflammation. Despite its alternative name, Hailey–Hailey disease has nothing to do with autoimmune pemphigus and immunofluorescence is negative.
▶ **Diagnostic approach:** Clinical examination, biopsy; family history often positive.
▶ **Differential diagnosis:** Usually misdiagnosed at first as candidiasis or intertrigo. In some instances, can appear very similar to Darier disease. Pemphigus vegetans also involves flexures but has thicker (vegetating) lesions.
▶ **Therapy:** Systemic acitretin is best choice but not as reliably effective as in Darier disease. Methotrexate 5–15 mg weekly can be tried. Both topical disinfectants and systemic antibiotics useful. Surgery just as in Darier disease, but easier to do, as worst areas are usually flexural areas which can be excised and covered with split-thickness graft.

Transient Acantholytic Dermatosis

▶ **Synonym:** Grover disease.
▶ **Definition:** Acquired intensely pruritic papular eruption with same histology as Darier disease.
▶ **Epidemiology:** Most patients are older men; often more severe in winter months with drier environment.

▶ **Pathogenesis:** Unknown.

▶ **Clinical features:** 1–2 mm pruritic red papules, sometimes juicy, occasionally with tiny vesicle; favor the trunk.

▶ **Histology:** Usually very similar to Darier disease; in other cases may have primarily acantholysis and resemble Hailey–Hailey disease or pemphigus foliaceus; immunofluorescence always negative.

▶ **Diagnostic approach:** Clinical examination, biopsy.

▶ **Differential diagnosis:** Folliculitis, dermatitis herpetiformis, prurigo simplex subacuta, scabies.

▶ **Therapy:** Phototherapy (PUVA or narrow band 311 nm) is most effective; also topical antipruritic agents. If drying seems to be a factor, then aggressive lubrication. Topical corticosteroids under occlusion briefly may help with itch..

Porokeratosis

▶ **Definition:** Group of probably unrelated disorders with same distinctive histologic appearance featuring cornoid lamellae.

▶ **Classification:**

- *Porokeratosis Mibelli:*
  - Erythematous hyperkeratotic to atrophic plagues with distinctive border; usually one or few plaques.
  - More common in immunosuppressed patients, suggesting some may be viral.
  - Small risk of development of squamous cell carcinoma.

- *Linear porokeratosis:* Probably variant of linear epidermal nevus with histology of porokeratosis, as grouped smaller lesions follow Blaschko lines.

- *Disseminated superficial actinic porokeratosis (DSAP):* Multiple 1–2 cm atrophic patches with distinctive border on arms or legs in older individuals with sun damage; sometimes provokes by light (Fig. 21.7).

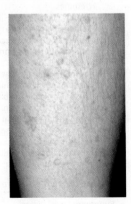

Fig. 21.**7** · Disseminated superficial actinic porokeratosis.

- *Porokeratosis punctata palmoplantaris:* Multiple 1–2 mm papules on palms and soles; autosomal dominant inheritance. Columnar parakeratosis.

- *Porokeratosis palmaris et plantaris disseminata:* Usually starts with multiple punctate lesions on palms and soles with onset in adolescence. Similar to porokeratosis punctata palmoplantaris but may also involve rest of body. Lesions fancifully compared to spines on a music box wheel. May have facial sebaceous hyperplasia as well.

- *Unilateral porokeratosis:* Lesions restricted to one side of body.

► **Histology:** The border should be biopsied, ideally with a small spindle-shaped piece of tissue with a long axis perpendicular to the prominent rim. This makes it easiest to identify the pathognomonic *cornoid lamella*—a focal area of disruption of the granular layer with a column of parakeratotic cells in the stratum corneum.

► **Diagnostic approach:** Clinical examination, biopsy.

► **Differential diagnosis:** Multiple lesions can be mistaken for psoriasis, lupus erythematosus, pityriasis rubra pilaris, or verrucous lichen planus. Solitary lesions often misinterpreted as tinea, warts, or actinic keratoses. The palmoplantar lesions are hard to diagnosis clinically; one can consider nevoid basal cell carcinoma syndrome, Cowden syndrome, punctate palmoplantar keratoderma, arsenical keratoses, and warts; only the biopsy provides the answer.

► **Therapy:** Cryotherapy or other destructive measures for limited lesions; otherwise, consider acitretin or PUVA (except for DSAP). Regular use of sunscreens; monitor for possible development of squamous cell carcinoma.

Erythrokeratodermia

► **Definition:** Group of uncommon disorders with both erythroderma and keratotic lesions.

► **Erythrokeratodermia variabilis (Mendes da Costa):**
- MIM code: 133200.
- Autosomal dominant inheritance; involves mutation in either connexin 30.3 or 31, both located at 1p35.1. The connexins are involved in gap junctions between cells.
- Two distinct types of lesions:
  - Relatively stable psoriasiform with bizarre configurations, usually on extremities.
  - Rapidly changing erythematous macules and patches on trunk.
  - Relation between two types of lesions unexplained.
- No tendency to improvement.

► **Erythrokeratodermia symmetrica progressiva (Gottron):**
- MIM code: 602036.
- Autosomal dominant inheritance. Mutation in loricrin gene at 1q21; loricrin is major component of cornified cell envelope.
- Psoriasiform plaques on backs of hands and feet, spreading to shins; sometimes compared to stockings and gloves; quite stable but can involve other areas.

► **Histology:** Not diagnostic in either case; marked hyperkeratosis with acanthosis and parakeratosis in the case of the Gottron type.

► **Diagnostic approach:** Clinical examination, biopsy; family history often positive.

► **Differential diagnosis:** Confused with psoriasis or pityriasis rubra pilaris.

► **Therapy:** Systemic acitretin; otherwise keratolytics and other psoriatic regimens.

Hyperkeratosis Lenticularis Perstans

► **Synonym:** Flegel disease.

► **MIM code:** 144150.

► Rare disorder with flat keratotic papules on the extensor surfaces of the feet and hands. Histology shows focal hyperkeratosis with dermal lichenoid inflammatory infiltrate. Differential diagnostic considerations include acrokeratosis verruciformis and acrokeratoelastoidosis. Treatment difficult; try keratolytics or cryotherapy.

21.4 Palmoplantar Keratoderma

Overview

▶ **Definition:** Diffuse or localized hyperkeratotic lesions on palms and soles; either hereditary or acquired. Tylosis means callus, but is used as a synonym.

▶ **Diagnostic approach:** Clinical examination (diffuse, localized, punctate; transgrediens or not (extending away from palms and soles); history (congenital or acquired); biopsy (epidermolytic hyperkeratosis or not); associated findings.

▶ **Classification:**

- *Hereditary palmoplantar keratoderma:*
  - Diffuse nontransgrediens palmoplantar keratoderma.
  - Diffuse transgrediens palmoplantar keratoderma.
  - Localized and punctate palmoplantar keratoderma.

- *Hereditary palmoplantar keratoderma associated with other syndromes:*
  - Erythrokeratodermia.
  - Bullous congenital ichthyosiform erythroderma.
  - Some forms of epidermolysis bullosa (EB), especially EB simplex Dowling–Meara.
  - Hidrotic ectodermal dysplasia.
  - Darier disease.

- *Acquired palmoplantar keratoderma:*
  - Paraneoplastic marker.
  - Pregnancy, menopause.
  - Many forms of dermatitis, secondary syphilis, tinea manuum, crusted scabies, psoriasis, hyperkeratotic lichen planus, Sézary syndrome.
  - Clavi, calluses.
  - Myxedema, lymphedema with reactive verrucous changes.

▶ **Therapy:** All keratodermas are treated the same. Mechanical debridement (pumice stone, sanding) following by keratolytic ointments; vitamin D analogues useful; retinoids not.

Diffuse Nontransgrediens Palmoplantar Keratoderma

▶ **Diffuse palmoplantar keratoderma (Vörner–Unna–Thost):**
- *Synonym:* Epidermolytic palmoplantar keratoderma (EPPK).
- *MIM code:* 144200.
- *Pathogenesis:* Most common palmoplantar keratoderma; usually mutation in keratin 9 gene on 17q12–21; autosomal dominant inheritance.
- *Clinical features:* Diffuse palmoplantar hyperkeratosis with sharp border; often fissures and rhagades (Fig. 21.**8a**).
- *Histology:* Epidermis shows epidermolytic hyperkeratosis; the original idea that Unna–Thost keratoderma was separate and had no epidermolytic hyperkeratosis was mistaken. Often multiple biopsies needed.

▶ **Diffuse nonepidermolytic palmoplantar keratoderma:** Several rare syndromes exist that are clinically similar to Vörner but do not show epidermolytic hyperkeratosis. They likely represent other keratin mutations.

▶ **Tylosis with esophageal cancer:**
- *Synonym:* Howel–Evans syndrome.
- *MIM code:* 148500.
- *Pathogenesis:* Rare disorder; autosomal dominant inheritance; gene defect located at 17q25 but gene product unknown.

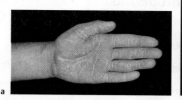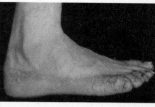

Fig. 21.8 · Diffuse palmoplantar keratoderma. **a** Vörner–Unna–Thost type (nontransgrediens). **b** Mal de Meleda (transgrediens).

- *Clinical features:* Diffuse palmoplantar keratoderma appears in childhood along with benign leukokeratosis; affected patients have almost 100% risk of squamous cell carcinoma of the esophagus as adults (sometimes five decades after developing keratoderma).
- *Differential diagnosis:* Acquired palmoplantar keratoderma may accompany a variety of carcinomas; it appears in temporal connection with the tumor.

▶ **Naxos syndrome:**
- *MIM code:* 601214.
- Located at 17q21; gene for plakoglobin.
- Combination of cardiac myopathy with arhythmia, palmoplantar keratoderma, and woolly hair.
- Autosomal recessive inheritance; reported on Greek island of Naxos.

▶ **Schöpf–Schulz–Passarge syndrome:**
- *MIM code:* 224750.
- Genetic basis unclear; autosomal recessive inheritance.
- Palmoplantar keratoderma, apocrine hidrocystomas of the eyelids, hypodontia, hypotrichosis.

▶ **Olmsted syndrome:**
- Rare syndrome; genetic basis not understood.
- Combination of severe mutilating palmoplantar keratoderma and periorificial plaques (perioral, then later genital).

Diffuse Transgrediens Palmoplantar Keratoderma

▶ **Mal de Meleda:**
- *MIM code:* 248300.
- *Pathogenesis:* Autosomal dominant inheritance. Initially described among residents of the Adriatic island of Meleda. Mutation in *SLURP1* gene at 8qter, a transmembrane signaling protein.
- *Clinical features:*
  - Keratoderma with peripheral erythema that frequently extends onto dorsal aspects of hands and feet (Fig. 21.**8 b**).
  - Associated subungual hyperkeratosis, hyperhidrosis, nail dystrophy, and shortened digits.

▶ **Papillon–Lefèvre syndrome:**
- *Synonym:* Palmoplantar keratoderma with periodontitis.
- *MIM code:* 245000.
- *Pathogenesis:* Inherited in autosomal recessive fashion; mutation in cathepsin C gene (*CTSC*) at 11q14.1-q14.3; essential for neutrophil function.

- *Clinical features:* Severe periodontal disease, palmoplantar keratoderma and psoriasiform plaques on knees and elbows.
- *Haim–Munk syndrome* (MIM code 245010) is mutation in same gene but with a leukocyte adhesion defect in addition to the mucocutaneous findings.
- *Therapy:* Acitretin helps on occasion.

▶ **Vohwinkel syndrome:**
- *Synonym:* Mutilating palmoplantar keratoderma.
- *Pathogenesis:* Two different mutations produce similar clinical picture:
  - MIM code 124500; 13q11-q12; mutation in *GJB2* gene coding for connexin 26; autosomal dominant inheritance.
  - MIM code 604117; 1q21; mutation in loricrin (part of cornified envelope); autosomal dominant inheritance (also known as Camisa syndrome).
- *Clinical features:* Diffuse palmoplantar keratoderma plus pseudoainhum (constricting bands of digits) and peculiar starfish-pattern hyperkeratoses over flexures; those with loricrin mutation have ichthyosis; those with connexin mutation, deafness.

▶ **Sclerotylosis:**
- *Synonym:* Huriez syndrome.
- *MIM code:* 181600.
- *Pathogenesis:* Gene defect located at 4q23 but not further characterized; autosomal dominant inheritance.
- *Clinical features:* Diffuse palmoplantar keratoderma with atrophy, nail dystrophy, and increased incidence of cutaneous squamous cell carcinomas.

Localized and Punctate Palmoplantar Keratoderma

▶ **Punctate palmoplantar keratoderma:**
- *Synonym:* Buschke–Fischer–Brauer palmoplantar syndrome.
- *MIM code:* 148600.
- *Pathogenesis:* Etiology unclear; autosomal dominant inheritance.
- *Clinical features:* Many small (2–8 mm) keratotic lesions; coalesce over pressure points; onset in adolescence.
- *Differential diagnosis:*
  - Punctate lesions of the palmoplantar creases are common in blacks; probably not related to the diffuse form.
  - Often misdiagnosed as warts and incorrectly treated.

▶ **Porokeratosis punctata palmaris et plantaris** (p. 343).

▶ **Richner–Hanhart syndrome:**
- *Synonyms:* Tyrosine transaminase deficiency, tyrosinemia type II.
- *MIM code:* 276660.
- *Pathogenesis:* Gene located at 16q22.1-q22.3; codes for tyrosine transaminase.
- *Clinical features:* Painful punctate palmoplantar keratoderma, as well as corneal ulcers.
- *Therapy:* Low phenylalanine-low tyrosine diet.

▶ **Striate palmoplantar keratoderma:**
- *Synonym:* Brunauer–Fohs–Siemens syndrome.
- *Pathogenesis:* Three mutations identified, all with autosomal dominant inheritance:
  - MIM code 148700; 18 q12.1-q12.2; desmoglein 1.
  - MIM code 125647; 6p21; desmoplakin (also associated with woolly hair and cardiac myopathy as autosomal recessive variant).
  - MIM code 139350; 12q11-q12; keratin 1.

- *Clinical features:* Linear hyperkeratotic plaques run the length of the fingers and onto the palm; can be very disabling.
► **Hereditary painful callosities:**
  - *MIM code:* 114140.
  - Limited to feet, even in manual laborers.
  - Histology shows epidermolytic hyperkeratosis, but not further clarified.
► **Focal palmoplantar and marginal gingival hyperkeratosis:**
  - *MIM code:* 148730.
  - Focal hyperkeratotic lesions both on palms and soles and mouth, especially marginal gingiva.
► **Acrokeratoelastoidosis (Costa):**
  - *MIM code:* 101850.
  - *Pathogenesis*: Unclear; both autosomal dominant inheritance and solar damage have been implicated.
  - *Clinical features:* Distinct; white-yellow coalescent papules and plaques limited to lateral aspects of palms and soles.
  - *Histology*: Marked damage to elastic fibers.
  - *Differential diagnosis:* Punctate porokeratosis and *focal acral hyperkeratosis,* which is clinically identical but shows no elastic fiber defects on biopsy.

21.5 Linear or Striped Lesions

The usual explanation for linear or striped lesions is *mosaicism*—a common genetic phenomenon. During human development, the skin moves in a peculiar fashion to cover the growing trunk and limbs, producing a pattern known as *Blaschko lines*. Any time there is a mutation in a somatic gene during the early stages of development, linear lesions are produced, whether it be epidermal nevi (mutations in keratins or other epidermal growth control genes), large pigmented nevi, or others. Every female is a mosaic, because of the process of lyonization or random inactivation of one or other X chromosome during early embryonic life. Diseases such as incontinentia pigmenti, which are inherited in an x-linked dominant manner and caused by mutations in crucial genes, are fatal to those male embryos who only express the abnormal gene, and always produce clinical mosaics in women. Other mosaic lesions often not thought of as genetic include Becker nevus and its associated syndrome, nevus spilus, and linear and whorled hypermelanosis.

Incontinentia Pigmenti (IP)

► **Synonym:** Bloch–Sulzberger disease.
► **MIM code:** 308310.
► **Definition:** Uncommon syndrome with progressive linear lesions and associated ocular, skeletal, and CNS abnormalities.
► **Pathogenesis:** Mutation in the *NEMO* gene, modulator of NFκB, at Xq28; NEMO inhibits apoptosis, so IP patients have been described as pro-apoptotic. X-linked dominant inheritance; transmission from mother to daughter; mutation is lethal in males (except for Klinefelter syndrome).

▶ **Clinical features:**
- *Cutaneous findings:* Four phases of lesions all following peculiar linear and streaked pattern (100%):
  - At birth, vesicular stage with numerous eosinophils and associated urticarial plaques; also peripheral blood eosinophilia (Fig. 21.9).
  - In infancy, warty plaques, most often acral.
  - As adults, bizarre hyperpigmentation (*Chinese letter sign*) on trunk; blue-gray to brown shades.
  - Also white atrophic scars on legs, which neither tan nor sweat.
  - About 25% have aplasia cutis congenita (see below).

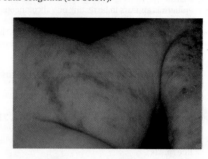

Fig. 21.**9** · Incontinentia pigmenti with linear erythematous and bullous lesions.

- *Dental anomalies* (50%): Delayed dentition, missing teeth (upper canines and premolars typically).
- *Ocular anomalies* (30%): Strabismus, optic nerve atrophy, blindness.
- *CNS anomalies* (25%): Mental retardation, delayed motor development, paraplegia.

▶ **Histology:** Blisters are rich in eosinophils; warty lesions show peculiar dyskeratotic keratinocytes; hyperpigmentation is result of incontinence of pigment.

▶ **Diagnostic approach:** Clinical examination, history of miscarriages, check mother's trunk and legs.

▶ **Differential diagnosis:**
- *Hypomelanosis of Ito.* Also known as IP achromians, incorrectly described as the "reverse image" of IP; white streaks on a dark normal background (p. 374).
- *Linear and whorled nevoid hypermelanosis:* Macular hyperpigmentation along Blaschko lines without underlying defects (p. 379).

▶ **Therapy:** Cutaneous lesions require no therapy; excellent dental and ophthalmologic care; monitor for developmental problems.

Focal Dermal Hypoplasia

▶ **Synonym:** Goltz syndrome.
▶ **MIM code:** 305600.
▶ **Definition:** Disorder limited almost exclusively to women, with multiple ectodermal and mesenchymal defects.
▶ **Pathogenesis:** Exact gene still controversial.

► **Clinical features:**
- Linear skin lesions along Blaschko lines.
- Areas with almost no dermis and outpouchings of fat.
- Hypo- and hyperpigmented streaks and telangiectases.
- Aplasia cutis congenita.
- Periorificial papillomas.
- Skeletal anomalies, most classic finding claw or lobster hand.
- Dental anomalies.
- Occasionally mental retardation.

► **Histology:** Striking finding; dermis is often only 1–2 cell layers thick, so that epidermis appears to be resting on subcutaneous fat.

► **Diagnostic approach:** Clinical examination, biopsy, radiography of long bones shows osteopathia striata (longitudinal streaks) in the metaphyses.

► **Differential diagnosis:** The individual fatty lesions can be confused with nevus lipomatosus; otherwise clinically distinctive.

Other X-linked Dominant Genodermatoses

► **MIDAS syndrome:** Combination of **mi**crophthalmia, **d**ermal **a**plasia, and **s**clerocornea.

► **Conradi–Hünermann–Happle syndrome (p. 339).**

► **CHILD syndrome: C**ongenital **h**emidysplasia with **i**chthyosiform nevus and **l**imb **d**efects; peculiar large psoriasiform plaques, which often stop abruption at midline (p. 414).

Aplasia Cutis Congenita

► **Definition:** Congenital absence of skin and often subcutaneous tissue; may be solitary or associated with a long list of rare syndromes.

► **Pathogenesis:** Probably represents somatic mosaicism, as lines often follow Blaschko lines.

► **Clinical features:**
- Most common presentation is punched-out ulcer on vertex of scalp (60%); 1–2 cm with erythematous base. Usually birth trauma is suspected, so documentation is crucial to avoid misunderstandings (and lawsuits). Heals with scarring and permanent alopecia.
- Other sites include extremities and trunk; multiple lesions may be seen.

► **Diagnostic approach:** When other sites or multiple lesions present, likelihood of associated syndrome increases.

► **Therapy:** Disturbing lesions can usually be excised later in life.

Other Linear Lesions

► **Epidermal nevi** (p. 410) are also mosaics and thus usually linear. In some instances they are associated with underlying defects (epidermal nevus syndromes).

► **Lichen striatus (p. 289).**

► **"Blaschkitis":** A number of inflammatory dermatoses (psoriasis, lichen planus, graft-versus-host disease) can follow Blaschko lines; the proposed explanation is that the patient's skin shows somatic mosaicism and only a part of the keratinocytes are susceptible to whatever triggers or modulates the dermatosis.

21.6 Ectodermal Dysplasias

Hundreds of diseases are listed as ectodermal dysplasias, defined as defects in one or more of the following structures: skin, adnexal glands, hair, nails, teeth. Many of the diseases discussed in this section qualify as ectodermal dysplasias. Only two common disorders are considered here as examples.

Anhidrotic Ectodermal Dysplasia

▶ **MIM codes:** 305100 (X chromosome); 224900 (autosomal recessive).
▶ **Definition:** Rare disorder with two causative genes both leading to defects in hair, teeth, and eccrine sweat glands.
▶ **Pathogenesis:** Defects in ectodysplasin binding are the problem. This member of the TNF family comes in two isoforms: EDA1, which binds to the EDAR receptor on chromosome 22a11-q13, and EDA2, which binds to XEDAR on the X chromosome.
▶ **Clinical features:**
  • *Classic triad:* Reduced sweating, hypotrichosis, hypo- or adontia.
  • *Typical facies (Popeye look):* Prominent forehead, saddle node, sunken cheeks, large ears, and thin hair. Mental retardation in 30–50%.
▶ **Diagnostic approach:** Clinical examination, check pedigree for consanguinity and check mother for focal areas of decreased sweating (mosaic pattern for carrier).
▶ **Therapy:** Supportive care; caution in hot weather because of inability to sweat.

Hidrotic Ectodermal Dysplasia

▶ **Synonym:** Clouston syndrome.
▶ **MIM code:** 129500.
▶ **Definition:** Disorder with defects in nails and hair, as well as palmoplantar keratoderma; autosomal dominant inheritance.
▶ **Pathogenesis:** Mutation in *GJB6* gene coding for connexin 30; located at 13q12.
▶ **Clinical features:** All patients have thickened, slowly growing yellow nails, often with paronychia. Transgrediens palmoplantar keratoderma with keratoses over the knees and elbows. Thin, easily broken hair. Teeth not involved. Normal sweating.
▶ **Diagnostic approach:** Clinical examination, family history usually positive.
▶ **Differential diagnosis:** Consider other syndromes with nail defects (p. 519).
▶ **Therapy:** File nails; treat keratoderma as on p. 345.

21.7 Epidermolysis Bullosa (EB)

Overview

▶ **Definition:** Group of disorders with mechanical defects leading to easy blistering, caused by defective structural proteins.
▶ **Classification:** Based on level of defect:
  • *EB simplex (epidermolytic EB):* Defects in keratins, other epidermal proteins.
  • *Junctional EB:* Defects in structures of the dermoepidermal junction.
  • *Dystrophic EB (dermolytic EB):* Defects in type VII collagen.
▶ **Diagnostic approach:** Clinical examination and family history can only point to possible diagnosis. Work together with specialized centers. Final diagnosis based on antigen mapping of skin biopsy and identification of genetic defect.

EB Simplex

Least disturbing form of EB; patients tend to easily develop blisters from minor mechanical trauma such as crawling on knees and elbows or (later in life) walking (Fig. 21.**10**). The first three disorders listed below all involve mutations in keratins 5 and 14, which are paired and expressed low in the epidermis, either in the basal layer or just above. All have autosomal dominant inheritance except the form associated with muscular dystrophy. In most instances, patients learn how to avoid and treat blisters and thus are able to cope well with life.

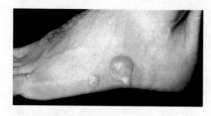

Fig. 21.**10** · Epidermolysis bullosa simplex.

▶ **EB simplex, Köbner type:**
  • Mutations in keratin 5 or 14.
  • Starts at birth of soon after; can appear anywhere on body.
  • No milia, scarring, or nail loss.
▶ **EB simplex, Weber–Cockayne:**
  • Mutations in keratin 5 or 14.
  • Onset of signs and symptoms in first two decades.
  • Problems limited to palms and soles; worse in summer, associated with hyperhidrosis; can scar.
  • Treating hyperhidrosis sometimes helps.
▶ **EB herpetiformis, Dowling–Meara:**
  • Mutations in keratin 5 or 14.
  • Onset just after birth; slight mortality rate.
  • Herpetiform, sometimes hemorrhagic blisters on trunk; later palmoplantar keratoderma, nail dystrophy, mucosal erosions.
▶ **EB simplex with mottled hyperpigmentation:**
  • Rare disease with keratin 5 mutation, generalized blisters, heals with hypopigmentation; corneal dystrophy, mental retardation.
▶ **EB simplex, Ogna:**
  • Mutation in plectin 1 gene; found in Scandinavia, Germany.
  • Blisters on extremities.
▶ **EB simplex with muscular dystrophy:**
  • Autosomal recessive inheritance; also involves plectin 1 mutation. Plectin is found in both hemidesmosomes and muscular fibers.
▶ **Other EB simplex subtypes:**
  • Autosomal recessive variant; also involves keratin 14 mutation.
  • EB simplex superficialis; perhaps collagen XVII.
  • EB simplex Jonkman; palmoplantar blisters, nail dystrophy; mutation in integrin β_4.

Junctional EB

▶ Mutations involve proteins involved in the formation of the dermoepidermal junction; all have autosomal recessive inheritance. Tend to scar.

▶ **Junctional EB, Herlitz type:**
- Mutations in different subunits of laminin 5.
- Formerly called lethal EB, but molecular biological studies have revealed a range from mild to severe involvement. Onset at birth. Progressive form is often fatal; characterized by distinctive vegetations on nape, axillae, periorificial locations. In the localized and inverse (limited to axilla, groin) subtypes, recurrent blisters but with better outlook. Oral blisters, dental anomalies, growth retardation.

▶ **Generalized atrophic benign EB (GABEB) (Hinter–Wolff type):**
- Heterogenous; mutations in collagen XVII (bullous pemphigoid antigen 2), laminin 5 or integrin β_4.
- Onset at birth, widespread blisters; nail loss, scarring alopecia, modest mucosal involvement; often improve over time.
- Benign only in comparison to Herlitz.

▶ **Other forms of junctional EB:.**
- Associated with pyloric atresia; mutations in integrin α_6 or β_4.
- Localized mutations in collagen XVII.

Dystrophic EB

▶ Most severe form; mutations in type VII collagen, the main component of the anchoring fibrils in the papillary dermis; invariable scarring, often mutilating.

▶ **Dominant dystrophic EB:**
- *Hyperplastic type, Cockayne–Touraine:*
  - MIM code: 131705.
  - Onset at birth; widespread blisters, heal with scars and milia. Also form hyperkeratotic lesions.
- *Albopapuloid type, Pasini:*
  - MIM code: 131800.
  - Onset at birth; widespread blisters heal with scars and milia; mutilation of fingers and toes.
  - White papular scars on trunk.
- Some sources no longer divide Cockayne–Touraine and Pasini as they have considerable overlap. There are also some minor variants in this group:
  - Pretibial dominant dystrophic EB.
  - EB pruriginosa.
  - Transient bullous dermolysis of the newborn.

▶ **Recessive dystrophic EB, Hallopeau–Siemens:**
- MIM code: 226500.
- Onset at birth; widespread blisters heal with scars and milia; mutilation of fingers and toes, clinically similar to severe dominant dystrophic forms.
- Other finings include marked mucosal involvement, dental anomalies, scarring alopecia, anemia, growth retardation.
- ▣ *Note:* Two disastrous complications:
  - Scarring of hands and feet leads to formation of socks and mittens, as the skin grows together over the digits enclosing them in translucent sheets (Fig. 21.11).
  - Greatly increased risk of squamous cell carcinoma of the skin and mucosa.

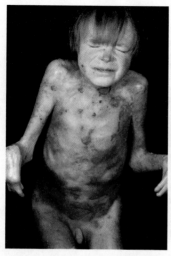
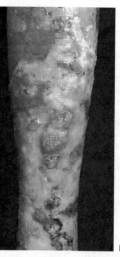

Fig. 21.**11** · **Dystrophic epidermolysis bullosa. a** With scarring and mitten formation of hands. **b** With scarring and erosions—a fertile ground for the development of squamous cell carcinomas.

Therapy

Patients with junctional and dystrophic EB are major therapeutic challenges. They are best treated in specialized centers. The only real therapy for such patients will be genetic manipulation to restore the missing proteins. In the meanwhile, perfect nursing care provided initially by experienced nurses who simultaneously teach the parents is the only approach. Modern dressings have technically made things easier, but even in developed countries, insurance companies sometimes refuse to pay the high costs associated with nursing care and bandaging material.

21.8 Diseases of Connective Tissue

Lipoid Proteinosis

► **Synonyms:** Urbach–Wiethe syndrome, hyalinosis cutis et mucosae.
► **MIM code:** 247100.
► **Definition:** Rare disease with deposits of hyaline material in skin and other tissues; autosomal recessive inheritance.
► **Epidemiology:** Uncommon, but large pedigrees exist in Sweden and South Africa, due to founder effect.
► **Pathogenesis:** Mutations in the *ECM1* (extracellular matrix protein) gene at 1q21, leading to deposition of type IV collagen and lipids; same mutation in lichen sclerosus (p. 217).

▶ **Clinical features:**
- Initial finding often a hoarse voice because of vocal cord and tongue deposits.
- Cutaneous lesions include waxy papules along edges of eyelids, which are thickened and have often lost their lashes.
- Papules and nodule on face and trunk; sometimes plaques resembling morphea as well as hyperkeratoses over knees and elbows.
- Seizures not uncommon.

▶ **Histology:** Deposits of PAS-positive amorphous material in the upper dermis.

▶ **Diagnostic approach:** Clinical examination, family history, biopsy.

▶ **Differential diagnosis:** Resembles erythropoietic protoporphyria but no photo-sensitivity and negative porphyrin studies.

▶ **Therapy:** Disturbing deposits can be removed from vocal cords; superficial destructive measures sometimes help skin lesions.

Ehlers–Danlos Syndrome

▶ **Definition:** Group of genetic disorders of collagen synthesis; see classification in Table 21.1.

Table 21.1 · Classification of Ehlers–Danlos syndrome

Type	Old code	Clinical findings	Inheritance	Defective protein
Classical	I, II	Hyperextensible skin, easy bruising, gaping scars, joint hypermobility, prematurity	AD	Type V collagen, tenascin
Hypermobility	III	Joint hypermobility, few skin findings	AD	Unknown
Arterial	IV	Thin skin with prominent veins, easy bruising, small joint hypermobility; risk of rupture of arteries, uterus, or bowel	AD	Type III collagen
Kyphoscoliosis	VI	Intraocular bleeding, severe scoliosis, marked skin and joint involvement	AR	Lysyl hydroxylase
Arthrochalasis	VIIA, VIIB	Marked joint involvement with subluxations, scoliosis, minimal skin involvement, growth retardation	AD	Type I collagen
Dermatosparaxis	VIIC	Marked skin fragility, bruising	AR	Procollagen-*N*-peptidase
Other	V, VIII, IX, X	See text		

AD = autosomal dominant; AR = autosomal recessive.

► **Epidemiology:** Incidence 1:5000.
► **Pathogenesis:** Collagen synthesis is complex, as collagen fibers consist of 3 chains that must be manufactured, modified, and combined. There are at least 25 different kinds of collagen. The situation is further complicated by the interactions between collagens, elastin, and the extracellular matrix. In Ehlers–Danlos syndrome the defects are either in collagen or in the enzymes needed to process it.
► **Clinical features:**
  • The features of classic Ehlers–Danlos syndrome are hyperextensible skin, easy bruising, gaping thin scars, and joint hypermobility. Hematomas are common and may heal as fibrotic pseudotumors. Patients with other varieties of Ehlers–Danlos syndrome have distinguishing features, such as scoliosis or growth retardation, which usually allow them to be identified quickly.
  • Patients with classic Ehlers–Danlos syndrome are at risk for premature birth and should be carefully monitored.
  • The only form associated with a shortened life span is arterial or type IV Ehlers–Danlos syndrome with mutations in type III collagen. These patients have thin skin so that the vessels and sebaceous glands are easily seen; the yellow sebaceous glands are often mistaken for the chicken skin of pseudoxanthoma elasticum (see below). They are at risk of fatal ruptures of arteries, uterus, or gastrointestinal tract.
  • The older groups of type V (X-linked), type VIII (periodontal), type X (fibrinonectin), and type XI (hypermobile large joints) are extremely rare and have not been clearly characterized. Old type X is now classified as a form of cutis laxa (see below).
► **Diagnostic approach:** Based on clinical examination and then detailed genetic evaluation. Histology is of no benefit; recent work has shown that the old clinical classification was often wrong.
► **Differential diagnosis:** Often patients with hypermobile joints are identified, for example among ballet dancers, gymnasts, or circus performers. In many instances these individuals have no other defects and in the absence of genetic testing should not be considered as having Ehlers–Danlos syndrome.
► **Therapy:** Avoid trauma, warn surgeons of need for meticulous suture work, monitoring during pregnancy, genetic counseling.

Marfan Syndrome

► **MIM code:** 305600.
► **Definition:** Disorder with defect in fibrillin leading to skeletal, cardiac, ocular, and cutaneous abnormalities; autosomal dominant inheritance.
► **Epidemiology:** Incidence 1:75000; occasionally identified unexpectedly in tall athletes following cardiac problems.
► **Pathogenesis:** Defect in fibrillin 1, a major component of elastic fibers.
► **Clinical features:**
  • *Skeletal:* Arachnodactyly, taller than average, arm span often greater than height, hyperextensible joints (easily injured), pectus excavatum, pes valgus. Characteristic elongated facies.
  • *Ocular:* Ectopia lentis (50–70%), myopia, heterochromic irises, retinal detachment.
  • *Cardiac:* Aortic valve insufficiency, aortic aneurysms, aortic rupture in first three decades is main threat to survival.
  • *Skin:* Many problems, but all minor; striae, elastosis perforans serpiginosa.
► **Diagnostic approach:** Cardiologic and ophthalmologic examination; genetic studies.

- **Differential diagnosis:** Congenital contractural arachnodactyly is similar but caused by mutation in fibrillin 2. Patients with MEN2B and homocystinuria are often described as marfanoid.
- **Therapy:** Monitoring of ocular and cardiac status; β-blockers and prompt surgery with aortic graft.

Cutis Laxa

- **Definition:** Group of disorders with defective elastic fibers leading to characteristic skin changes, as well as cardiac and pulmonary disorders.
- **Classification:** There are three types of inherited cutis laxa as well as acquired types:
  - *Autosomal recessive cutis laxa* (MIM code 219100): mutation in fibulin 5 gene at 14q32.1. Fibulin 5 is an elastic binding protein found on the surface of elastic fibers; severe systemic and cutaneous manifestations.
  - *Autosomal dominant cutis laxa* (MIM code 123700); mutations in either elastin gene at 7q11.2 or fibulin 5; primarily cutaneous manifestations.
  - *X-linked recessive cutis laxa* (MIM code 304150; formerly type IX Ehlers–Danlos syndrome or occipital horn disease); mutation in *ATP7A* gene coding for Cu^{2+} transport protein, also involved in Menkes syndrome; minimal skin changes.
  - *Acquired cutis laxa:* Very rare, may follows inflammatory dermatoses and be associated with monoclonal gammopathies; sometimes evidence for antibodies against elastic fibers.
  - *Penicillamine-induced cutis laxa:* Complication of treatment with long-term penicillamine for Wilson syndrome or cystinuria.
- **Clinical features:**
  - Unflatteringly described as "basset hound look." Patients have droopy skin, making them appear far older than their chronological age. Often ectropion.
  - Systemic problems include aortic dilation, pulmonary emphysema, pulmonary artery stenosis, and a tendency to multiple hernia and diverticula.
- **Histology:** Biopsy when stained for elastic fibers shows marked destruction or absence of these structural elements throughout the skin.
- **Diagnostic approach:** Clinical examination, biopsy.
- **Differential diagnosis:** Nothing else really looks like cutis laxa. *Mid-dermal elastolysis* is an acquired disease with fine wrinkling of the skin and loss of elastic fibers in the mid-dermis.
- **Therapy:** Monitor cardiac and pulmonary status; be alert to gastrointestinal complications; skin can be helped somewhat by cosmetic surgery as progression continues.

Anetoderma

- **Synonym:** Dermatitis maculosa atrophicans.
- **Definition:** Disorder with focal loss of dermal elastic fibers.
- **Pathogenesis:** Anetoderma is secondary to inflammation and destruction of classic fibers. Sometimes it follows an obvious disorder such as syphilis, lymphoma, or acne. More often, the initial disorder is unclear and the disease is subdivided into three types based on apparent precursor stage:
  - *Jadassohn type:* Initially erythematous lesions that later fade.
  - *Pellizari type:* Initially urticarial lesions.
  - *Schweninger–Buzzi type:* Anetoderma lesions develop without a visible precursor.

► **Clinical features:** The hallmark lesion is a 5–20 mm atrophic area which when palpated almost resembles a hernia, so that one can push the tip of the little finger into the depression. Lesions often hypopigmented.
► **Histology:** Normal epidermis, loss of elastin in dermis.
► **Diagnostic approach:** Clinical examination, often wise to take biopsy as ellipse with long axis including both normal and abnormal skin.
► **Differential diagnosis:**
   • White depressed lesions: morphea, lichen sclerosus et atrophicus, scars.
   • Histologic loss of elastin:
      – Acquired cutis laxa (clinically not macular).
      – Granulomatous slack skin (granulomatous inflammation, T-cell lymphoma).
► **Therapy:** Nothing good; disturbing individual lesions can be excised.

Pseudoxanthoma Elasticum

► **Definition:** Rare genodermatosis with calcification of elastic fibers in skin, eyes and cardiovascular system.
► **Epidemiology:** Incidence 1:160 000.
► **Pathogenesis:** Inheritance usually autosomal recessive (MIM code 264800), but rarely and controversially reported as autosomal dominant. Mutation in *ABCC6* gene, which codes MRP6, a transporter protein primarily expressed in kidneys and liver, not skin and eyes. The working hypothesis is that it is needed to break down substances that damage elastin; when it fails to function, elastic fiber damage occurs. Pseudoxanthoma elasticum is also associated with thalassemia and sickle cell anemia, as well as amyloid elastosis and chronic renal failure. Penicillamine, L-tryptophan, and saltpeter can cause cutaneous pseudoxanthoma elasticum, but not systemic disease.
► **Clinical features:** Two main clinical features and confirmatory histology required for diagnosis:
   • *Cutaneous lesions:* 1–5 mm yellow flat-topped papules, resembling xanthomas coalesce to produce patches in the flexural areas (neck, antecubital and popliteal fossae, axillae, groin). Skin in these areas folded and stiff. Occasionally periumbilical involvement. Sometimes discharge of chalky material from crusted lesions. Often elastosis perforans serpiginosa.
   • *Angioid streaks:* Classic retinal changes seen in 99% of patients; red-orange streaks reflecting tears in Bruch membrane. Also seen in sickle cell anemia, idiopathic thrombocytopenic purpura, acromegaly, some forms of Ehlers–Danlos syndrome, lead poisoning, Paget disease of bone.
   • Involvement of the ocular vessels leads to leakage and hemorrhage with resultant neovascularization, scarring. and visual loss. Even minor trauma to the orbit accelerates the process.
   • Involvement of medium-sized arteries in the limbs causes claudication; cardiac involvement leads to early myocardial infarcts; also hypertension and involvement of gastrointestinal and articular vessels.
► **Histology:** Twisted disrupted basophilic elastic fibers; von Kossa stain reveals marked calcification. On occasion, the calcified elastic fibers are discharged through defects in the epidermis (*perforating pseudoxanthoma elasticum*).
► **Diagnostic approach:** Clinical examination, consultation with ophthalmology and vascular surgery, skin biopsy usually most accessible. If pseudoxanthoma elasticum is considered but there are no skin findings, biopsy of a scar may reveal the same histologic changes in elastic fibers.
► **Differential diagnosis:** The neck changes may be confused with the thin skin and prominent sebaceous glands of type IV Ehlers–Danlos syndrome. Otherwise clini-

cally distinct. Perforating pseudoxanthoma elasticum is usually periumbilical, often in multiparous black patients or renal dialysis patients, and may be seen without any other stigmata of the disease.

▶ **Therapy:** No treatment for skin lesions; avoid trauma (contact sports) to reduce risk of ocular injury and hemorrhage; careful monitoring for cardiovascular disease.

21.9 Perforating Dermatoses

The concept of perforating dermatoses is fascinating but confusing. The idea that the skin can discharge undesirable dermal accumulations such as damaged collagen or elastic fibers, or any calcified tissues, through the epidermis seems logical. On the other hand, the idea that keratin can penetrate into the dermis in the absence of trauma is hard to fathom. Dermatologists have long memorized lists of perforating dermatoses; we consider the phenomenon to be more limited, as shown in Table 21.2.

*Table 21.2 · **Perforating dermatoses***

Diseases with unquestioned perforation	Elastosis perforans serpiginosa
	Perforating pseudoxanthoma elasticum (see above)
	Perforating granuloma annulare (p. 292)
	All forms of cutaneous calcification
Diseases with folliculitis and/or epidermal defects	Perforating disease of renal dialysis (p. 330) and its variants:
	Perforating folliculitis
	Kyrle disease
	Reactive perforating collagenosis (p. 360)

Elastosis Perforans Serpiginosa

▶ **MIM code:** 130100.

▶ **Definition:** Dermatosis in which damaged elastic fibers are eliminated through the epidermis.

▶ **Pathogenesis:** Most patients have connective tissue defect (pseudoxanthoma elasticum, Marfan syndrome, Ehlers–Danlos syndrome) or Down syndrome. Also occurs in those taking penicillamine for Wilson disease; here different pattern to elastic fibers (*bramble bush branching*). Also occurs sporadically but most likely from fruste of pseudoxanthoma elasticum.

▶ **Clinical features:** Usually appears in adolescence; small delled papules arranged in a linear, annular or serpiginous pattern; usually located on neck, nape, or shoulders.

▶ **Histology:** Epidermal hyperkeratosis; channels through epidermis containing damaged elastic fibers, which also accumulate in the dermis.

▶ **Diagnostic approach:** Clinical examination, biopsy.

▶ **Differential diagnosis:** Porokeratosis of Mibelli, perforating granuloma annulare, perforating pseudoxanthoma elasticum.

▶ **Therapy:** Curettage or cryotherapy may help to flatten lesions; if small, excise.

Reactive Perforating Collagenosis

► **Definition:** Disease in which the spontaneous elimination of defect collagen occurs.
► **Pathogenesis:** Both inherited and familial forms have been identified; no genetic defect is known. We believe this disease does not exist, but is simply the result of many types of epidermal damage exposing the dermis. The two most recent papers in Germany have identified exuberant curettage of seborrheic keratoses and excessive use of keratolytics as possible causes. If the familial form exists, it features crusted lesions out of proportion to identifiable trauma.
► **Clinical features:** Crusted, inflamed papules and nodules, usually on the extremities. In some patients, there is so much crusting that the term *verrucous perforating collagenoma* is employed. Usually nearby scars from previous lesions.
► **Histology:** Epidermal defect; inflammation; collagen fibers in exposed dermis and among debris; identified with van Gieson or other collagen stains.
► **Differential diagnosis:** Lichen simplex chronicus, prurigo nodularis; artifacts.
► **Therapy:** Topical antibiotics, occlusive dressings to eliminate further manipulation.

21.10 Poikiloderma

Overview

► **Definition:** Poikiloderma is the combination of telangiectases, hypo- and hyperpigmentation, and atrophy, producing a mottled appearance. It is present in many disorders. Often the definition is stretched to include disorders with only some of these features. Poikilos is the Greek word for varied.
► **Classification:** There is no widely accepted classification, but a useful one is presented in Table 21.**3**. Differential diagnosis listed on p. 706.

Dyskeratosis Congenita

► **Synonym:** Zinsser–Cole–Engman syndrome.
► **MIM code:** 305000.
► **Definition:** Rare syndrome with poikiloderma, nail dystrophy, and oral leukoplakia with risk of squamous cell carcinoma.
► **Pathogenesis:** X-linked recessive manner inheritance; mutation in dyskeratin at Xq28; protein involved in ribosomal function. Also even rarer forms with autosomal recessive and autosomal dominant inheritance.
► **Clinical features:**
  • Nail dystrophy is first sign, usually before age 5; by age 10, most nails lost.
  • Poikiloderma, primarily mottled hypo- and hyperpigmentation with some telangiectases, on neck and thighs (dirty neck sign).
  • Oral leukoplakia with common development of squamous cell carcinoma
  • Pancytopenia, which is the usual cause of death.
► **Diagnostic approach:** Clinical examination; limited to males.
► **Differential diagnosis:** Fanconi syndrome is similar with reticulate hyperpigmentation and pancytopenia, but has skeletal defects and at least eight different genetic types.
► **Therapy:** Monitor oral lesions for malignant change; management by hematology; may benefit from bone marrow transplantation (ironically, skin changes look just like graft-versus-host disease).

Table 21.3 · Classification of poikiloderma

Disease	Comments
Congenital poikiloderma	Syndromes dominated by poikiloderma
Rothmund–Thomsen syndrome	Cataracts, photosensitivity, acral keratoses
Dyskeratosis congenita (see below)	Dystrophic nails, leukoplakia, squamous cell carcinoma, pancytopenia
Kindler syndrome	Poikiloderma plus epidermolysis bullosa-like fragility and blisters; mutation in kindlerin gene
Poikiloderma with blisters (Brain, Braun–Falco, Marghescu)	Blisters, keratoses
Hereditary acrokeratotic poikiloderma	Acral keratoses
Hereditary sclerosing poikiloderma	Prominent acral sclerosis
Syndromes with poikilodermoid features	
Bloom syndrome	Dwarfism, photosensitivity, lymphoma, leukemia
Ataxia-telangiectasia	Neurological findings, ocular and facial telangiectases
Xeroderma pigmentosum	Photosensitivity, multiple cutaneous malignancies; in some types, mental retardation
Fanconi syndrome	Multiple genes; reticulate hyperpigmentation, pancytopenia, skeletal defects
Acquired poikiloderma	
Radiation dermatitis	The prototype!
Mycosis fungoides	Some early lesions (poikiloderma atrophicans vasculare)
Parakeratosis variegata	Variant of mycosis fungoides with papules, telangiectases, reticular pattern but no atrophy.
Chronic graft-versus-host disease	Obvious history

21.11 Neurofibromatoses

Overview

The neurofibromatoses are a group of disorders having in common the presence of cutaneous neurofibromas. The most common member of the group is classical neurofibromatosis, also known as neurofibromatosis 1 or von Recklinghausen syndrome. Neurofibromatosis 2 features bilateral acoustic neuromas; other forms may be localized or linear.

Pathogenesis

The *NF1* gene on chromosome 17 encodes neurofibromin, a tumor suppressor gene most extensively expressed in neural and glial tissue. Its absence leads to the disturbance in the GTP/Ras signal transduction pathway. The gene responsible for NF2 is merlin or schwannomin, located on chromosome 22, which binds membrane proteins to the cytoskeleton. In both instances, loss of heterozygosity is usually responsible for the development of tumors.

Neurofibromatosis 1 (NF1)

▶ **MIM code:** 162200.
▶ **Synonym:** von Recklinghausen disease.
▶ **Definition:** Disorder with multiple malformations and tumors involving skin, nervous system, and skeleton; autosomal dominant inheritance.
▶ **Epidemiology:** Common genodermatosis; incidence 1:3000; about 50% of cases are new mutations. Male:female ratio = 1.
▶ **Clinical features:**
  ☐ *Note:* NF1 is characterized by three pathognomonic clinical findings: café-au-lait macules, neurofibromas, Lisch nodules of the iris.
  • *Hyperpigmentation* (99%):
    – *Café-au-lait macule* (99%). Tan, irregular, sharply bordered patches, usually several centimeters in diameter (Fig. 21.**12a**) (p. 378). Six or more café-au-lait macules > 1.5 cm in an adult are one criterion for NF1. Lesions usually present at birth or develop in first year of life.
    – Axillary freckles (*Crowe sign*): Multiple small lentigines usually in axilla or groin; appear later than café-au-lait macules.
    – Large pigmented macules overlying plexiform neurofibromas.
  • *Multiple neurofibromas* (100%):
    – Always present on skin; may also involve nerves or internal organs.
    – Well-circumscribed soft fleshy papules or nodules, millimeters to centimeters in size, either cutaneous or subcutaneous. The tumors can usually be pushed into the subcutis (*door bell* or *buttonhole sign*) (Fig. 21.**12b**).
    – Not present at birth; start to develop in second decade, flaring with puberty and pregnancy; continue to develop throughout adult life.
    – Typically pruritic; may be tender or painful.
    – Malignant change very rare; usually in larger tumors.
  • *Lisch nodules* (95%):
    – Pigmented hamartomas on the iris that develop in early childhood (Fig. 21.**12c**); present before 6 years of age in 30%; in 95% of adults. Asymptomatic.
    – May be seen in patients with neurofibromin mutation and no skin findings.
▶ **Other findings (< 50%):**
  • *Skeletal changes:*
    – Reduced body size (50%).
    – Macrocephaly, both relative and absolute (30%).
    – Kyphoscoliosis (2%): S-shaped rotation scoliosis with prominent anterior angulation; early therapy mandatory.
    – Congenital *pseudoarthrosis* (0.5–1.0%). About half of all congenital pseudarthroses are caused by NF1; usually involve tibia or radius and more common in boys. (Pseudarthrosis is a nonhealing fracture that leads to the formation of a false joint.).

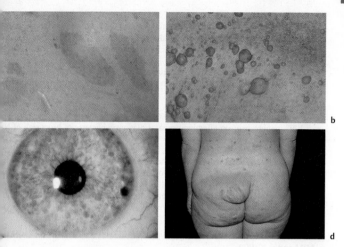

g. 21.**12** · **Neurofibromatosis 1. a** Café-au-lait macule. **b** Bultiple neurofibromas. **c** Lisch
odules. **d** Plexiform neurofibroma.

- *Nervous system tumors:*
  - CNS tumors (5–10%): Optic nerve glioma, astrocytoma, neurilemmoma, meningeoma, neurofibroma. Always search for optic nerve gliomas in patients with NF1.
- ☐ *Note:* No acoustic neuromas; they are a sign of NF2.
- *Other skin findings:*
  - *Pruritus:* Usually not limited to neurofibromas; can be extremely disturbing.
  - *Juvenile xanthogranuloma* (p. 469): If present, always exclude NF1; may be marker for increased risk of leukemia.
  - *Plexiform neurofibromas:* Congenital malformation consisting of masses of intersecting nerves (sack of worms on palpation); favor orbit periorbital region, nape, retropharyngeal, cervical, and mediastinal areas (Fig. 21.**12 d**). Often associated with segmental hypertrophy or large pendulous tumors; overlying skin often hyperpigmented. Risk of malignant transformation.
  - *Malignant neural tumors:* Generic name of *malignant peripheral nerve sheath tumor* probably best; features of both malignant neurofibroma and schwannoma. Most malignant neural tumors arise in NF1.
  - *Other tumors* (1–2%): Wilms tumor, rhabdomyosarcoma, leukemia (especially juvenile myelomonocytic leukemia), pheochromocytoma (always suspect if NF1 patient is hypertensive at early age).
  - ☐ *Note:* Malignant tumors reduce life expectancy; the effect is greater in women.
  - *Mental retardation (30%):* Usually mild, trouble with speaking or reading.

Segmental neurofibromatosis: Somatic mosaic; typically one segment of body, strictly respecting midline, features café-au-lait macules as well as cutaneous and systemic neurofibromas.

► **Diagnostic approach:**
  • The patient must be completely evaluated at the time of the initial diagnosis. Recommended tests include EEG, audiometry, ophthalmologic examination, CT of the skull and orbits, 24 hour urine for catecholamines and their metabolites, intelligence testing.
  ☒ *Note:* Each of these tests has consequences for 5–10% of patients.
  • Later yearly evaluation to identify potential problems and insure prompt referral to other specialties.
► **Genetic counseling:**
  • *Patient with NF1:* Each child has 50% chance of having NF; both sexes at risk; 100% penetrance; no effective prenatal diagnosis because of huge size of NF gene.
  • *First-degree relatives:* Brother, sister, or child of NF patient who has no clinical signs of NF by 20th birthday has almost no risk of having an affected child.
► **Therapy:** No curative treatment. Neurofibromas that are bothersome can be excised and ablated with CO_2 laser. Ketotifen is often helpful for pruritus. Plexiform neurofibromas should be monitored for malignant change. Many systemic problems (scoliosis, hypertension) can be treated.

Neurofibromatosis 2 (NF2)

► **MIM code:** 101000.
► **Definition:** Syndrome featuring bilateral acoustic neuromas as well as other neural tumors; autosomal dominant inheritance.
► **Epidemiology:** Much less common that NF1; incidence 1:40000; also high degree of penetrance; male:female ratio = 1.
► **Clinical features:**
  • *Bilateral acoustic neuromas:* Schwann cell tumors that usually start in the vestibular nerve; signs and symptoms usually start after puberty with hearing loss (usually unilateral at first), loss of equilibrium and headache.
  • *Other neural tumors:* Schwann cell tumors of cranial and peripheral nerves, usually sensory branches. Meningiomas in skull and spinal canal. Gliomas usually low-grade; also plexiform neurofibromas.
  • *Cutaneous lesions:* About 50% have café-au-lait macules, axillary freckles, neurofibromas or sometimes cutaneous schwannomas. All skin changes less prominent than in NF1.
  • *Ophthalmologic findings:* Juvenile posterior or subcapsular cortical *cataracts* in > 50%; these may appear before acoustic neuromas and are usually helpful in evaluating family members at risk. No Lisch nodules.
► **Diagnostic approach:** Dermatologists or ophthalmologists may be able to make the diagnosis first. Patients should be carefully followed for the development of acoustic neuromas. Gadolinium-enhanced MRI is considered gold standard in searching for these tumors.
► **Differential diagnosis:** Rare patients have multiple schwannomas (schwannomatosis) without clear evidence for NF2. They may be mosaics, or have other mutations.
► **Therapy:** Surgery for acoustic neuromas is not without risk; often residual disease (hearing loss or balance problems). Long-term follow-up required.

21.12 Tuberous Sclerosis

Overview

....

- **Synonyms:** Bourneville–Pringle disease, epiloia.
- **MIM codes:** 191100, 191092.
- **Definition:** Genodermatosis involving multiple organ systems including skin and CNS; autosomal dominant inheritance. Classical triad is adenoma sebaceum, epilepsy, and mental retardation.
- **Epidemiology:** Incidence 1:15000; most cases are spontaneous mutations as many patients become institutionalized and do not have families.
- **Pathogenesis:** Two different genes are involved; hamartin for TSC1 and tuberin for TSC2. Both interact in the intracellular signaling pathway by encoding two subunits of a heterodimer signal transduction protein. Best example of how genetic studies identified (to everyone's surprise) two genes producing same clinical features.
- **Clinical features:**
  - *Neurological findings:*
    - Almost 100%; initially localized seizures, later generalized. The tubers are cortical and subcortical hamartomas; presumed focus for seizure activity.
    - Mental retardation (90%); severity highly variable; most common genodermatosis in institutionalized patients.
  - *Dermatologic findings:*
    - *Angiofibromas:* Present in > 90%. The facial angiofibromas are known as adenoma sebaceum—erroneously, as they are not sebaceous gland tumors but connective tissue tumors. Erythematous smooth papules favoring nasolabial fold and chin (Fig. 21.**13 a**). Often initially mistaken for acne if no other stigmata present. The subungual angiofibromas are known as Koenen tumors (Fig. 21.**13 b**). Also gingival angiofibromas.
    - *Connective tissue nevi.*
    - *Shagreen patch:* Patch usually in lumbosacral region, fancifully compared to pebbled pigskin surface of an American football (Fig. 21.**13 c**). Shagreen is a French leather with a similar appearance. Histologically proliferation of collagen.
    - *Forehead plaque:* Less common than shagreen patch; usually in more severely affected individuals; several cm erythematous elevated plaque.
    - *Hypopigmentation:*
    - *Ash-leaf macule:* Oval to pointed patches of hypopigmentation; caused by impaired transfer of melanosomes to keratinocytes. Present in infants. Best seen with Wood's light.
    - ▶ *Note:* Wood's light examination is indicated for all infants with unexplained seizures to exclude tuberous sclerosis.
    - Confetti-like and linear hypopigmentation less common.
  - *Visceral lesions:* CNS hamartomas (tubers), retinal hamartomas, calcified glial nodules, enamel defects, renal angiomyolipomas, cardiac rhabdomyomas; hyperostosis of inner table of skull.

Therapy: No specific therapy possible. Neurologists most important in management for seizure control. Early educational testing and guidance to maximize opportunities. Angiofibromas can be treated with laser ablation or dermabrasion; tend to recur but can be re-treated.

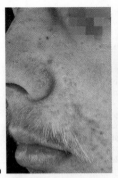 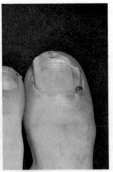

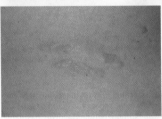

Fig. 21.**13** · **Tuberous sclerosis. a** Facial angiofibromas (adenoma sebaceum).
b Nailfold angiofibroma (Koenen tumor).
c Connective tissue nevus (shagreen patch).

21.13 Cancer-associated Genodermatoses

Overview

► There are a number of syndromes in which cutaneous findings provide early clue to the possible development of systemic malignancies (Table 21.**4**).

▶ *Note:* Patients with multiple cutaneous tumors (adnexal or neural) should be suspected of having a genodermatosis and carefully evaluated. In addition, first degree relatives should be checked.

Cowden Syndrome

► **Synonym:** Multiple hamartoma syndrome.
► **MIM code:** 158350.
► **Definition:** Genodermatosis with high risk of carcinoma of the breast with characteristic cutaneous findings and many associated systemic findings; autosomal dominant inheritance.
► **Epidemiology:** Very uncommon; incidence around 1:200000 in Western Europe.
► **Pathogenesis:** The involved gene is *PTEN* at 10p22–23; it plays a role in the phosphatidyl-inositol signaling pathway enhancing apoptosis; mutations in *PTEN* are seen in many disorders including juvenile polyposis, Lhermitte–Duclos syndrome (cerebellar "dysplasia"), and Bannayan–Riley–Ruvalcaba syndrome (rare cutaneous hamartoma syndrome). These disorders reflect artificially fixed points in a changing spectrum. *PTEN* is also mutated in many spontaneous carcinoma.

Table 21.4 · Cancer-associated genodermatoses

Genodermatosis	Clinical findings	Malignant tumors
Autosomal dominant inheritance		
Nevoid basal cell carcinoma syndrome	Multiple basal cell carcinomas, palmoplantar pits	Medulloblastoma, basal cell carcinoma
Birt–Hogg–Dubé syndrome	Multiple fibrofolliculomas	Renal cell carcinomas
Carney syndrome	Lentigenes, blue nevi, myxomas	Cardiac myxomas, testicular carcinomas
Cowden syndrome	Trichilemmomas, oral papules, acral fibromas	Carcinoma of breast, thyroid, GI tract
Familial melanoma-pancreatic carcinoma syndrome	Melanocytic nevi, often dysplastic	Malignant melanoma of skin and uvea, carcinoma of pancreas
Gardner syndrome	Epidermoid cysts, osteomas, fibromas, pigmented retinal epithelium	Carcinoma of colon; many others but uncommon
Howel–Evans syndrome	Palmoplantar keratoderma, leukokeratosis	Carcinoma of esophagus
Multiple leiomyomas	Multiple painful red-brown papules and nodules	Renal cell carcinoma, uterine leiomyomas
MEN1	Angiofibromas, connective tissue nevi (similar to tuberous sclerosis)	Parathyroid, pancreas, and pituitary tumors
MEN2B	Mucosal neuromas	Medullary thyroid carcinoma, pheochromocytoma
Muir–Torre syndrome	Sebaceous tumors and keratoacanthomas	GI, urogenital, and lung carcinomas; often multiple primary tumors
Neurofibromatosis 1	Café-au-lait macules, axillary freckles, neurofibromas	Malignant peripheral nerve sheath tumors, other rare soft tissue tumors, leukemia
Peutz–Jeghers syndrome	Periorificial lentigines	Intestinal, ovarian, and testicular carcinomas
Autosomal recessive inheritance		
Ataxia-telangiectasia	Ocular and facial telangiectases, severe ataxia, multiple infections	Leukemia, lymphoma, breast carcinoma, others
Bloom syndrome	Photosensitivity, telangiectases, dwarfism	Leukemia, lymphoma
Chediak–Higashi syndrome	Albinism	Lymphoma
Dyskeratosis congenita	Nail dystrophy, leukokeratosis, poikiloderma	Squamous cell carcinoma of mouth, leukemia
Fanconi anemia	Poikiloderma	Leukemia
Werner syndrome	Premature aging, growth retardation	Lymphoma

► **Clinical features:**
- *Cutaneous findings:*
  - Multiple trichilemmomas (smooth to warty papules located primarily on face); type of adnexal tumor (p. 432).
  - Similar papules on oral mucosa, can coalesce producing cobblestone pattern.
  - Acral papules and fibromas.
  - All of these changes are likely part of a spectrum—not distinct lesions. Highly variable histology.
- *Systemic findings:*
  - Macrocephaly, mild mental retardation, cerebellar changes (*Lhermitte–Duclos syndrome*).
  - *Gastrointestinal polyposis:* Hamartomatous, very low risk of malignant change.
  - *Breasts:* More than 75% of female patients have fibrocytic changes with at least 25% lifetime risk of carcinoma. Risk also increased in male patients.
  - *Thyroid gland:* 50% have adenomas or multinodular goiters; 3–10% risk of thyroid carcinoma.

► **Therapy:** Prophylactic mastectomy often recommended; otherwise close monitoring of breasts and thyroid gland, as well as colonoscopic monitoring.

Gardner Syndrome

► **Synonym:** Gardner syndrome is one manifestation of the familial polyposis syndrome.
► **MIM code:** 175100.
► **Definition:** Genodermatosis with a very high risk of carcinoma of the colon, as well as multisystem involvement; autosomal dominant inheritance.
► **Epidemiology:** Incidence of 1:15 000 in Holland; 25% new mutations.
► **Pathogenesis:** Mutations in *APC* (adenomatous polyposis of colon) gene, which is tumor suppressor gene controlling β-catenin.
► **Clinical features:**
- *Skin:* Multiple epidermoid cysts (p. 407), sometimes with histological features of pilomatricomas (p. 432), favoring head and neck region. Sometimes massive. Usually appear in childhood. Also other soft tissue tumors, such as fibromas and lipoma. No malignant degeneration.
- Osteomas (primarily mandibula, maxilla, petrous bone).
- **C**ongenital **h**ypertrophy of **r**etinal **p**igment **e**pithelium (CHRPE) is earliest clinical sign.
- Desmoid tumors, especially after abdominal surgery.
- Intestinal polyposis, concentrated on colon but involving entire gastrointestinal tract; usually present in young adult life.
- *Malignant tumors:*
  - 100% lifetime risk of carcinoma of the colon; may be multiple if prophylactic colectomy not performed.
  - Much less commonly carcinomas of liver, biliary tree, thyroid, and others.

► **Diagnostic approach:** History, presence of multiple epidermoid cysts or osteomas (dental radiographs); confirmed on colonoscopic examination.
► **Therapy:** Prophylactic colectomy; aspirin or NSAIDs may reduce development of new polyps; cysts and osteomas can be excised; desmoids following abdominal surgery are major problem with no effective treatment. Family members at risk should be followed.

Muir–Torre Syndrome (MTS)

- **MIM code:** 158320.
- **Definition:** Genodermatosis which is part of the hereditary nonpolyposis colon cancer (HNPCC) syndrome; combination of multiple sebaceous tumors and keratoacanthomas with multiple internal malignancies; autosomal dominant inheritance.
- **Epidemiology:** HNPCC is relatively common but MTS is rare; in other words, only a small number of HNPCC patients have cutaneous findings. The cancer family syndrome (Lynch syndrome) is an older term for the same disorder.
- **Pathogenesis:** Defects in a number of related DNA mismatch repair genes; the most common mutation in HNPCC syndrome is in MLH-1, but MSH-2 is more common in MTS. Somatic inactivation of second normal allele leads to microsatellite instability, a marker for genetic instability, and tumor growth.
- **Clinical features:**
  - *Skin:* Multiple sebaceous neoplasms and keratoacanthomas; often hard to clinically separate; papules and nodules, often with central dell or plug, favor midface (Fig. 21.14). Cystic sebaceous tumor, usually on back, is almost specific for MTS. Sebaceous carcinomas extremely rare.
  - *Malignant tumors:* Carcinoma of colon is most common (50%) but carcinomas involving lungs, urogenital tract, and other organs also possible. Tumors appear earlier than sporadic lesions, but have better prognosis. Most patients develop multiple tumors.
  - ☐ *Note:* These patients do not have intestinal polyposis, making monitoring for colonic tumors more challenging.

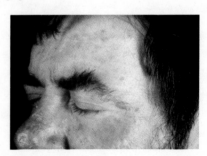

Fig. 21.**14** · Muir–Torre syndrome with multiple facial sebaceous tumors.

- **Diagnostic approach:** History, complete physical examination including gynecologic evaluation, colonoscopic examination; patients with multiple sebaceous tumors or keratoacanthomas should be carefully studied. Absence of specific gene products can be shown in skin biopsies, confirming diagnosis.
- **Therapy:** Appropriate treatment and follow-up for all tumors; screening and follow-up of family members at risk.

Peutz–Jeghers Syndrome

- **MIM code:** 175200.
- **Definition:** Genodermatosis featuring multiple lentigines, intestinal polyposis, and increased risk of carcinomas; autosomal dominant inheritance.

▶ **Pathogenesis:** Mutation in *STK11*, encoding a serine-threonine kinase growth control gene.

▶ **Clinical features:**
- *Skin:* Multiple lentigines, usually periorificial (lips, oral mucosa, perinasal, periorbital, anogenital) as well as acrally. Appear early in life but often overlooked as freckles. Associated with pigmented nail streaks and occasionally hyperpigmented palmoplantar creases.
- *Intestinal polyposis:* Jejunum is most often (90%) involved, but stomach, colon, rectum also affected (50%). Hamartomatous polyps with a small risk of malignant change. Main problems are intussusception and bleeding.
- *Malignant tumors:*
  - Tumors of testes and ovaries most common; often peculiar histologic types
  - Gastrointestinal tumors less common.

▶ **Diagnostic approach:** History, endoscopic examination, and follow-up; regular gynecologic or urologic examinations.

▶ **Differential diagnosis:** Many possibilities for multiple lentigines and systemic findings; exclude LEOPARD syndrome and Carney complex.

▶ **Therapy:** Surgical management as indicated; radical surgery rarely needed; examination and follow-up of family members at risk.

22 Disorders of Pigmentation

22.1 Overview

Definitions

- **Hyperpigmentation:** Increase in pigmentation.
- **Melanosis, hypermelanosis:** Increase in pigmentation due to excess melanogenesis.
  - ▶ *Note:* Hyperpigmentation and hypermelanosis are generally used as synonyms, although technically hyperpigmentation can result from other pigments in the skin.
- **Hypopigmentation, depigmentation:** Reduction (hypo-) or total loss (de-) of pigmentation.
- **Hypomelanosis, amelanosis:** Congenital reduction (hypo-) or total loss (a-) of pigmentation because of abnormal melanogenesis.
- **Leukoderma:** Hypo- or depigmentation following an inflammatory skin disease.
- **Pseudoleukoderma:** Less increase in pigmentation in diseased skin as compared to normal skin, following exposure to UV irradiation or exogenous pigments, producing a hypopigmented area (psoriatic leukoderma).
- **Dyschromatosis:** Literally, any abnormality in color of the skin; often refers to combination of hyper- and hypopigmentation; others use it to refer to pigmentary changes not related to melanocytes and melanin.
- **Poikiloderma:** Combination of atrophy, telangiectases, and hypo- as well as hyperpigmentation; classic example is radiation dermatitis.
- Unfortunately, these terms are not always used precisely. The critical distinctions are between:
  - *Congenital* and *acquired* changes.
  - *Hyperpigmentation:*
    - Excess melanin or other pigments (iron, silver, tattoos). If other pigments, then endogenous vs. exogenous.
    - Increased melanin production and transfer (café-au-lait macule) vs. increased number of melanocytes (lentigines, melanocytic nevi, malignant melanoma).
  - *Hypopigmentation:*
    - Loss of melanin (albinism) vs. loss of melanocytes (vitiligo).
- ◤ *Note:* Examine the entire skin surface in patients with pigmentary abnormalities; use of the Wood's lamp helps to identify changes more readily.

Classification

- **Hypopigmentation:**
  - *Entire body:*
    - *Congenital:* Albinism, Chédiak–Higashi syndrome, Hermansky–Pudlak syndrome, phenylketonuria, homocystinuria, histidinemia.
    - *Acquired:* Panhypopituitarism.
  - *Widespread areas:*
    - *Congenital:* Piebaldism, Waardenburg syndrome, hypomelanosis of Ito (incontinentia pigmenti achromians).
    - *Acquired:* Vitiligo, postinflammatory hypopigmentation, idiopathic guttate hypomelanosis, systemic sclerosis (confetti hypopigmentation).

- *Localized:*
  - *Congenital:* Nevus depigmentosus, tuberous sclerosis (ash-leaf macules).
  - *Acquired:* Vitiligo, chemically induced depigmentation (cleansing compounds), postinflammatory hypopigmentation, halo nevus.
► **Brown hyperpigmentation:**
  - *Diffuse:*
    - *Metabolic:* Hemochromatosis, Wilson disease, porphyria, hepatic failure, renal failure, Addison disease, tumors producing MSH or ACTH, ACTH therapy.
    - *Drugs or chemicals:* ACTH, amiodarone, antimalarials, arsenic, chlorpromazine, estrogens, minocycline, phenytoin, phenothiazine, psoralens (with UV); chemotherapy agents (busulfan, 5-fluorouracil, cyclophosphamide).
    - *Disease-related:* Systemic sclerosis, Whipple disease, mycosis fungoide, Sézary syndrome (melanoerythroderma).
  - *Localized:*
    - *Tumors and nevi:* Freckle, lentigo, syndromes with lentigines (p. 385), café au-lait macule, seborrheic keratosis, melanocytic nevus, Becker nevus, linear and whorled nevoid hypermelanosis, urticaria pigmentosa, acanthosis nigricans, epidermal nevus (some cases).
    - *Melasma.*
    - *Phototoxic dermatitis:* Berloque and meadow grass dermatitis.
    - *Medications:* Bleomycin (flagellate streaks), 5-fluorouracil (over veins).
    - *Burns, ionizing radiation, trauma.*
    - Postinflammatory hyperpigmentation following dermatoses or trauma.
► **Gray or blue hyperpigmentation:**
  - *Diffuse:* Hemochromatosis, metastatic melanoma with circulating melanin, bismuth, silver, gold, systemic ochronosis.
  - *Localized:* Nevus of Ota, nevus of Ito, mongolian spot, blue nevus, incontinentia pigmenti (late stage), macular amyloidosis, fixed drug reaction, erythema dyschromicum perstans, exogenous ochronosis.

22.2 Hypopigmentation

Albinism

► **Definition:** Family of disorders with disturbances in either melanin production or formation and transfer of melanosomes; typically affect skin and eyes; patient initially classified on clinical features but today defined by genetic studies. All inherited in autosomal recessive manner.
► **Epidemiology:** Overall incidence 1:20000; all races affected.
► **Tyrosinase-negative albinism**.
  - *MIM code:* 203100.
  - *Pathogenesis:* Mutation in tyrosinase gene; melanosomes contain no melanin.
  - *Clinical features:* Most severe form of albinism:
    - *Skin:* White hair, white to pale pink skin, no pigmented nevi, risk for UV-induced tumors (actinic keratoses, squamous cell carcinomas).
    - *Eyes:* Gray translucent iris, red reflex, photophobia, nystagmus, loss of vision.
  - *Diagnostic approach:* Hair bulb negative for tyrosine, ophthalmologic examination.
  - *Therapy:* Absolute sun avoidance or protection, dark glasses, regular dermatologic and ophthalmologic examinations.

▶ **Tyrosinase-positive albinism**.
- *MIM code:* 203200.
- *Pathogenesis:* Most common form of albinism; tyrosinase presence; melanin formed and melanosomes start to form but rarely mature completely.
- *Clinical features:*.
  - *Skin:* White skin and hair at birth; later slight pigmentation, often yellow-red hair; may have few freckles.
  - *Eyes:* Some pigment presence; defects less severe than above.
- *Diagnostic approach:* Hair bulb positive for tyrosinase, ophthalmologic examination.
- *Therapy:* Sun protection and regular monitoring.

▶ **Yellow albinism**.
- *MIM code:* 203100.
- *Pathogenesis:* Lack of eumelanin synthesis with reduced pheomelanin synthesis.
- *Clinical features:* Pale skin, freckles, can have pigmented nevi; pale yellow hair; iris with radial pigmentation; slight photophobia and nystagmus.
- *Diagnostic approach:* Hair bulb positive for tyrosinase, ophthalmologic examination.
- *Therapy:* Sun protection and regular monitoring.

▶ **Hermansky–Pudlak syndrome**.
- *MIM code:* 203300.
- *Pathogenesis:* Disease of diluted melanosomes, caused by mutations in at least seven different genes. Most common mutation is in *HPS1* gene; 1:20 Puerto Ricans are heterozygotes.
- *Clinical features:* Blond hair, blue eyes, freckling, multiple melanocytic nevi. Nystagmus and photophobia. Bleeding disturbance because of lack of dense bodies in platelets. Patients with *HPS1* mutation have pulmonary fibrosis, granulomatous colitis, and renal insufficiency.
- *Diagnostic approach:* Electron microscopy of platelets, identification of *HPS1* mutation or more complex studies if negative.
- *Therapy:* Sun protection and regular monitoring. Should be managed by physician experienced with problem.
- ⚠ *Caution:* Aspirin is contraindicated.

▶ **Chédiak–Higashi syndrome**.
- *MIM code:* 214500.
- *Pathogenesis:* Mutation in *LYST*, a gene controlling lysosome trafficking on chromosome 1q42.1–42.2. Giant lysosomes found in many cells including neutrophils, monocytes, hepatocytes and renal epithelial cells. Giant melanosomes in melanocytes.
- *Clinical features:* Pale skin with silvery hair and blue-violet or light brown irises. Course complicated by multiple infections and risk of lymphoma (accelerated reaction); most die in first decade.
- *Diagnostic approach:* Giant lysosomes can be identified in peripheral blood.
- *Therapy:* Prompt treatment of infections; if donor is available, bone marrow transplantation.

▶ **Ocular albinism:** At least four types, inherited in several patterns. Pattern has ocular findings similar to oculocutaneous albinism but minimal skin findings. Still unclear why changes are limited to melanocytes of retinal pigment epithelium.

▶ **Phenylketonuria**.
- *MIM code:* 261600.
- *Definition:* Common metabolic disturbance in phenylalanine metabolism inherited in autosomal recessive manner.

- *Pathogenesis:* Because of mutations in phenylalanine hydroxylase, phenylalanine is not converted to tyrosine, but instead accumulates, blocking tyrosinase. This has two effects: (1) failure to produce adequate melanin, (2) toxic effects of increased phenylalanine.
- *Clinical features:*
  - Pale skin, blond hair, blue eyes.
  - Pseudo-scleroderma: diffuse areas of sclerosis.
  - Growth retardation.
  - Mental retardation; variety of neurological problems.
- *Diagnostic approach:* Prenatal screening is standard is most countries. Diagnosis can be made on cord blood (Guthrie test) or even diaper urine. Prenatal diagnosis possible.
- *Therapy:* Low-phenylalanine diet as soon as diagnosis is made; most defects not reversible.

► **Nevus depigmentosus**.
  - *Definition:* Localized area of depigmentation, usually following Blaschko lines; caused by aberrant transfer of melanosomes.
  - *Clinical features:* Sharply demarcated permanent area of depigmentation present at birth, which grows with child; usually respects midline.
  - *Diagnostic approach:* History, clinical examination.
  - *Differential diagnosis: Nevus anemicus* is pharmacologic nevus, which is pale because of vasoconstriction; thus nevus depigmentosus becomes red with rubbing; nevus anemicus does not.
  - *Therapy:* Camouflage cosmetics or staining, as for vitiligo.

► **Hypomelanosis of Ito**.
  - *Synonyms:* Incontinentia pigmenti achromians, pigment mosaic—Ito type.
  - *Pathogenesis:* Not a single disease, but a manifestation of genomic mosaicism and thus associated with wide variety of underlying defects, including mental retardation and severe neurological defects.
  - *Clinical features:* Widespread areas of hypopigmentation following Blaschko lines; individual lesions identical to nevus depigmentosus.
  - *Diagnostic approach:* History, extensive physical examination, cytogenetic testing.
  - *Therapy:* None available.

► **Piebaldism**.
  - *MIM code:* 172800.
  - *Definition:* Uncommon genodermatosis with circumscribed hypomelanosis; autosomal dominant inheritance.
  - *Epidemiology:* Incidence of 1: 20000; more common among Hopi Indians.
  - *Pathogenesis:* Mutation in *KIT* gene on chromosome 4q12; *KIT* codes for the transmembrane receptor of a mast cell-stem cell growth factor.
  - *Clinical features:*
    - Permanent and nonprogressive hypopigmented area involving forehead and upper chest and back, as well as extremities. Areas may develop freckles or lentigines.
    - White forelock (poliosis) and white medial eyebrows, usually noticed at birth.
    - No other systemic signs and symptoms.
  - *Diagnostic approach:* History, complete physical examination; the Hopi patients were first diagnosed as having albinism as they were reluctant to disrobe for examiners.
  - *Differential diagnosis:* Vitiligo, which is acquired.
  - *Therapy:* None available.

- *Associated syndromes:* There are several forms of Waardenburg syndrome associated with piebaldism:
  - *Waardenburg syndrome I:* (MIM code 193500; mutation in *PAX3* gene with lateral displacement of the inner canthi (dystopia canthorum), broad nasal bridge, heterochromia irides (one blue eye, one brown eye), congenital deafness because of lack of migration of melanocytes to inner ear.
  - *Waardenburg syndrome IIA:* Lacks dystopia canthorum; otherwise similar.

Vitiligo

MIM code: 193200.

Definition: Acquired localized depigmentation of skin, hair, and occasionally mucosa, of unknown etiology, characterized by complete loss of melanocytes.

Epidemiology: Prevalence around 1%; more obvious, but not more common, in dark-skinned individuals. Onset before 20 years of age in 50%; around $1/3$ of patients have affected family members.

Pathogenesis: Etiology not well understood. Theories include:
- Autoimmune destruction of melanocytes.
- Neural pathways, because of relation to stress.
- Metabolic abnormalities: accumulation of toxic metabolites.
- "Self-destruct" action because of aberrant tetrahydrobiopterin and catecholamine synthesis.

Clinical features:
- Typical macule is oval or round, sharply circumscribed but with irregular border (Fig. 22.**1**). Size may range from a few mm to several cm. The border usually has the same color as normal skin; occasionally it is red or hyperpigmented. Early lesions may have areas of hypopigmentation rather than depigmentation (*trichrome vitiligo*).
- Palms and soles are frequently involved; hairs less often.

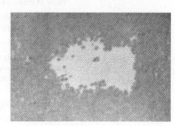

Fig. 22.**1** · Vitiligo: sharply bordered, irregular, completely depigmented macule.

Classification: Degree of involvement highly variable, ranging from a few macules to almost complete depigmentation. The following classification is useful:
- *Localized:*
  - *Focal:* One or more patches in the same area.
  - *Segmental:* Limited to a dermatome or Blaschko lines.
  - *Mucosal:* Only affected mucous membranes (rare).
- *Generalized:*
  - *Acrofacial:* Distal extremities and facial, especially periorificial.
  - *Vulgaris (common):* Disseminated lesions without region predilection.
  - *Universal:* Complete or almost complete depigmentation.

Associated diseases: Many autoimmune diseases are associated with vitiligo: either patients with vitiligo are more likely to be affected, or patients with the disease are more likely to have vitiligo. They include: hyperthyroidism, hypothyroidism, pernicious anemia, Addison disease, diabetes mellitus, alopecia areata, myasthenia gravis, uveitis (Vogt–Koyanagi–Harada syndrome), morphea, systemic sclerosis, halo nevus, malignant melanoma.

▶ **Prognosis:** Course highly variable and unpredictable. Spontaneous repigmentation that is cosmetically satisfactory for the patient occurs only rarely. Speckled repigmentation in a patch indicates that melanocytes from the outer root sheath of the hair follicle are producing melanin. Important to establish if the vitiligo is stable or progressive, as this influences choice of therapy.

▶ **Diagnostic approach:** See Table 22.**1**.
▶ **Differential diagnosis:** See Table 22.**2**.
▶ **Therapy:** The established therapy of vitiligo can be generously described as unsatisfactory. Table 22.**3** offers suggested approaches based on the patient's age.

Table 22.1 · **Vitiligo: diagnostic checklist**	
History	Skin type?
	How long has depigmentation been present?
	Was there inflammation or other skin lesions prior to depigmentation?
	Any triggers—stress, systemic illnesses, sunburn, other skin trauma—occurring 2–3 months before depigmentation?
	Course—stable or progressive? Repigmentation?
	History of photosensitivity?
	How severe is emotional impact of vitiligo?
	Köbner phenomenon, halo nevi, or poliosis?
	Visual or ocular problems?
	Industrial or hobby exposure that could have caused chemically induced depigmentation?
	Family history of vitiligo?
	Personal or family history of premature graying (< 30 years of age) alopecia areata, thyroid disease, juvenile diabetes mellitus, pernicious anemia, connective tissue diseases, Addison disease, atopy?
	History of melanocytic nevi which have regressed?
	Medications (β-blockers can worsen vitiligo)
	Previous treatment effectiveness, side effects?
Physical examination	Wood's light examination including mucosal surfaces.
	Documentation of degree of involvement (whole body photography or diagrams; number of lesions < 5, > 20, > 100).
	Classification: Look for poliosis, achromotrichosis (white hairs in vitiligo patch), halo nevi, inflammatory border to lesions
	Ophthalmologic examination (40% of patients have subclinical retinal pigmentary abnormalities)
Laboratory evaluation	Thyroid function tests including autoantibodies, anti-parietal cell antibodies, total IgE, ANA, glucose

Table 22.2 · **Differential diagnosis of vitiligo**

Diagnosis	Clinical features	Melanocyte abnormality
Nevus anemicus	Pale area because of vasoconstriction	None
Nevus depigmentosus	Localized hypomelanosis present since birth	Impaired transfer of melanosomes
Piebaldism	White forelock and depigmented areas	No melanocytes
Waardenburg syndrome	White forelock, depigmented areas, iris heterochromia, facial dysmorphism, deafness	No melanocytes, also missing in inner ear; autophagocytosis of melanocytes
Incontinentia pigmenti achromians	Hypopigmentation along Blaschko lines; often neurological abnormalities	Reduced melanocytes, abnormal melanosomes
Tuberous sclerosis	Ash-leaf macules, confetti depigmentation, adenoma sebaceum, connective tissue nevi, epilepsy, mental retardation	Normal numbers of melanocytes, abnormal transfer of melanosomes
Pityriasis alba	Facial depigmentation in atopic dermatitis	Normal numbers of melanocytes, abnormal transfer of melanosomes (reversible)
Postinflammatory hypopigmentation	Hypopigmentation following inflammatory dermatoses	Normal numbers of melanocytes, abnormal transfer of melanosomes (reversible); residual signs of inflammatory disease
Postinfectious leukoderma	After syphilis, lepra, pinta, yaws; white macules evolve from inflammatory lesions	Normal numbers of melanocytes, abnormal transfer of melanosomes (reversible); residual granulomatous inflammation
Pityriasis versicolor	Hypopigmented scaly macules; *Malassezia* spp. in skin	Normal numbers of melanocytes, abnormal transfer of melanosomes (reversible); hyphae and spores in stratum corneum (spaghetti and meatballs)
Systemic sclerosis	Confetti hypopigmentation	Reduced numbers of melanocytes
Idiopathic guttate hypomelanosis	Hypopigmented tiny macules on arms and legs in older individuals	Reduced numbers of melanocytes, photodamage
Chemically induced hypopigmentation	Appropriate history; hypo- or depigmented patches	Reduced to absent melanocytes

▶ *Note:* Complete depigmentation is possible, using 20% monobenzyl ether of hydroquinone. The patient must be given detailed advice on lifelong use of sunscreens and irreversibility of action. The product is no longer available in the USA because it was too often used for localized hyperpigmentation and caused widespread, distressing depigmentation.

Table 22.3 · **Treatment of vitiligo**

Age	Clinical type	First choice	Options
<5 years	Focal (<5%)	Topical corticosteroids	None
	Segmental	None	None
	Widespread (<5%)	Topical corticosteroids (+UVA)	UVB (311 nm), topical PUVA
>5 years, adults	Focal (<5%)	Topical corticosteroids (+UVA)	UVB (311 nm), topical PUVA, oral PUVA (>12 years), minigrafts (if stable)
	Segmental	Minigrafts	Stains, self-tanning agents
	Widespread (>5%)	UVB (311 nm)	Oral PUVA (>12 years), topical corticosteroids (+UVA), L-phenylalanin (+UVA), minigrafts (if stable)
Adults	Eyelids, lips, nipples, penis	Minigrafts	Stains, tanning agents
	Resistant, involving >80%	Total depigmentation	Stains, tanning agents

22.3 Brown Hyperpigmentation

▶ *Note:* The major differential diagnostic consideration for all focal brown hype
pigmentation is a melanocytic nevus or malignant melanoma, as discussed in th
next chapter. The lesions discussed below all feature increased melanin primaril
in the basal layer of the epidermis. They are sometimes grouped together a
melanotic macules.

Café-au-lait Macule

▶ **Definition:** Circumscribed tan macule, usually present at birth.
▶ **Clinical features:** Irregular tan macules and patches varying in size from 1 t
many cm. More than five café-au-lait macules >1.5 cm suggest neurofibromat
sis 1, but the macules can be sporadic or associated with a variety of syndromes
▶ **Histology:** Increased pigment in basal layer, normal number of melanocyte
giant melanosomes.

Syndromes with Café-au-lait Macules

▶ **Neurofibromatosis 1** (p. 362).
▶ **Neurofibromatosis 2** (p. 364).
▶ **Albright syndrome** (MIM code: 174800): Polyostotic fibrous dysplasia; e
docrine abnormalities; and giant, more regular, pigmented patches reflectir
mosaicism.
▶ **Watson syndrome** (MIM code: 193520): Mental retardation, pulmonic stenos
axillary freckling.

Ataxia-telangiectasia: (p. 453).
Bloom syndrome: (p. 306).

phelides

Synonym: Freckles.
Definition: Localized hyperpigmentation caused by sun exposure; waxes and wanes with seasons.
Clinical features: Much more common in skin types I and II; especially among redheads. Usually appear in childhood, flaring each summer; irregular brown macules of varying shades of tan and brown.
Histology: Increased melanin, normal to reduced numbers of melanocytes.
Differential diagnosis: Lentigines have an increased number of melanocytes and are permanent. Some patients with multiple lentigines (Carney complex) also have ephelides. Hyperpigmented plane warts occasionally mistaken for ephelides, but palpable.
Therapy: Sunscreens, light avoidance, as freckles are marker for increased risk of skin cancers.

ecker Nevus

More than a melanotic macule, although it clinically falls in this category until hypertrichosis appears at puberty. Best considered an organoid nevus (p. 412).

inear and Whorled Nevoid Hypermelanosis

Although nevoid hypomelanosis (nevus depigmentosus) is common, nevoid hypermelanosis usually following Blaschko lines is uncommon. Extensive lesions may be linear and whorled, but often one or two patches accompanied by a few macules is all that the patient displays. Search for underlying abnormalities warranted. Laser ablation of pigment possible.

ucosal Melanotic Macules

Irregular tan macules can be seen on the lips, penis, or labia. Harmless, but often confused with melanocytic nevi or malignant melanoma. On the genitalia, they often cause great concern. Biopsy is diagnostic, as there is only basal layer increase in melanin, without a proliferation of melanocytes. Once the diagnosis is secure, no treatment is needed, but patients may prefer excision or laser ablation.

elasma

Synonyms: Chloasma, mask of pregnancy.
Definition: Combined epidermal and dermal hyperpigmentation of forehead, cheeks, and perioral area.
Epidemiology: Common problem, almost exclusively limited to women; extremely prevalent in Latin America, among patients with mixed Indian/Spanish background. Pathogenesis: Risk factors include:
- Sun exposure.
- Pregnancy.
- Use of oral contraceptives (or tumors secreting estrogens).
- Rarely caused by phenytoin.

► **Clinical features:** Irregular brown hyperpigmentation, sometimes with blu
tones, often speckled. Sometimes mask-like pattern. Typically worsens with su
exposure.
► **Histology:** Biopsy not needed, but shows increased epidermal melanin as with in
continence of pigment in papillary dermis.
► **Differential diagnosis:** Topical photosensitivity reactions can mimic melasma
sometimes both occur together, as when contact dermatitis develops to a sur
screen. Typical causes are berloque dermatitis (perfumes) and phenolate
petrolatum.
► **Therapy:** Eliminate triggers (such as contraceptives), maximum sun protectior
avoidance using physical screens, bleaching with 2–4% hydroquinone, azelai
acid, or topical retinoids (combinations possible).

Berloque Dermatitis

► **Definition:** Type of phytophotodermatitis caused by combination of phototoxi
agent and sunlight.
► **Pathogenesis:** Berloque refers to the use of bergamot oil in perfumes; simila
furocoumarins are present in many plants.
► **Clinical features:** Initially acute dermatitis following light exposure; the
development of often bizarre hyperpigmented patches and streaks. When pe
fume is responsible, dripping streaks on neck and behind ear are classic.
► **Diagnostic approach:** Striking clinical picture usually gives answer.
► **Differential diagnosis:** Melasma.
► **Therapy:** Avoid triggers, maximum sun avoidance or protection, mild bleachir
with azelaic acid.

Cronkhite–Canada Syndrome

► **MIM code:** 175500.
► Rare sporadic syndrome, most common in East Asia, featuring generalize
gastrointestinal polyposis associated with malabsorption and wasting. Patien
have brown hyperpigmentation of face, nape, nipples, and distal extremities, z
well as nail dystrophy and alopecia. Cutaneous findings usually follow the sy
temic problems, which determine the management and course.

Acral Melanosis

► Rare acral hyperpigmentation seen in newborns; usually remains localized, bi
can later be more widespread.

22.4 Blue and Gray Hyperpigmentation

Erythema Dyschromicum Perstans

► **Synonym:** Ashy dermatosis.
► **Definition:** Poorly understood dermatosis with inflammatory phase and la
postinflammatory dermal melanosis.
► **Epidemiology:** Almost limited to mixed-race individuals in Latin America.
► **Pathogenesis:** Divided opinions whether form of lichen planus or idiopathic de
matosis.

Clinical features: Early lesions are erythematous macules favoring the trunk; they slowly evolve into blue-gray (ashy) macules with indistinct borders, often coalesce. Totally asymptomatic.

Histology: Dermal deposits of melanin in macrophages.

Differential diagnosis: Other forms of postinflammatory hyperpigmentation.

Therapy: Nothing well established; both chloroquine and PUVA have proponents.

Alkaptonuria

Synonym: Ochronosis.

MIM code: 203500.

Definition: Metabolic disturbance associated with arthritis and discoloration of cartilage and skin; autosomal recessive inheritance.

Pathogenesis: Mutation in HGD (homogentisate 1,2 dioxygenase) leads to accumulation of homogentisic acid in urine and tissues.

Clinical features:

- Discoloration of tissues including cartilage by accumulations of homogentisic acid, leading to arthritis.
- Discolored sclerae, auricular cartilage and nasal cartilage, giving blue tinge to overlying skin. Sometimes diffuse blue color.

Diagnostic approach: Clinical examination; urine darkens dramatically on standing.

Differential diagnosis: *Acquired ochronosis* is caused by abuse of hydroquinone bleaching agents, using either for too long or in too high a concentration; skin becomes darkened rather than lighter and dermal collagen is clumped and discolored.

Therapy: Symptomatic management of arthritis; avoidance of sunlight, which exaggerates pigmentary changes.

Diffuse Melanosis with Metastatic Melanoma

Rarely patients with metastatic malignant melanoma (p. 400) produce so much melanin in their tumors that it can be released into the circulation and settle out in all tissues, imparting a diffuse blue-gray color to the skin, as well as urine. A sign that death is near.

Deposition of Metallic Salts

A number of heavy metals can be deposited in the skin, usually imparting various shades of blue and gray. The most common agents are shown in Table 22.4.

Argyria

Definition: Deposition of silver in the skin and other tissues.

Pathogenesis: Localized argyria results from the topical application of silver to skin or mucous membranes. Systemic argyria results from the ingestion of silver-containing medications or massive abuse of topical agents; 2–4 g of silver are required to cause problems. A number of topical and systemic agents containing silver are available in Germany, some over the counter. The most commonly used silver product, silver sulfadiazine or "burn butter," almost never causes argyria.

Clinical features: Localized or diffuse blue-gray discoloration of skin.

Histology: The silver particles are best found in the basement membrane of sweat glands.

Therapy: No effective form of removal available.

Table 22.4 · Hyperpigmentation caused by heavy metals

Metal	Sources	Disorder
Silver	Nose drops, silver nitrate sticks	Argyria
Gold	Arthritis medication	Chrysiasis
Iron	Multiple blood transfusions, excessive ingestion	Siderosis
Arsenic	Fowler solution, skin tonics, old insecticides	Arsenical melanosis
Mercury	Topical bleaches or ophthalmic ointments	Hydrargyria: blue-gray discoloration, especially palmar creases
	Systemic exposure to fumes (hatters in past)	Gingival hyperpigmentation
Lead	Paints with lead; in distant past, topical use of lead salts	Plumbism with gingival hyperpigmentation
Bismuth	Antacids; old syphilis medications	Bismuthism with stomatitis and dermatitis

Hyperpigmentation Caused by Medications

▶ **Amiodarone:** Diffuse blue-gray hyperpigmentation in sun-exposed areas, especially face (lipofuscin deposits).
▶ **Minocycline:** Following long-term use:.
  • Dark blue to black macules in acne scars or over cysts.
  • Hyperpigmented patches in light-exposed areas (slowly reversible); on occasion, diffuse disease.
  • Hyperpigmentation of mucosal surfaces, especially mouth.
  • Combination of both interaction with melanocytes and iron complexes.
▶ **Chemotherapy agents:**
  • *Generalized hyperpigmentation:* 5-fluorouracil, busulfan.
  • *Localized hyperpigmentation:* Adriamycin, bleomycin, cyclophosphamide, other alkylating agents, mithramycin, actinomycin D, various hormones.
  • *Lineare hyperpigmentation:* 5-Fluorouracil and many others (over veins), bleomycin (flagellate, presumably following scratching).
  • *Nail hyperpigmentation:* Adriamycin, cyclophosphamide, 5-fluorouracil, dacarbazine, mechlorethamine.
▶ **Antimalarials:** Chloroquine and hydroxychloroquine may cause gray hyperpigmentation, especially facial and pretibial, as well as on gingiva and palate. Quinacrine causes diffuse gray-yellow discoloration.

22.5 *Reticular Hyperpigmentation and Dyschromatosis*

Definitions

- **Reticular hyperpigmentation**: Net-like or lacy.
- **Dyschromatosis:** Combines hypo- and hyperpigmentation without the atrophy or telangiectases of poikiloderma.

Localized Reticular Hyperpigmentation

- **Acropigmentatio reticularis (Kitamura):** Rare disorder, primarily seen in Japan, with dominant inheritance; depressed reticulate macules on backs of hands and feet, palmoplantar pits, interrupted hieroglyphics; later spread centrally.
- **Dowling–Degos disease (reticular pigmented anomaly of the flexures):** Similar to Kitamura disease, but involves primarily axillae and groin; also inherited in autosomal dominant manner. Increased basal layer melanin.
- **Galli–Galli disease:** Similar to Dowling–Degos but with acantholysis histologically; also apparently has autosomal dominant inheritance.
- **Erythema ab igne:** Result of local exposure to heat (hand warmers, heating pads, sitting in front of heat source); combination of reticulate hyperpigmentation and livid vascular network. Melanin is dermal.

Generalized Reticular Hyperpigmentation

- **Naegeli–Franceschetti–Jadassohn syndrome** (MIM code: 161000): Rare disorder with autosomal dominant inheritance; reticulate hyperpigmentation of nape, axillae, groin, associated with palmoplantar keratoderma, hypohidrosis, and dental anomalies.
- **Dermatopathia pigmentosa reticularis** (MIM code: 125595): Extremely rare genodermatosis with autosomal dominant inheritance; atrophic reticulate hyperpigmentation of trunk and extremities, associated with nonscarring alopecia. Nail dystrophy and occasionally hypohidrosis.
- **Confluent and reticulated papillomatosis (Gougerot–Carteaud):** Pigmented patches and papules, sometimes with reticulated pattern, mainly on trunk: perhaps variant of pityriasis versicolor, as *Malassezia* spp. have been identified and lesions sometimes clear with antimicrobials.

Dyschromatoses

- **Dyschromatosis symmetrica hereditaria (Dohi)** (MIM code: 127400): Another Japanese genodermatosis with hypo- and hyperpigmented macules, believed to have autosomal dominant inheritance; prevalence of 1:100000. Usually involves just the dorsal aspects of the extremities; about 20% have truncal lesions.
- **Dyschromatosis symmetrica universalis hereditaria** (MIM code: 127500): Variant of Dohi disease with widespread involvement.

23 Melanocytic Tumors

23.1 Benign Melanocytic Tumors

Overview

The first step in analyzing pigmented lesions is to decide if:

► **Only increased melanin is present:** Then one must think of brown hyperpigmentation (p. 378) including café-au-lait macule, freckles, Becker nevus, and mucosal pigmented macules. Sometimes the term *melanotic macule* is applied to this entire group, which is discussed in the preceding chapter on pigmentation.

► **Increased numbers of melanocytes are present:** This indicates lentigo, melanocytic nevus, or malignant melanoma.

23.2 Lentigenes

Lentigo Simplex

► **Definition:** Localized hyperpigmentation secondary to increase in melanocytes at the dermoepidermal junction.

► **Clinical features:** Sharply circumscribed, uniformly pigmented tan to dark brown macules; no relation to sun exposure (unlike freckles).

► **Histology:** Increased numbers of melanocytes at dermoepidermal junction; no nests. If nests (accumulations of more than three melanocytes) are seen, then preferred term is *nevoid lentigo, nevus incipiens* or, if more advanced, *junctional melanocytic nevus.*

► **Diagnostic approach:** It is not essential to know if a lesion is a lentigo or melanotic macule; a biopsy is not needed. If multiple lentigines are present, a variety of syndromes should be considered.

   ◨ *Note:* Lentigines are permanent lesions and usually uniformly pigmented; ephelides (freckles) are paler, more irregular and vary with sun exposure, becoming more prominent in the summer.

► **Therapy:** None needed; if bothersome, cryotherapy or laser ablation, usually with erbium or ruby laser.

PUVA Lentigo

PUVA therapy induces a number of flat small irregular melanocytic lesions that persist for months or years after therapy. Histologically they show a proliferation of melanocytes at the dermoepidermal junction. The melanocytes are often atypical and occasionally PUVA lentigenes may evolve into malignant melanoma. The lentigenes in xeroderma pigmentosum (p. 304) are very similar. Older adults may also develop irregular pigmented macules in sun-exposed skin, with proliferation of atypical melanocytes.

Syndromes with Lentigines

The following disorders should be considered in patients with multiple lentigines:
▸ **Multiple lentigines without associated findings.**
▸ **Multiple lentigines in mosaic pattern.**
▸ **LEOPARD syndrome** (MIM code 151100): Autosomal dominant inheritance; **l**entigines, **E**KG abnormalities, **o**cular hypertelorism, **p**ulmonary stenosis, **a**bnormal genitalia, **r**etarded growth, **d**eafness.
▸ **Carney syndrome** (MIM code: 160980): Autosomal dominant inheritance; also known as NAME syndrome: **n**evi (lentigines, blue nevi), **a**trial myxoma, **m**yxoid cutaneous tumors and **e**phelides (freckles). Two different responsible genes: CNC1 at 17q23, *PRKAR1A* gene encoding a protein kinase, and CNC2 at 2p16 with unknown product; patients may also have Cushing syndrome, as well as testicular and neural tumors.
▸ **Peutz–Jeghers syndrome** (p. 369).
▸ **Axillary freckles** (also genital, perianal): Also known as Crowe sign; marker for neurofibromatosis.
▸ **Lentiginosis perigenito-axillaris of Korting:** Similar to axillary freckles, but no associated diseases.
▸ **Centrofacial lentiginosis of Touraine** (MIM code 151000): Autosomal dominant inheritance; association of midfacial lentigenes with mental retardation.
▸ **Mid-facial lentigenes in blacks:** common finding in light-colored, red-haired blacks; may also include freckles; no associated findings. May also be seen in whites as incidental finding.

Solar Lentigo

Terminology is very confusing, but we consider these lesions to be flat seborrheic keratoses, which are discussed under benign epidermal tumors (p. 416).

23.3 Melanocytic nevi

Congenital Melanocytic Nevus

▸ **Synonyms:** Large lesions often called *bathing trunk nevus* or *giant hairy nevus*.
▸ **Definition:** Melanocytic nevus present at birth.
▸ **Epidemiology:**
- 1% of newborns have melanocytic nevus; 1:20000 have lesion > 10 cm; 1:500000 have giant melanocytic nevus.
- Smaller (< 1.5 cm) lesions with histological features of congenital melanocytic nevus can appear in infancy: tardive congenital melanocytic nevus.
▸ **Clinical features:**
- Lesions are subdivided by size (Fig. 23.1): *Small:* < 1.5 cm diameter; *medium:* 1.5–20 cm diameter; *large:* > 20 cm diameter; the giant or bathing trunk lesions involve an entire body segment.
- Most congenital melanocytic nevi are heavily pigmented, have a papillomatous surface and contain hairs. Few if any acquired melanocytic nevus have these features. At birth, the nevi may be less heavily pigmented or not have prominent hairs.
▸ **Histology:** Always junctional and dermal component; the junctional changes at birth are quite atypical and suggest a malignant melanoma until the history is

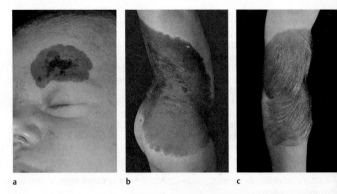

a   b   c

Fig. 23.**1** · **Congenital melanocytic nevus. a** Medium-sized. **b** Giant. **c** Nevus pigmentosus et pilosus.

known; the dermal component usually extends deeply, often following adnexal structures.

▶ **Diagnostic approach:** Clinical examination; then dermatoscopy and photo documentation.

▶ **Differential diagnosis:** Clinically unique when dark and hairy; at birth if tan, consider café-au-lait macule, nevus spilus, and early epidermal nevus.

▶ **Prognosis:** There is a risk of developing malignant melanoma, varying with the type of congenital melanocytic nevus:

- *Large congenital melanocytic nevus:* Risk of malignant melanoma is around 10% (5–30%); tumors often develop in childhood as irregular, frequently amelanotic nodules in the midst of the tumor. They often arise deep and cannot be readily appreciated so prognosis is grim.

- *Medium and small congenital melanocytic nevus:* Risk is much lower, clearly less than 5%. Change occurs in adult life. When a malignant melanoma develops within a preexisting nevus, often the precursor lesion was a small congenital lesion.

▷ *Note:* Despite this worrisome information, do not forget that the vast bulk of malignant melanoma develop spontaneously, rather than from a preexisting lesion.

▶ **Therapy:**

- Two goals: (1) Avoid malignant melanoma; (2) cosmetic improvement, as patients with large disfiguring nevi have marked psychosocial problems.

- Small and medium lesions can be excised, either in a single step or as part of staged excision. If larger, skin expanders can be helpful to facilitate closure. Since the risk of malignant melanoma becomes higher in adult life, the procedure can be delayed until the child can cooperate.

- Large lesions are a treatment problem. Often staged excision is not even an option because of the size. Early dermabrasion or curettage removes much of the melanocyte load and improves cosmetic appearance. Whether it reduces the risk of malignant melanoma remains controversial.

- Patients should be followed yearly. Parents and then patients instructed in self-examination. Any new nodules are highly suspicious and should be excised.

Neurocutaneous Melanosis

▶ **Clinical features:** Patients with extensive or multiple congenital melanocytic nevi are at risk of having leptomeningeal involvement with drastic consequences:
- Increased intracranial pressure and hydrocephalus.
- Impingement on brain or spinal column with functional impairments.
- Development of leptomeningeal malignant melanoma, which is almost invariably fatal.

▶ **Diagnostic approach:** Patients with extensive lesions crossing midline or in head and neck region should be subjected to imaging studies and then followed with ophthalmology and neurology.

Nevus Spilus

▶ **Synonym:** Speckled lentiginous nevus.
▶ **Definition:** Congenital lesion consisting of café-au-lait macule speckled with small melanocytic nevi.
▶ **Clinical features:** Irregular tan patch, several cm in diameter, with numerous small dark macules (lentigenes) or papules (melanocytic nevi) (Fig. 23.2). Rarely associated with systemic findings: *nevus spilus syndrome* with ipsilateral neurological findings such as hyperhidrosis or *phacomatosis pigmentokeratotica* (associated with nevus sebaceus).

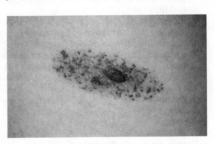

Fig. 23.**2** · Nevus spilus.

▶ **Histology:** The background skin contains increased melanin, while the darker spots have increased melanocytes, sometimes in nests.
▶ **Differential diagnosis:** Early in life, may be confused with Becker nevus or multiple lentigines in mosaic pattern; later distinctive.
▶ **Therapy:** Small lesions can be excised; otherwise follow and remove any darker component that is changing. The risk of malignant melanoma is very low.

Acquired Melanocytic Nevus

▶ **Definition:** Benign proliferation of melanocytes; most common human tumor.
▶ **Epidemiology:** Everyone has melanocytic nevi; lesions appear first at age 2–3 and their number usually stabilizes at about 30 years of age. Then some lesions may regress.
▶ **Pathogenesis:** Even though melanocytic nevi are so common, their pathogenesis is poorly understood. Accepted trigger factors include early sun exposure (uncommon in areas covered by two layers of clothing), hormones (puberty and pregnancy), and immunosuppression (flares following chemotherapy or in HIV/AIDS).

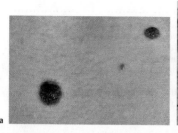
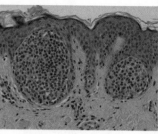

Fig. 23.**3** · **a** Acquired melanocytic nevi. **b** Microscopic picture of junctional melanocytic nevus with nests of melanocytes in basal layer.

▶ **Clinical features:**
- Average patient has 20–40 melanocytic nevi.
- Start as homogenous tan macules, which gradually darken but almost never exceed 6 mm. Later become papules or nodules (Fig. 23.**3 a**).
- Color varies from patient to patient, and from lesion to lesion, ranging from skin-colored to tan to red-brown to almost black. In general, older nevi tend to lose their color.
- Surface may vary from papillomatous to smooth.
  ▷ *Note:* Size > 1 cm or hair suggests a congenital melanocytic nevus.

▶ **Histology:** Traditionally divided into three types:
- *Junctional:* Nests of melanocytes at dermoepidermal junction; nests are round to oval and all about the same size (Fig. 23.**3 b**).
- *Compound:* Nests of melanocytes both at the dermoepidermal junction and through the dermis with varying patterns and degree of dermal involvement.
- *Dermal:* No increase in melanocytes at dermoepidermal junction; limited to the dermis; older lesions may have areas with neuroid pattern, fat, or fibrosis.
  ▷ *Note:* Nonetheless, early nevi are usually junctional and old nevi most often dermal.

▶ **Diagnostic approach:** Careful clinical examination. If many lesions or atypical lesions are present, then photo-documentation and regular follow-up. Instruct patient on ABCDE rules (p. 389).

▶ **Differential diagnosis:** In most instances, the patient can make the diagnosis. The issue is always: Is there any reason to be suspicious of malignant melanoma? Older nonpigmented nevi may be mistaken for skin tags or neurofibromas.

▶ **Prognosis:** Patients with >50 melanocytic nevi have 5-fold increased melanoma risk; with >100, 10-fold increase.

▶ **Therapy:** Lesions that are likely to be traumatized, as well as those about which the patient is either worried or cosmetically bothered, can be excised.

Halo Nevus

▶ **Synonym:** Sutton nevus.
▶ **Definition:** Melanocytic nevus surrounded by hypopigmentation.
▶ **Pathogenesis:** A prominent host lymphocytic response attacks the nevus and may be responsible for its disappearance; at the same time, melanocytes and melanin in the adjacent epidermis are also destroyed. Often multiple; sometimes triggered by sunburn.

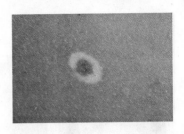

Fig. 23.4 · Halo nevus.

▶ **Clinical features:** Papular melanocytic nevus surrounded by white halo (Fig. 23.**4**). Later nevus may fade or even disappear. Later, pigmentation comes back.

▶ **Histology:** Dense lymphocytic infiltrate that often obscures the residual melanocytes.

▣ *Note:* Halo nevi may also be the result of a host response to malignant melanoma. All patients with halo nevi should be checked for other suspicious pigmented lesions. In adults, ophthalmologic and genital examinations are indicated, along with total body examination.

▶ **Therapy:** Excision if desired; if multiple lesions, only excise those in which the nevus is atypical.

Dysplastic Nevus

▶ **Synonym:** Atypical nevus.

▶ **Definition:** Melanocytic nevi with irregular border, larger size, and collection of distinctive histological features.

▶ **Epidemiology:** 2–8% of whites have dysplastic nevi. They begin developing during puberty and continue to appear through out life. Dysplastic nevi may be sporadic or have autosomal dominant inheritance (dysplastic nevus syndrome).

▶ **Pathogenesis:** Hormones and sun exposure appear to be the major etiologic factors.

▶ **Clinical features:**
- Dysplastic nevi (Fig. 23.**5 a**)and early malignant melanomas can be identified by the **ABCDE rule**; the criteria are most pronounced in melanoma.
  - **A**symmetry.
  - **B**order: irregular border, leakage of pigment.
  - **C**olor: multiple colors, best appreciated with dermatoscopy.
  - **D**iameter: >6 mm.
  - **E**levating or **E**nlarging: a papule nevus is usually harmless; a flat nevus that grows or develops a nodular component is suspicious.
- Dysplastic nevi may have a "fried egg" appearance: broad flat nevi (white of egg) with raised central portion (yolk).
- Sporadic dysplastic nevi are commonly found on the palms, soles, breast, umbilicus, genital, and perianal regions.

▶ **Histology:** The histological features of dysplastic nevi are highly controversial. They include:
- Junctional proliferation of melanocytes extending beyond the dermal component of the nevus (shoulder effect) often with fusion of adjacent nests (bridging).
- Melanocytes in nests are often spindle-shaped.

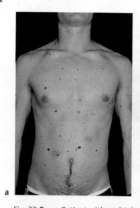
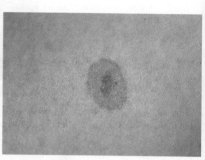

Fig. 23.5 · **a** Patient with multiple dysplastic nevi. **b** Dysplastic or atypical nevus.

- Fibrosis around the nests (lamellar fibrosis).
- Lymphocytic infiltrates.
- Atypia of melanocytes: most controversial point; some groups say no atypia; others grade degree of atypia (mild, moderate, severe).
  - ▣ *Note:* Many studies have shown that these criteria, greatly simplified here, are not reproducible, even between expert observers, or even by the same observer over a period of time. Almost every flat melanocytic nevus shows some of these features under the microscope.
- ▶ **Differential diagnosis:** Banal melanocytic nevus, malignant melanoma.
- ▶ **Therapy:** If a patient has only one or a small number of dysplastic nevi, excision is the simplest approach.

Dysplastic Nevus Syndrome

- ▶ **Synonyms:** B-K mole syndrome, familial atypical mole malignant melanoma syndrome, melanoma pancreas carcinoma syndrome.
- ▶ **MIM codes:** 155600, 606719.
- ▶ **Definition:** Syndrome with multiple dysplastic nevi, increased risk of malignant melanoma, and in some pedigrees increased risk of carcinoma of the pancreas or ocular malignant melanoma. Either familial or sporadic.
- ▶ **Epidemiology:** In contrast to sporadic dysplastic nevi, patients with multiple nevi are uncommon and those with a family history of melanoma even less common.
- ▶ **Pathogenesis:**
  - A number of genes have been associated with familial melanoma syndromes. The most common are mutations in *CDKN2A* (p16), a cyclin-dependant kinase inhibitor at 9p21, or in *CDK4*, a cyclin-dependent kinase, at 12q13. Both of these products help control the cell growth cycle. Some patients with p16 mutations also have an increased risk of pancreatic cancer; in well-established families, the risk of malignant melanoma is around 50% and pancreatic cancer, 17%. Many other loci and potential genes have been identified.
  - Still no consensus if multiple dysplastic nevi are markers for a predisposition to develop malignant melanoma or precursor lesions, likely to evolve into malignant melanoma. Most recent work points surprisingly more in the direction of marker than precursor.

▪ *Note:* Not all families with an increased likelihood of malignant melanoma have dysplastic nevi.

▶ **Clinical features:** These patients have many, many dysplastic nevi—often more than 100, most common on the trunk, but also on protected sites such as scalp, breast, and bathing trunks area (Fig. 23.**5 b**).

▶ **Histology:** Identical to sporadic dysplastic nevus.

▶ **Therapy:**
- Family history of atypical moles or malignant melanoma.
- Complete body examination; dermatoscopic evaluation of atypical nevi.
- Excision and histologic examination of especially large, irregular or changing nevi.
- Documentation: Total body photographs, ideally digital; can be combined with computer-supported dermatoscopic examination in many systems, such as Dermascan or Fotofinder.
- Follow-up every 6–12 months with excision of suspicious lesions.

▶ **Patient education:**
- Self-examination.
- Avoidance of excessive sun exposure.
- Offer to examine first-degree relatives.

▪ *Note:* :
- Dermatoscopy with photodocumentation has proved to be most useful in identifying suspicious or changing dysplastic nevus.
- Even the most aggressive surgeon cannot cure patients with dysplastic nevus syndrome; many of their malignant melanomas develop de novo, not from preexisting nevi.

Spitz Nevus

▶ **Synonym:** Spindle and epithelioid cell nevus.

▶ **Definition:** Variant of benign melanocytic nevus with distinctive histologic pattern that features considerable atypia and is easily confused with malignant melanoma.

  ▪ *Note:* When Sophie Spitz described these nevi over 50 years ago, she used the term "benign juvenile melanoma," showing just what a histologic challenge these lesions present.

▶ **Epidemiology:** The vast bulk of Spitz nevi occur in children; about 1 % of histologically examined melanocytic nevi are Spitz nevi.

▶ **Clinical features:** Red-brown papule or nodule, often on face or upper trunk (Fig. 23.**6 a**). History of sudden growth. In adults, no typical appearance.

▶ **Histology:** Junctional or compound nevus with spindle cell and/or epithelioid pattern; symmetrical but with cellular and architectural atypia, including mitoses. Cells more normal at base with mitoses uncommon. Eosinophilic bodies at junction (*Kamino bodies*).

▶ **Differential diagnosis:** Two classic differential diagnostic considerations are mast cell tumor and juvenile xanthogranuloma; other possibilities include adnexal tumor, hemangioma, arthropod bite reaction, ordinary melanocytic nevus.

▶ **Therapy:** Excision.

▪ *Note:* Atypical Spitz nevus describes lesions which cannot be separated with certainty from melanoma. They should be treated as would be a melanoma.

Melanocytic Tumors

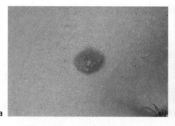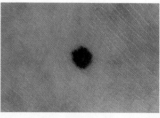

a

Fig. 23.**6** · **a** Spitz nevus. **b** Pigmented spindle cell nevus (Reed nevus).

Pigmented Spindle Cell Nevus

- ▶ **Synonym:** Reed nevus.
- ▶ **Definition:** Superficial heavily pigmented melanocytic nevus, sharing some features of Spitz nevus.
- ▶ **Clinical features:** Dark flat or slightly raised papule usually on extremities of young adults; more common in women (Fig. 23.**6 b**).
- ▶ **Histology:** Nests of spindle cells at the dermoepidermal junction with horizontal orientation parallel to skin surface. Marked melanin both in macrophages and in the epidermis, including stratum corneum.
- ▶ **Diagnostic approach:** Very distinctive starburst pattern on dermatoscopy.
- ▶ **Differential diagnosis:** Dysplastic nevus, malignant melanoma.
- ▶ **Therapy:** Excision.

Congenital Dermal Melanosis

There are a number of congenital lesions in which there are spindled melanocytes and melanin in the dermis, imparting a blue-gray color:
- ▶ **Mongolian spot:** Blue-gray sacral patch; common in black and Asian children; usually resolves by 5 years of age (Fig. 23.**7**). No biopsy needed, but very subtle presence of spindle-shaped melanocytes.
- ▶ **Nevus of Yamamoto:** Mongolian spot in extrasacral location, such as hands and feet; rare, and tends not to resolve.
- ▶ **Nevus of Ota (nevus fuscoceruleus ophthalmomaxillaris):** Common in Japanese; most often involves women; affects area served by 1st and 2nd branches of trigeminal nerve; sclera also pigmented. Usually present at birth; rare development of malignant melanoma. Major cosmetic problem in Japan, where it is relatively common.
- ▶ **Nevus of Hori:** Bilateral acquired nevus of Ota.

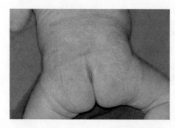

Fig. 23.**7** · Mongolian spot.

- **Nevus of Ito (nevus fuscoceruleus deltoideoacromalis):** Same as nevus of Ota, but affects shoulder girdle.
- **Therapy:** Ruby and alexandrite lasers are most helpful for destroying the dermal melanin.

Blue Nevus

- **Definition:** Benign tumor consisting of dermal proliferation of spindle-shaped melanocytes.
- **Clinical features:** Firm blue-gray to almost black flat-topped 1–2 cm papule; often acral or on face (Fig. 23.8 a). Cellular variant usually on buttocks, and larger.
- **Histology:**
  - *Ordinary blue nevus:* Spindle-shaped cells, varying degrees of melanin, sometimes in melanophages; junctional changes uncommon (Fig. 23.8 b).
  - *Cellular blue nevus:* Plump epithelioid cells and neuroid area, in deep dermis and often into subcutaneous fat; sometimes with satellite lesions. Mitoses and necrosis suggest a malignant blue nevus.
  - *Combined nevus:* Usually combination of blue nevus and compound nevus; no special clinical considerations.
  - *Deep penetrating nevus:* Variant or relative of blue nevus with both junctional nests and a spindle-cell proliferation that extends deep into the dermis, often along adnexal structures, or may involve subcutaneous fat.
- **Differential diagnosis:** Clinical: malignant melanoma, pigmented dermatofibroma, traumatic tattoo; histological: malignant melanoma, especially melanoma metastasis.
- **Therapy:** Excision.

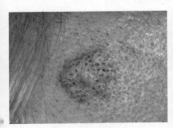 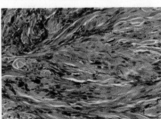

b

Fig. 23.8 · **a** Blue nevus. **b** Micrograph of blue nevus with marked melanin and spindle-shaped cells.

23.4 Malignant Melanoma

Overview

- **Synonym:** Melanoma (both terms used throughout this book).
- **Definition:** Malignant tumor of melanocytes.
- **Epidemiology:**
  - The lifetime risk of malignant melanoma for white Europeans increased dramatically from 1:1500 in 1935 to 1:75 in 2000, representing a doubling of incidence every 10–15 years (Fig. 23.9). In Australia and Southwestern USA, lifetime risk is 1:25. Uncommon in blacks and Asians (annual incidence 2–4/million).

Lifetime risk of melanoma in Germany

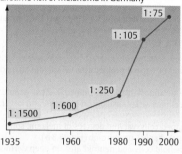

Fig. 23.**9** · Increasing incidence of malignant melanoma.

- Male:female ratio 1:1.5; uncommon in children; most occur between 30–70 years of age; varies with type.
- ► **Pathogenesis:** Risk factors include (up to 10%):
  - Genetic predisposition (familial melanoma syndromes) (up to 10%).
  - Excessive sun exposure and sunburns < 20 years of age, especially as infants.
  - Number of melanocytic nevi (> 50), which correlates with childhood sun exposure.
  - Presence of atypical melanocytic nevi.
  - Skin types I and II (p. 50).
  - About $^2/_3$ of malignant melanomas develop novo; $^1/_3$ arise in melanocytic nevi.
- ► **Biology:** Melanomas have two relatively distinct growth phases:
  - *Horizontal or radial phase:* Melanoma starts with abnormal junctional melanocytes; expands laterally in most instances for long period of time; number of different clones can establish themselves with differing growth capabilities. Tumors in this phase rarely metastasize.
  - *Vertical phase:* Tumor cells break through the basement membrane and begin to grow down into the dermis. Once the basement membrane has been bridged, the melanoma has the potential to metastasize.
- ► **Prevention:**
  - Melanomas should be preventable tumors, as they develop in full sight of the patient and family in most cases.
  - Two steps are essential for early detection of malignant melanoma:
    - Patients must learn how to identify suspicious melanocytic nevi and then to present promptly for evaluation and treatment.
    - Every physician must have an appreciation of the morphology of early malignant melanomas so that every visit to the doctor is a form of screening examination.

Clinical Features

There are four clinico-pathologic subtypes:
- ► **Superficial spreading melanoma (SSM):**
  - Most common type; 60%; age peak 40–60 years.
  - Irregularly pigmented, poorly circumscribed, often polycyclic macule or plaque; usually > 6 mm; over time frequently develops hypopigmented areas of tumor regression, as well as new nodules representing invasive tumors (vertical growth phase) (Fig. 23.**10**).

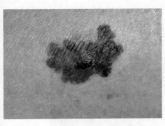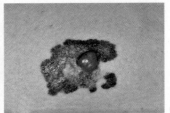

b

Fig. 23.**10** · **a** Superficial spreading melanoma. **b** Nodule and area of regression of the tumour shown in **a**.

- Described by Fitzpatrick as "red, white, and blue" tumor.
- Usually on trunk in men; lower legs in women.
- *Differential diagnosis:* Pigmented Bowen disease, pigmented flat seborrheic keratosis, dysplastic nevus.

► **Nodular melanoma (NM):**
- About 20%; age peak 40–60 years.
- Dark-brown papule or nodule; rarely pink or skin-colored (amelanotic); frequently ulcerated (outgrows vasculature and is traumatized) (Fig. 23.**11 a**). Circumscribed, with little hint of peripheral spread.
- Prototype of vertical growth phase with very short period of horizontal spread.
- Prognosis usually worst because diagnosed at a thicker stage.
- **⚠ *Caution:*** Nodular melanomas can be less than 6 mm in diameter.
- *Differential diagnosis:* Pigmented basal cell carcinoma, irritated seborrheic keratosis, porocarcinoma, pigmented squamous cell carcinoma, thrombosed vascular tumor (senile angioma), angiokeratoma, pyogenic granuloma, especially if nail fold and amelanotic, angiosarcoma.

► **Lentigo maligna melanoma (LMM):**
- About 10%; peaks > 60 years with increasing incidence until death.
- Areas of chronic light exposure; most often face.
- Large irregularly pigmented macule, often with areas of regression; as long as confined to epidermis, known as *lentigo maligna melanoma in situ.*
- When clinical nodule develops or tumor is found in dermis on microscopic examination, then LMM (Fig. 23.**11 b**).
- Better prognosis because of very long radial growth phase.
- *Differential diagnosis:* Pigmented actinic keratosis, solar lentigo (flat seborrheic keratosis).

► **Acral-lentiginous melanoma (ALM):**
- 5%; most common melanoma in dark-skinned individuals.
- Occurs on areas without hair follicles; otherwise resembles SSM or NM.
- Several clinical variants:
  - *Subungual melanoma:* May present as dark streak in nail, with streaks of pigment in nail fold (*Hutchinson sign*) and extension to finger tip; when amelanotic, may be mistaken for pyogenic granuloma (Fig. 23.**11 c**).
  - *Digital melanoma:* Typical on tips of toes or less often fingers; or less often palmoplantar; later lesions can be confused with tinea nigra (p. 121).

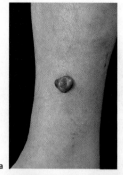

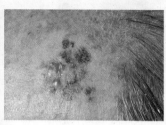

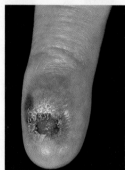

Fig. 23.**11** · **a** Nodular malignant melanoma.
b Lentigo maligna melanoma. **c** Acral-lentiginous
melanoma.

Melanoma and Preexisting Nevi

► About 25% of melanomas show histological signs of preexisting melanocytic nevus.
► Of these nevi, 40% are congenital, 60% dysplastic.
► Giant congenital melanocytic nevi undergo malignant change early in life; smaller lesions much later.

Special Variants of Melanoma

► **Amelanotic malignant melanoma:** Skin-colored or pink; more often nodular or subungual, but any melanoma can be amelanotic. Extremely difficult to recognize; differential diagnostic considerations include vascular tumors, Spitz nevus, basal cell carcinoma.
► **Verrucous or polypoid malignant melanoma:** May at same time be amelanotic; verrucous, or papillomatous surface; almost always confused with seborrheic keratosis or verrucous nevus.
► **Mucosal melanoma:** Can involve mouth, pharynx, trachea, genitalia, and anorectal region; variants of ALM; usually recognized late in course and thus with dismal prognosis. Differential diagnostic considerations include benign racial hyperpigmentation, amalgam tattoos, and mucosal melanotic macules.

▶ **Uveal melanoma:** About 5% of melanomas; relatively good prognosis.
▶ **Meningeal melanoma:** Rare, occurs in patients with neurocutaneous melanosis.
▶ **Gastrointestinal melanoma**.
▶ **Metastatic malignant melanoma:** Metastases can be extremely hard to identify, as clinically they may be amelanotic or erythematous, while histologically they may be epidermotropic. When multiple lesions are present in a known melanoma patient (Fig. 23.**12**), the diagnosis is easier.
▶ **Occult melanoma:** Presents as metastatic disease with no evidence of primary tumor. Assumption is that primary melanoma has either undergone complete regression or was internal. Even at autopsy, mystery sometimes remains. Accounts for 5–8% of patients in referral centers.
▶ **Desmoplastic/neurotrophic melanoma:** Usually presents as LM of face or arms, but evolves into scar- or keloid-like lesion; diagnosis first made histologically.
　 ⚠ Caution: Be suspicious of facial keloid following removal of any poorly defined pigmented lesion.
▶ **Other histologic variants:** Melanomas may resemble ordinary or Spitz nevi under the microscope; making this diagnosis simply indicates a degree of uncertainty in the diagnosis. Balloon cell nevi and melanomas have large cells with clear cytoplasm; they are only identified histologically.

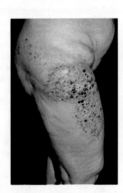

Fig. 23.**12** · Widespread cutaneous metastases from malignant melanoma.

Histology

The distinction between melanoma and atypical nevus is the most difficult one in dermatopathology. Some of the features favoring melanoma are:
▶ More single melanocytes than nests at the dermoepidermal junction.
▶ Atypical melanocytes at all levels of the epidermis.
▶ Atypical melanocytes in dermis.
▶ Mitoses, especially abnormal mitoses, in all levels of tumor; most worrisome at base.
▶ Lack of maturation of melanocytes in deeper levels.
▶ Asymmetry because of overall pattern, as well as variations in cell size, color and nature of infiltrate.
▶ **Immunohistochemistry:** No one specific melanoma marker. S100 has highest sensitivity but identifies melanocytes of all types and many other cell lines. HMB-45 and Melan A/Mart 1 are more specific (>90%) for malignant melanoma. Proliferation markers such as Ki-67/MIB 1 also useful.

Diagnostic Approach

▸ Clinical examination, dermatoscopy, and photo-documentation.

▸ Employ the ABCDE rules (see p. 389) to identify suspicious nevi and early malignant melanomas.

▸ Pruritus, bleeding, and ulceration are worrisome signs in nevi, but usually occur too late in the evolution of a melanoma to be of much help in improving outlook.

▸ Perform excisional biopsy if any suspicion of malignant melanoma exists; incisional biopsies should be reserved for rare cases of LMM that are too large for excision.

▸ As diagnostic certainty increases, more and more often the tentative diagnosis of malignant melanoma is made and the lesion excised with appropriate margins, avoiding a re-excision. Ultrasonography with a 20–50 MHz head can be used for preoperative assessment of tumor thickness but plays no role in diagnosing malignant melanoma.

Dermatoscopy

The principles of dermatoscopy are discussed in Chapter 2, but expanded here. Dermatoscopic examination usually make it possible to rapidly separate melanocytic lesions from other pigmented tumors such as pigmented basal cell carcinoma, dermatofibroma, seborrheic keratosis, and vascular tumors. It is also the most useful way to distinguish between benign and malignant melanocytic tumors, and certainly the most reliable way to monitor atypical pigmented lesions for changes over time, using computer-assisted photodocumentation and analysis.

The clinical criteria used for identifying melanoma, such as symmetry, border, and color, are partly transferable to a dermatoscopic examination (Tables 23.**1**, 23.**2**), but the dermatoscopy criteria are much more detailed and specific, so considerable experience and training is required (Figs. 23.**13–16**).

Differential Diagnosis

▸ The greatest clinical difficulties are provided by melanocytic lesions, especially dysplastic nevus, pigmented spindle cell nevus, Spitz nevus, blue nevus.

▸ Nonmelanocytic lesions may also be troublesome; they include pigmented actinic keratosis, pigmented basal cell carcinoma, irrigated seborrheic keratosis, pyogenic granuloma, thrombosed hemangioma, angiokeratoma, dermatofibroma.

Staging

▸ Once the diagnosis of malignant melanoma has been established, the following procedures are routinely employed for lesions > 1.00 mm in thickness and can be employed in selected cases for thinner lesions:

• Routine laboratory evaluation.

• Chest radiograph.

• Sonography of regional lymph nodes, abdomen, pelvis, and retroperitoneum.

• Sentinel lymph node biopsy.

• In higher risk patients (stage IIB and higher), imaging studies (CT, MRI, PET) and tumor marker levels may be helpful.

▸ **Prognostic parameters:** The most important prognostic parameters are obtained from the histological interpretation of the excisional biopsy (T). The tumor thickness according to Breslow is reproducible and of prognostic significance, as is the presence or absence of ulceration. The Clark level is only rarely independently use-

Table 23.1 · Dermatoscopic criteria for melanoma

Pigment network

Irregular	Irregular meshwork, with tumor progression—loss of network
Thickened trabeculae	Parts of the network become thickened

Other criteria

Branched streaks	At the border of the lesion, the meshwork falls apart, leaving thickened dark brown-black remnant Histological equivalent: confluent pigmented melanocytic nests
Radial streaks and pseudopods	Further continuation of process with pigmented streaks extending into normal skin as residua of irregular pigment network. When thickened distally, known as pseudopods Histological equivalent: irregular pigmented nests at junction in periphery ⚠ *Caution:* When radial streaks and pseudopods form a star burst pattern around tumor, diagnosis is usually pigmented spindle cell tumor (Reed tumor).
Black dots	Very dark, round-oval structures about 0.1 mm in diameter, mainly in periphery Histological equivalent: melanocytes or melanin in the stratum corneum
Veil	White veil-like areas over a dark background Histological equivalent: orthokeratosis or hyperkeratosis
Gray-blue areas	Gray-blue to gray-black areas are typically areas of regression in a melanoma Histological equivalent: areas of regression with melanophages in papillary dermis

Table 23.2 · Dermatoscopic risk estimation for melanocytic tumors (after Kenet and Fitzpatrick)

Risk group	Dermatoscopic criteria
Low risk	Regular pigment network, with no other melanoma criteria
Medium risk	Irregular pigment network, more prominent at periphery, with no other melanoma criteria
High risk	Irregular pigment network with other criteria (branched streaks, radial streaks, pseudopods, black dots, veil, and gray-blue areas)

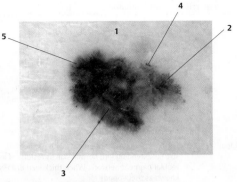

Fig. 23.**13** · **Dermatoscopy of malignant melanoma. 1** Asymmetry in all axes. **2** Atypical network. **3** Blue-white veil. **4** Irregular dots. **5** Irregular streaks at periphery (Image courtesy of Prof. Dr. Helmut Kerl MD, Graz, Austria.)

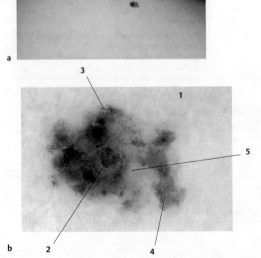

Fig. 23.**14** · **Malignant melanoma. a** Lesion on back. **b** Dermatoscopy of malignant melanoma shown in **a**: **1** Asymmetry in all axes. **2** Blue-white structures. **3** Irregular streaks. **4** Atypical network. **5** Dotted vessels. (Images courtesy of Prof. Dr. Helmut Kerl MD, Graz, Austria.)

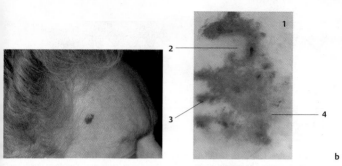

Fig. 23.**15** · **Malignant melanoma. a** Lesion on temple. **b** Dermatoscopy of malignant melanoma shown in a: **1** Asymmetry in all axes. **2** White structures. **3** Asymmetrically pigmented follicles. **4** Annular granular structures. (Images courtesy of Prof. Dr. Helmut Kerl MD, Graz, Austria.)

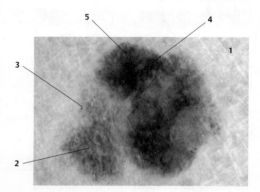

Fig. 23.**16** · **Dermatoscopy of malignant melanoma**. **1** Asymmetry in all axes. **2** Blue-white veil. **3** Irregular dots and globules. **4** Irregular blotches. **5** Irregular streaks. (Image courtesy of Prof. Dr. Helmut Kerl MD, Graz, Austria.)

ful, such as in selected body sites for tumors < 1.00 mm in thickness (Figs. 23.**17**, 23.**18**).

▶ When evaluating lymph nodes, the number of positive nodes and the degree of involvement (clinically apparent vs. clinically occult) are significant, as well as the presence of ulceration in primary tumor (N). In considering metastases (M), visceral metastases have a worse prognosis than cutaneous. See Tables 23.**3** and 23.**4**..

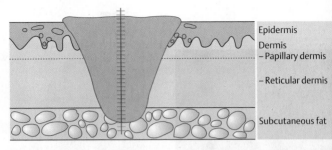

Fig. 23.**17** · Measuring the thickness of a tumor with an ocular micrometer to determine the Breslow depth. The measurement is taken from the stratum granulosum to the deepest point; melanoma cells extending along hair follicles are not measured.

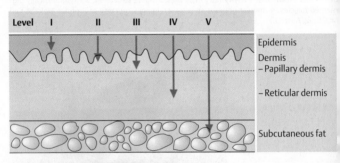

Fig. 23.**18** · Clark levels of malignant melanoma.

Table 23.3 · **TNM classification of malignant melanoma**		
Primary tumor (T)		
T1	≤1.00 mm	a) without / b) with—ulceration or Clark level IV/V
T2	1.01–2.00 mm	a) without / b) with—ulceration
T3	2.01–4.00 mm	a) without / b) with—ulceration
T4	>4.00 mm	a) without / b) with—ulceration
Lymph nodes (N)		
N1a	Involvement of 1 LN with micrometastasis	
N1b	Involvement of 1 LN with macrometastasis	
N2a	Involvement of 2–3 LN with micrometastasis	
N2b	Involvement of 2–3 LN with macrometastasis	
N2c	Satellite or in-transit metastases without LN involvement	
N3	4 or more involved LN or satellite or in-transit metastases with LN involvement, or ulcerated primary tumor with LN involvement	

Table 23.3 · Continued

mph nodes (N)	
Micrometastasis	LN involvement detected with histologic examination, such as after sentinel LN dissection
Macrometastasis	Clinically palpable LN involvement or identified during surgical procedure

Distant metastases	
M1	Distant metastases in skin, LN, or subcutaneous fat with normal LDH
M2	Pulmonary metastases with normal LDH
M3	All other metastases, or any metastases with elevated LDH

LN = lymph node.
Based on American Joint Committee on Cancer (AJCC) criteria, 2002.

Table 23.4 · Staging of malignant melanoma with pathologic criteria

Stage	T	N	M	Criteria
	Tis	N0	M0	Tis in situ melanoma
A	T1a	N0	M0	T = 1.00 mm without ulceration
B	T1b	N0	M0	T = 1.00 mm with ulceration or Clark level IV–V
	T2a	N0	M0	T 1.01–2.00 mm without ulceration
A	T2b	N0	M0	T 1.01–2.00 mm with ulceration
	T3a	N0	M0	T 2.01–4.00 mm without ulceration
B	T3b	N0	M0	T 2.01–4.00 mm with ulceration
	T4a	N0	M0	T > 4.00 mm without ulceration
C	T4b	N0	M0	T > 4.00 mm with ulceration
IA	T1–4a	N1a	M0	All T1–4a and 1 LN with micrometastasis
	T1–4a	N2a	M0	All T1–4a and 2–3 LN with micrometastasis
IB	T1–4a	N1b	M0	All T1–4a and 1 LN with macrometastasis
	T1–4a	N2b	M0	All T1–4a and 2–3 LN with macrometastasis
	T1–4b	N1a	M0	All T1–4b (with ulceration) and 1 LN with micrometastasis
	T1–4b	N2a	M0	All T1–4b (with ulceration) and 2–3 LN with micrometastasis
	T1–4a/b	N2c	M0	All T ± ulceration and in-transit or satellite metastases without LN involvement

Continued ▶

Table 23.4 · Continued				
Stage	T	N	M	Criteria
IIIC	T1–4b	N1b	M0	All T1–4b (with ulceration) and 1 LN with macro-metastasis
	T1–4b	N2b	M0	All T1–4b (with ulceration) and 2–3 LN with macro-metastasis
	Any T	N3	M0	Any T with 4 or more LN with macrometastasis or any T with ulceration and macroscopic or in-transit metastases
IV	Any T	Any N	M1	Distant metastases

LN = lymph node.
Based on American Joint Committee on Cancer (AJCC) criteria, 2002.

Sentinel Lymph Node Biopsy

► Procedure recommended for tumors > 1 mm thickness.
► Sentinel lymph node is the first node in the regional drainage basin.
► Radioactive colloid injected about tumor with lymph node scintigraphy; then after period of time (4–24 hours), patent blue dye injected about tumor; scintigraph and visual inspection for blue dye used to identify sentinel node (or nodes).
► Histologic status of sentinel lymph is of great prognostic importance; regardless c tumor thickness:
  • Negative SLN → 85% 5-year survival.
  • Positive SLN → 30% 5-year survival.
  • If SLN biopsy is positive, regional lymph node dissection is carried out.
☐ *Note:* SLN biopsy is still a staging procedure; many studies are in progress to deter mine if it contributes to an improved survival..

Therapy

Malignant Melanoma

► Curable when recognized early and excised. When lymph node involvement c distant metastases occur, the prognosis is grave, although new therapeutic ad vances have increased the survival time for patients in this group.
► **Primary tumor:**
  • Excision is treatment of choice.
  • Margin of safety:
    – Tumors ≤ 1 mm thickness → 1 cm excision margin.
    – Tumors > 1 mm thickness → 2 cm excision margin.
► Melanomas on the face or in acral or anogenital sites may be excised using micro scopic control of margins.
► **Adjuvant therapy:**
  • There is no proven increased survival for patients with any category of malig nant melanoma following adjuvant chemotherapy, radiation therapy, or hyper thermic limb perfusion with chemotherapy agents.
  • All patients with high-risk melanomas (stage IIB or higher) should be offere adjuvant immunotherapy as part of a clinical study. The most promising agen is interferon-α_2, but the most effective regimen has yet to be determined.

Metastatic Malignant Melanoma

▶ Dismal outlook, with 6–9 months mean survival time.

▶ In-transit or satellite metastases should be surgically removed as far as possible. If multiple inoperable metastases are confined to a limb, hyperthermic perfusion with chemotherapy agents (for example with melphalan and TNF α) achieves a high remission rate (80%) but is fraught with complications and does not prolong life. Other possibilities include cryotherapy, laser ablation, topical immunotherapy.

▶ If LN metastases are identified, radical LN dissection is required. Adjuvant immunotherapy should be offered.

▶ **Radiation therapy** is the treatment of choice for bone and brain metastases. Isolated inoperable brain metastases ($< 3–5$) should be irradiated individually with sterotactic convergence radiation. In addition, fotemustine $100 \, mg/m^2$ i. v. can be added. Dexamethasone should also be administered to reduce brain edema.

▶ If there are multiple brain metastases, then whole brain irradiation can combined with chemotherapy including fotemustine $100 \, mg/m^2$ i. v. on days 1, 8, and 15; then 5 week pause, combined with temozolomide $150–200 \, mg/m^2$ orally every 4 weeks. Both agents cross the blood–brain barrier well.

▶ **Distant metastases:**
- Dacarbazine (DTIC) $800 \, mg/m^2$ i. v. every 4 weeks until progression occurs is the standard approved monotherapy, with about 20% response rate.
- Polychemotherapy (many different regimens available) offers slightly higher response rates (20–30%) but with considerably more side effects.
- High-dose interleukin (IL)-2 is a potential first line therapy in patients in good general health (high Karnofsky score).
- Combined chemo- and immunotherapy (for example, DTIC, cisplatin, interferon-α and IL-2) achieves response rates as high as 50%. In individual cases, complete, long-lasting remissions are achieved. Such treatment should only be offered as part of a clinical study; with more than 1500 patients already treated, analysis shows a clear advantage over chemotherapy alone.
- Solitary brain, liver, and lung metastases can be removed by surgery; 5-year survival up to 20% if truly only one metastasis.
- Histamine increases the effect of IL-2 on liver metastases.

▶ **Experimental therapy:** Because of the dismal outlook for metastasis malignant melanoma, many experimental therapies are in development. Dendritic cell vaccination and gene therapy protocols are available, as well as administration of tumor-infiltrating lymphocytes and lymphokine-activated killer cells. All such approaches must be offered as part of clinical studies.

▶ **Follow-up:**
- Clinical evaluation should be carried out every 3–6 months for 10 years, depending on the stage of the primary tumor. The current German guidelines are shown in Table 23.**5**.
- ☒ *Note:* Dermatologic evaluation must be part of all malignant melanoma follow-up, because patients with malignant melanoma have an increased risk of developing a second melanoma.

▶ **Early diagnosis of LN metastases:** Routine sonography (7.5–14 MHz) of in-transit area and regional nodes, coupled with fine needle aspiration, improves sensitivity.

▶ **Tumor markers:** S100, tyrosinase, and MIA all have been proposed as markers for recurrent disease. They may be better for following response to therapy than for discovering early metastases. In addition, false-positive results cause considerable anxiety and expense.

Table 23.5 · Follow-up of patients with malignant melanoma

Stage	Thickness	Clinical examination		LN sono-graphy	Laboratory	Other imaging
		Years 1–5	Years 6–10			
I	<1 mm	q. 6 mo.	q. 12 mo.	–	–	–
I + II	>1 mm	q. 3 mo.	q. 6 mo.	q. 6 mo.	q. 6 mo.	–
III[a]		q. 3 mo.	q. 6 mo.	q. 3–6 mo.	q. 3–6 mo.	q. 6 mo.
IV[b]		prn	prn	prn	prn	prn

LN = lymph node.
a Frequency can be reduced after 3 years.
b All investigations for stage IV patients must be individualized.

▶ **Oncologic terminology:** The terms oncologists use to describe responses to therapy are often not known to patients and physicians. Some of the most common terms are shown in Table 23.**6**.

Table 23.6 · Oncologic terms for therapeutic responses

Complete remission (CR)	Disappearance of all signs of tumor for 4 weeks
Partial remission (PR)	Tumor reduction >50% for 4 weeks
No change (NC) or stable disease	Tumor reduction <50% or tumor progression <25% or no change in parameters
Duration of remission	Period of time between achieving remission and recurrence of tumor
Total survival	Period of time between onset or therapy and death of patient
Recurrence-free survival	Period of time between tumor-free status and recurrence

24 Cysts and Epidermal Tumors

24.1 Cysts

Epidermoid Cyst

▸ **Synonyms:** Infundibular cyst, epidermal inclusion cyst, sebaceous cyst (common term, but completely incorrect).

▸ **Definition:** Cyst whose wall consists of stratified epithelium with stratum corneum.

▸ **Pathogenesis:** Most arise from the infundibulum, the upper part of the hair follicle above the site of entry of the sebaceous duct. Some are true inclusion cysts following trauma, usually to palms or soles, where a fragment of epidermis is embedded in dermis; others follow severe acne.

▸ **Clinical features:** Slowly growing, skin-colored, firm cystic structures, usually with visible central pore, ranging in size from 0.5 to 5.0 cm (Fig. 24.1). Most commonly on face or trunk. Two clinical variants include:
  - *Scrotal cysts:* Multiple epidermal cysts on scrotum, often calcified.
  - *Gardner syndrome* (p. 368): May present with multiple epidermoid cysts in childhood.

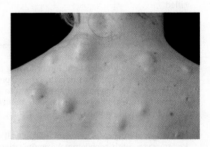

Fig. 24.1 · Multiple epidermoid cysts.

▸ **Histology:** Cyst wall resembles normal epidermis with granular layer, inner layers thinner than basal layer, and stratum corneum; cyst contents are keratin arranged in layers. If cyst ruptures, keratin induces foreign body reaction with giant cells containing slivers of keratin (*cornflakes sign*).

▸ **Differential diagnosis:** Trichilemmal cyst.

▸ **Therapy:** Simple excision or extraction where small incision is made with scalpel or punch and then cyst contents extruded and cyst wall removed with curved forceps.

  ☐ *Note:* If the cyst wall is not completely removed, recurrences are more likely.

Milia

▸ **Definition:** Tiny variant of epidermoid cyst.

▸ *Pathogenesis:* Milia may be primary or secondary:
  - *Primary milia:* Tiny retention cysts of vellus hair follicle or rarely eccrine glands. Occasionally multiple and grouped: *plaque-like milia.*

- *Secondary milia:* Develop following trauma (dermabrasion) or subepiderma blistering diseases (bullous pemphigoid, porphyria cutanea tarda, junction and dystrophic epidermolysis bullosa), presumably from small fragments c epithelium landing in dermis.
► **Clinical features:** 1–2 mm dome-shaped white-yellow papules, favoring fac (cheeks, temples, periorbital).
► **Histology:** Exactly like epidermoid cyst; just smaller, except in rare cases of ec crine milia when sweat gland remnants can be seen.
► **Differential diagnosis:** Plane warts, xanthomas, syringomas.
► **Therapy:** Incision and expression of contents; laser ablation.

Trichilemmal Cyst

► **Synonyms:** Pilar cyst, isthmus-catagen cyst, wen.
► **Definition:** Cyst arises deeper in hair follicle with wall showing keratinizatio pattern without flattening of cells or granular layer.
► **Pathogenesis:** Often familial tendency; suggestion of autosomal dominant inher itance.
► **Clinical features:** Most lesions are on scalp (90%); rest on face, neck, upper trun 70% multiple; 30% solitary. Firmer than epidermoid cyst, no central pore; conten compact keratin with cheesy nature and smell.
► **Histology:** Keratinocytes in cyst wall show no tendency to flattening; abrup transition to homogenous glassy keratin (trichilemmal keratinization). Often ca cified.
► **Therapy:** See epidermoid cyst.

Proliferating Trichilemmal Cyst

► **Synonym:** Proliferating pilar tumor.
► **Definition:** Poorly understood tumor arising in connection with trichilemma cysts. Some view tumor as benign; others consider it an extremely low-grad squamous cell carcinoma growing initially into a cyst cavity.
► **Clinical features:** Slow-growing nodule, sometimes eroded or ulcerated. Mor common in elderly women. Sometimes accompanied by other banal trichilemma cysts. Can reach monstrous size.
► **Histology:** In early cases, remnants of cyst wall with atypical nests and strands c keratinocytes with trichilemmal keratinization extending into or toward cys lumen. Later obliteration of cystic structure and appearance of squamous cell car cinoma.
► **Differential diagnosis:** Squamous cell carcinoma, pilomatrical carcinoma, basa cell carcinoma, malignant cylindroma.
► **Therapy:** Excision; follow-up as squamous cell carcinoma.

Dermoid Cyst

► **Definition:** Embryologic epidermal cyst containing adnexal structures; no rela tion to the benign ovarian teratoma known by the same name.
► **Pathogenesis:** Result of abnormal embryonic fusion, usually in midventral loca tions, leading to entrapment of epidermis in dermis.
► **Clinical features:** Midline cyst 1–4 cm present at birth; most common site is be tween eyes.
► **Histology:** Cyst wall shows normal epidermis with hairs, sweat glands, and rarel bone or even teeth.

- **Differential diagnosis:** Epidermoid or trichilemmal cyst; in newborn, ectopic neural tissue, vascular tumors.
- **⚠ Caution:** Before surgery, consult an expert and carry out imaging studies on all suspected dermoid cysts to exclude ectopic neural tissue (nasal glioma, meningioma).
- **Therapy:** Excision.

Steatocystoma

- **Synonym:** True sebaceous cyst.
- **Definition:** Epithelial cyst whose wall contains small sebaceous glands.
- **Pathogenesis:** Multiple lesions may be inherited in autosomal dominant manner.
- **Clinical features:** Three clinical settings:
  - *Steatocystoma simplex:* Solitary often flaccid cyst, clinically identical to epidermoid cyst.
  - *Steatocystoma multiplex:* Multiple flaccid yellow cysts appearing usually at puberty favoring anterior chest, neck, axillae, genitalia.
  - *Oldfield syndrome:* Rarely steatocystoma are associated with intestinal polyposis, analogous to Gardner syndrome (p. 368); relationship controversial.
- **Histology:** Cyst wall usually collapsed and crenulated (notched) with tiny sebaceous glands.
- **Differential diagnosis:** *Eruptive vellus hair cysts* appear very similar, are usually somewhat smaller and more papular; they contain numerous vellus hairs as well as sebaceous glands. Some feel two conditions are part of a spectrum. *Keratocysts* are usually part of nevoid basal cell carcinoma syndrome (p. 435), but can also be sporadic. Identical to steatocystoma with crenulated cyst wall, but no sebaceous glands found.
- **Therapy:** Excision or laser ablation; systemic isotretinoin produces improvement in multiple lesions, usually short-lived when therapy is discontinued.

Ganglion

- **Synonym:** Digital mucous cyst (for special variant).
- **Definition:** Benign cyst arising from joint capsule or tendon, consisting of fibrous capsule containing mucinous material.
- **Pathogenesis:** Ganglion cysts can be viewed as herniations of synovial tissue.
- **Clinical features:** A true ganglion cyst is a soft tissue lesion occurring most commonly about the wrist. The ganglion variant familiar to dermatologists is the *digital mucous cyst*, a shimmering blue cystic structure almost always at the proximal border of a finger or toe nail. The associated nail is often distorted.
- **Histology:** A ganglion is a true cyst. The digital mucous cyst is a pseudocyst, as the mucinous joint fluid is surrounded by granulomatous response, not a cyst wall.
- **Diagnostic approach:** Larger cysts can be transilluminated. Digital cysts can be punctured; a clear gelatinous material oozes out.
- **Differential diagnosis:** The larger cysts over joints may be confused with lipomas, neuromas, chondromas, and exostoses. The digital lesion is clinically distinctive.
- **Therapy:** Ganglion cysts are usually removed by orthopedic or hand surgeons. The connection to a joint space is established with dye injection and then the connection tied off. The same procedure is often necessary for the digital mucous cyst, as other approaches such as drainage, intralesional corticosteroids, and superficial ablation often produce only short-term improvement.

Mucocele

Oral pseudocyst; results from bite or other trauma interrupting minor salivary gland duct with extravasation of mucinous material and histiocytic reaction. Presents a glistening dome-shaped nodule, usually as site of bite trauma. On histology, no cyst wall. Easily excised or otherwise destroyed. A *sialolith* or salivary duct stone may temporarily block off a duct, causing a mucocele-like swelling that resolves spontaneously as the obstruction clears.

24.2 Epidermal and Organoid Nevi

Epidermal Nevus

▶ **Synonym:** Verrucous nevus, nevus verrucosus.
▶ **Definition:** Focal area of abnormal epidermal development following Blaschko lines and having a variety of histologic patterns, sometimes associated with systemic abnormalities (*epidermal nevus syndrome*).
▶ **Pathogenesis:** There is considerable overlap between epidermal and organoid nevi, so both are considered together. A true epidermal nevus has an abnormal pattern of keratinization. Any mutation that can cause diffuse disturbances in keratinization (epidermolytic hyperkeratosis, Darier disease) or isolated lesions (porokeratosis) can also present as an epidermal nevus, the result of somatic mosaicism occurring early in embryonic life. Organoid nevi feature both epidermal and adnexal structures.
▶ **Clinical features:** An epidermal nevus is always present at birth, but sometimes not recognized as it may be flat, perhaps slightly pigmented, and only later become hyperkeratotic (Fig. 24.2). Soft and hard epidermal nevi can be distinguished; the former is papillomatous, similar to a skin tag or fleshy melanocytic nevus, while the latter is warty. Both may range in color from pale tan to dark brown. Most typical locations are face, neck, upper trunk.
▶ **Histology:** Typically, papillomatosis and varying degrees of hyperkeratosis.
▶ **Diagnostic approach:** History (present at birth), clinical examination; biopsy for confirmation.

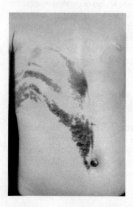

Fig. 24.**2** · Epidermal nevus.

- **Differential diagnosis:** Other epidermal nevi, other linear lesions. In the absence of history, a large seborrheic keratosis cannot be separated with certainty from a small epidermal nevus.
- **Therapy:** Excision (often serial excisions if large); dermabrasion, cryosurgery, and laser ablation may be successful for more superficial lesions.

ILVEN

- **Synonym:** ILVEN is an acronym for **i**nflammatory **l**inear **v**errucous **e**pidermal nevus.
- **MIM code:** 163200.
- **Epidemiology:** Women more often affected.
- **Pathogenesis:** ILVEN is exceptional in that it appears later in life. The suggestion is that there is a mutation in mosaic pattern, which predisposes certain areas of the skin to develop a dermatitic response.
- **Clinical features:**
  - Linear psoriasiform or dermatitic streaks, usually on extremities.
  - Appears later in life; not visible at birth.
  - ILVEN syndrome possible, association with other developmental anomalies.
- **Histology:** Without a history, easily mistaken for psoriasis or psoriasiform dermatitis with acanthosis, hyperkeratosis, and a dermal inflammatory cell infiltrate with exocytosis.
- **Differential diagnosis:** Other linear lesions especially lichen striatus.
- **Therapy:** Excision; treatment with antipsoriatic measures such as vitamin D analogues sometimes helpful.

Acantholytic Dyskeratotic Nevus

- **Synonym:** Segmental Darier disease, segmental Hailey–Hailey disease.
- **Pathogenesis:** Mosaic with mutation in *ATP2A2* gene (responsible for Darier disease) or *ATP2C1* gene (responsible for Hailey–Hailey disease). Described as type I mutation by Happle, as abnormal skin arises on background of normal skin. A type II segmental Darier disease, for example, occurs when a patient with Darier disease experiences loss of their normal allele in a mosaic pattern and develops even more severe skin disease in this location.
- **Clinical features:** Cannot be clinically separated from other epidermal nevi.
- **Therapy:** Excision when possible; otherwise, retinoids sometimes help, as they do for the systemic disorder.

Nevus sebaceus

- **Synonym:** Organoid nevus, Jadassohn nevus.
- **Definition:** Prototype of organoid nevus with increase in all epithelial components, especially the sebaceous glands.
- **Pathogenesis:** Once again, somatic mosaic with lesion following Blaschko lines.
- **Clinical features:** Nevus sebaceus is one of the few epidermal nevi that is clinically distinct (Fig. 24.**3**):
  - At birth, hairless yellow-orange plaque usually on scalp or temple.
  - At puberty, becomes thicker, nodular or verrucous.
  - Variety of tumors develop within nevus:
    - Trichoblastoma is most common.
    - Syringocystadenoma papilliferum also typical.
    - Basal cell carcinoma can occur, but extremely rare.

Cysts and Epidermal Tumors

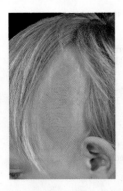

Fig. 24.**3** · Nevus sebaceus.

▶ **Histology:** Biopsies taken before puberty are relatively nondistinct, showin small sebaceous glands and sometimes abundant eccrine glands. When thickened lesion is biopsied, then numerous sebaceous, eccrine, and apocrin glands, as well as abortive hairs, are seen beneath a papillomatous epidermis.

▶ **Diagnostic approach:** History, clinical examination; biopsy only needed if lesio is changing.

▶ **Differential diagnosis:** Other epidermal nevi, especially if not on scalp.

▶ **Therapy:** Excision.

Becker Nevus

▶ **Synonym:** Melanosis neviformis Becker.

▶ **Definition:** Type of organoid nevus with hyperpigmentation, increased hairs, an often increased smooth muscles.

▶ **Epidemiology:** Relatively common malformation.

▶ **Pathogenesis:** Type of organoid nevus involved hairs and smooth muscle marked increase in androgen receptors explains flare at puberty. More easily rec ognized in men because of response to androgens. No increase in melanocytes.

▶ **Clinical features:**

• Large patch or plaque; present at birth, but usually ignored. First sign is hyper pigmentation, but most dramatic change is growth of hairs during pubert (Fig. 24.**4**). Usually on trunk.

• Hairs may become erect with rubbing if there is an associated *smooth musc hamartoma* at base.

• Area is hormonally sensitive; sometimes acne occurs, confined to nevus.

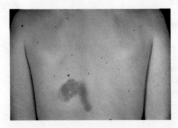

Fig. 24.**4** · Becker nevus.

- *Becker nevus syndrome:* Combination of one or more Becker nevi with ipsilateral breast hypoplasia, skeletal anomalies (ipsilateral shoulder girdle or arm hypoplasia, scoliosis, vertebral anomalies) and other cutaneous malformations.
- **Histology:** Increased basal layer melanin, normal number of melanocytes. Thick mature but normal hairs. In many cases, proliferation of arrector pili (smooth muscle).
- **Differential diagnosis:** Usually misdiagnosed as some form of melanocytic nevus; other possibilities include café-au-lait macule (early), nevus spilus, atypical dermal melanosis.
- **Therapy:** None needed; generally too large for excision.

Other Epidermal and Organoid Nevi

- **Hair follicle nevus:** Area of hypertrichosis with multiple hairs, often in immature stages and in peculiar groupings. When an accessory tragus (cartilaginous rest anterior to ear) is sectioned tangentially, it is often misinterpreted as hair follicle nevus.
- **Angora hair nevus:** Similar to hair follicle nevus, but with long hypopigmented hairs; not described as solitary finding but just in angora hair nevus syndrome.
- **Apocrine nevus:** Similar to nevus sebaceous but contains only excess apocrine glands.
- **Eccrine nevus:** Similar to nevus sebaceous but contains only excess eccrine glands.
- **Eccrine angiomatous hamartoma:** Linear lesion usually on legs, patients complain of localized hyperhidrosis; on biopsy, increased eccrine glands and small vessels.
- **Porokeratotic eccrine nevus:** Clinically multiple spines and plugs, which histologically show a parakeratotic column filling the eccrine duct ostia.
- **Nevus comedonicus:** Lesion with thick comedone-like epidermal invaginations but without inflammatory lesions of acne.
- **Munro nevus:** Local area of acne; contains same mutation in FGFR2 (fibroblast growth factor receptor) as in Apert syndrome (craniosynostosis, skeletal defects, and severe acne often involving extremities).

Epidermal Nevus Syndromes

The epidermal nevus syndromes feature some of the above mentioned nevi, in association with skeletal, neurological, and other developmental defects. They reflect somatic mosaicism, with mutation presumably occurring at an earlier embryonic stage leading to involvement of multiple systems.

Schimmelpenning–Feuerstein–Mims Syndrome

- **Synonym:** Nevus sebaceus syndrome.
- **MIM code:** 163200.
- **Definition:** Prototype of epidermal nevus syndrome with generalized nevus sebaceus and multiple anomalies.
- **Clinical features:**
  - Multiple nevus sebaceus, favoring scalp, but widespread, usually unilateral.
  - Pigmentary changes including café-au-lait macules and lentigines.
  - Ocular, cardiac, and skeletal anomalies; epilepsy; growth retardation.
- **Diagnostic approach:** Multidisciplinary diagnosis; skin biopsy may help confirm.
- **Differential diagnosis:** Proteus syndrome, other epidermal nevus syndromes.
- **Therapy:** Symptomatic depending on manifestations; nevus sebaceus can be excised.

Proteus Syndrome

▶ **MIM code:** 176920.
▶ **Definition:** Complex malformation syndrome; Proteus was a Greek god who could assume many different appearances.
▶ **Pathogenesis:** Lethal mutation that is viable only in the mosaic state. Still controversy over which gene is involved.
▶ **Clinical features:**
• Ordinary epidermal nevi, but often extensive.
• Large connective tissue nevi (p. 438), typically involving hands and feet.
• Areas of hypoplasia of dermis or fat.
• Vascular malformations and lipomas.
• Disproportionate overgrowth of bone and soft tissue producing misshapen hands and feet.
• Many other abnormalities, involving almost every organ system.
  ▣ *Note:* Joseph Merrick, the "Elephant Man," had Proteus syndrome, not neurofibromatosis.
▶ **Differential diagnosis:** A full-blown case is easy to diagnose; when only a few features are present, may be confused with vascular malformation syndromes.
▶ **Therapy:** Symptomatic; some problems amenable to surgical correction.

CHILD Syndrome

▶ **Mim code:** 308050.
▶ **Definition:** **C**ongenital **h**emidysplasia with **i**chthyosiform nevus and **l**imb **d**efects.
▶ **Pathogenesis:** Defect in *NHDSL* gene involved in sterol synthesis; located at X28. X-linked dominant inheritance, so only women are affected.
▶ **Clinical features:** Rare epidermal nevus syndrome with striking ichthyosiform or psoriasiform epidermal nevi which strikingly represent the midline, usually associated with ipsilateral skeletal defects. Favor body folds (*ptychotropism*). May wax and wane, so that some formerly considered the CHILD nevus a type of ichthyosis. Ipsilateral skeletal defects, as well as a variety of other systemic problems.
▶ **Histology:** Often very reminiscent of psoriasis; dermal papillae may contain foamy cells (*verruciform xanthoma*, p. 315).
▶ **Therapy:** Cutaneous lesions may improve with antipsoriatic therapy, such as vitamin D analogues.

Other Epidermal Nevus Syndromes

Systemic involvement has also been reported with Becker nevus, phacomatosis pigmentokeratotica (nevus spilus and nevus sebaceus), and angora hair nevus.

24.3 Benign Epidermal Tumors

Seborrheic Keratosis
....

▶ **Synonym:** Verruca seborrhoeica.
▶ **Definition:** Common verrucous pigmented tumor, usually after 40 years of age.
▶ **Epidemiology:** Very common; almost every 60-year-old has at least one seborrheic keratosis.
▶ **Pathogenesis:** Unknown; despite histologic similarities, not caused by human papillomavirus.

▶ **Clinical features (Fig. 24.5):**

- *Flat type:* Smooth flat waxy plaques 0.5 to several cm on trunk; vary from tan to dark brown, sometimes with visible punctate inclusions *(horn pseudocysts)*.
- *Acanthotic type:* Elevated dome-shaped, usually smooth, often heavily pigmented *(melanoacanthoma)* nodule with inclusions.
- *Verrucous type:* Paler 0.5–1.5 cm tumor with warty surface but without the punctate papillary hemorrhage so typical of viral warts.
- *Stalked type:* Pedunculated tags with surface changes of seborrheic keratosis, often in flexures or periorbital.
- *Irritated seborrheic keratosis:* Inflamed or irritated keratosis, secondary to trauma, irritation, or infection; tend to be smoother and less pigmented, so difficult to recognize.
- *Stucco keratoses:* Pale, small keratoses typical on shins and back of feet, but occasionally on forearms and hands. Usually mistaken for warts.
- *Dermatosis papulosa nigra:* Heavily pigmented small papules on the cheeks of blacks; present in over 40% of individuals (who rarely have multiple seborrheic keratoses elsewhere). Not seen in whites.
- *Leser–Trélat sign:* Sudden appearance of multiple small seborrheic keratoses and skin tags in adult is a variant of acanthosis nigricans (p. 485) and should raise the possibility of an underlying malignancy. Extremely rare; in adults with multiple seborrheic keratoses there is no cause for concern about cancer without a history of sudden eruption.
- ▣ *Note:* Seborrheic keratoses grow in crops; very unusual to see a solitary lesion. If a lesion is atypical (very dark, inflamed), look for other, more normal variants in the area.

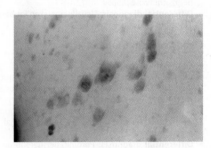

Fig. 24.5 · Multiple seborrheic keratoses.

▶ **Histology:** Unifying features are exophytic growth, acanthosis, and horn pseudocysts (epidermal invaginations filled with keratin). Degree of pigmentation varies. Some lesions very papillomatous with church spires (stucco keratosis, for example). Others show clonal proliferation of keratinocytes *(Borst–Jadassohn effect)*.

▶ **Diagnostic approach:** Clinical examination; if questions, dermatoscopy is helpful.

▶ **Differential diagnosis:** Usually no differential diagnosis; sometimes common warts; if smooth or ulcerated, basal cell carcinoma; if heavily pigmented, melanocytic tumors.

▶ **Therapy:** Curettage is simplest; cryotherapy, dermabrasion and laser ablation are alternatives. Cryotherapy should be avoided for dark-skinned patients, such as those with dermatosis papulosa nigra, as postinflammatory hyperpigmentation is common.

Solar Lentigo

► **Synonyms:** Senile lentigo, actinic lentigo, old-age spot, liver spot.
► **Definition:** Common acquired lesion in older adults; number of synonyms makes it clear that there is lack of agreement on its exact nature. We few it as flat seborrheic keratosis in sun-exposed skin.
► **Clinical features:** Usually multiple, tan or brown macules with irregular shape on sun-exposed areas, especially backs of hands. Often a cosmetic problem. *Ink spot lentigo* is a variant with fine lines of pigment in skin folds, as if a drop of ink had been spilled on skin.
► **Histology:** Flat seborrheic keratosis with increased basal layer pigment (*dirty feet*), but no striking increase in melanocytes and definitely no nests.
► **Diagnostic approach:** If not clear with clinical examination and dermatoscopy biopsy may be needed.
► **Differential diagnosis:** Pigmented actinic keratosis, Bowen disease, lentigo maligna melanoma in situ.
► **Therapy:** Cryotherapy, curettage, camouflage; laser ablation.

Lichenoid Keratosis

► **Clinical features:** Smooth erythematous papule or plaque, typically on décolletage, neck, or beneath breast.
► **Histology:** Dense lichenoid infiltrate at dermoepidermal junction; sometimes remnants of flat seborrheic keratosis or actinic keratosis.
► **Diagnostic approach:** Very difficult to diagnose clinically; dermatoscopy may help; otherwise biopsy.
► **Differential diagnosis:** Usually mistaken for basal cell carcinoma.
► **Therapy:** Excision.

Clear Cell Acanthoma

► **Synonym:** Degos tumor.
► **Clinical features:** Scaly plaque or nodule almost always on the shin of older individuals. Usually solitary, with no tendency to regress. No malignant potential.
► **Histology:** Numerous glycogen-rich keratinocytes give the epidermis a clear appearance and the tumor its name. Sharp transition from normal to clear epidermis Also acanthosis and sometimes intraepidermal neutrophils, so confusion with psoriasis possible.
► **Differential diagnosis:** Poroma, dermatofibroma and old wart are most likely considerations; an amelanotic malignant melanoma must be excluded. Diagnosis always microscopic; some eccrine tumors, such as hidroacanthoma simplex, look quite similar.
► **Therapy:** Excision.

Cysts and Epidermal Tumors

24.4 Carcinoma in situ

A carcinoma in situ is a neoplasm in which the tumor cells are confined to the epithelium of origin, without invasion of the basement membrane. If left untreated, progression to invasive carcinoma may occur.

Actinic Keratosis

▸ **Synonym:** Solar keratosis.
▸ **Definition:** UVB-induced carcinoma in situ.
▸ **Pathogenesis:** Mutations in a variety of genes including telomerase (delayed apoptosis, prolonged life) and TP53 (delayed apoptosis, accumulation of genetic damage).
▸ **Clinical features:**
  • 0.5–2.0 cm multiple sharply bordered irregular erythematous patches and papules with adherent scale, always in sun-exposed areas, more common in type I skin (Fig. 24.6).
  ◨ *Note:* It is often easier to palpate actinic keratoses as "rough spots" than to try and see them.

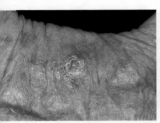 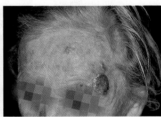

b

Fig. **24.6** · **a** Actinic keratosis. **b** With squamous cell carcinoma.

  • Early lesions (erythematous type) are 1–2 mm, with fine telangiectases only; the hykeratosis comes later.
  • Individual lesions may become irritated or inflamed (*lichenoid actinic keratosis*).
  • About 1% of actinic keratoses yearly are expected to change into invasive squamous cell carcinoma.
▸ **Histology:** Epidermis usually atrophic with hyperkeratotic scale, marked variation in size, and nuclear features of keratinocytes. Characteristic *pink and blue* as the hair follicles and eccrine ducts tend not to be involved so their keratin stains blue, while the intervening abnormal epidermis has pink, often parakeratotic keratin. Lichenoid actinic keratosis shows an intense dermoepidermal junction infiltrate. Bowenoid actinic keratosis shows more striking individual cell keratinization and atypia.
▸ **Diagnostic approach:** Strictly a clinical diagnosis; overdiagnosis results in an unneeded but harmless treatment; underdiagnosis is established at the regular follow-up all patients with actinic keratoses require.
▸ **Differential diagnosis:** In sun-exposed skin, few options. A flat pale seborrheic keratosis is identical clinically; hyperkeratotic lesions may be confused with warts.

▶ *Note:* Actinic keratosis is the most common lesion underlying cutaneous horn. Other possibilities include squamous cell carcinoma, wart and seborrheic keratosis, but almost any tumor can be present at the base. Histological diagnosis always needed.

► **Therapy:**
- Freezing with liquid nitrogen, ideally using a spray device and freezing for 5–10 seconds; you will soon acquire a feel for how long to freeze, depending on lesion thickness and location (more acrally and on scalp). In either case, lesions become necrotic and then peel or scab off.
- Curettage with electrodesiccation or cautery, requires local anesthetic.
- Excision, especially if thick, resistant to therapy or suspicious of squamous cell carcinoma.
- *For numerous lesions:*
  - Topical 5-fluorouracil cream b.i.d. for 10–14 days; lesions become inflamed and red, then crust and peel off. All residual lesions (survivors) must be otherwise treated. Can be combined with topical tretinoin.
  - Topical imiquimod 3× weekly for 6 weeks.
  - Several other topical products available in USA: hyaluronic acid, masoprocol.
  - Trichloracetic acid peels, usually > 30%, and dermabrasion are more aggressive approaches.
- *Photodynamic therapy:* Topical application of photosensitizing substance (usually methyl δ-aminolevulinic acid) followed by irradiation at a wavelength absorbed by agent. Can be used to identify and then to treat lesions that more readily absorb the photosensitizer.

Arsenic and Radiation Keratoses

These lesions arise in distinct clinical settings, tend to be more hyperkeratotic than actinic keratoses, and are generally more likely to progress to squamous cell carcinoma. They appear years after exposure to the carcinogen, but associated with arsenical melanosis or radiation dermatitis. Treatment is the same as for actinic keratosis.

Bowen Disease

► **Definition:** Squamous cell carcinoma in situ on the skin.
► **Pathogenesis:** Formerly most common triggers were radiation and arsenic; nowadays human papillomavirus (HPV) seems to be usual cause.
► **Clinical features:**
- *Bowen disease:* Typically 1–3 cm slightly raised patch, tan to red-brown with variable scale. Most often truncal but can be anywhere (Fig. 24.**7**).
- Over years, Bowen disease evolves into an invasive squamous cell carcinoma known as *Bowen carcinoma.*
- Lengthy debate over association of Bowen disease with internal malignancies, usually explained by linkage with past arsenic exposure.
► **Diagnostic approach:** Clinical examination, biopsy.
► **Differential diagnosis:**
- Often mistaken for patch of dermatitis. Other possibilities include tinea, psoriasis, warts, actinic keratosis, superficial basal cell carcinoma, extramammary Paget disease.
- Bowenoid papulosis (p. 71) is HPV-induced squamous cell carcinoma in situ of the genitalia; typically hyperpigmented; may undergo spontaneous regression.
► **Therapy:** Excision, curettage and electrodesiccation, laser ablation, or cryosurgery.

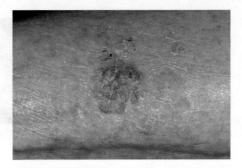

Fig. 24.**7** · Bowen disease.

Erythroplasia of Queyrat

▶ **Pathogenesis:** Exactly the same as Bowen disease, but confined to mucous membranes.
▶ **Clinical features:** Velvety red patch typically on penis, vulva, perianal area, or mouth. Speckled leukoplakia in mouth is the combination of erythroplasia with dyskeratotic areas. Speckled red and white speckled pattern.
▶ **Diagnostic approach:** Clinical examination, biopsy.
▶ **Differential diagnosis:** Zoon balanitis, other forms of balanitis, psoriasis, lichen planus, fixed drug eruption.
▶ **Therapy:** Excision, superficial destruction; topical 5-fluorouracil under occlusion can be used in hair-free areas when surgery is not desired.

24.5 Malignant Epidermal Tumors

Squamous Cell Carcinoma (SCC)

▶ **Definition:** Malignant epidermal tumor arising from keratinocytes, with potential for local spread and metastasis.
▶ **Epidemiology:** Incidence 100:100000 in men; 50:100000 in women; increasing in frequency yearly. All statistics are distorted by how many actinic keratoses (SCC in situ) are counted.
▶ **Pathogenesis:** The main factor is UVB exposure, but there are many other factors including HPV (certainly types 16 and 18; others also implicated include 31, 33, and 38), radiation therapy, arsenic exposure, chemical carcinogens (tar, pitch), and immunosuppression (iatrogenic, HIV/AIDS).
▶ **Clinical features:** Usually present as hyperkeratotic papule or plaque, often with crust or ulceration (Fig. 24.**8**). Difficult to separate from precursor lesions. Growth rate and risk of metastasis are highly variable (Table 24.**1**); outlook is best for lesions on skin arising from actinic keratoses; worst for lip, penis, and vulva SCC.
▶ **Histology:** Keratinocytes are in disarray, with marked variation in cell size and nuclear features. Individual cell keratinization. Degree of keratinization reflects degree of differentiation and is used in staging schemes for some tumors such as

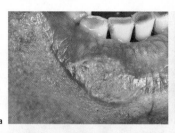
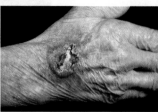

Fig. 24.**8** · **Squamous cell carcinoma. a** Early disease of lip. **b** Hand.

Table 24.1 · Risk of metastasis for squamous cell carcinoma	
Form	Risk of metastasis (%)
Cutaneous, from actinic keratosis	0.1
Cutaneous, from Bowen disease	2 – 10
Mucous, from erythroplasia	20 – 40

oral cavity SCC. Downward growth of atypical keratinocytes into dermis and development of islands of atypical cells free from epidermis are unequivocal signs of progression to SCC.

▶ **Diagnostic approach:** Clinical examination and biopsy.

   ◩ *Note:* Any actinic keratosis or other carcinoma in situ that is resistant to therapy or ulcerated should be suspected of being an SCC.

▶ **Differential diagnosis:** Keratoacanthoma, irritated seborrheic keratosis, basal cell carcinoma, warts, adnexal tumors as well as established precursor lesions such as actinic keratosis, Bowen disease, and erythroplasia, where question is— Has invasion occurred?.

▶ **Therapy:**

   • Excision with histologic control of margins. All other approaches are less than ideal; they include radiation therapy, photodynamic therapy, laser ablation, and cryosurgery. Some flexibility is reasonable when treating small actinic keratoses that show histologic invasion but are not clinically alarming, as their risk of spread is almost immeasurable. Utmost caution required when treating lip or genital lesions.

   • Inoperable or metastatic SCC are usually treated with palliative protocols borrowed from head and neck oncology programs. Typical agents include methotrexate or cisplatin combined with doxorubicin or 5-flurouracil.

▶ **Follow-up:** Patients should be checked every 3–6 months for 5 years, with the interval depending on risk of metastasis. Follow-up also includes checking for developing of additional tumors, as most patients have multiple SCC precursor lesions.

Verrucous Carcinoma

▶ **Definition:** Well-differentiated SCC with variety of clinical patterns and extremely low risk of metastasis.

▶ **Pathogenesis:** Few tumors have been more poorly understood. Verrucous carcinomas were long considered to be pseudocarcinomas, as their malignant potential is so low. In addition, they were described as "warty" but not virally induced. Now well established that they are low-grade cancers induced by HPV.

▶ **Clinical features:** Four distinct clinical forms:
- *Ackerman tumor*: Indolent thick oral tumor; when multiple, *florid oral papillomatosis* is preferred term.
- *Buschke–Löwenstein tumor* or *giant condyloma:* Large persistent destructive genital wart, involving scrotum, penis, vulva, vagina, cervix, or anus.
- *Epithelioma cuniculatum*: Persistent destructive plantar wart usually on heel; cuniculatum refers to rabbit burrows, describing the invasive nature of the tumor.
- *Papillomatosis cutis carcinoides (Gottron)*: Irregular nodules usually over shins; relationship to HPV not as clear as with other forms.

▶ **Histology:** Proliferation of keratinocytes, often with clear cytoplasm, sometimes papillomatous, with islands of keratinization and downward-pushing tumor masses; mitoses uncommon.

▶ **Diagnostic approach:** Clinical examination; any persistent verrucous lesion should be biopsied, especially in these locations. Often multiple biopsies and expert pathologic consultation required.

▶ **Differential diagnosis:** Large warts and other forms of SCC.

▶ **Therapy:** Surgical exesion; laser ablation for florid oral papillomatosis.
   ⚠ *Caution:* Laser smoke plume may contain HPV particles.
- For advanced disease, treat as any other SCC.

Keratoacanthoma

▶ **Definition:** Peculiar tumor of keratinocytes, which often shows spontaneous regression but has histologic features of an SCC.

▶ **Epidemiology:** Tumor of elderly people.

▶ Pathogenesis: Rapid growth suggests viral etiology, but no HPV type definitely incriminated; other triggers include UVB, ionizing radiation, and chemical carcinogens. Expression of TP53 reduced. Most have follicular features, suggesting that a keratoacanthoma may involute just as the normal hair follicle does.

▶ **Clinical features:**
- Usually on sun-exposed sites in fair-skinned individuals. Usually solitary.
- Starts as innocuous papule; over weeks grows into characteristic delled nodule 1–3 cm in diameter with prominent central plug. Sharply defined; adjacent tissue always normal (Fig. 24.**9**).
- Can evolve in cutaneous horn (p. 417).
- Over months, most keratoacanthomas resolve spontaneously with scarring; unfortunately, some do not but behave as SCC.

▶ **Variants:**
- *Giant keratoacanthoma*: Rare lesions reach several cm in size.
- *Keratoacanthoma centrifugum marginatum:* Slowly expanding giant keratoacanthoma with prominent border and little tendency for regression.
- Keratoacanthomas of nailbed and mucous are more likely verrucous carcinomas.

Cysts and Epidermal Tumors

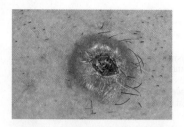

Fig. 24.**9** · Keratoacanthoma.

▶ **Histology:** Invaginated keratinocytic tumor with ground-glass cytoplasm, frequent mitoses, sometimes islands of tumor at base; most dermatopathologists hedge on the histologic diagnosis, suggesting that keratoacanthoma is likely, but that a SCC cannot be excluded with certainty.

▶ **Diagnostic approach:** If clinical suspicion is high, excisional biopsy is usually preferable. Punch biopsy not helpful.

▶ **Differential diagnosis:** Early stage: verruca or molluscum contagiosum; later, basal cell carcinoma, squamous cell carcinoma (less sharply defined).

▶ **Therapy:**
  • Observation rarely practiced because of risk of persistence and destructive behavior.
  • Simple excision most appropriate.
  • Laser ablation or cryosurgery also possible, if diagnosis has been histologically confirmed (as mentioned, difficult on biopsy).
  • Intralesional 5-fluorouracil (0.2–0.3 mL of 50 mg/mL, weekly for 6 weeks) is effective; intralesional methotrexate or bleomycin are alternatives.
  • For multiple keratoacanthomas:
    – Single dose of methotrexate 0.5 mg/ kg orally.
    – Acitretin 1 mg/kg daily for 4 weeks.

Multiple Keratoacanthomas
....

There are several syndromes with multiple keratoacanthomas:
▶ **Ferguson–Smith syndrome** (MIM code 132800): Rare syndrome with autosomal dominant inheritance, initially described in Scotland, in which patients develop hundreds of keratoacanthomas. Almost every patient has at least one invasive SCC. Also known as *multiple self-healing epithelioma syndrome*, but the name is misleading.

▶ **Eruptive keratoacanthomas (Gryzbowski):** Multiple eruptive keratoacanthomas over entire body; small (2–5 mm) papules, often without central plug; tend to heal with scarring and in some instances ectropion; some patients have immune defects.

▶ **Multiple keratoacanthomas (Witten–Zak):** Poorly defined group with multiple keratoacanthomas.

▶ **Muir–Torre syndrome** (p. 369): 30% of patients have multiple keratoacanthomas; many patients with Witten–Zak syndrome may fall into this group, as not all have accompanying sebaceous neoplasms.

  ◘ *Note:* Always monitor patients with multiple keratoacanthomas for the development of internal malignancies.

Merkel Cell Carcinoma

▶ **Synonyms:** Merkel cell tumor, neuroendocrine carcinoma, trabecular carcinoma.
▶ **Definition:** Dermal or subcutaneous tumor apparently related to epidermal Merkel cell with rapid growth pattern.
▶ **Epidemiology:** Uncommon tumor, affecting elderly almost exclusively in sun-exposed skin. Female predominance.
▶ **Pathogenesis:** Tumor cells have many similarities to the epidermal neuroendocrine Merkel cells, so Merkel cell carcinoma is regarded as likely epidermal tumor.
▶ **Clinical features:** Rapidly growing blue-red nodules often with telangiectases; usually on face. Less than 10% truncal. Highly aggressive course, with 30–50% metastasizing and 10–20% leading to death (Fig. 24.10).
▶ **Histology:** Infiltrate of monomorphous indistinct (murky) blue-gray cells, often arranged in strands or trabeculae. Numerous mitoses. Neuron-specific enolase is positive; in contrast to metastatic small-cell tumor of the lung (which is otherwise identical), Merkel cell carcinomas expressed cytokeratin 20, as well as cytokeratins 8 and 18.
▶ **Differential diagnosis:** First recognize as separate tumor in the 1970s, previously diagnosed as anaplastic lymphoma; other possibilities include metastasis, sweat gland carcinoma, and amelanotic malignant melanoma.
▶ **Therapy:** Excision with 3 cm margins or micrographic surgery. Sentinel lymph node biopsy and postoperative radiation therapy are both becoming widely used. Metastases are treated with protocols similar to those employed for small-cell carcinoma of the lung, but with little success.

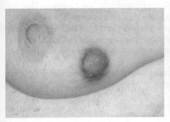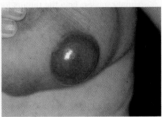

Fig. 24.**10** · **a** Merkel cell carcinoma. **b** Same patient three months later, having declined therapy.

25 Adnexal Tumors

25.1 Overview

► **Histogenesis:** The skin adnexal structures—eccrine, apocrine or sebaceous glands, hair follicles—can give rise to a baffling array of tumors, mimicking almost every cell and stage of adnexal development. The most common malignant human tumor, the basal cell carcinoma, usually shows signs or markers suggesting hair follicle differentiation, so it is included as a malignant adnexal tumor.

► **Localization:** The distribution of the different adnexal tumors follows that of the various normal structures; for example, eccrine tumors are expected on the palms and soles; follicular tumors are not. The classic tumor is a red-brown papule or nodule in the head and neck region.

► **Genetics:** Solitary adnexal tumors are sporadic events; most patients with multiple adnexal tumors have an autosomal dominant mutation that may lead to other cutaneous or even systemic abnormalities and can be transmitted to future generations. For example, a single trichilemmoma means little; multiple tumors suggest Cowden syndrome and a high risk of breast cancer.

► **Histology:** The tumor should be examined for clues to the line of differentiation:
- *Eccrine:* Clear cells, myoepithelial cells, pores.
- *Apocrine:* Decapitation secretion.
- *Sebaceous:* Holocrine secretion, foamy cells.
- *Follicular:* Hair germs, mimics of follicular structures.
- When terms such as "resembling" or "derived from" are used below, they simply suggest how the tumors look microscopically. We recognize that the tumors may arise from stem cells and only share features with specific structures. There is also considerable controversy over the type of differentiation; for example, eccrine spiradenomas and cylindromas are caused by the same mutation in the Brooke–Spiegler syndrome, but one is considered eccrine; the other, follicular or apocrine.

► **Differential diagnosis:** In most instances, the differential diagnosis is other adnexal tumors and basal cell carcinoma. Only exceptions to this rule will be stated.

► **Therapy:** In almost every case, the treatment is excision.

25.2 Benign Tumors with Eccrine Differentiation

Eccrine Hidrocystoma
....

► **Definition:** Cyst derived from dermal component of eccrine duct.

► **Clinical features:** Translucent yellow or light blue cystic tumor, typically around eyes (Fig. 25.**1**). More common in women. Occasionally appear in crops suddenly, but then more likely reactive with ductal occlusion.

► **Histology:** Small cyst with colorless contents whose wall is composed of ductal cells.

► **Differential diagnosis:** Apocrine hidrocystoma.

► **Therapy:** Excision.

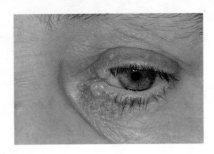

Fig. 25.**1** · Eccrine hidrocystoma.

Eccrine Poroma

▶ **Definition:** Tumor derived from the intraepidermal and/or upper dermal component of the eccrine duct.
▶ **Clinical features:** Skin-colored or erythematous solitary papule or nodule typically on soles (60%), palms (20%) or scalp (Fig. 25.**2**). Tends to be painful (because of location) and bleed (highly vascularized tumor). Usually appears in middle-aged adults.
▶ **Histology:** Strands of uniform cuboidal basaloid tumor cells arising from epidermis, containing ductal elements; if totally intraepidermal (*hidroacanthoma simplex*), if no epidermal connections (*dermal duct tumor*).
▶ **Differential diagnosis:** On the palms and soles, often mistaken for a wart; on the scalp, usually diagnosed as a vascular tumor.
▶ **Therapy:** Excision.

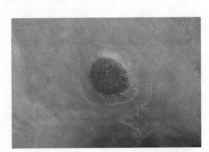

Fig. 25.**2** · Eccrine poroma on sole.

Syringoma

▶ **Definition:** Benign tumor that resembles the eccrine dermal duct.
▶ **Clinical features:**
  • More common in women, starting in puberty. Usually multiple skin-colored to yellow papules (Fig. 25.**3**). Most common site is periorbital, although axillae, umbilicus, and genital region also seen. Rarely on scalp, but then with alopecia.
  • *Eruptive syringomas:* Sudden onset of multiple papules usually on trunk; usually in young women. Sometimes spontaneous regression occurs. Occasionally inherited in autosomal dominant manner.

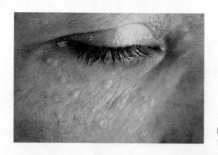

Fig. 25.**3** · Multiple syringomas in typical periorbital location.

▶ **Histology:** Small tubular structures in dermis surrounded by thickened connective tissue; thin epithelial strands (fancifully compared to tadpoles) also present.
▶ **Differential diagnosis:** Xanthelasma, other xanthomas, plane warts; on trunk, disseminated granuloma annulare, eruptive vellus hair cysts.
▶ **Therapy:** In most instances, best left alone; if cosmetically disturbing, a variety of destructive measures including laser ablation, dermabrasion or electrosurgery is possible. Recurrences are the rule.

Eccrine Spiradenoma

▶ **Definition:** Tumor from secretory component of eccrine sweat duct.
▶ **Epidemiology:** More common in women; may be multiple (Brooke–Spiegler syndrome).
▶ **Clinical features:** 0.3–5.0 cm intradermal solitary nodule with red-brown color; usually painful. Most often head, neck, upper trunk.
▶ **Histology:** Dense nests of basaloid epithelial cells associated with larger less dense cells producing rosette pattern.
▶ **Differential diagnosis:** Painful skin tumors; ANGEL mnemonic (p. 714).
▶ **Therapy:** Excision.

Clear Cell Hidradenoma

▶ **Synonym:** Eccrine acrospiroma.
▶ **Definition:** Solid-cystic eccrine tumor, dominated by secretory clear cells.
▶ **Clinical features:** 0.5–2.0 cm solid tumor; no favored sites.
▶ **Histology:** Nodules composed of clear tumor cells (glycogen-rich cells which have lost their content during fixation), admixed with small blue cells and myo-epithelial cells.
▶ **Therapy:** Excision.

Mixed Tumor

▶ **Synonym:** Chondroid syringoma.
▶ **Definition:** Adnexal tumor with either eccrine or apocrine differentiation, ductal structures, and a prominent chondroid stroma.
▶ **Clinical features:** Typically 0.5–3.0 cm firm nodule in head and neck region.
▶ **Histology:** Ductal structures embedded in cartilage-like stroma; if decapitation secretion is seen, apocrine; otherwise, eccrine.
▶ **Therapy:** Excision.

25.3 Benign Tumors with Apocrine Differentiation

Accessory Nipple

▶ **Definition:** Congenital malformation with additional nipples formed along milk line; often erroneously considered a tumor and thus included here.
▶ **Pathogenesis:** Polythelia (multiple nipples) sometimes associated with Wilms tumor.
▶ **Clinical features:** Red-brown papules located along lines extending from axillae through nipples to groin. Soft brown asymptomatic papule; rarely identified clinically. Rarely may be tender, have discharge, or fluctuate with menstrual periods.
▶ **Histology:** Increased amount of smooth muscle fibers coupled with excessive mammary glands which are of apocrine origin.
▶ **Differential diagnosis:** Dermatofibroma, melanocytic nevus.
▶ **Therapy:** Excision.

Apocrine Hidrocystoma

▶ **Definition:** Cyst whose wall shows apocrine differentiation.
▶ **Clinical features:** Solitary cystic tumor, usually periorbital. May be dark blue to black (*hydrocystome noire*). On lid, may arise from glands of Moll.
▶ **Histology:** Cyst wall with apocrine secretion; may have hemorrhage or lipofuscin imparting color.
▶ **Differential diagnosis:** Eccrine hidrocystoma, thrombosed hemangioma, blue nevus, basal cell carcinoma.
▶ **Therapy:** Excision.

Hidradenoma Papilliferum

▶ **Definition:** Papillomatous adenoma with apocrine differentiation.
▶ **Clinical features:** Dermal nodule, usually on labia, generally asymptomatic, appears after puberty.
▶ **Histology:** Complex nodule of interlacing strands of glandular epithelium with decapitation secretion.
▶ **Differential diagnosis:** Endometriosis, Bartholin gland cyst, epidermoid cyst.
▶ **Therapy:** Excision.

Syringocystadenoma Papilliferum

▶ **Definition:** Papillomatous adenoma of distal apocrine duct, often with connection to epithelium.
▶ **Clinical features:**
  • Papule or plaque; usually red-brown, generally with central pore or erosion; 70% are on head.
  • Can be present at birth in linear arrangement.
  • Second most common tumor to development in nevus sebaceus (p. 411); 30% seen in this setting.
▶ **Histology:** Compound papilliferous tumor with stroma rich is plasma cells and almost always epidermal connection. Otherwise similar to hidradenoma papilliferum.
▶ **Therapy:** Excision.

Cylindroma

▶ **Synonym:** Turban tumor.
▶ **Definition:** Complex adenoma whose pattern of differentiation is disputed.
▶ **Clinical features:** Two separate patterns:
- *Solitary cylindroma:*
  - Negative family history.
  - Several cm firm hairless tumor on scalp or less often face.
  - *Histology:* Nodules of basaloid tumor cells surrounded by a dense PAS-positive hyaline membrane.
  - *Therapy:* excision.
- *Multiple cylindromas:*
  - Brooke–Spiegler syndrome.
  - Mutation in *CYLD1*, tumor suppressor gene, autosomal dominant inheritance.
  - Three different adnexal tumors may be present in same patient: cylindroma, spiradenoma, and trichoepithelioma.
  - *Clinical features:* On scalp, numerous flesh-colored to pink nodules, hairless; when numerous, fancifully compared to a turban (Fig. 25.**4**). Often trichoepithelioma in the midface and scattered spiradenoma; clinical distinction impossible with overlaps both clinically and histologically.
  - *Differential diagnosis:* Other multiple adnexal tumors; nevoid basal cell carcinoma syndrome; on scalp, trichilemmal cysts, metastases.
  - *Therapy:* Extremely difficult, complex surgical procedures (scalpectomy with grafting; dermabrasion, extensive laser ablation).

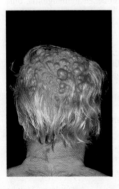

Fig. 25.**4** · Multiple cylindromas.

Nipple Adenoma

▶ **Synonyms:** Papillary adenoma, erosive adenomatosis of nipple, florid papillomatosis of nipple, subareolar duct papillomatosis.
▶ **Definition:** Adenoma of the milk ducts, usually associated with surface erosion.
▶ **Epidemiology:** Uncommon, usually in middle-aged women.
▶ **Clinical features:** Unilateral crust or erosion of nipple; often tender or burning.
▶ **Diagnostic approach:** Biopsy mandatory to exclude Paget disease.
▶ **Histology:** Cohesive mass in disarray composed of normal ductal and glandular elements.
▶ **Differential diagnosis:** Paget disease, Bowen disease, nipple dermatitis, psoriasis.
▶ **Therapy:** Excision.

Paget Disease of Breast

▶ **Definition:** Intraductal carcinoma of the breast extending to involve nipple with invasion of epidermis by malignant cells.
▶ **Epidemiology:** Almost exclusively limited to women.
▶ **Clinical features:** Unilateral sharply bordered area of crusting or erosion on nipple. Generally no underlying mass can be palpated.
▶ **Histology:** Epidermis contains numerous clear cells positive for carcinoembryonic antigen (CEA) and generally above the basal layer. Underlying intraductal tumor seen only rarely in biopsy.
▶ **Diagnostic approach:** Biopsy, breast examination, appropriate imaging studies.
▶ **Differential diagnosis:** Nipple adenoma, Bowen disease, nipple dermatitis, psoriasis; histologically, superficial spreading melanoma.
▶ **Therapy:** Surgery and follow-up management following guidelines for carcinoma of the breast.

Extramammary Paget Disease

▶ **Definition:** Intraepidermal growth of malignant adnexal tumor or underlying carcinoma, not located on the nipple.
▶ **Clinical features:** Most common site is anogenital region, where urogenital and rectal carcinomas must be excluded. Less often periumbilical (gastrointestinal carcinoma), axillary (breast carcinoma or apocrine carcinoma), external ear canal (ceruminous carcinoma).
▶ **Histology:** Identical to Paget disease of nipple.
▶ **Diagnostic approach:** Biopsy, search for underlying tumor.
▶ **Differential diagnosis:** Chronic dermatitis, Bowen disease.
▶ **Therapy:** Excision; often difficult to provide curative surgery because of extent of lesion, unclear margins and underlying tumor. Laser ablation and photodynamic therapy useful for palliation.

25.4 Benign Tumors with Sebaceous Differentiation

Ectopic Sebaceous Glands

▶ **Definition:** Sebaceous glands found on hairless surfaces.
▶ **Clinical features:** Most common are *Fordyce glands* or spots on lips: tiny yellow papules that are totally asymptomatic but sometimes annoy patient. Other common sites are nipple (*Montgomery tubercle*) and genitalia (labia and penis, where known as *Tyson glands*).
▶ **Therapy:** None needed.

Sebaceous Hyperplasia

▶ **Synonym:** Senile sebaceous hyperplasia.
▶ **Definition:** Most common sebaceous lesion; accumulation of enlarged, otherwise normal glands around a central follicle.
▶ **Clinical features:** Clinically distinctive, rosette of yellow tiny papules just beneath skin surface, arranged around a dilated hair follicle with central dell. Usually multiple, <5 mm in size. More common in renal dialysis patients.

▶ **Differential diagnosis:** Basal cell carcinoma is usual mistake, but clinically distinctive.
▶ **Therapy:** None needed; excision is cosmetically disturbing; laser ablation possible. Some patients have hundreds; then systemic retinoids may provide some help.

Sebaceous Adenoma

▶ **Definition:** Dermal tumor comprised of normal sebocytes with some disarray in glandular organization.
▶ **Clinical features:** Solitary tumor, usually on head and neck region, frequently crusted; yellow color often not appreciated.
▶ **Histology:** Enlarged sebaceous lobules with an increased basaloid or undifferentiated peripheral zone; usually have connection to surface.
▶ **Differential diagnosis:** Basal cell carcinoma.
▶ **Therapy:** Excision.

Sebaceoma

▶ **Synonym:** Sebaceous epithelioma.
▶ **Definition:** Benign sebaceous tumor with marked loss of lobular pattern.
▶ **Clinical features:** No clinically distinct features; usually facial nodule in older adult.
▶ **Histology:** Basaloid tumor masses with at least foci of sebocytes and with no unequivocal signs of basal cell carcinoma.
▶ **Differential diagnosis:** Basal cell carcinoma, sebaceous adenoma.
  ☐ *Note:* Unusual or multiple sebaceous tumors, especially cystic tumors, suggest Muir–Torre syndrome (p. 369).
▶ **Therapy:** Excision.

25.5 Benign Tumors with Hair Follicle Differentiation

Trichofolliculoma

▶ **Definition:** Organoid hair follicle tumor.
▶ **Clinical features:** One of the few adnexal tumors with distinctive clinical features: firm nodule with central pore through which pokes a bundle of wispy, fine hairs. Usually on scalp or face.
▶ **Histology:** Thickened dilated hair follicle with budding extending into dermis; some buds differentiate into complete follicles.
▶ **Differential diagnosis:** Melanocytic nevus, basal cell carcinoma.
▶ **Therapy:** Excision.

Trichoblastoma

▶ **Definition:** Recently defined group of hair follicle tumors, all featuring hair germs and matrical cells in varying patterns.
▶ **Clinical features:** No distinctive features; dermal nodule, usually in head and neck region.

▶ **Histology:** Crucial feature is basaloid tumor islands without peripheral palisading and without cleft formation (two hallmarks of basal cell carcinoma). Lesions may have large or small tumor nodules with lacy or sieve-like pattern, or with predominance of stromal proliferation (*desmoplastic trichoblastoma*). Adamantinoid trichoblastoma is clear cell tumor with rich lymphocytic infiltrate; also known as lymphadenoma.

▶ **Differential diagnosis:** Basal cell carcinoma; Ackerman has renamed BCC as trichoblastic carcinoma.

▶ **Therapy:** Excision.

Trichoepithelioma

▶ **Synonym:** Superficial trichoblastoma; if multiple, epithelioma adenoides cysticum.

▶ **Definition:** Most common benign hair follicle tumor; incomplete differentiation toward hair follicle.

▶ **Clinical features:**

- *Solitary trichoepithelioma:*
  - Facial papule or nodule; not distinct.
  - *Histology:* Basaloid tumor strands and nests with small follicular cysts and without definite features of basal cell carcinoma.
  - *Differential diagnosis:* Overlaps with basal cell carcinoma.
  - *Therapy:* Excision.

- *Desmoplastic trichoepithelioma:*
  - Flat-topped facial papule or plaque; very often on chin.
  - *Histology:* Similar to solitary lesion but with prominent desmoplastic stroma, thinner tumor stands.
  - *Differential diagnosis:* Clinically always mistaken for basal cell carcinoma; histologically shares features with syringoma and microcystic adnexal carcinoma.
  - *Therapy:* Excision.

- *Multiple trichoepitheliomas:*
  - Brooke syndrome (part of Brooke–Spiegler syndrome [p. 428]) with mutation in *CYLD* gene but at different point.
  - Onset in puberty of multiple firm papules in perinasal and midface region; can also involve scalp, neck, and trunk.
  - Sometimes basal cell carcinomas develop amidst the otherwise benign lesions.
  - *Differential diagnosis:* Tuberous sclerosis, nevoid basal cell carcinoma syndrome, multiple syringomas, other adnexal tumors.
  - *Therapy:* Dermabrasion or laser ablation; recurrences common. If single lesion is worrisome, excision.

Trichoadenoma

▶ **Synonym:** Nikolowski tumor.

▶ **Definition:** Rare tumor, seemingly composed of many tiny trichilemmal cysts.

▶ **Clinical features:** Plaque or nodule, usually on head or neck; rarely buttocks.

▶ **Histology:** Dermal tumor with many tiny cystic spaces whose lining resembles follicular infundibulum.

▶ **Differential diagnosis:** Basal cell carcinoma, microcystic adnexal tumor, other adnexal tumors.

▶ **Therapy:** Excision.

Fibrofolliculoma/Trichodiscoma

▶ **Synonym:** Mantleoma.
▶ **Definition:** Benign tumors arising from mantle zone—perifollicular connective tissue just above entry of sebaceous duct.
▶ **Clinical features:**
  • Usually numerous 2–4 mm flesh-colored papules on face and trunk; solitary lesions hard to recognize.
  • Multiple lesions suggest Birt–Hogg–Dubé syndrome (p. 367).
▶ **Histology:** Fibrofolliculomas (or perifollicular fibromas) have a normal follicle with lacy branches surrounded by dense connective tissue stroma. A trichodiscoma represents the late stage of a fibrofolliculoma and has simply dermal fibrosis. The initial suggestion that a trichodiscoma was related to the hair disk (Haarscheibe) sensory organ common in animals was incorrect, but the name has been retained.
▶ **Diagnostic approach:** Patients with multiple tumors at risk for renal carcinoma.
▶ **Therapy:** Dermabrasion or laser ablation.

Pilomatricoma

▶ **Synonym:** Calcifying epithelioma of Malherbe; also written pilomatrixoma.
▶ **Definition:** Common cystic tumor with differentiation toward hair follicle matrix.
▶ **Epidemiology:** One of the most common childhood tumors, except for epidermoid cysts and lipomas, but also seen in adults.
▶ **Clinical features:** Firm 0.5–5.0 cm dermal nodule, almost always head and neck, location especially anterior to ear or in eyebrows (Fig. 25.5). If superficial, has blue-red tones, may ulcerate and discharge pathognomonic chalky granules.
▶ **Histology:** Distinctive histological picture: dermal nodule with basaloid tumor cells, bland matrix with empty spaces (ghost cells), and usually calcification and peripheral inflammation.
▶ **Differential diagnosis:** Infected epidermoid cyst, actinomycosis, cutaneous osteoma, other adnexal tumors.
▶ **Therapy:** Excision.

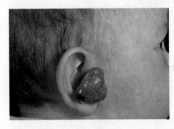

Fig. 25.**5** · Pilomatricoma.

Trichilemmoma

▶ **Definition:** Benign tumor with differentiation pattern suggesting outer root sheath.
▶ **Pathogenesis:** HPV implicated in solitary trichilemmomas, which may be old warts.
▶ **Clinical features:** Solitary warty tumor, usually facial; when multiple, consider Cowden syndrome (p. 367).

▶ **Histology:** Papillomatous tumor with thickened follicle containing numerous clear cells with basaloid band at periphery.
▶ **Differential diagnosis:** Wart, other adnexal tumors.
▶ **Therapy:** Excision.

25.6 Malignant Adnexal Tumors

▶ **Pathogenesis:** The only common malignant adnexal tumor is basal cell carcinoma. All others are very uncommon. Some appear to be malignant equivalents of benign tumors; *eccrine porocarcinoma* is one of the most common members of the group. Controversial if such tumors arise from benign tumor or are malignant from start with similar differentiation. Other malignant sweat duct tumors do not seem to have a benign equivalent. The malignant tumors are often very difficult to distinguish from squamous cell carcinoma and should be treated as such, with a risk for metastasis.

▶ Several malignant adnexal lesions have already been considered because they fit didactically better elsewhere; included in this group are proliferating trichilemmal cysts as well as Paget disease and extramammary Paget disease.

Basal Cell Carcinoma (BCC)

▶ **Synonym:** Basal cell epithelioma.
▶ **Definition:** Heterogenous group of low-grade malignant cutaneous tumors, characterized by differentiation markers usually associated with hair follicle development, locally aggressive but almost never metastatic.
▶ **Epidemiology:** Most common malignancy in humans: incidence 200/100000 in men, 100/100000 in women but gap narrowing. Incidence has doubled over past two decades. Most patients are > 50 years of age.
▶ **Pathogenesis:** The cell of origin of BCC has long been argued. Since it is the most common human malignancy, the question is not insignificant. Most BCC arise from epidermal cells differentiated in the direction of the primitive hair bulb. Thus the term *trichoblastic carcinoma* has been proposed but has not won acceptance. The main trigger appears to be UVB, but this is not the only factor, because BCCs are extremely uncommon on the backs of the hands where actinic keratoses are frequent. The underlying genetic mutations in BCC frequently involve the *PATCH* gene or other members of the sonic hedgehog signaling pathway, resulting in overexpression of transcription factor Gli1, as suggested by research in nevoid BCC syndrome.
▶ **Clinical features:**
   ☐ *Note:* Key unifying clinical features of BCC include pearly nodules and telangiectases; always look for these (Fig. 25.**6 a**).
   • Most common site is face; 80% arise above the line connecting the corner of mouth to the ear lobe. Multiple lesions are more common on trunk. No mucosal lesions.
   • *Nodular BCC:* Most common variant, pearly, telangiectatic dome-shaped nodule or ring of papules; often with central ulceration (Fig. 25.**6 b,c**).
      – *Differential diagnosis:* Adnexal tumors.
   • *Superficial or multicentric BCC:* Flat, tan to red-brown patch, often with scaly and with a pearly border when carefully examined; usually on trunk; often a history of arsenic or radiation exposure (Fig. 25.**6 d**).
      – *Differential diagnosis:* Dermatitis, Bowen disease, extramammary Paget disease, psoriasis, tinea corporis.

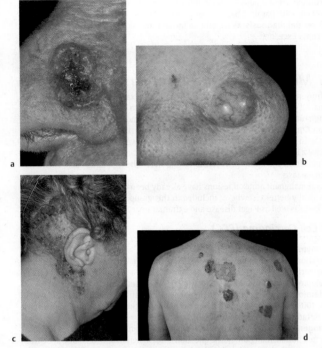

Fig. 25.**6** · **Basal cell carcinoma. a** On nose, showing typical pearly border. **b** Nodular BCC. **c** Large ulcerated BCC. **d** Multiple superficial BCC secondary to arsenic exposure.

- *Pigmented BCC:* Both nodular and superficial BCCs can be pigmented; melanin accumulates in tumor cells. More common in dark-skinned individuals. Rarely occurs in people with blue eyes.
  - *Differential diagnosis:* Malignant melanoma (dermatoscopy), melanocytic nevus, blue nevus, pigmented seborrheic keratosis, angiokeratoma.
- *Sclerosing (sclerodermiform) BCC:* Atrophic plaque, often with telangiectases or ulcer, but no other stigmata of BCC. Typically in lines of embryonic fusion around nose or ears. Desmoplastic dermal response far exceeds the proliferation of tumor cells. Margins difficult to determine clinically, causing treatment problems.
  - *Differential diagnosis:* Scar, desmoplastic trichoepithelioma, morphea.
- *Rodent ulcer:* Older name for predominantly ulcerated BCC usually on forehead or scalp, but sometimes in midface.
- *Ulcus terebrans:* Extremely aggressive BCC invading underlying structures such as large vessels, bones, even meninges; frequently fatal but mercifully rare. Causes of death include uncontrolled bleeding and infection.

▶ **Histology:** The histologic spectrum is as wide as the clinical. The unifying feature is collections of basaloid tumor cells with peripheral palisading and stromal retraction. The tumors may mimic many aspects of hair follicle differentiation:

- *Nodular BCC:* Large tumor islands, sometimes with cystic degeneration, analogous to holocrine secretion.
- *Keratotic BCC*: Hair follicle differentiation with keratinization.
- *Adenoid BCC:* Glandular elements mimicking apocrine glands.
- *Adamantinoid BCC:* Clear cell differentiation resembling enamel organ.
- *Superficial or multicentric BCC:* Tiny buds arise from basal layer, mimicking primitive hair germ.
- *Pigmented BCC:* Typical pattern but with excess melanin; no proliferation of melanocytes.
- *Sclerosing (sclerodermiform) BCC:* Thin strands of basaloid tumor cells surrounded by thickened bundles of collagen.

▶ **Diagnostic approach:** Clinical examination and biopsy. Dermatoscopy is also helpful for pigmented or otherwise puzzling BCC. Fortunately BCC is a straightforward pathological diagnosis, even when clinical questions exist.

▶ **Therapy:** The aim is complete removal and thus a 100% cure, and as good a cosmetic result as can be obtained. There are many ways to achieve this gratifying goal:

- Surgical excision with histologic control and cosmetic closure is the treatment of choice. Micrographic surgery should be employed for recurrent, sclerosing, or otherwise difficult BCC. Recurrence rate should be less than 5%, in expert hands.
- Alternatives all have somewhat higher recurrence rates. They include:
  - *Cryosurgery:* Suitable for superficial BCC. Two freeze–thaw cycles should be used. Cryosurgery for nodular lesions is also possible, but requires a thermocouple so that tumor-killing parameters can be obtained. Disadvantages include lack of histologic control, recurrences, and scarring.
  - *Radiation therapy:* Best for elderly patients with numerous lesions or in difficult locations. Often recommended for lid lesions. 60–70 Gy, fractionate in 3–5 Gy administered 3–5× weekly. For deeper lesions, consult radiation therapy regarding electron beam therapy.
  - ◢ *Note:* Even around the eyes, surgical procedures now usually achieve better results than radiation therapy.
  - *Photodynamic therapy:* Useful for superficial and small lesions; new procedure, so long-term recurrence rates not well-established.
  - *Curettage and electrodesiccation or cautery:* Formerly widely used for superficial or small lesions; scarring and high recurrence rate limit its use today to exceptional situations.
  - *Laser ablation:* Lack of histologic control gives laser therapy the same disadvantages as curettage.
  - Topical imiquimod or 5-fluorouracil can be used over a long period of time, usually 3× weekly for 6 weeks, for superficial BCC.
- There is no effective chemotherapy regimen for the rare cases of metastatic BCC. A standard approach is cisplatin 100 mg/m^2 every 3 weeks, perhaps combined with 5-fluorouracil. Fluids should be forced and 12.5 g of mannitol given just prior to cisplatin. Other regimens incorporate systemic retinoids.

▶ **Follow-up:** Every patient with BCC is likely to develop several more. Thus, at a bare minimum patients should be checked yearly; in the sunbelt of the USA, every 6 months is standard. New lesions can be identified and promptly treated at the same time as previous sites are monitored for recurrences.

Nevoid Basal Cell Carcinoma Syndrome

▶ **Synonyms:** Basal cell nevus syndrome, Gorlin–Goltz syndrome.
▶ **MIM code:** 109400.
▶ **Definition:** Genodermatosis with numerous BCC and multiple developmental anomalies; autosomal dominant inheritance.
▶ **Epidemiology:** One of more common tumor syndromes; incidence around 1:50000. About 25% of patients presenting with a BCC before 20 years of age will have this disorder.
▶ **Pathogenesis:** The defect is a mutation in the *PATCH* gene at 9q22.3, an important signal transduction gene involved in segmental regulation of embryologic growth and later of controlling hair follicle differentiation, explaining the combination of developmental defects and BCC.
▶ **Clinical features:**
  • Multiple BCC, often starting in childhood. Earliest lesions often on neck, resembling skin tags. Later lesions can take all forms of BCC; most common site is face.
  • *Palmoplantar pits:* Tiny hyperkeratotic lesions with a definite defect in epidermis. On careful inspection, appear different than palmoplantar keratoderma.
  • Epidermoid cysts are more common (especially acral ones), as are lipomas.
  • Developmental anomalies include odontogenic cysts of maxilla and mandible, dental defects, bifid ribs, scoliosis, hypertelorism, and frontal bossing.
  • Peculiar radiologic finding is calcification of the corpus callosum.
  • Most patients are normal, although both EEG abnormalities and mental retardation may occur.
  • Tumors include:
    – *Medulloblastoma:* Occurs in 5% of patients but accounts for less than 1% of childhood medulloblastomas. Appears before any other stigmata of syndrome. Patients require radiation therapy, which induces 1000s of BCC in the radiation fields.
    – Ovarian fibromas and cardiac fibromas.
    – Mesenteric lymphatic cysts.
▶ **Diagnostic approach:** History (well over 50% have positive family history, as syndrome has little effect on reproduction), clinical examination; earliest clues are pits. Dental radiographs usually identify one or more cysts; other screening approaches; specialist consultation.
▶ **Differential diagnosis:** When complete, none; otherwise multiple BCC sporadically or after arsenic exposure. Rare syndromes with multiple adnexal tumors may also be similar.
▶ **Therapy:** Careful monitoring and prompt treatment of BCC when small. All the methods discussed above are appropriate except for radiotherapy, which must be avoided. Imiquimod appears useful for superficial lesions. Systemic retinoids may reduce the development of tumors, but have too many side effects for lifelong usage.

Microcystic Adnexal Carcinoma

▶ **Synonym:** Malignant syringoma.
▶ **Definition:** Carcinoma of eccrine ducts with characteristic tubular pattern and prominent stromal desmoplasia.
▶ **Clinical features:** Slowly growing deep nodule, usually lip or chin.
▶ **Histology:** Superficial component resembles syringoma with tiny cysts, while deeper component has basaloid strands of tumors often with perineurial entrapment. Little cytologic atypia or other features of malignancy.

⚠ *Caution:* Be extremely skeptical of the diagnosis of a solitary syringoma when the clinical lesion is a deep nodule; always re-excise.

► **Differential diagnosis:** Scar, sclerosing BCC.

► **Therapy:** Excision with control of margins; careful follow-up because of high risk of recurrence and slight risk of metastasis.

Eccrine Porocarcinoma

► **Clinical features:** Appear to develop from eccrine poroma; most common on feet; risk of regional lymph node involvement and distant metastasis. Generous excision and close follow-up mandatory. Metastatic disease treated as squamous cell carcinoma.

Other Malignant Adnexal Tumors

Table 25.1 · Other malignant adnexal tumors

Tumor	Derivation	Comments
Mucinous carcinoma	Eccrine	Periorbital tumor; tiny eccrine tumor islands in mucinous stroma
Aggressive digital papillary adenocarcinoma	Eccrine	Cystic tumor on fingers or toes; often requires amputation
Malignant spiradenoma	Eccrine	Only arises in background of Brooke–Spiegler syndrome
Adenoid cystic carcinoma	Apocrine	Red nodule usually on scalp; Swiss cheese pattern on histology; identical to salivary gland adenoid cystic tumor secondary metastasis must be excluded
Malignant cylindroma	Apocrine	Only arises in background of Brooke–Spiegler syndrome.
Apocrine carcinoma	Apocrine	Usually axilla; can have intraepidermal spread similar to extramammary Paget disease
Sebaceous carcinoma	Sebaceous	Two forms: Eyelid: frequent intraepidermal spread Trunk: nodular tumor
Pilomatrical carcinoma	Hair follicle	Does not develop from pilomatricoma; usually in adults
Lymphoepithelioma-like carcinoma	Hair follicle?	Remnants of adnexal structures with extensive lymphocytic infiltrate; keratin stains identify tumor stroma; treat as squamous cell carcinoma

26 Soft Tissue Tumors

26.1 Connective Tissue Tumors

Connective Tissue Nevus

- **Definition:** Localized lesion with increased amounts of collagen and/or elastin.
- **Epidemiology:** Uncommon solitary malformation; often associated with tuberous sclerosis (p. 365), MEN1 (p. 367), Proteus syndrome (p. 414), or Buschke–Ollendorff syndrome.
- **Clinical features:** Present at birth; sometimes first prominent after a few years. Usually a plaque over the lumbosacral region, unilateral, consisting of numerous 5–10 mm skin-colored papules and nodules.
- **Histology:** One of the few lesions where normal skin is needed for comparison; often useful to biopsy contralateral normal skin or include a tag of normal skin in elliptical biopsy. On H&E stain, dermis looks thickened; special stains confirm increase in collagen, elastin or both.
- **Differential diagnosis:** Often overlooked; only serious differential diagnostic consideration is organoid nevus (p. 410).
- **Therapy:** If small, excision; otherwise, none.

Buschke–Ollendorff Syndrome

- **Synonym:** Dermatofibrosis lenticularis disseminata.
- **MIM code:** 166700.
- **Definition:** Rare genodermatosis with multiple connective tissue nevi and bony changes; autosomal dominant inheritance.
- **Clinical features:**
  - *Dermatofibrosis lenticularis:* Multiple widely distributed small yellow-white papules.
  - *Skeletal system: Osteopoikilosis* features stippling and sclerotic foci in the epiphyses and metaphyses of long bones; asymptomatic, only detected by chance on radiologic examination.
- **Histology:** Skin lesions are connective tissue nevi, usually dominated by elastic fibers.
- **Diagnostic approach:** Skin biopsy and radiography of long bones.
- **Differential diagnosis:** Pseudoxanthoma elasticum.
- **Therapy:** None.

Elastofibroma Dorsi

- **Definition:** Subcutaneous tumor in adults with increased amounts of elastic fibers.
- **Pathogenesis:** Poorly understood; seems a result of trauma, as it is more common in manual laborers. New elastin may come from the periosteum; familial cases reported.
- **Clinical features:** Usually overlooked and found on autopsy; slow-growing firm nodules between scapula and thoracic wall in older adults.
- **Histology:** Indistinct nodule rich in elastic fibers and collagen bundles.
- **Differential diagnosis:** Clinically specific; histologically confused with keloid or connective tissue nevus.
- **Therapy:** None or excision.

Soft Fibroma

▶ **Synonyms:** Skin tag, acrochordon, fibroepithelial polyp, fibroma molle, fibroma pendulans.

  ◪ *Note:* As is so often the case, the least important lesions have the most names.
▶ **Definition:** Harmless outpouching of epidermis and dermis.
▶ **Clinical features:** Some distinguish between three sizes of soft fibromas:
  • *Tiny:* Skin tags: 1–2 mm skin-colored stalked papules around eyes, neck, axillae (Fig. 26.**1**).
  • *Medium:* Roughly 5–10 mm stalked papule; no site of predilection.
  • *Large* (fibroma pendulans): 1–5 cm stalked soft tumor.
▶ **Histology:** The small lesions share some similarities with seborrheic keratoses and may have such surfaces changes. The medium and larger lesions are often older nevi and may contain a few nests of melanocytes. Otherwise, normal epidermis and dermis with increased vessels in a polypoid pattern.
▶ **Differential diagnosis:** Seborrheic keratosis, melanocytic nevus, neurofibroma.
▶ **Therapy:** Small lesions can be snipped off without anesthesia; medium and larger lesions are likely to have a central vessel that bleeds, so should be anesthetized and then removed by standard or scissor excision.

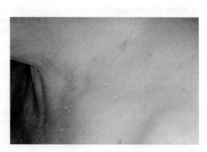

Fig. 26.**1** · Multiple skin tags.

Angiofibroma

▶ **Definition:** Benign proliferation of connective tissue and vessels; many different clinical lesions have same microscopic pattern:
  • *Fibrous papule of the nose:* Solitary flat-topped skin-colored 5–10 mm papule on distal aspect of nose.
  • *Adenoma sebaceum:* These marker lesions of tuberous sclerosis (p. 365) are actually angiofibromas.
  • Associated with *MEN1* (p. 367).
  • *Isolated angiofibromas:* 1–3 mm red papules on nose, nasolabial folds, and cheeks.
    ◪ *Note:* Always check for tuberous sclerosis and MEN1, but isolated lesions far more common.
  • *Acquired digital fibrokeratoma:* Digital angiofibroma that acquires a unique collarette scale because of acral location.
  • *Pearly penile papules:* Tiny harmless angiofibromas at the base of glands in the coronal sulcus; often mistakenly treated as condylomata.
  • *Hirsuties vulvae:* Similar lesions forming fringe at line of transition from labia minor to vagina.

► **Histology:** Increased vessels and dermal fibrosis; can be subtle changes; biopsy is usually taken to exclude other possibilities, such as melanocytic nevus, wart, or basal cell carcinoma.
► **Therapy:** Genital lesions require no therapy. Solitary facial or digital lesions can be tangentially excised. Multiple lesions may be treated with dermabrasion or laser ablation, but recurrences common.

Perifollicular Fibroma

This term is synonymous with fibrofolliculoma and simply represents one stage in the evolution of tumors of the hair mantle region (p. 432). Marker for Birt–Hogg–Dubé syndrome (p. 367).

Dermatofibroma

► **Synonyms:** Histiocytoma, fibrous histiocytoma, sclerosing hemangioma, fibroma durum, nodular subepidermal fibrosis.
► **Definition:** Extremely common reactive fibrous proliferation.
► **Pathogenesis:** Two most common triggers appear to be arthropod assault and folliculitis.
► **Clinical features:** 5–10 mm firm tumor; almost always on legs (Fig. 26.2). Color varies from skin-colored through tan to red-brown or even dark brown. When one compresses a dermatofibroma from the sides, the lesion becomes depressed, rather than protruding as would a melanocytic nevus (*dimple sign* or *Fitzpatrick sign*).
  ▶ *Note:* Multiple dermatofibromas, especially on other body sites, can be associated with systemic lupus erythematosus.
► **Histology:** The histologic spectrum of dermatofibroma is enormous and continuously being expanded. The classic lesion has a proliferation of fibroblasts with entrapment of collagen at the periphery, foci of hemosiderin, macrophages (histiocytoma), thickened vessels (sclerosing hemangioma), and reactive epidermal changes including acanthosis, increased melanin, and hair germs budding down from basal layer. The subcutaneous fat is usually not involved.
  ▶ *Note:* A basal cell carcinoma over a dermatofibroma is almost always a mistaken diagnosis—instead, reactive proliferating hair germs are seen.

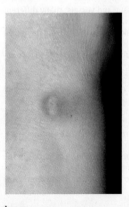

Fig. 26.2 · Dermatofibroma.

► **Variants** include cellular changes (epithelioid, giant, granular, myxoid, desmo-plastic or ossifying cells) as well as unusual patterns (giant or deep penetrating). The latter two patterns are associated with an increased recurrence rate and are sometimes described as fibrous histiocytomas.

🗹 *Caution:* Cellular dermatofibroma, cellular neurothekeoma, and plexiform fibro-histiocytic tumor are three dermatofibroma variants that require careful histo-logic control of margins and follow-up.

Dermatomyofibroma

► **Synonyms:** Plaque-like dermal fibromatosis, Hügel tumor.
► **Definition:** Benign proliferation of myofibroblasts limited to dermis.
► **Clinical features:** Difficult to recognize; typically around shoulder girdle where it presents as large dermal plaque 1–2 cm in size of varying colors; some lesions 10–15 cm. Can also be palmoplantar.
► **Histology:** Proliferation of spindle cells (myofibroblasts) in dermis; poorly cir-cumscribed and may impinge on subcutaneous fat but does not extend along fat septa; cells are usually actin-positive, suggesting smooth muscle or myofibroblas-tic differentiation.
► **Differential diagnosis:** Because of location and site, most important considera-tion is dermatofibrosarcoma protuberans. Other histologic possibilities: dermato-fibroma, hypertrophic scar, keloid, leiomyoma; clinically larger lesions have been confused with morphea.

Hypertrophic Scars and Keloids

► **Definition:** Excessive connective tissue proliferation following an injury; a *hyper-trophic scar* remains confined to the boundaries of the original insult, while a *keloid* proliferates beyond these limits.
► **Pathogenesis:** Predisposing factors include:
  • *Ethnic factors:* Far more common in blacks.
  • **Location:** Sternum, shoulders, neck (after thyroid operation), ear lobes (pierc-ing), ankles, shins, over clavicle, edge of chin, and other sites where skin tension is generally increased.
  • **Type of injury:** Burns and infections more often form keloids, leading to con-tractures and impaired function, as well as considerable cosmetic defects.
  • The biologic reasons for the excess proliferation remain unclear, although most recent data shows that epidermal cytokines drive the dermal reaction.
► **Clinical features:** Firm skin-colored to red nodules and plaques rich in telangiec-tases. Keloids have irregular "fingers" growing at the periphery. Both may be tender, painful, or pruritic (Fig. 26.**3**).
► **Histology:**
  • *Normal scar:* Fibroblasts arranged in loose myxoid stroma; as healing proceeds, collagen fibers are laid down parallel to epidermis.
  • *Hypertrophic scar:* Fibroblasts scattered, admixed between myxoid stroma and dense collagen bundles.
  • *Keloid:* Similar to hypertrophic scar, but large amorphous bundles of eosinophilic collagen; later hyalinized.
► **Therapy:**
  • *Hypertrophic scar:* Improvement with time can be expected; cryotherapy may speed involution.
  • *Keloid:* No good therapy. Never make any bold promises of success. Possibilities include:

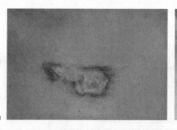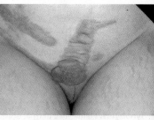

Fig. 26.3 · **Keloids. a** Hypertrophic scar with transition to keloid. **b** Large keloids.

- Injection of corticosteroids, ideally using a needleless injection system; use 2.5–5.0 mg triamcinolone/mL; inject every month for 6 months and re-assess.
- Injections can be combined with cryotherapy; freezing the lesion 5 minutes before injection makes injecting physically easier and may have an additive effect.
- Pressure dressing with pressure > 24 mm Hg is useful for fresh wounds and especially for burn scars as prophylactic measure. Variety of pressure suits and wraps available.
- Tangential debulking excision can be combined with intralesional steroids, cryotherapy, and pressure dressings.
- Debulking can also be combined with postoperative radiation therapy; usually 10–20 Gy are given in 3–5 divided doses.
- Excision and coverage with skin graft can be considered only if it is certain that the new wound can heal under less skin tension with exogenous pressure applied and that the graft donor site can be placed under prophylactic pressure.
- ▶ *Note:* Simple re-excision almost never works and often worsens the problem greatly.
- Silicon gel sheeting for at least 12 hours daily; early studies were promising but recent ones less so.

Fibromatoses

▶ **Definition:** Confusing group of benign fibrous proliferations, which can be locally aggressive and tend to recur, but are not capable of metastasis.
▶ **Classification** (based on Enzinger and Weiss):
  • *Superficial fibromatoses* (arise in fascia, grow slowly, relatively small):
    - Dupuytren contracture (palmar fibromatosis).
    - Ledderhose contracture (plantar fibromatosis).
    - Peyronie disease (penile fibromatosis).
    - Infantile digital fibromatosis.
    - Torticollis.
    - Gingival fibromatosis.
  • *Deep fibromatoses* (desmoid tumors, arise from muscle aponeuroses, growing rapidly, are locally aggressive, but do not metastasize):
    - Extra-abdominal fibromatosis.
    - Abdominal fibromatosis.
    - Intra-abdominal fibromatosis.

- Pelvic fibromatosis.
- Mesenteric fibromatosis.
- Desmoids in Gardner syndrome (p. 368).
- Retroperitoneal fibromatosis (Osmond disease).

- **Clinical features:** The superficial lesions are characterized by firms nodules, bands, and strands of fibrous tissue, leading to tissue deviation (Peyronie disease or torticollis) or contractions (Dupuytren or Ledderhose disease).
- **Histology:** Irregular proliferations of myofibroblasts and fibroblasts; superficial variants usually parallel to the skin surface; deeper variants more cellular and highly irregular.
- **Differential diagnosis:** All connective tissue proliferations and tumors must be considered. The superficial lesions are clinically diagnosable; the deeper ones usually present as a mass and are harder to suspect.
- **Therapy:** All are hard to treat; infantile digital fibromatosis often resolves spontaneously. Fortunately, none are the direct responsibility of dermatologists.

Nodular Fasciitis

- **Definition:** Rapidly growing, histologically atypical reactive fascial proliferation.
- **Pathogenesis:** Trauma often appears to be trigger.
- **Clinical features:** More common in young adults; presents as rapidly growing tender nodule typically on ulnar aspect of forearm; variant in children on scalp (*cranial fasciitis*). Usually grows over 4–6 weeks, is larger than 3 cm, firm, and adherent to fascia. Spontaneous regression over 2 years.
- **Histology:** Myxoid stroma containing whorled arrangements of fibroblasts, some of which may be bizarre; periphery often contains inflammatory infiltrate.
- **Differential diagnosis:** Clinically lipoma usual consideration; histologically misdiagnosed as fibrosarcoma until entity firmly established.
- **Therapy:** None needed, but not clinically relevant, as excisional biopsy is done for diagnostic purposes.

Dermatofibrosarcoma Protuberans

- **Definition:** Low-grade malignant fibrous tumor always presenting in the skin.
- **Epidemiology:** Only common cutaneous sarcoma; prevalence 1/100 000.
- **Pathogenesis:** Usually specific reciprocal translation (17;22) (q22;q13) forming a ring chromosome; gene for type $1\alpha1$ collagen is placed under control of platelet-derived growth factor (PDGF), leading to excessive collagen deposition.
- **Clinical features:** Firm, slowly growing skin-colored or erythematous tumor, usually around shoulder girdle; resembles a scar (Fig. 26.4). Gradually develops multiple nodules and bizarre configuration.
  - ◨ *Note:* If a lesion looks like a scar but patient denies trauma or surgery, always consider dermatofibrosarcoma protuberans and sclerosing basal cell carcinoma.
- **Variants** include pigmented form (*Bednar tumor*) and juvenile form (*giant cell fibroblastoma*).
- **Histology:** Small bundles of fibroblasts and fibrocytes with storiform or radial pattern; infiltrate subcutaneous fat creating thickened septae and also have irregular peripheral spread. Mitoses uncommon. Tumor cells CD34-positive.
- **Diagnostic approach:** Adequate biopsy specimen essential; even if excision biopsy is impossible, provide a generous ellipse.
- **Differential diagnosis:** Deep or atypical dermatofibroma, leiomyosarcoma, myofibroblastic sarcoma.

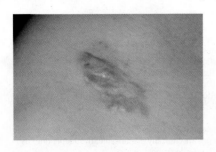

Fig. 26.**4** · Dermatofibrosarcoma protuberans.

► **Therapy:** Best chance for cure is a complete initial excision with a 3 cm margin of safety. The excision should include the underlying fascia. Micrographic surgery is very useful in this setting, coupled with CD34 staining. Follow-up should be every 6 months.

Myofibroblastic Sarcoma

► **Definition:** Low-grade sarcoma usually involving the skin or less often subcutaneous connective tissue.
► **Clinical features:** Favors extremities, relatively well-circumscribed painless nodule without distinguishing features; rarely ulcerated. Can be locally aggressive; occasionally rapidly growing forms may metastasize.
► **Histology:** Fascicles of tumor cells, sometimes storiform or herringbone pattern with varying degrees of nuclear atypia. The myofibroblasts are positive for smooth muscle actin and muscle-specific actin (HHF35), but usually negative for CD34.
► **Differential diagnosis:** Higher grade fibrosarcomas, dermatofibrosarcoma protuberans, leiomyosarcoma.

Malignant Fibrous Histiocytoma (MFH)

► **Definition:** Malignant soft tissue tumor with varying histologic patterns presumably derived from connective tissue elements.
► **Pathogenesis:** Controversial. For years it was considered the most common soft tissue tumor of adults, but now many of its variants have been reestablished as other sarcomas.
► **Clinical features:** Subcutaneous or deep soft tissue tumor; most common sites thighs and buttocks. Frequently recurs and can metastasize; cutaneous metastases occasionally seen.
► **Histology:** The best established variant is the myxoid MFH, also known as myxofibrosarcoma. Other patterns include inflammatory, xanthomatous, giant cell, and angiomatoid variants. Nuclear atypia and mitoses are common.
► **Differential diagnosis:** Other sarcomas.
► **Therapy:** Generous excision and follow-up every 6 months.

Atypical Fibroxanthoma

► **Definition:** Superficial malignant fibrous histiocytoma; dermal tumor with bizarre histologic pattern and low-grade malignant behavior.
► **Clinical features:** Usual lesion develops rapidly in sun-exposed skin of older patients; 1–2 cm erythematous, crusted lesion. Much less commonly similar le-

sions appear in younger patients without extensive sun exposure; these tend to grow slowly but achieve a greater size.

▶ **Histology:** Mixture of extremely bizarre spindled and epithelioid cells with wildly irregular nuclei embedded in fibrous stroma. Formerly considered a pseudomalignancy (*too bizarre to be malignant*), but now acknowledged as a low-grade malignancy.

▶ **Differential diagnosis:** Basal cell carcinoma, amelanotic melanoma, poorly differentiated squamous cell carcinoma, other sarcomas. Immunohistochemistry allows the exclusion of other possibilities, but there are no stains specific for atypical fibroxanthoma.

▶ **Therapy:** Complete excision; yearly follow-up.

Epithelioid Sarcoma

▶ **Definition:** Highly malignant sarcoma of uncertainty differentiation.

▶ **Clinical features:** Most patients are young adults; most typical sites are extremities and scalp. Firm subcutaneous nodules, sometimes ring-shaped and occasionally ulcerated. Recurrences and metastases are common, even years after removal of primary tumor.

▶ **Histology:** Cellular nodules with oval, polygonal, spindled, or epithelioid nuclei. Often necrosis with peripheral palisading, as well as hemorrhage and cyst formation. Vascular invasion common.

▶ **Differential diagnosis:** Early lesions often mistaken for granuloma annulare (annular, necrosis with peripheral palisading) or infections; later other sarcomas, especially synovial sarcoma, are the main consideration.

▶ **Therapy:** Generous excision is required; when limited to a distal limb, amputation is often required for cure.

26.2 Smooth Muscle Tumors

Overview

▶ **Definition:** Leiomyomas are benign smooth muscle tumors. They are often tender or painful; see ANGEL list (p. 714). Their classification is shown in Table 26.**1**.

Piloleiomyoma

▶ **Clinical features:** Usually start in puberty; red-brown 1–2 cm papules, usually multiple and on extremities; often tender.

▶ **Histology:** Bundles of dermal smooth muscle, resembling arrector pili muscles, but larger; nuclei are blunted or cigar-shaped.

▶ **Differential diagnosis:** Clinically mast cell tumor, Spitz nevus, adnexal tumor; histologically, neurofibroma.

▶ **Therapy:** Solitary or few lesions can be excised; unfortunately, usually so many that surgery is not an option. Phenoxybenzamine (10 mg 3–6 × daily) combined with nifedipine (10 mg t.i.d.) may relieve pain by relaxing smooth muscle fibers.

▶ **Multiple cutaneous leiomyomas** (MIM code 160800) have mutation in fumarate hydratase on chromosome 1q; also present in some solitary tumors. Such patients should be evaluated for leiomyomas elsewhere. Hereditary leiomyomatosis (MIM code 605839) has mutations in the same gene, but also uterine leiomyomas and leiomyosarcomas as well as papillary renal cell carcinomas.

Table 26.1 · Classification of cutaneous leiomyomas

Type	Frequency (%)	Origin
Piloleiomyoma	60	Arrector pili muscle
Genital leiomyoma	20	Dartos, other genital smooth muscle; may also arise from erectile muscle of nipple
Angioleiomyoma	20	Smooth muscle of vessel wall

Genital Leiomyoma

▶ **Clinical features:** Flat plaques, rarely larger than 2 cm.
▶ **Histology:** Same microscopic features as piloleiomyoma.
▶ **Differential diagnosis:** Cyst, fibroma; nipple adenoma.
▶ **Therapy:** Excision.

Angioleiomyoma

▶ **Clinical features:** Usually on the legs of middle-aged women; 1–2 cm painful subcutaneous nodule.
▶ **Histology:** Circumscribed nodular tumor consisting of bundles of smooth muscle surrounding thick-walled vessels.
▶ **Differential diagnosis:** Other subcutaneous masses—cysts, lipomas, fibromas.
▶ **Therapy:** Excision.

Cutaneous Leiomyosarcoma

▶ **Epidemiology:** Patients usually middle-aged; both sexes affected.
▶ **Clinical features:** Usually on trunk arising from arrector pili or extremities arising from vascular smooth muscle. Less often on breast or genitalia. Generally asymptomatic low-growing nodule, rarely ulcerated. Often overlooked.
▶ **Histology:** Same pattern as leiomyoma, but more nuclear atypia and mitoses. Very difficult histologic diagnosis.
▶ **Differential diagnosis:** Dermatofibrosarcoma protuberans, malignant fibrous histiocytoma; main problem is corresponding leiomyoma.
▶ **Therapy:** Excision with 1–2 cm safety margin and microscopic control of margins.
▶ **Prognosis:** Excellent prognosis for cutaneous and subcutaneous leiomyosarcomas; > 95 % 5-year survival. Follow-up every 6 months.

26.3 Tumors of Fat

Nevus Lipomatosus Superficialis

▶ **Synonym:** Hoffmann–Zurhelle nevus.
▶ **Definition:** Congenital malformation with islands of fat high in dermis.
▶ **Clinical features:** Grouped papules or plaque, usually around buttocks, with yellow tones (Fig. 26.**5**).
▶ **Histology:** Islands of normal fat in the dermis, often almost impinging on the epidermis; not uncommonly associated with melanocytic nevus.

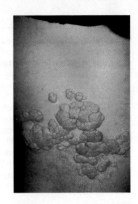

Fig. 26.**5** · Nevus lipomatosus.

▶ **Differential diagnosis:** Connective tissue nevus; histologically, focal dermal hypoplasia.
▶ **Therapy:** Smaller lesions can be excised.

Lipoma

▶ **Definition:** Most common benign soft tissue tumor; accumulation of mature fat cells.
▶ **Clinical features:** Soft, lobulated, freely movable round or oval subcutaneous mass; usually appears in adult life; rarely symptomatic. Variants include:
  • *Angiolipoma:* Usually painful (see ANGEL p. 714), rich in small vessels that may have thromboses.
  • *Spindle cell lipoma:* Almost always on nape of older men; painless; bands of spindled fibrous cells admixed with fat cells.
  • *Mobile lipoma:* Usually on forearm; moveable over several cm; microscopically encapsulated; probably posttraumatic.
  • *Lumbosacral lipoma:* Congenital, often associated with spina bifida.
  • *Pleomorphic lipoma:* Clinically banal; histologically features giant cells and even lipoblasts.
▶ **Histology:** Normal fat tissue surround by a wispy fibrous capsule; variants as described above.
▶ **Differential diagnosis:** Cysts, other subcutaneous tumors.
▶ **Therapy:** Excision. In most cases, one can make an incision and manipulate out the lipoma; in other instances, complete excision required.

Multiple Lipomas

Two main groups:
▶ **Familial multiple lipomas** (MIM code 151900): Multiple lipomas, can be painful or disfiguring; possible association with diabetes mellitus. Individual troublesome lesions can be excised.
▶ **Dercum disease (adiposis dolorosa):** Puzzling condition with painful lipomas; limited to middle-aged women, often overweight. Lesions often angiolipomas.

Lipomatoses

► **Definition:** Multiple localized accumulations of fat, which may be symmetric or asymmetric.
► **Benign symmetric lipomatosis of Launois–Bensaude** (MIM code: 151800).
  • Type I: Cervical (Madelung neck).
  • Type II: Shoulder girdle; weightlifter form.
  • Type III: Pelvic (Engels).
  • Often associated with alcoholism and liver disease. Patients look muscular and healthy, but have paradoxical excess fatty deposits with other profound metabolic problems. No good treatment.
► **Proteus syndrome** (p. 414) often with multiple lipomas.
► **Michelin tire baby syndrome** (MIM code 156610): Extremely rare syndrome in which children develop multiple folds of skin resembling the advertising figure for Michelin tires; sometimes underlying fat tissue; in other instances fibrous tissue or smooth muscle. Often associated with mental retardation and other problems.

Hibernoma

► **Definition:** Benign tumor of embryonal brown fat.
► **Clinical features:** Tumor of young adults (not newborns); slowly growing asymptomatic tumor on trunk; can be large (5–10 cm).
► **Histology:** Fat cells are filled with many small vacuoles, typical of brown fat, which is also found in hibernating mammals.
► **Differential diagnosis:** Lipoma, liposarcoma.
► **Therapy:** Excision.

Liposarcoma

► **Definition:** Uncommon malignant tumor of fatty tissues.
► **Epidemiology:** Usually appear after age 40; do not develop from lipomas. Liposarcomas are the most common sarcoma, but are extremely rare in the skin.
► **Classification:** Based on histologic features: well-differentiated, myxoid, round cell and pleomorphic, with prognostic differences. Well-differentiated and myxoid have much better 5-year survival figures.
► **Clinical features:** Mass in deep soft tissues, retroperitoneum; about 5% of myxoid liposarcomas are cutaneous. Slowly growing subcutaneous mass; never clinically distinct.
► **Histology:** Useful in typing and thus in prognosis.
► **Therapy:** Radical excision.

26.4 Vascular Malformations and Tumors

Overview

Vascular embryogenesis is a complex process with many different types of aberrant vessel formation leading to *malformations*. Vascular *tumors* or new proliferations of vessels after birth are typically lobular and generally benign, although malignant and borderline variants are occasionally seen. The following primarily histopathological classification is useful, although we have varied from it slightly to group clinically similar disorders together:

➤ Malformations.
  ● Capillary.
  ● Venous.
  ● Lymphatic.
➤ Dilated vessels.
➤ Hemangiomas and benign tumors.
➤ Tumors of glomus cells and pericytes.
➤ Borderline (low grade) malignant tumors.
➤ Malignant tumors.

Malformations

Nevus Flammeus
➤ **Synonym:** Port wine stain.
➤ **Definition:** Congenital localized vascular malformation consisting of dilated capillaries.
➤ **Classification:**
  ● *Medial form:* Usually nape or forehead (stork bite nevus).
  ● *Lateral form:* Follows peripheral or cranial nerve.
➤ **Clinical features:**
  ● Circumscribed, flat pink or deeper red area; present at birth; grows with child. In adult life, tendency to thicken, develop papules.
  ● Median lesions may regress during infancy; lateral ones do not.
  ● Median lesions are not associated with other abnormalities; lateral ones may be.
➤ **Diagnostic approach:** Children with lateral lesions should be followed for vascular, neurologic, or orthopedic problems. Biopsy not needed.
➤ **Therapy:** Camouflage; capillaries can be destroyed with pulsed dye or copper vapor laser; later papules destroyed with Nd:YAG laser.

Sturge–Weber Syndrome
➤ **MIM code:** 185300.
➤ **Clinical features:**
  ● Unilateral nevus flammeus in distribution of 1st or 2nd branch of trigeminal nerve with ipsilateral vascular abnormalities of meninges or cortex (Fig. 26.**6**).
  ● Epilepsy (80 %), mental retardation, contralateral hemiparesis, and muscle atrophy. CNS lesions may calcify.
  ● Glaucoma, especially when 1st branch is involved.
➤ **Diagnostic approach:** Multidisciplinary approach with neurologic and ophthalmologic follow-up.
➤ **Therapy:** Nevus flammeus can be treated as outlined above.

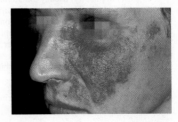

Fig. 26.**6** · Sturge–Weber syndrome.

Klippel–Trénaunay–Weber Syndrome
► **MIM code:** 149000.
► **Clinical features:**
  • Nevus flammeus involving a limb, with hypertrophy of underlying bones and muscles.
  • Frequent associated arteriovenous fistulas, potentially leading to high-output cardiac failure.
► **Diagnostic approach:** Angiologic evaluation to exclude shunts.
► **Therapy:** Many measures tried to limit distorted blood flow: ligation of anastomoses, microembolization, laser coagulation; in milder cases, compression stockings.

Venous Malformation
► **Synonym:** Cavernous hemangioma.
► **Clinical features:** Venous malformations are deeper, softer and unlikely to regress spontaneously. They are readily compressible. Because of their slow flow, venous malformations are subject to thromboses and thus can be painful. Thromboses almost unheard of in capillary and arterial malformations. Color of the overlying skin determined by depth of vascular structures.
► Multiple venous malformations may be familial.
► **Diagnostic approach:** Imaging studies to exclude arteriovenous shunts, thromboses, and internal malformations.
► **Differential diagnosis:** Hemangioma, nevus flammeus.
► **Therapy:** If limited to a limb, compression therapy and perhaps anticoagulants. Best active treatment is sclerotherapy, followed by surgery.

Congenital Lymphedema
► **Pathogenesis:** A "negative" vascular malformation, associated with defective or absent lymphatics leading to swollen limbs.
► **Clinical features:**
  • *Familial congenital lymphedema:*
    – *Synonym:* Nonne–Milroy syndrome.
    – *MIM code:* 153100.
    – *Pathogenesis:* Mutation in VEGF receptor 3 gene; autosomal dominant inheritance.
    – *Clinical features:* Lymphedema present at birth or infancy; usually involves both legs; associated with pleural effusions and ascites.
  • *Familial lymphedema praecox:*
    – *Synonym:* Meige syndrome.
    – *Pathogenesis:* Mutation in transcription factor in the forkhead family (*FOXC2*); autosomal dominant inheritance.
    – Onset in puberty; usually unilateral without other findings.
  • *Sporadic primary lymphedema:* No family history.
► **Differential diagnosis:** Much more common is lymphedema secondary to obstruction. Causes include filariasis, lymph node dissection, irradiation or involvement by metastatic disease, recurrent erysipelas.
► **Therapy:** Early and aggressive use of compression bandages or stockings; in more extreme cases, home compression machine is essential.

Lymphangiomas
► **Definition:** Group of lymphatic malformations and proliferations involving skin and soft tissue.

Clinical features:

- *Lymphangiectases:* Small dilated primarily clear vesicles; also known as cutaneous chylous reflux. Appear secondary to lymphatic obstruction or chronic lymphedema.
- *Lymphangioma circumscriptum:* Congenital lesion that may first become apparent in childhood; multiple grouped vesicles, clear to red-blue, usually described as resembling frogspawn. Usually on extremities. Generally connect to deeper lymphatic vessels, so excision is often followed by recurrences. Smaller lesions can be treated with laser ablation or contact cryotherapy.
- *Cystic hygroma:* Congential deep unilocular lymphatic malformation; typically involves soft tissue of face, neck; less often axilla or groin. Can be deforming. Surgery is difficult, but usually the most effective approach.

Caution: Patients with lymphangiomas and lymphedema are predisposed to cellulitis.

Dilated Vessels

Nevus Araneus

- **Synonym:** Spider nevus.
- **Definition:** Acquired vascular lesion consisting of central dilated arteriole and radiating capillaries.
- **Clinical features:**
  - 2–4 mm red papule from which extend fine telangiectases (thus spider nevus) (Fig. 26.**7**).
  - Usually face or décolletage.
  - Associated with pregnancy, liver disease, and CREST syndrome (p. 219).
- **Diagnostic approach:** If multiple lesions or sudden onset, search for cause.
- **Therapy:** Destruction of central vessel with laser or intense pulsed light source (IPL).

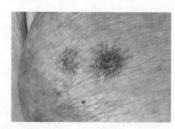

Fig. 26.**7** · Spider nevus.

Arteriovenous Fistula

- **Synonym:** Cirsoid aneurysm.
- Uncommon nodular vascular lesion, usually follows trauma. Often on forehead or distal extremities. Typically 1–2 cm nodule, which may pulsate or have auditory thrill. Histology shows vessels with extremely thick walls. Excision curative.

Venous Lake

- Common lesion on lips. Compressible, dome-shaped blue-pink nodule. When darker, occasionally mistaken for pigmented lesion. Harmless, but easily excised or ablated.

Telangiectases

► **Definition:** Irreversible dilation of cutaneous capillaries and postcapillary venules.
► **Classification (p. 706):**
- *Primary telangiectases* (congenital or without obvious cause):
  – Generalized essential telangiectases.
  – Unilateral nevoid telangiectasia syndrome.
  – Poikiloderma syndromes.
  – Ataxia-telangiectasia.
  – Hereditary benign telangiectases.
  – Hereditary hemorrhagic telangiectases.
  – Telangiectasia macularis eruptiva perstans (combination of telangiectases and mast cell disease).
- *Secondary telangiectases:*
  – Mycosis fungoides (poikiloderma vasculare atrophicans variant).
  – Rosacea.
  – Dermatomyositis.
  – Systemic sclerosis, especially CREST syndrome.
  – Lupus erythematosus.
  – Xeroderma pigmentosum.
  – Sun-damaged skin.
  – Erythema ab igne.
  – Portal hypertension.
  – Carcinoid syndrome.

Generalized Essential Telangiectases

► **Clinical features:** Common, usually found in middle-aged women, primarily on legs. Depending on severity. ranges from minor nuisance to major cosmetic problem. No associated findings.

Unilateral Nevoid Telangiectasia Syndrome

► **Clinical features:** Unilateral distribution of multiple spider nevi with prominent halos; usually starts in the shoulder girdle or upper arm region. May be congenital or acquired; latter usually in women and estrogen-driven (pregnancy, oral contraceptives). If troublesome in postmenopausal women, can be treated with antiestrogens; otherwise, laser destruction of individual lesions.

Hereditary Benign Telangiectases

► **MIM code:** 187260.
► **Clinical features:** Telangiectases with slight atrophy; often larger and thus venous. No associated hemorrhage or systemic problems. Likely autosomal dominant inheritance, but with expression primarily in women.

Hereditary Hemorrhagic Telangiectasia

► **Synonym:** Osler–Weber–Rendu syndrome.
► **MIM code:** 187300.
► **Definition:** Inherited disorder with cutaneous and mucosal telangiectases with tendency to bleeding.
► **Pathogenesis:** Autosomal dominant inheritance. Two well-established mutations in genes that interact with transforming growth factor-β to regulate small vessel growth: *HHT1* codes for endoglin gene at 9q34.1 while *HHT2* codes for activin receptor kinase 1 at 12q13. Other rarer genes also under consideration.

▶ **Clinical features:**
- Most common presenting feature frequent nosebleeds in childhood.
- During puberty, development of telangiectases, favoring oral and nasal mucosa, as well as internal organs; also on face, hands.
- Internal complications include gastrointestinal bleeding (from telangiectases) and pulmonary arteriovenous fistulas, which serve as source of septic emboli for CNS.

▶ **Diagnostic approach:** History, physical examination including gastrointestinal studies, pulmonary imaging.

▶ **Differential diagnosis:** Fabry disease and other causes of multiple angiokeratomas.

Ataxia-telangiectasia

▶ **Synonym:** Louis–Bar syndrome.

▶ **MIM code:** 208900.

▶ **Definition:** Syndrome with profound neurological and immune defects associated with telangiectases.

▶ **Epidemiology:** Frequency 1: 40000; autosomal recessive inheritance. Carriers appear to have higher risk for internal malignancies.

▶ **Pathogenesis:** Mutation in *ATM* gene at 11q22.3, responsible for DNA surveillance and repair.

▶ **Clinical features:**
- *Progressive cerebellar ataxia:* Major problem; children usually bedridden as infants.
- *Telangiectases:* Almost always conjunctival at first, later facial or more widespread.
- Other skin findings include café-au-lait macules, premature graying, sclerodermoid changes, and peculiar aggressive form of necrobiosis lipoidica.
- Combined immune defect with defects in both humoral and cellular immunity, leading to multiple infections.
- Endocrine problems—early-onset insulin-resistant diabetes mellitus.
- Patients who survive infections have 100-fold increased incidence of malignancies, especially lymphoma and leukemia.

▶ **Prognosis:** Dismal; few survive childhood.

▶ **Therapy:** Bone marrow transplantation; if not available, then supportive care. Must be done early to minimize neurological defects.

Cutis Marmorata Telangiectasia Congenita

▶ **Synonyms:** Van Lohuizen syndrome, congenital generalized phlebectasia.

▶ **MIM code:** 219500.

▶ **Pathogenesis:** Sporadic disorder; cause unknown.

▶ **Clinical features:**
- Present at birth; dilated vessels with striking marbled pattern that varies little with temperature. Most improve slowly over time. Can be associated with necrosis and ulcerations.
- Midline nevus flammeus is sometimes marker.
- About 30% of patients have systemic findings including limb hypo- or hypertrophy, craniofacial anomalies, glaucoma, and mental retardation.

▶ **Diagnostic approach:** History, clinical examination.

▶ **Therapy:** Nothing effective.

Angiokeratomas

▶ **Definition:** Capillary-lymphatic malformation in upper dermis associated with hyperkeratotic epidermis.
▶ **Clinical features:** Several clinically distinct forms:
- *Solitary angiokeratoma:* Multihued or black hyperkeratotic papule, usually on legs of children; differential diagnostic considerations include melanocytic nevus and malignant melanoma (Fig. 26.**8**).

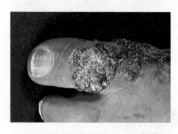

Fig. 26.**8** · Angiokeratoma.

- *Angiokeratoma circumscriptum*: Verrucous blue-black plaque usually on extremities; present at birth, grows with patient. Can also be mistaken for malignant melanoma.
- *Angiokeratoma of Mibelli*: Small blue-black hyperkeratotic papules of distal extremities, usually in children with acrocyanosis or cold injury; differential diagnosis including warts.
- *Angiokeratoma Fordyce*: Tiny violet papules on scrotum or labia of older adults; differential diagnosis includes senile angioma when nongenital.
- *Fabry disease:*
  - *Synonym:* Angiokeratoma corporis diffusum.
  - *MIM code:* 315500.
  - Pathogenesis: Mutation in *GLA* gene at Xq22 coding for α-galactosidase; X-linked recessive inheritance; lyosomal storage disorder.
  - *Clinical features:* Multiple angiokeratomas, typically starting around umbilicus; acral paresthesias, hypohidrosis, heat intolerance. Corneal dystrophy. Renal, cardiac, and CNS vascular problems.
  - *Differential diagnosis:* Osler–Weber–Rendu syndrome, senile angiomas.
  - *Therapy:* Enzyme replacement therapy possible.
- Other metabolic diseases including fucosidosis, Kanzaki syndrome, and Spangler syndrome; check pediatric genetic sources.
▶ **Diagnostic approach:** Despite this puzzling list, the clinical pictures are usually quite distinct. A solitary or plaque-like lesion will usually be biopsied to exclude a pigmented lesion. Multiple scrotal or vulvar lesions are clear. Porokeratosis of Mibelli is usually overlooked. The metabolic disorders usually present with other findings, so the dermatologist rarely has the chance to make the diagnosis.
▶ **Therapy:** Individual small lesions can be destroyed with lasers; large plaques are best excised.

Hemangioma

▶ **Synonym:** Capillary hemangioma.
▶ **Definition:** Benign vascular tumor, which typically appears at birth or just thereafter.

Pathogenesis: Sporadic event; angiogenesis is very active in utero and presumably perturbations in vascular growth control mechanisms are responsible.

Clinical features:

- Raised red to purple soft nodules that can become very large. About 30% can be seen at birth, but most appear later and all continue to grow (Fig. 26.**9**). Tumors can be compressed, but do not disappear with diascopy.

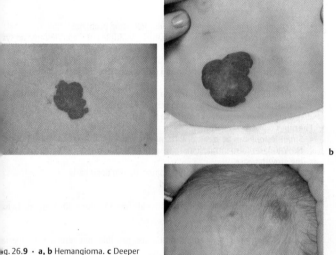

g. 26.**9** · **a, b** Hemangioma. **c** Deeper emangioma without bright red color, erhaps in regression.

- Those which appear after birth are 2–5 × more common in girls.
- Congenital hemangiomas typically are large nodules with a rim of dilated vessels; they are divided into rapidly involuting and noninvoluting forms. No sex predilection.
- Old distinction of capillary versus cavernous hemangioma rarely made today. The deeper vessels in cavernous lesions are usually venous malformations and do not regress.
- Telangiectatic hemangiomas may mimic nevus flammeus, but continue to grow.
- Complications include:
  - Obstruction of vital structures: eyes, nose, mouth.
  - *Bleeding:* Serious events surprisingly rare.
- During the first months of life, hemangiomas can continue to grow. After about years of age, no further growth is anticipated and regression starts. It may take many years and often leaves behind scar or loose skin.

Diagnostic approach: Clinical diagnosis:

  ☐ *Note:* Three questions to separate hemangioma from malformation are listed in Table 26.**2**.

Table 26.2 · Separating hemangioma from malformation

Question	Hemangioma	Malformation
Present at birth?	Usually no; appears in first weeks of life	Yes
Growing?	Yes	No
Regressing?	Yes	No

- If multiple lesions are present, consider following problems:
  - Generalized eruptive hemangiomatosis: Multiple cutaneous lesions; no systemic involvement.
  - Diffuse neonatal hemangiomatosis: Multiple cutaneous lesions, plus cardiac, gastrointestinal, hepatic and pulmonary hemangiomas. Probably with hemorrhage, cardiac failure.
  - *PHACES syndrome:* **P**osterior fossa malformation, **h**emangiomas (mainly facial); **a**rterial, **c**ardiac, **e**ye, and **s**ternal anomalies.
  - Blue rubber bleb nevus syndrome (p. 458).
- ► **Therapy:**
  - Small lesions can be treated with intense pulsed light source, pulsed dye or Nd:YAG laser (also intralesional); treatment should be started early, not awaiting growth phase.
  - Contact cryotherapy is alternative approach; also done early.
  - Residual lesions or scars best excised.
  - Aggressive periorificial lesions:
    - Intralesional or systemic corticosteroids (prednisolone 20–30 mg daily for 2–3 weeks).
    - Interferon-α2 (systemic).
    - Sclerosing therapy or embolization also possible, but reserved for special centers.
  - ◪ *Note:* The effectiveness of IPL and lasers has shifted the trend toward treating hemangiomas. Nonetheless, some parents may prefer to allow nature to take its course, especially for small truncal lesions, and they should be offered this option.

Senile Angioma
- ► **Synonym:** Cherry angioma.
- ► **Definition:** Common small capillary proliferation, usually appears in middle-aged adults.
- ► **Clinical features:** Small smooth ruby-red papules, usually on trunk and multiple. No associated findings.
- ► **Differential diagnosis:** Clinically distinct; if thrombosed, can be confused with pigmented lesions.
- ► **Therapy:** None needed; laser destruction easy if desired.

Pyogenic Granuloma
- ► **Synonym:** Eruptive hemangioma.
- ► **Definition:** Rapidly growing capillary hemangioma usually developing after trauma (Fig. 26.**10**).
- ► **Clinical features:**
  - Typically eroded, often weeping or friable tumor that reaches several cm in size over week; history of trauma.

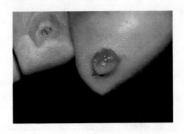

Fig. 26.**10** · Pyogenic granuloma.

- Many different clinical patterns:
  - Common on digits, especially nail folds.
  - Next most likely site is interdental gingiva, common during pregnancy (epulis of pregnancy).
  - Satellite lesions are common, as are satellite recurrences (central lesion removed; many small peripheral lesions recur).
  - Deeper pyogenic granulomas are often intravenous.
► **Histology:** Eroded epidermis; lobular proliferation of new vessels in dermis associated with neutrophilic infiltrate.
► **Diagnostic approach:** Sudden history, clinical appearance, histology.
► **Differential diagnosis:** Usually clinically distinct; nail lesions should always be studied histologically to exclude amelanotic malignant melanoma. Polypoid lesions on feet can be confused with Kaposi sarcoma. Satellite lesions usually cause concern; confused with metastases. In patients with HIV/AIDS, also consider bacillary angiomatosis.
► **Therapy:** Excision, cryotherapy, or any other destructive measures.

Tufted Angioma
► Uncommon lesion that clinically looks like bruise, but is persistent and slowly progressive. Histologic pattern very similar to pyogenic granuloma with multiple proliferative nodules. Associated with Kasabach–Merritt syndrome. Treatment difficult; options include surgery, laser ablation, and even ionizing radiation.

Acroangiodermatitis
► **Synonym:** Mali disease, pseudo-Kaposi sarcoma.
► **Definition:** Reactive dilated veins in areas of chronic venous insufficiency produce cutaneous nodules.
► **Clinical features:** Almost exclusively limited to ankles, dorsal aspect of feet; dark red to brown lichenoid papules and plaques, which may become confluent or ulcerate.
► **Histology:** Thickened epidermis over lying dermal proliferation of thick-walled vessels associated with hemosiderin deposition and fibrosis.
► **Diagnostic approach:** Usually obvious, if one appreciates the presence of chronic venous insufficiency. If any questions, biopsy.
► **Differential diagnosis:** Sporadic Kaposi sarcoma.
► **Therapy:** Compression therapy, possible excision.

Acquired Progressive Lymphangioma
► Another rare lesion that can cause differential diagnostic problems.
► Clinically resembles a slowly expanding bruise. Microscopically shows delicate vascular slits very similar to early Kaposi sarcoma.
► Treatment is excision or other destructive measures.

Blue Rubber Bleb Nevus Syndrome

► **MIM code:** 112200.
► **Definition:** Association of multiple cutaneous and gastrointestinal venous mal formations.
► **Pathogenesis:** Most cases sporadic, but autosomal dominant inheritance.
► **Clinical features:**
  • Compressible blue nodules often tender (see ANGEL list, p. 714); present in infancy; involve trunk and extremities.
  • Associated gastrointestinal lesions usually bleed, leading to abdominal pain anemia.
► **Diagnostic approach:** Gastrointestinal evaluation.
  ☒ *Note:* Always search for gastrointestinal bleeding in patients with vascular lesions and anemia.
► **Therapy:** Individual painful lesions can be excised; sclerotherapy and laser ablation also possibilities.

Maffucci Syndrome

► **MIM code:** 166000.
► **Definition:** Combination of lymphatic–venous malformations and endochondromas.
► **Pathogenesis:** Mutations in *PTHR* gene at 3p22-p21.1; exact genetics unclear.
► **Clinical features:**
  • Multiple venous and lymphatic malformations, often favoring the extremities.
  • Vascular neoplasms, especially spindle cell hemangioendothelioma.
  • Endochondromas with a 20% risk of chondrosarcoma.
  • Short stature.
► **Diagnostic approach:** Careful monitoring for malignant change.
► **Therapy:** Vascular lesions treated as for venous malformations.

Glomus Tumor

► **Definition:** Benign tumor arising from the cutaneus glomus or Sucquet–Hoyer anastomosis; group of contractile cells responsible for arteriovenous shunting, especially in digits.
► **Epidemiology:** More common in men, although subungual more common in women.
► **Pathogenesis:** Usually sporadic; multiple lesions may be autosomal dominant inheritance.
► **Clinical features:**
  • Solitary lesions are tender red-blue tumors, often subungual or acral
  • Multiple lesions (*glomus malformations* or *glomangiomas*) are larger, compressible (more clearly associated with vessel spaces) and less likely to be painful (Fig. 26.11).
► **Histology:** Nests of small blue cuboidal cells in dermis, sometimes associated with vascular spaces. *Glomangiomyomas* have spindled rather than cuboidal cells.
► **Diagnostic approach:** Solitary lesions: see ANGEL list for painful tumors (p. 714); multiple lesions, gastrointestinal survey.
► **Therapy:** Excision.

Hemangiopericytoma

► **Clinical features:** Tumor of deep soft tissues with little dermatologic relevance.
► **Histology:** Classic histological picture of spindle cells and staghorn vessels; today felt to be reaction pattern seen in fibrous, neural, and smooth muscle tumors with different biological behaviors.

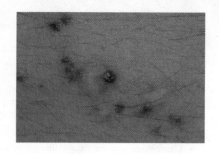

Fig. 26.11 · Multiple glomus tumors.

▶ *Note:* If confronted clinically with a tumor alleged to be hemangiopericytoma, seek expert dermatopathologic consultation.

Hemangioendotheliomas

- **Definition:** Vascular tumors of intermediate-grade biologic behavior; low-grade angiosarcomas.
- **Classification:** All are rare but some of dermatologic significance:
  - *Kaposiform hemangioendothelioma:* Spindle cell tumor of childhood; despite its rarity, most common tumor for Kasabach–Merritt syndrome (platelet consumption coagulopathy).
  - *Dabska tumor (malignant intravascular papillary angioendothelioma):* Head and neck tumor in children with intravascular tumor islands.
  - *Retiform hemangioendothelioma:* Tumor with hobnail endothelial cells; usually on distal extremities with slow, locally aggressive growth pattern.

Malignant Vascular Tumors

Angiosarcoma

- **Definition:** Sarcoma arising from vascular and lymphatic structures.
- **Pathogenesis:** Often caused by ionizing radiation, toxins (especially for hepatic angiosarcoma) or chronic lymphedema. Most recent studies show that lymphatic origin is likely.
- **Clinical features:** Several distinct clinical settings:
  - *Angiosarcoma of scalp:* Initially subtle, but relentless tumor of scalp; early lesions mistaken for vascular malformation; later nodules, ulceration; always extends far beyond apparent clinical margins, so difficult to cure.
  - *Angiosarcoma secondary to chronic lymphedema (Stewart–Treves syndrome):* Mostly common in edematous arm following mastectomy.
  - Postradiation angiosarcoma.
- **Histology:** Highly variable, ranging from benign lobular proliferations to spindle-cell rich areas to epithelioid areas with high mitotic rate and nuclear atypia. New vessels insinuate between strands of collagen.
- **Diagnostic approach:** Must think of disease and then biopsy.
- **Differential diagnosis:** Clinically, many ulcerated tumors such as malignant melanoma; histologically, Kaposi sarcoma.
- **Therapy:**
  - The only chance for cure is complete surgical excision, usually followed by consolidation radiation therapy.
  - Careful margin control; tumor often extends far beyond imagined borders; micrographic surgery valuable.

- Palliative radiation therapy if inoperable.
- Neither chemotherapy and interleukin-2 (intralesional and/or intravenous) ha helped much.
► **Prognosis:** Five-year survival around 10%; both lymphatic and hematogenou spread.

Kaposi Sarcoma

► **Definition:** Virally induced, usually multifocal tumor with many clinical forms.
► **Pathogenesis:** Caused by human herpesvirus 8 (HHV-8); exact mechanism o tumor induction unclear but HHV-8 encodes many growth control genes. HHV- present in all forms of Kaposi sarcoma.
► **Clinical features:**
- *Classic Kaposi sarcoma*: Usually affects elderly men of Jewish or Mediterranea background; slowly growing red-brown patches and plaques on feet or leg (Fig. 26.**12**); when advanced, nodules, ulceration and rarely systemic involve ment. Excellent prognosis.
  ☑ *Note:* Patients tend to die with, rather than from, classic Kaposi sarcoma.

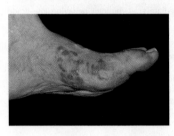

Fig. 26.**12** · Kaposi sarcoma—classic typ

- *Endemic (African) Kaposi sarcoma:* Several types:
  - Lymphadenopathic: Usually in children; resembles lymphoma; usually fata
  - Chronic localized or benign: Similar to classic.
  - Locally aggressive: Ulcerated cutaneous lesions; infiltration of bone.
  - Florid disseminated: Skin and visceral involvement.
- *Iatrogenic Kaposi sarcoma:* Associated with immunosuppression; resolves if im mune status can be restored. Usually diffuse subtle lesions, but can resembl HIV-associated Kaposi sarcoma.
- *HIV-associated Kaposi sarcoma:* Disseminated Kaposi sarcoma, usually in mer often oral involvement or facial involvement, but can occur anywhere. Early le sions oval macules and papules that follow skin tension lines.
► **Diagnostic approach:**
- Biopsy to confirm diagnosis; then evaluate depending on clinical scenario.
- Exclude HIV infection; check HLA-DR status.
- Routine laboratory parameters and chest radiograph.
- Abdominal and lymph node sonography.
- Gastrointestinal examination as directed by signs and symptoms.
- Immune status.
► *Differential diagnosis:*
- Classic Kaposi sarcoma: Acroangiodermatitis, spindle cell hemangiom Kaposiform hemangioendothelioma, leiomyosarcoma.
- HIV-associated Kaposi sarcoma: Bacillary angiomatosis.

Therapy: Varies greatly with form:

- *Local:*
  - Excision.
  - Cryotherapy (better for macular lesions).
  - Intralesional vincristine or vinblastine; also bleomycin.
  - Interferon-α.
  - Fractionated radiation therapy (20–30 Gy in 8–10 sessions).
  - Photodynamic therapy or laser ablation.
- *Systemic:*
  - HAART.
  - Interferon-α 9 million IU subq. 3× weekly; watch for bone marrow toxicity.
  - Etoposide 100 mg/m^2 daily for 3 days; repeat every 28 days.
  - Liposomal doxorubicin 20 mg/m^2 every 28 days.
  - Polychemotherapy with doxorubicin 20 mg/m^2 and vincristine 2 mg every 2–3 weeks.

6.5 Neural Tumors

verview

eural tumors encompass a wide range of lesions, including:

- Malformations and hamartomas.
- Reactive processes.
- Benign neoplasms.
- Malignant neoplasms.

ney may be sporadic or associated with systemic diseases such as neurofibromato-
s or MEN2B.

asal Glioma

Definition: Embryologic herniation of CNS tissue.
Clinical features: Nodule present at birth, usually at root of nose (nasion), flesh-colored, representing outpouching of CNS with incomplete midline closure.
Histology: Glial tissue with astrocytes; no neurons.
Diagnostic approach: Careful evaluation prior to surgery.
⚠ *Caution:* All midline congenital lesions should be evaluated in multidiscipli-
nary fashion with imaging studies to exclude connection to underlying neural
structures. Cutting unprepared in neural tissue is not a pleasant experience.
Differential diagnosis: Vascular malformation, dermoid cyst, lipoma.
Therapy: Excision by neurosurgery.

utaneous Meningioma

Definition: Benign tumor of meningeal tissue.
Pathogenesis: In contrast to glioma, no brain tissue is involved, just meninges.
Clinical features: Three forms:

- *Primary cutaneous meningioma* (*ectopic meningothelial hamartoma*): Present at
  birth; located on scalp, forehead (then similar to nasal glioma), or paravertebral
  region. Highly vascular; can be mistaken for angiosarcoma. Good prognosis.
- *Secondary cutaneous meningioma:* Local spread of CNS meningioma either via
  erosion of skull or following surgery to involve skin. Outlook that of underlying
  tumor.

- *Peripheral meningioma* (*ectopic meningioma*): Meningeal remnants along th tracts of cranial or peripheral nerves; usually in adults. Typical sites includ scalp, perinasal, periauricular, and periorbital. Troublesome because of con pression and destruction of vital structures.
- In each case, dermal or subcutaneous plaques, 2–10 cm, on scalp or followir nerves.
▶ **Diagnostic approach:** Once again, exclude underlying defects.
▶ **Therapy:** Excision.

Neurofibroma

▶ **Definition:** Benign tumor of peripheral nerve sheath.
▶ **Pathogenesis:** Neurofibromas can be solitary or when multiple associated wit neurofibromatosis 1 (p. 362).
▶ **Clinical features:** A solitary neurofibroma is a soft compressible tumor, usual identified in young adult.
▶ **Histology:** Dermal spindle cell tumor, nuclei are long and wavy, often rich in ma cells.
▶ **Diagnostic approach:** Histology; then exclude neurofibromatosis.
▶ **Differential diagnosis:** Usually mistaken for weakly pigmented melanocyt nevus or skin tag.
▶ **Therapy:** Excision.

Neurilemmoma

▶ **Synonym:** Schwannoma.
▶ **Definition:** Benign tumor of Schwann cells.
▶ **Pathogenesis:** Both neurofibroma and neurilemmoma are Schwann cell tumo why they look so different is unclear.
▶ **Clinical features:** Neurilemmomas can be sporadic, associated with neurofibr matosis 2 (p. 364), or multiple without other findings (*schwannomatosis*).
- They are associated with a nerve, most commonly the acoustic nerve.
▪ *Note:* Bilateral acoustic nerve neuromas always suggest neurofibromatosis 2
- Confusingly, neurilemmomas are also seen in neurofibromatosis 1. Sporad neurilemmomas are usually on the extensor aspects of the extremities a sociated with peripheral nerves. Typically 2–5 cm firm nodule, sometim tender.
▶ **Histology:** Circumscribed tumor with orderly array of nuclei (*Antoni patter* sometimes surrounding accumulations of collagen (*Verocay bodies*). Usually ner associated with specimen.
▶ **Diagnostic approach:** Histology; exclude neurofibromatosis 2.
▶ **Differential diagnosis:** Other painful tumors (see ANGEL list p. 714); lipom epidermoid cyst, neurofibroma, rheumatoid nodule.
▶ **Therapy:** Excision.

Granular Cell Tumor

▶ **Synonym:** Abrikosov tumor; granular cell myoblastoma no longer appropriate; infants, congenital epulis.
▶ **Definition:** Benign Schwann cell tumor with characteristic granular cytoplasm
▶ **Clinical features:**
- In infants, tumor of oral mucosa, usually palate.
- In adults, solitary tumor most commonly on tongue, frequently associated w overlying pseudoepitheliomatous hyperplasia leading to mistaken diagnosis squamous cell carcinoma.

- As solitary cutaneous lesion, no site of predilection; 1–2 cm skin-colored nodule; simply a surprise when histologic report comes back.
▶ **Histology:** Dermal tumor with nests and strands of epithelioid cells with granular cytoplasm.
▶ **Therapy:** Excision.

Perineurioma

▶ **Synonym:** Nerve sheath myxoma.
▶ **Definition:** Benign tumor of perineurium—fibrous component of nerve sheath.
▶ **Clinical features:** Solitary asymptomatic tumor, usually in adult women; often acral. Painless; no connection to neurofibromatosis.
▶ **Histology:** Combination of cut-onion pattern and myxoid areas in circumscribed dermal tumor.
▶ **Therapy:** Excision.

Traumatic Neuroma

▶ **Definition:** True neuroma, resulting from trauma to peripheral nerve.
▶ **Clinical features:** Dermal tumor, usually asymptomatic, but can be tender. Several clinical variants including:
- *Morton neuroma:* Painful tumor between metatarsal bones.
- *Pacinian neuroma:* Painful tumor on distal aspect of fingers; microscopically rich in Pacinian corpuscles (pressure receptors).
- *Rudimentary digit:* Following intrauterine autoamputation of accessory digit, sometimes neuroma remains on lateral aspect of 5th digit.
▶ **Histology:** Benign neural fibers in fibrous stroma, sometimes with obvious scar formation.
▶ **Differential diagnosis:** If painful, see ANGEL list p. 714).
▶ **Therapy:** Excision.

Mucosal Neuromas

▶ **Definition:** True neuroma associated with MEN2B syndrome (p. 367).
▶ **Clinical features:** Multiple soft nodules on tongue, lips; enlarged conjunctival nerves may lead to spontaneous lid eversion (Gorlin or everted lid sign).
▶ **Histology:** Circumscribed submucosal neural tissue.
🚺 *Caution:* Be suspicious of diagnosis of traumatic neuroma in the mouth. Oral trauma usually leads to bite fibroma, not bite neuroma. Always check patients for MEN2B because of risk of medullary thyroid carcinoma and phaeochromocytoma.
▶ **Therapy:** Excision if painful or troublesome.

Soft Tissue Ependymoma

▶ **Definition:** Soft tissue tumor arising from ependymal rests; potentially malignant.
▶ **Clinical features:** Slowly growing mass, almost always over sacrum or coccyx in child or young adult, associated with spina bifida and other signs of incomplete spinal closure. About 20% behave in malignant fashion with metastases; rest are locally aggressive.
▶ **Histology:** Poorly circumscribed myxoid-papillary dermal tumor.
▶ **Differential diagnosis:** Often mistaken for pilonidal cyst or sinus.
▶ **Therapy:** Generous excision and careful monitoring.

Malignant Peripheral Nerve Sheath Tumor

▶ **Synonyms:** Neurofibrosarcoma, malignant schwannoma, MPNST.
▶ **Pathogenesis:** Half of MPNST arise in patients with neurofibromatosis; th
 tumors arise from plexiform neurofibromas, not from ordinary cutaneous neurofi
 bromas; most common in men in their 30s. Sporadic MPNST occur in an olde
 population without gender predilection. Trunk and head are most common site
 Rarely following ionizing radiation.
▶ **Clinical features:** Deep, aggressive tumor without distinctive clinical features un
 less neurofibromatosis is present.
▶ **Histology:** Pleomorphic tumor, sometimes with residua of benign precursor
 often with myxoid areas and frank nuclear atypia.
▶ **Therapy:** Generous excision and careful monitoring; five-year survival less tha
 50% with better outlook for sporadic tumors.

27 Other Cutaneous Tumors

27.1 Mast Cell Disorders

Overview

Mast cells are derived from the bone marrow and then populate many organs, including the skin. They are typically in a perivascular location and release a variety of mediators in response to both immune and nonimmune stimulation. Mast cells contain granules; the main mediators in these organelles are histamine and heparin. In addition, a variety of cytokines and prostaglandins are released. Most cutaneous mast cell disease is limited to the skin; in rare instances, the bone marrow or other organs are involved. Many cases of mast cell proliferation are caused by mutations in the c-*kit* gene.

Classification

- **Cutaneous mastocytosis:**
  - Mastocytoma.
  - Urticaria pigmentosa.
  - Diffuse cutaneous or bullous mastocytosis.
  - Telangiectasia macularis eruptiva perstans.
- **Systemic mastocytosis:**
  - Extracutaneous mastocytoma.
  - Indolent systemic mastocytosis, with variant of smoldering mastocytosis.
  - Systemic mastocytosis with associated hematologic non–mast cell lineage disorder.
  - Aggressive systemic mastocytosis.
  - Mast cell leukemia.
  - Mast cell sarcoma.

Mastocytoma

- **Definition:** Localized mast cell accumulation, usually in dermis.
- **Epidemiology:** Often present at birth, but can appear in childhood.

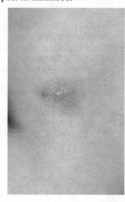

Fig. 27.**1** · Mastocytoma.

▶ **Clinical features:** Red-brown papule or nodule; may urticate or blister whe rubbed (*Darier sign*) (Fig. 27.**1**). Occasionally multiple lesions.

▶ **Histology:** Dermal nodule of uniform cuboidal cells whose granules can be see with Giemsa or toluidine blue staining. Histologically can be confused with derma nevus.

▶ **Differential diagnosis:** Spitz nevus, juvenile xanthogranuloma.

▶ **Therapy:** None needed; if troublesome, excision.

Urticaria Pigmentosa

▶ **Definition:** Multiple mast cell lesions in the skin; may be associated with systemi mast cell disease.

▶ **Clinical features:** Red-brown 1–5 mm disseminated macules or papules; Darie sign positive as lesions easily urticate releasing mast cell mediators (Fig. 27.**2** Sometime release severe enough to cause systemic signs and symptoms (hypoten sion, tachycardia, headache, dizziness). In children, likelihood of spontaneous re mission; in adults usually permanent with risk of systemic disease.

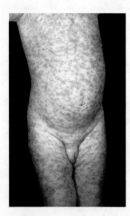

Fig. 27.**2** · Urticaria pigmentosa.

▶ **Histology:** Increased dermal mast cells, usually perivascular, but smaller accumu lations than mastocytoma.

▶ **Differential diagnosis:** When patients describe signs and symptoms, mistake diagnosis of allergic urticaria often made. Careful clinical examination usuall points in the right direction.

▶ **Therapy:** Trial of PUVA; if effective, maintenance therapy needed. Systemic anti histamines and high-potency topical corticosteroids under occlusion.

Diffuse Cutaneous Mastocytosis

▶ Rare form usually seen in infants < 3 years of age; may present as erythroderma o widespread bullae. Clinically can be very alarming, but usually resolves spon taneously.

Telangiectasia Macularis Eruptiva Perstans

▶ Another rare variant, seen in adults, with diffuse red-brown macules and multiple telangiectases. Patients have significant risk of systemic involvement.

Indolent Systemic Mastocytosis

▶ **Definition:** Mast cell proliferation in multiple organs, usually coupled with urticaria pigmentosa.
▶ **Clinical features:** Main symptoms are usually produce by histamine release. A number of medications, such as codeine, can cause mast cell degranulation. The following organ systems most like to be involved:
  • *Gastrointestinal tract:* Nausea, vomiting, diarrhea, duodenal ulcer. Endoscopy and biopsy usually needed for diagnosis.
  • *Bone:* Pain and osteoporosis main findings; bone biopsy or scintigraphy.
  • *Bone marrow:* Proliferation of mast cells or other marrow elements.
  • Hepatosplenomegaly or lymphadenopathy may also be seen.
▶ **Therapy:** Combined treatment with H1 and H2 blockers; oral cromolyn sodium, a mast cell stabilizer, may help gastrointestinal manifestations but is not absorbed to benefit other organs. If indications of mast cell leukemia or other hematologic involvement, refer to a hematology center with special interest in mast cell disease.

27.2 Histiocytoses

The histiocytoses include two separate lineages of diseases—Langerhans cell histocytosis and macrophage disorders. Both Langerhans cell and macrophages are derived from the bone marrow but fulfill different functions. Langerhans cells are dendritic cells involved primarily in antigen presentation, while macrophages are phagocytic cells. There are overlaps both among normal cells and the different disease states. The different histiocytoses can be readily separated with a small battery of special stains, as shown in Table 27.**1**.

Table 27.1 · Simple classification of histiocytoses

Disease	S100[a]	CD1a[a]	CD68[b]	EM (BG)[c]
Langerhans cell disease	+	+	–	+
Sinus histiocytosis with massive lymphadenopathy	+	–	–	–
Macrophage disorders (xanthogranulomas)	–	–	+	–

a S100 and CD1a are reliable markers for Langerhans cells.
b CD68 is the best macrophage marker but others are available.
c Electron microscopy to search for Birbeck granules was formerly the gold standard for identifying Langerhans cells.

Langerhans Cell Histiocytosis (LCH)

▶ **Synonym:** Langerhans cell disease; formerly known as histiocytosis X.
▶ **Definition:** Group of disorders featuring proliferation of Langerhans cells with varying degrees of systemic involvement.

- ▶ **Epidemiology:** All forms of LCH are rare; incidence is around 4/1 000 000.
- ▶ **Pathogenesis:** The proliferations of Langerhans cells are clonal, but in many instances, spontaneous regression occurs, so LCH is somewhere between a malignancy and a reactive proliferation.
- ▶ **Clinical features:** There are four clinical forms with extensive overlap:
  - *Hashimoto–Pritzker disease (congenital self-healing reticulohistiocytosis):* Nodules present at birth, which almost always regress; differential diagnostic considerations include TORCH disorders (p. 65), mastocytoma, congenital leukemia.
  - *Letterer–Siwe disease:* Widespread disease; most common in infants and children; purpuric scaly papules, favoring scalp, seborrheic areas and flexures (Fig. 27.3). High likelihood of systemic involvement. Can appear in adult life.

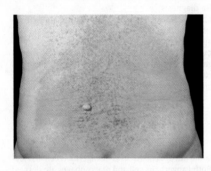

Fig. 27.3 · Langerhans cell histiocytosis, Letterer–Siwe form

  - *Hand–Schüller–Christian disease:* Classic triad of diabetes insipidus, exophthalmos, and bony defects; usually self-limited.
  - *Eosinophilic granuloma:* Single or limited number of lesions usually involving bone; more common in adults.
- ▶ **Histology:** All have same microscopic picture; infiltrate of large epidermotropic cells with kidney-shaped nuclei, often admixed with eosinophils; S100 and CD1 positive. Identification of Birbeck granules no longer required for diagnosis.
- ▶ **Diagnostic approach:** Clinical examination, biopsy. The prognosis depends on the number of organs with functional impairment; most crucial are bone marrow, liver, lungs and spleen. Isolated pulmonary LCH occurs in adult smokers and rarely has any cutaneous findings.
- ▶ **Differential diagnosis:** In infants, seborrheic dermatitis, diaper dermatitis or candidiasis; later Darier disease.
  - ◼ *Note:* Always biopsy infants with purpuric diaper dermatitis or seborrheic dermatitis not responsive to treatment.
- ▶ **Therapy:** Mild or localized disease responds to topical steroids, topical nitrogen mustard is effective but generally avoided in children. Localized lesions are sensitive to radiation therapy or curettage. Systemic disease treated with standard regimen of vinblastine and corticosteroids, or under protocol (consult tertiary centers).
- ▶ **Prognosis:** 30% clear completely; 60% resolve with residua, and 10% die.

ndeterminate Cell Histiocytosis (ICH)

n the past, patients with LCH who did not have Birbeck granules were described as aving ICH. Today, the indeterminate cell is no longer recognized and electron microscopy is rarely performed. ICH is now used to describe cases with overlapping histological features of LCH and macrophage disorders; usually clinically the cases represent widespread xanthogranulomas.

inus Histiocytosis with Massive Lymphadenopathy

- **Synonym:** Rosai–Dorfman disease.
- **Definition:** Uncommon disorder, usually affecting children with massive lymphadenopathy.
- **Pathogenesis:** Etiology unknown.
- **Clinical features:** Most striking presenting finding is massive lymphadenopathy. About 10% of these patients has cutaneous red-brown papules and nodules. The skin and soft tissues are the most common sites of nonnodal SHML.
- **Histology:** Appearance likened to "lymph node within the skin"; proliferation of lymphocytes and large clear sinus histiocytes that ingest the lymphocytes (*emperipolesis*).
- **Differential diagnosis:** Cutaneous lesions not clinically distinct; if solitary, possibilities include juvenile xanthogranuloma, Spitz nevus, mastocytoma, melanocytic nevus.
- **Therapy:** No established treatment for systemic disease; about 10% of patients succumb. Individual skin lesions can be excised.

Macrophage Disorders

The prototypical macrophage disorder is juvenile xanthogranuloma. The rest of the diseases are very uncommon; they may be divided into solitary and local variants, and further classified on what type of macrophage (foamy, ground glass, spindle) dominates. This entire group is sometimes referred to as non-Langerhans cell histiocytosis.

uvenile Xanthogranuloma

- **Epidemiology:** Most common in infants and small children, but can appear in adults.
- **Clinical features:** Yellow to red-brown nodules; favors scalp, trunk or flexures. Number may range from 1 to >20. In children, almost always resolve spontaneously. Variants include plaque-like, disfiguring, and subcutaneous forms. Occasionally ocular involvement with hemorrhage and glaucoma.
  - ◪ *Note:* It is wise to refer all children with juvenile xanthogranuloma to the ophthalmologist.
- **Histology:** Infiltrate of small macrophages, CD68 positive and CD1a negative; occasionally focal S100 positivity. Touton giant cells almost always present (larger wreathed giant cells with lipids inside wreath), as well as eosinophils.
- **Diagnostic approach:** Rare association between juvenile xanthogranuloma, neurofibromatosis 1, and juvenile myelomonocytic leukemia. Check all patients for café-au-lait macules.
- **Differential diagnosis:** Spitz nevus, mastocytoma.

Multicentric Reticulohistiocytosis

► **Epidemiology:** Rare disease, most common in middle-aged women.
► **Clinical features:** Skin-colored to red-brown papules and nodules over joints, resembling rheumatoid nodules; sometimes tiny papules along nail fold (*coral bead sign*). Destructive arthritis, associated autoimmune diseases (lupus erythematosus) as well as occasional paraneoplastic marker.
► **Histology:** Infiltrate of multinucleated giant cells with haphazardly arranged nuclei and ground glass cytoplasm; same changes may be seen in synovium.
► **Differential diagnosis:** Sarcoidosis, rheumatoid arthritis, tuberous and tendinous xanthomas.
► **Therapy:** No satisfactory treatment; methotrexate usually employed; anti-TNF biologicals show promise.

Other Rare Macrophage Disorders
Other diseases with a similar histologic profile are listed in Table 27.**2**. In each instance, solitary lesions can be excised while multiple lesions are not easily influenced..

Table 27.2 · **Rare macrophage disorders**

Disease	Comments
Benign cephalic histiocytosis	Multiple small xanthogranulomas in mid-face of small children; resolves spontaneously
Generalized eruptive histiocytosis	Multiple small red-brown papules which wax and wane; may evolve into other members or group or serve as paraneoplastic marker
Solitary reticulohistiocytoma	Variant of xanthogranuloma with ground class giant cells; not associated with systemic signs and symptoms
Papular xanthoma	Solitary or limited number of foamy xanthogranulomas with normal serum lipid studies; normolipemic xanthoma
Xanthoma disseminatum	Multiple normolipemic xanthomas
Spindle cell xanthogranuloma	Large nodule usually mistaken histologically for dermatofibroma
Progressive nodular histiocytosis	Patients with multiple spindle cell and papular xanthomas; extremely rare

28 *Cutaneous Lymphomas and Leukemia*

28.1 *Benign Lymphocytic Infiltrates*

Overview

Definition: Benign reactive lymphocytic infiltrate, which must be distinguished from a lymphoma.

Classification: The old term "pseudolymphoma" only causes confusion. Many of the lesions formerly diagnosed as pseudolymphoma have turned out to be low-grade B-cell lymphomas; one example is marginal zone lymphoma. There are nonetheless several situations where benign lymphocytic infiltrates do occur in the skin. All lesions are clinically similar, presenting as red-brown nodules.

- *Lymphadenosis cutis benigna:* Proliferation associated with *Borrelia burgdorferi* infection (p. 94). Nodules, often involving earlobe or nipple, resolve with antibiotic therapy. Infiltrate of CD20+ B cells with both ϰ and λ light chains and regular germinal centers.
- *Lymphocytic infiltration of Jessner–Kanof:* Erythematous nodules and plaques, often facial, which on biopsy show abundant CD4+ helper T cells and mucin. In many instances, this disease is actually lupus tumidus (p. 206) and may respond to corticosteroids or antimalarials.
- Reactions to arthropod assaults (tick bites, nodular scabies) and viral infections (molluscum contagiosum) can be misinterpreted as lymphomas if the history is not available; mixed collection of lymphocytes, often with eosinophils (p. 130).
- Vascular tumors may have such an intense lymphocytic infiltrate that the underlying abnormal vessels are obscured; two dramatic examples are:
  - *Angiolymphoid hyperplasia with eosinophilia*: Typically facial nodules featuring vessels lined by thick epithelioid (hobnail) endothelial cells, associated with a dense infiltrate of lymphocytes and eosinophils.
  - ▶ *Note:* This disorder is sometimes erroneously designated *Kimura disease*; the latter is a systemic disease found in the Far East which rarely has cutaneous findings and is not relevant for Western physicians.
  - **A**cral **p**seudolymphomatous **a**ngiokeratoma of **ch**ildren (*APACHE syndrome*): Acral papules in children; mixed lymphocytic infiltrate around superficial vessels.
  - Rarely drugs, foreign bodies, or allergic contact dermatitis may induce a lymphocytic infiltrate, but such lesions are much less common than the other categories.

Differential diagnosis: The most important exclusion is a true lymphoma. Molecular biologic analysis including clonality studies can be crucial, if a typical history is not available. Other possibilities include polymorphous light eruption, tinea, leukemic infiltrates, Kaposi sarcoma, angiosarcoma, adnexal tumors.

28.2 Primary Cutaneous Lymphomas

Overview

▶ Primary cutaneous lymphomas manifest themselves primarily in the skin and a▪ confined there initially without evidence of nodal or systemic involvement. The▪ may be either B-cell or T-cell lymphomas, presumably with skin-specific homin▪ mechanisms.

▶ **Epidemiology:** Very rare; incidence 1–2/100 000, but has increased in rece▪ years.

▶ **Pathogenesis:** Many different factors appear involved, including persistent a▪ tigen stimulation (*Borrelia burgdorferi, Helicobacter pylori* for intestinal tumor▪ for B-cell lymphomas and transforming viruses (HTLV1, Epstein–Barr virus) for ▪ cell lymphoma. Genetic instability, immunosuppression, and carcinogens all pl▪ a role.

Classification

▶ Recently a working committee unified the classifications used by the Wor▪ Health Organization (WHO) and European Organization for Research and Trea▪ ment of Cancer (EORTC), as shown in Table 28.**1**. We will follow this classificati▪ and not attempt to cross-reference to older or alternate schemes.

▶ The frequency and 5-year survival for the most common cutaneous lymphomas ▪ the WHO/EORTC classification are shown in Table 28.**2**.

Table 28.1 · **WHO-EORTC classification of cutaneous lymphomas**

Cutaneous T-cell and NK-cell lymphomas

Mycosis fungoides
MF variants and subtypes
   Folliculotropic MF
   Pagetoid reticulosis
   Granulomatous slack skin

Sézary syndrome
Adult T-cell leukemia/lymphoma
Primary cutaneous CD30+ lymphoproliferative disorders
   Primary cutaneous anaplastic large cell lymphoma
   Lymphomatoid papulosis

Subcutaneous panniculitis-like T-cell lymphoma*
Extranodal NK/T-cell lymphoma, nasal type
Primary cutaneous peripheral T-cell lymphoma, unspecified
   Primary cutaneous aggressive epidermotropic CD8+ T-cell lymphoma (provisional)
   Cutaneous γ/δ T-cell lymphoma (provisional)
   Primary cutaneous CD4+ small/medium-sized pleomorphic T-cell lymphoma (provisional)

Table 28.1 · Continued

Cutaneous B-cell lymphomas

Primary cutaneous marginal zone B-cell lymphoma
Primary cutaneous follicle center lymphoma
Primary cutaneous diffuse large B-cell lymphoma, leg type
Primary cutaneous diffuse large B-cell lymphoma, other
  Intravascular large B-cell lymphoma

Precursor hematologic neoplasm

CD4+/CD56+ hematodermic neoplasm (blastic NK-cell lymphoma) †

Table 28.2 · Relative frequency and disease-specific 5-year survival of 1905 primary cutaneous lymphomas

WHO/EORTC classification	Number	Frequency (%)	Disease-specific 5-year survival (%)
Cutaneous T-cell lymphoma			
Indolent clinical behavior			
Mycosis fungoides	800	44	88
Folliculotropic MF	86	4	80
Pagetoid reticulosis	14	<1	100
Granulomatous slack skin	4	<1	100
Primary cutaneous anaplastic large cell lymphoma	146	8	95
Lymphomatoid papulosis	236	12	100
Subcutaneous panniculitis-like T-cell lymphoma	18	1	82
Primary cutaneous CD4+ small/medium pleomorphic T-cell lymphoma †	39	2	75
Aggressive clinical behavior			
Sézary syndrome	52	3	24
Primary cutaneous NK/T-cell lymphoma, nasal type	7	<1	NR
Primary cutaneous aggressive epidermotropic CD8+ T-cell lymphoma †	14	<1	18
Primary cutaneous γ/δ T-cell lymphoma †	13	<1	NR
Primary cutaneous peripheral T-cell lymphoma, unspecified #	47	2	16
Cutaneous B-cell lymphoma			
Indolent clinical behavior			
Primary cutaneous marginal zone B-cell lymphoma	127	7	99
Primary cutaneous follicle center lymphoma	207	11	95

Continued Table 28.3 ▶

Table 28.2 · Continued

WHO/EORTC classification	Number	Frequency (%)	5-year survival (%
Cutaneous B-cell lymphoma (Continued)			
Intermediate clinical behavior			
Primary cutaneous diffuse large B-cell lymphoma, leg type	85	4	55
Primary cutaneous diffuse large B-cell lymphoma, other	4	< 1	50
Primary cutaneous intravascular large B-cell lymphoma	6	< 1	65

NR indicates not reached. * Data are based on 1905 patients with a primary cutaneous lymphoma reg
tered at the Dutch and Austrian Cutaneous Lymphoma Group between 1986 and 2002.
† Primary cutanous peripheral T-cell lymphoma, unspecified excluding the three provisional entities in
cated with a double dagger (#).

28.3 Primary Cutaneous T-cell Lymphomas

Mycosis Fungoides

▶ **Definition:** An epidermotropic cutaneous T-cell lymphoma characterized by
proliferation of small to medium-sized CD4+ t cells with cerebriform nuclei.
▶ **Epidemiology:** Male:female ratio 2–3:1; typically starts after 50 years of age, b
can be seen in younger patients.
▶ **Clinical features:**
   • *Patch stage*: Macules and patches, slightly erythematous and scaly, often wi
     cigarette paper surface (wrinkled appearance, also called pseudoatrophy); sit
     of predilection include buttocks, trunk, upper thighs, upper arms (Fig. 28.1 a
     Less often involvement of flexures, scalp, and palms.
   ◘ *Note:* If confronted with erythematosquamous plaques with varying shades
     color, always think of mycosis fungoides.
   • *Plaque stage*: Gradual thickening of patches with increased scale (Fig. 28.1 b)
   • *Tumor stage*: Usually after many years, abrupt development of thick, ofte
     ulcerated tumors arising from the plaques (Fig. 28.1 c).
▶ **Variants:**
   • *Folliculotropic mycosis fungoides*: Malignant T cells are highly concentrated
     and about hair follicles; often mucinous deposits in follicles, which are then d
     stroyed producing alopecia; two synonyms are *mucinosis follicularis* and *alop
     cia mucinosa*.
   • *Granulomatous slack skin*: Granuloma formation and destruction of elast
     fibers leads to pendulous skin, especially in flexures; also seen with Hodgk
     lymphoma.
   • *Pagetoid reticulosis:* Two clinical patterns:
     – Classic *Woringer–Kolopp* pagetoid reticulosis: One or few acral plaque
       sharply bordered, scaly, stable.
     – Disseminated *Ketron–Goodman* pagetoid reticulosis: Widespread plaque
       without patch stage lesions or pruritus; most do not distinguish this for
       from mycosis fungoides.

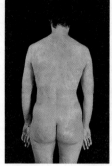
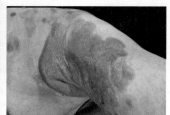
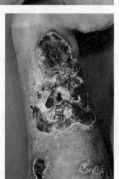

28.1 · Mycosis fungoides. a Multiple patches and ghtly raised plaques. **b** Obviously raised plaques. Ulcerated tumors.

Histology:

- *Patch stage:* Perivascular or confluent subepidermal infiltrate of lymphocytes, some with atypical cerebriform nuclei. Some cells enter the epidermis and may form small collections (*Pautrier microabscess*). The cells are usually T-helper cells of memory type (CD3+, CD4+, CD8-, CD45 RO+, CD30-). Rarely CD8+ tumor cells.
- *Plaque stage:* Dermal infiltrate is thicker and more pleomorphic, with lymphocytes, histiocytes, eosinophils and sometimes plasma cells. Epidermotropism is more prominent.
- *Tumor stage:* Nodular dermal infiltrate of clearly atypical cerebriform lymphocytes with other cells admixed.
- *Granulomatous slack skin:* Destructive granulomas with loss of elastic fibers; infiltrates of malignant T cells.
- *Pagetoid reticulosis:* More epidermotropism of atypical T cells, thus mimicking Paget disease.
- *Molecular biology*: Using PCR a clonal T-cell proliferation can be shown in the skin in 80% of cases and in the blood in >50%. Presence of a clone at time of diagnosis is associated with poorer prognosis.

Staging:

- Staging is based on a modified TNM (Bunn and Lamberg, 1979) shown in Tab. 28.**3**.
- *T (Skin):* The most advanced lesions are used for staging.

Table 28.3 · **Staging of mycosis fungoides (based on Bunn and Lamberg, 1979)**

Stage	TNM	Clinical features
IA	pT1 N0 M0	Patch and plaque lesions, < 10% of body surface
IB	pT2 N0 M0	Patch and plaque lesions, > 10% of body surface
IIA	pT1–2 N1 M0	Skin involvement as in I, but lymphadenopathy without histologic evidence of involvement
IIB	pT3 N0–1 M0	Tumors ± lymphadenopathy without histologic evidence of involvement
III	pT4 N0–1 M0	Erythroderma ± lymphadenopathy without histologic evidence of involvement
IVA	pT1–4 N2–3 M0	All skin involvement ± lymph nodes with histologic evidence of lymphoma
IVB	pT1–4 N0–3 M1	Visceral involvement; histologically proven

- *N (Lymph nodes):*
    - N1: clinically palpable nodes without specific lymphoma cells (*dermatopathic lymphadenopathy*).
    - N2: nodes contain lymphoma cells; need not be dramatically enlarged.
    - N3: nodal architecture destroyed by lymphoma cells; nodes usually enlarged.
    - Involvement of deeper lymph nodes (para-aortal, mediastinal) occurs late and is associated with short survival.
- *M (Metastases):* Histologically proven internal organ involvement.
▶ **Diagnostic approach:** The diagnosis of patch-stage mycosis fungoides is difficult. Often a certain diagnosis cannot be made even when clinical, histological, and molecular biological information is combined.
    - Patients should be checked every 4–12 months. Baseline skin biopsy, lymph node evaluation, and laboratory studies essential.
    - If skin lesions appear to thicken, re-biopsy is indicated.
    - Lymph nodes should be assessed with sonography and suspicious ones excised.
    - Once plaque or tumor stage is reached, chest radiography and abdominal sonography, as well as more directed imaging studies, become essential.
▶ **Differential diagnosis:**
    - *Patch stage:* Nummular dermatitis, tinea corporis, large-patch parapsoriasis.
    - *Plaque stage:* Psoriasis, subacute cutaneous lupus erythematosus, pityriasis lichenoides chronica.
    - *Tumor stage:* Other lymphomas, leukemic infiltrate.
    - *Pagetoid reticulosis: Clinical:* tinea corporis, psoriasis, Bowen disease, other papulosquamous diseases; *histological:* superficial spreading melanoma, Paget disease, Bowen disease.
▶ **Therapy:**
    - PUVA therapy; initially 4 × weekly, then once response has been seen, gradual reduction until complete clinical remission.
    - Interferon-α2a (9 million IU subq. 3 × weekly); in decreasing doses, for maintenance therapy.
    - When PUVA and interferon are combined, treatment time is reduced and longer remissions are induced.
    - Topical application of nitrogen mustard or BCNU is also highly effective and widely used in the USA.

- Solitary tumors can be irradiated (30 Gy fractionated into 2–3 Gy doses or electron beam).
- Biologicals such as cytokines (e.g., interleukin-12), traditional and new retinoids (bexarotene) and receptor-targeted cytotoxic fusion proteins (denileukin diftitox) are increasingly being used, but the exact role of these agents remains to be determined.
- Polychemotherapy should be considered in the case of unequivocal lymph node or internal organ involvement.

Prognosis: 5-year survival is 88%, but a more detailed view is instructive (Table 28.4).

- Patients with limited patch-stage mycosis fungoides have same survival as age-matched controls. Patients can rapidly progress after years of stable mild disease. Outlook in tumor stage is dismal.

Table 28.4 · Survival of patients with mycosis fungoides

Stage	Median survival (years)
I	Normal
Ib/IIa	13
IIb/III	4
IV	1.5

Sézary Syndrome

Definition: Leukemic form of cutaneous T-cell lymphoma with triad of erythroderma, generalized lymphadenopathy, and abnormal circulating T cells in peripheral blood (< 1000 Sézary cells/mm³ and/or expanded T-cell population with aberrant phenotypes).

Clinical features: Erythroderma accompanied by intense pruritus, alopecia, palmoplantar hyperkeratosis, and alopecia.

Histology: Most cases shows same changes as plaque stage mycosis fungoides. Infiltrate more monotonous and usually epidermotropic, but rarely only perivascular infiltrate with atypical cells. Lymph nodes show extensive replacement of normal architecture by atypical T cells.

- *Peripheral blood:* Standard for diagnosis is presence of > 1000 Sézary cells/mm³, FACS analysis with CD4+/CD8+ ratio > 10:1, expanded T-cell population with loss of CD2, CD3, or CD5 and proof of clonality. Some Sézary cells can be found in peripheral blood in a patient with severe atopic dermatitis and other inflammatory diseases.

Differential diagnosis: Other forms of erythroderma (p. 282).

Therapy: Extracorporeal photophoresis, methotrexate (0.3 mg/kg weekly), PUVA, combination therapy with chlorambucil and prednisolone for more advanced disease.

▶ *Note:* Do not forget symptomatic therapy of erythroderma: topical corticosteroids, wet dressings, oral antihistamines.

Prognosis: Dismal; median survival time 2–4 years.

Primary Cutaneous CD30-positive Lymphoproliferative Disorders

Primary Cutaneous Anaplastic Large Cell Lymphoma (C-ALCL)

► **Definition:** Low-grade cutaneous lymphoma in which most of the large malignant cells express CD30.
► **Clinical features:** One or more red-brown nodules, which are often ulcerated (Fig. 28.**2a**). About 20% with dissemination. Individual lesions may regress. Visceral involvement uncommon.
► **Histology:** Diffuse, nonepidermotropic infiltrates; tumor cell morphology varies from anaplastic to pleomorphic or immunoblastic. >75% of cells are CD30+, usually CD4+, CD8 –. Loss of typical T-cell markers (CD3, CD5) as well as expression of cytotoxic granules is common. Unlike systemic CD30+ lymphoma, most C-ALCL express cutaneous lymphoid antigen (CLA) but not epithelial membrane antigen (EMA) or anaplastic lymphoma kinase (ALK). Tumor cells usually clonal.
► **Diagnostic approach:** Clinical examination, histology, molecular biology. Once diagnosis is established, follow up every 3–4 months. Baseline and yearly staging (chest radiography, sonography of abdomen and lymph nodes) to exclude systemic involvement. Lymph node involvement alone is not poor prognostic sign.
► **Differential diagnosis:** Other lymphomas, skin metastases, leukemic infiltrates.
► **Therapy:** Excision or ionizing radiation for individual lesions; total dose 30 Gy. If more widespread, PUVA, interferon-α combination therapy. For advanced disease, polychemotherapy or denileukin diftitox.
► **Prognosis:** Good; 5-year survival 90%.

Lymphomatoid Papulosis

► **Definition:** Multifocal chronic, recurrent self-healing papulonecrotic or papulovesicular skin disease with histologic features suggesting a CD30+ lymphoma.
► **Clinical features:** Rapidly growing red-brown papules and nodules; sometimes papulonecrotic resembling pityriasis lichenoides et varioliformis acuta; picture varies from single large nodules to multiple lesions that may be pruritic; heal with atrophic scars (Fig. 28.**2b**).
► **Histology:** Three histologic types:
• A: mixed inflammatory infiltrate with nests of CD30+ T cells.
• B: resembles mycosis fungoides.
• C: resembles large cell, anaplastic T-cell lymphoma.

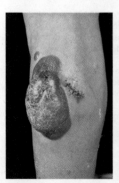
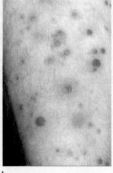

Fig. 28.**2** · **a** CD30+ cutaneous T-cell lymphoma. **b** Lymphomatoid papulosis.

a   b

- Molecular biology studies usually reveal a T-cell clone in the skin, sometimes also in peripheral blood.
- **Diagnostic approach:** Histologic picture most be combined with clinical history of regression. Multiple biopsies over time required to rule out associated lymphomas. If clinical history is clear, no staging required.
- **Differential diagnosis:** Other lymphomas, pityriasis lichenoides et varioliformis acuta.
- **Therapy:** PUVA; methotrexate 0.2–0.3 mg/kg weekly is amazingly effective, but often not appropriate for young patients.
- **Prognosis:** Excellent; 5-year survival about 95%.

ubcutaneous Panniculitis-like T-cell Lymphoma

- **Definition:** Cytotoxic T-cell lymphoma with presence of primarily subcutaneous infiltrates of pleomorphic cells of variable size, many macrophages and often the hemophagocytic syndrome.
- **Pathogenesis:** A more aggressive γδ and a more indolent αβ CD8+ subtype exist. The former is best classified under γδ lymphomas; only the latter αβ subtype is considered here.
- **Clinical features:** All ages are affected and both sexes are at equal risk. There are subcutaneous plaques and tumors, usually involving the legs (just as with inflammatory panniculitis) and sometimes with systemic signs and symptoms.
- **Histology:** Atypical pleomorphic T cells in the subcutaneous fat, often rimming individual lipocytes.
- **Therapy:** Systemic corticosteroids or doxorubicin-based chemotherapy.

xtranodal NK/T-cell Lymphoma, Nasal Type

- **Definition:** Lymphoma composed of small, medium or large cells with NK-cell phenotype, or more rarely of cytotoxic T cells.
- **Epidemiology:** Skin is second most common site after nose. Almost all cases are positive for Epstein–Barr virus.
- **Clinical features:** Involves nose, midface, upper airways (old *lethal midline granuloma*); cutaneous lesions usually nodules or plaques, which can become bullous or necrotic. Peripheral lymphadenopathy often absent.
  - Systemic involvement includes gastrointestinal tract, hepatosplenomegaly, lungs (lymphomatoid granulomatosis), bone marrow infiltration with pancytopenia.
  - Sometimes associated with hemophagocytic syndrome (*histiocytic medullary reticulosis*). Often "B symptoms" such as fever, weight loss.
- **Histology:** Highly variable; atypical lymphocytes of varying sizes, often angiocentric; CD56+, CD2+, CD3–, CD3ε in cytoplasm; express granzyme, perforin and TIA. Clonal population; TCR in germline configuration.
- **Differential diagnosis:** Varies with site; other lymphomas, pother forms of panniculitis, vasculitis (Wegener granulomatosis).
- **Therapy:** Polychemotherapy; usually CHOP, BACOP, or research protocols.
- **Prognosis:** Poor, but varies with disease type.

Other Primary Cutaneous T-cell Lymphomas

- **Primary cutaneous aggressive epidermotropic CD8+ cytotoxic T-cell lymphoma:** Proliferation of epidermotropic CD+ cytotoxic T cells with aggressive clinical behavior.
- **Cutaneous γδ+ T-cell lymphoma:** Proliferation of γδ+ t cells with development of ulcerated plaques and tumors, particular on extremities, with poor prognosis.
- **Primary cutaneous CD4+ small/medium-sized pleomorphic T-cell lymphoma:** Proliferation of small or medium-sized T cells without a history of mycosis fungoides. Mainly nodules or plaques with 5-year survival 60–80%.

28.4 Primary Cutaneous B-cell Lymphomas

Primary Cutaneous Follicle Center Cell Lymphoma

▶ **Definition:** Low-grade B-cell lymphoma of neoplastic follicle center cells, typically found on head and upper trunk.

▶ **Clinical features:** Picture variable; small nodules with erythema, red-brown plaques with little epidermal involvement, grouped papules (Fig. 28.3). On the trunk, tumors likely to be surrounded by erythema. Disseminated skin disease unusual.

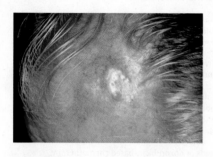

Fig. 28.3 · Follicle center cell lymphoma.

▶ **Histology:** Both follicular pattern and diffuse infiltrates without epidermotropism. Variable mixture of small centrocytes and centroblasts, sometimes admixed with larger centrocytes; also reactive T cells. Immunophenotype CD20 +, CD79a+; bcl-6+, bcl-2 –. λ/ϰ ratio usually shifted, but light chains not always expressed. Skin infiltrate usually clonal, but no clonality seen in peripheral blood.

▶ **Diagnostic approach:** Clinical features, histology, molecular biology; baseline and yearly imaging (chest radiograph, sonography of abdomen and lymph nodes; bone marrow examination at time of diagnosis and with any change in peripheral blood picture or suggestion of systemic involvement.

▶ **Differential diagnosis:** Dermatofibrosarcoma protuberans, other lymphomas, leukemic infiltrates.

▶ **Therapy:** Ionizing radiation (30 Gy in 10 fractions); excision of solitary lesions, anti-CD20 monoclonal antibody therapy, interferon-α2.

▶ Excellent; 5-year survival 95%.

Primary Cutaneous Marginal Zone Lymphoma

▶ **Definition:** Primary cutaneous lymphoma derived from the lymphocytes of the marginal zone surrounding the follicle; formerly immunocytoma or primary cutaneous plasmacytoma.

▶ **Clinical features:** Male:female ratio 10:1; usually >50 years of age; no systemic signs and symptoms. Single or multiple cutaneous or subcutaneous red-brown papules and nodules; favor the trunk (70%); associated with worse prognosis are involvement of the head and neck (20%) or disseminated disease (10%).

▶ **Histology:** Dermal infiltrate with sparing of the papillary dermis (*grenz zone*). Nodular or diffuse pattern with small lymphocytes, plasmacytoid cells, and plasma cells, often extending into subcutaneous fat. Involvement of sweat gland or hair follicles in 90%. About 50% have reactive follicles. Tumor cells are CD20+, CD79a+, CD5 –, CD10 –, bcl-2 –; λ/ϰ shift; monoclonality of heavy chain usually demonstrable; CD30+ cells at margin.

▶ **Diagnostic approach:** Clinical features, histology, molecular biology; baseline and yearly imaging (chest radiograph, sonography of abdomen and lymph nodes); bone marrow examination at time of diagnosis and with any change in peripheral blood picture or suggestion of systemic involvement.

▶ **Differential diagnosis:** Other lymphomas, metastases, leukemic infiltrates.

▶ **Therapy:** Excision if possible; otherwise ionizing radiation or electron beam (30 Gy total dose). Systemic therapy with anti-CD20 antibodies.

▶ **Prognosis:** Even with appropriate treatment, 30% relapse rate. 25% have extracutaneous involvement (parotid gland, subcutaneous fat, gastrointestinal tract, spleen, bone marrow, lymph nodes, orbit, thorax. Outlook excellent; 5-year survival 90%.

Primary Cutaneous Diffuse Large B-cell Lymphoma, Leg Type

▶ **Definition:** Aggressive cutaneous B-cell lymphoma with a predominance or confluent sheets of centroblasts and immunoblasts, almost always located on legs.

▶ **Clinical features:** Most patients are older women. Rapidly growing red-brown nodules and plaques on legs; often ulcerated (Fig. 28.**4**). Prompt lymph node involvement on same side and then systemic spread.

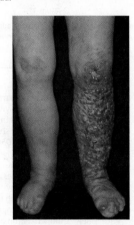

Fig. 28.**4** · Diffuse large B-cell lymphoma, leg type.

▶ **Histology:** Diffuse, nonepidermotropic infiltrate of large blasts with large nucleus and prominent central nucleolus; CD20+, CD79a+ and monotypic Ig expression. Bcl-2+, MUM–1+. No t(14;18) translocation as in noncutaneous large cell B-cell lymphoma. Tumor cells monoclonal.

▶ **Diagnostic approach:** Clinical examination, biopsy, extensive staging and close follow-up.

▶ **Differential diagnosis:** Other lymphomas, metastases, leukemic infiltrates. A comparison between primary cutaneous follicle center lymphoma and primary cutaneous diffuse large b-cell lymphoma, leg type is given in Table 28.**5**.

▶ **Therapy:** Polychemotherapy, usually anthracycline based; excision, ionizing radiation (30 Gy); radioactively labeled anti-CD20 antibodies (ibritumomab tiuxetan), or rituximab.

▶ **Prognosis:** Modest; 5-year survival 50%.

Table 28.5 · **Characteristic features of primary cutaneous follicle center lymphoma (PCFCL) and primary cutaneous diffuse large B-cell lymphoma (PCLBCL), leg type**

	PCFCL	PCLBCL, leg type
Morphology	Predominance of centrocytes that are often large especially in diffuse lesions. Centroblasts may be present but not in confluent sheets. Growth pattern may be follicular, follicular and diffuse, or diffuse (a continuum with distinct categories or grades)	Predominance of confluent sheets of medium-sized to large B cells with round nuclei, prominent nucleoli and course chromatin resembling centroblasts or immunoblasts. Diffuse growth pattern
Phenotype	Bcl-2: ∓ Bcl-6: + CD10: ∓ Mum-1: –	Bcl-2: + + Bcl-6: ± CD10: – Mum-1: +
Clinical features	Middle-aged adults. Localized lesions on head or trunk (90%); multifocal lesions rare	Elderly, especially women. Lesions localized to legs, usually below knees. Rare cases away from leg (10%).

CD4+, CD56+ Hematodermic Neoplasm (Blastic NK-cell Lymphoma).

▶ **Definition:** Blastic NK-cell lymphoma is a clinically aggressive neoplasm with a high incidence of cutaneous involvement and risk of leukemic dissemination.

▶ **Pathogenesis:** More recent studies suggest a plasmacytoid dendritic cell precursor; thus the names *CD4+, CD56+ hematodermic neoplasm*, and *early plasmacytoid dendritic cell leukemia/lymphoma* have been proposed.

▶ **Clinical features:** Blastic NK-cell lymphoma presents commonly in the skin with solitary or multiple nodules with or without extracutaneous disease. Moist patients, even if presenting with only cutaneous findings, rapidly develop involvement of bone marrow, lymph nodes, peripheral blood, and extranodal sites.

▶ **Histology:** Nonepidermotropic monotonous infiltrates of medium-sized cells with finely clumped chromatin. Immunophenotype is CD4+, CD56+, CD8-, CD7 ±, CD2∓, CD45RA+; the cells do not express surface and cytoplasmic CD3 or cytotoxic proteins. TCR is in germline configuration.

▶ **Therapy:** Systemic chemotherapy usually leads to complete remission but is soon followed by relapses that are not responsive. Median survival 14 months.

Hodgkin Lymphoma

▶ **Definition:** Hodgkin lymphoma (HL) is a common primarily nodal lymphoma with characteristic large tumor cells.

▶ **Pathogenesis:** Sometimes Epstein-Barr virus implicated.

▶ **Clinical Features:** HL rarely involves skin, and then usually secondary to either direct spread from involved lymph nodes or hematogenous spread. Primary cutaneous HL is extremely rare. Patients with HL often have pruritus and are predisposed to viral infections such as herpes zoster and warts.

▶ **Histology:** The distinctive tumor cell in HL is the Reed-Sternberg cell. Most often B-cell lineage although sometimes T-cell, then with overlaps with other CD30-

positive lymphoproliferative disorders. Inflammatory background and pattern variable.

▶ **Therapy:** Both radiation therapy and systemic chemotherapy are highly effective for nodal disease. Cutaneous lesions also respond well to ionizing radiation.

28.5 Leukemia and the Skin

Overview

In sharp contrast to lymphomas, no attempt is made to classify leukemias on the basis of cutaneous findings. Bone marrow examination and detailed cytological, immuno-histochemical, and molecular biologic analysis is required. Leukemias are divided into myeloid and lymphocytic types, with many subtypes. Some diseases, such as the hematodermic neoplasm mentioned just above or chronic lymphocytic leukemia (CLL) can be classified as either lymphomas or leukemias, depending on the manner of presentation. The cutaneous lesions associated with leukemia can represent either specific infiltrates with leukemic cells in the skin or nonspecific changes secondary to anemia, immunosuppression, and chemotherapy.

Leukemia Cutis

▶ **Clinical features:** Leukemic infiltrates are typically red-brown nodules, some-times with a blue hue, similar to other metastases but often with a more florid course. They may occasionally precede other signs and symptoms but more often herald failed therapy or a relapse. There are many distinctive clinical patterns to leukemic infiltrates, including:
  • Gingival infiltrates.
  • Bullous, ulcerated, and hemorrhagic lesions.
  • Leonine facies with symmetrical facial infiltrates, often in CLL.
  • Involvement of scars.
▶ **Granulocytic sarcoma:** Specific infiltrate of acute myeloid leukemia, which often precedes any other findings. Typically a facial, especially periorbital, mass in young adult. The biopsy surface, when cut in the pathology laboratory, develops a green color because of the presence of myeloperoxidase, so these tumors were ini-tially designated as *chloroma*.

Nonspecific Findings

▶ **Clinical features:** Almost all patients with leukemia have cutaneous findings at some point. Typical changes include:
  • Purpura, hemorrhage, and ecchymoses because of impaired bone marrow func-tion from disease and chemotherapy.
  • Wide variety of infections.
  • Atypical Sweet syndrome (p. 249) and pyoderma gangrenosum (p. 251).
  • Severe arthropod assault reactions.
  • Urticarial exanthems.
  • Broad spectrum of chemotherapy reactions because patients typically receive high-dose regimens. Examples include:
    – Mucositis.
    – Hair loss.
    – Acral erythema.
    – Lymphocyte recovery rash (occurs as lymphocytes begin to repopulate body after aggressive treatment).

▶ **Histology:** A standard problem is to determine if a maculopapular or urticarial rash represents a specific or nonspecific finding. Modern techniques have made it easier to identify leukemic cells in the skin, but the question remains: If a patient has >90% circulating leukemia cells and develops a drug reaction, the infiltrating cells in the skin will contain leukemic cells, but is the infiltrate is reactive or specific?

Signs of Selected Leukemias

The list is in Table 28.6 is not exhaustive, but indicates how some of the common leukemias may involve the skin.

Table 28.6 · Cutaneous signs of selected leukemias

Leukemia	Skin findings
Acute leukemias	
Acute myeloid leukemia	Leukemia cutis in 10% Oral infiltrates in >50% Granulocytic sarcoma in young adults
Acute juvenile myelomono-cytic leukemia	Association with neurofibromatosis; perhaps increased if juvenile xanthogranulomas are also present
Acute myelomonocytic leukemia	More likely to have fewer large nodules
Adult T-cell leukemia/lym-phoma	Papules and nodules in >50% Patches as in mycosis fungoides rare Infective dermatitis (severe recalcitrant disease with lym-phadenopathy in Jamaican children)
Acute lymphocytic leukemia	Leukemia cutis very uncommon
Chronic leukemias	
Chronic myeloid leukemia	Infiltrates uncommon; atypical Sweet and pyoderma gan-grenosum may herald blast crisis
Chronic lymphocytic leukemia	Infiltrates common; often leonine facies Exaggerated reaction to arthropod assault (often bullous, on shins, may mimic bullous pemphigoid)
Hairy cell leukemia	Atypical Sweet, pyoderma gangrenosum and vasculitis may be seen; infiltrates rare
Polycythemia vera	Pruritus after warm bath Erythromelalgia (pain in fingers with vasodilation) Hyperviscosity syndrome with vessel occlusion and in-farcts

29 *Paraneoplastic Disorders*

Overview

There ae a number of dermatologic conditions that should suggest the presence of an underlying malignancy. Some point to cancer-associated genodermatoses, others to acquired diseases associated with an increased incidence of malignancy (dermatomyositis or paraneoplastic pemphigus). Finally, there are conditions presumably caused by biologically active products manufactured by tumors. Schnyder established criteria for such conditions. They include:

► No other explanation for the skin finding.
► Skin changes improve with cancer treatment and may reappear if cancer recurs.
► Skin changes appear at about the same time as the systemic cancer; they may precede any clinical manifestations of the underlying malignancy.
► Statistical connection is shown.

Four of the most dramatic conditions are discussed below.

Acanthosis Nigricans

► **Definition:** Velvety hyperpigmentation of axilla, groin, and nape.
► **Pathogenesis:** Tumor-related acanthosis nigricans results from the secretion of insulin-like growth factor (IGF) or closely related proteins by the tumor; other forms involve abnormalities of IGF or insulin receptor.
► **Classification:**
  • *Malignant acanthosis nigricans:*
    – Usually involves adults > 40 years of age.
    – Sudden onset.
    – May also involve palms and soles (*tripe palms*) or mouth.
    – Most common tumor is carcinoma of the stomach (65%) or other gastrointestinal tumors.
    – Acanthosis nigricans typically improves with tumor therapy.
    – Possibly related findings:
    – *Leser–Trélat sign:* Eruptive skin tags and tiny seborrheic keratoses; similar mechanism, often occurs in same patient.
    – *Florid cutaneous papillomatosis:* Same changes but widespread rather than flexural.
► *Endocrine acanthosis nigricans:* Patients with insulin-resistant diabetes, because of acquired loss of function of insulin receptor, associated with collagen–vascular disorders and hyperandrogenism.
► *Syndromes with acanthosis nigricans:* Usually reflect abnormalities in insulin receptor or insulin-like growth factor secretion; often with associated lipodystrophy (p. 538).
► *Pseudo acanthosis nigricans:* Mild hyperpigmentation in obese individuals; more common in dark-skinned individuals and in the tropics.
► *Drug-induced acanthosis nigricans:* Most common trigger is nicotinic acid when used to treat hyperlipidemia.
► **Histology:** Not acanthotic and not hyperpigmented; microscopically looks like many small seborrheic keratoses.
► **Diagnostic approach:** Clinical examination, biopsy, always exclude diabetes mellitus. In adults without any obvious explanation, extensive tumor search is justified including imaging of gastrointestinal tract, CEA, α-fetoprotein;

▶ **Therapy:** Treat underlying problem, lose weight; topical retinoids may bring modest improvement in syndromic or endocrine acanthosis nigricans, but are irritating.

Erythema Gyratum Repens

▶ **Definition:** Characteristic migratory erythema with distinctive pattern.
▶ **Clinical features:** Rapidly changing "wood grain" pattern usually on trunk; extremely uncommon (Fig. 29.1). Not associated with any distinctive tumor.
▶ **Diagnostic approach:** Extensive tumor search always warranted.
▶ **Differential diagnosis:** Other figurate erythemas (p. 285).
▶ **Therapy:** No therapy possible.

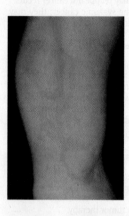

Fig. 29.**1** · Erythema gyratum repens.

Hypertrichosis Lanuginosa acquisita

▶ **Definition:** Generalized growth of lanugo hairs in an adult; obligate neoplastic marker.
▶ **Clinical features:** Extremely rare condition, more common in women. Relatively sudden onset of growth of thin silvery hairs. Often starts on face. The underlying tumor can precede, accompany, or follow the growth of hairs. Most common associated tumors are colon and rectal carcinomas (25%), bronchial carcinoma (25%), cervical carcinoma (10%).
▶ **Differential diagnosis:** Almost none; other causes of acquired diffuse hypertrichosis are discussed on p. 513.
▶ **Therapy:** Hairs can be removed with depilatories or shaving.

Necrolytic Migratory Erythema

▶ **Synonyms:** Glucagonoma syndrome, erythema necroticans migrans.
▶ **Definition:** Circinate and periorificial erythema and scaling associated with islet cell tumor of the pancreas producing glucagon.
▶ **Clinical features:** On trunk and extremities, 1–4 cm erythematous patches often with central blister or necrosis; in the flexures and about the mouth, erosions and crusts.

▶ **Histology:** High epidermal necrosis (reversal of staining) with neutrophilic infiltrate.
▶ **Diagnostic approach:** Clinical examination, biopsy; for screening, blood sugar; then glucagon level and imaging studies.
▶ **Differential diagnosis:** Acrodermatitis enteropathica (zinc levels may be reduced in both conditions); candidiasis.
▶ **Therapy:** Ideally surgery; unfortunately many tumors are discovered too late for curative surgery; palliative chemotherapy with variety of substances possible.

Other Cutaneous Markers of Malignancy

Many conditions that can on occasion indicate an underlying malignancy are listed in Table 29.1. They are less reliable markers than discussed above, but should never be overlooked. See also the cancer-associated genodermatoses (p. 367), as they are not repeated here.

Table 29.1 · Cutaneous markers of malignancy

Marker	Skin findings	Underlying malignancy	Strength of association[a]
Acanthosis nigricans	See above		
Bazex acrokeratosis	Psoriasiform lesions on fingers, toes, nose, ears	Carcinoma, usually upper airway	>95%
Dermatomyositis	Gottron papules, heliotrope eyelids, photosensitivity	Carcinoma, often ovarian	~15% in adults
Digital ischemia	Raynaud phenomenon, gangrene, other signs of cryoglobulinemia	Hematologic malignancies	Rare
Erythema annulare centrifugum	Slowly expanding annular erythematous plaques	Carcinomas, lymphomas	Rare
Erythema gyratum repens	See above		
Erythroderma	Diffuse erythema and widespread desquamation	Lymphomas (especially mycosis fungoides, Sézary syndrome); carcinomas	~25%
Florid cutaneous papillomatosis	Diffuse acanthosis nigricans-like changes	Carcinomas	>95%
Follicular mucinosis	Boggy plaques, usually on scalp	Mycosis fungoides (perhaps early lesion)	>75%
Flushing	Sudden diffuse erythema	Carcinoid tumors, other secretory carcinomas	Common
Hyperpigmentation	Diffuse or localized darkening	Metastatic melanoma with melanin in serum; rarely other tumors	Rare

Continued Table 29.1 ▶

Table 29.1 · Continued

Marker	Skin findings	Underlying malignancy	Strength of association[a]
Hypertrichosis lanuginosa acquisita	See above		
Leser–Trelat sign	Eruptive skin tags and small seborrheic keratoses	Carcinomas	> 95%
Necrobiotic xanthogranuloma	Red-yellow nodules, almost always periorbital	Gammopathy	> 95%
Necrolytic migratory erythema	See above		
Pachydermoperiostosis	Thickened digits, periostosis	Carcinoma of lung	Common
Panniculitis	Painful subcutaneous nodules, fat necrosis	Carcinoma of pancreas	Uncommon
Palmoplantar keratoderma	1) Acquired thickening and scaling of palms and soles	Carcinomas	Rare
	2) Congenital keratoderma and leukokeratosis (Howel–Evans syndrome)	Carcinoma of esophagus	> 95%
Paraneoplastic pemphigus	Oral erosions, cutaneous lesions that overlap between lichen planus and erythema multiforme	Lymphoma, Castleman tumor, thymoma	> 95%
Pruritus	Intense itching without explanation	Hodgkin lymphoma, many others	Rare
Pyoderma gangrenosum	Aggressive undermined ulcers without clear cause	Gammopathy (usually IgA)	< 25%
Sweet syndrome	Succulent red nodules and neutrophilia	Leukemia, especially hairy cell type	Unclear ~50%
Thrombophlebitis	Recurrent superficial thrombophlebitis (Trousseau sign)	Carcinoma of pancreas	> 25%
Tripe palms	Acute pebbly palms and soles; analogous to acanthosis nigricans	Carcinomas	> 95%
Xanthomas, diffuse plane	Large sheets of xanthomatous infiltration	Gammopathy	> 95%
Zoster	Severe or generalized zoster in young adult	Lymphoma, leukemia (HIV infection)	Uncommon

a This column refers only to the strength of the association, not to the frequency of the finding.
Based on Table 65.**3** in Braun-Falco O, Plewig G, Wolff HH, Burgdorf WHC. *Dermatology* (Springer, Berlin, 2000).

30 Diseases of the Lips and Oral Mucosa

30.1 Inflammation and Leukoplakia

Cheilitis

▶ **Definition:** Inflammation of the lips.
▶ **Clinical features:** Lip inflammation is similar to dermatitis elsewhere; features include erythema, scaling, and fissuring. The inflammation frequently involves the neighboring skin and is often impetiginized.
▶ **Classification:** There are many different causes of cheilitis; all appear quite similar.
  • *Irritant cheilitis:* Very common; result of repeated lip licking, biting or sucking; also caused by exposure to UV light, wind, and cold.
  • *Allergic contact cheilitis:* Most common causes are allergens in lipsticks (colophony).
  • *Atopic cheilitis:* Often worsened by lip licking and biting; characterized by frequent deep median fissures in lower lip.
▶ **Diagnostic approach:** Exclude atopy and allergic contact cheilitis; use special patch testing tray for typical lip allergens—lipsticks, topical medications (herpes ointments), fingernail polish, toothpastes, mouthwashes.
▶ **Differential diagnosis:** Lupus erythematosus, lichen planus, actinic cheilitis.
▶ **Therapy:** Avoid triggering factors and allergens; apply white petrolatum for protection; if severely inflamed, use corticosteroid ointment.

Angular Cheilitis

▶ **Synonym:** Perlèche.
▶ **Definition:** Inflammation at corners of mouth.
▶ **Pathogenesis:** In infants, usually from drooling; in children and young adults, infectious (*Candida albicans* or bacteria); other adults, poorly fitting dentures with drooling; all age groups, trauma during dental care; rarely vitamin or nutrient deficiency.
▶ **Clinical features:** Erythema, fissures, and maceration at corners of mouth.
▶ **Diagnostic approach:** Exclude candidiasis and bacterial infections; have dentures checked. Serum iron level and ferritin if other signs of bleeding or malnutrition.
▶ **Therapy:** Treat with protective (zinc oxide) or anticandidal paste.

Granulomatous Cheilitis

▶ **Definition:** Swelling of lip with granulomatous inflammation.
▶ **Pathogenesis:** Can be idiopathic or part of Melkersson–Rosenthal syndrome.
▶ **Clinical features:** Initially episodic swelling of lips; later more permanent. Rarely, swelling of other areas such as tongue, cheeks, eyelids, or forehead.
  • *Melkersson–Rosenthal syndrome*: Associated diagnostic features include Bell palsy (facial never paralysis) and furrowed tongue. Occasional lymph node involvement with granulomas (p. 291).

► **Histology:** Lymphocytic infiltrate, often rich in plasma cells; small granulomas can usually be detected.
► **Diagnostic approach:** Clinical triad, biopsy.
► **Differential diagnosis:** Sarcoidosis, recurrent erysipelas, herpes simplex, angioedema.
► **Therapy:** Intralesional corticosteroids (triamcinolone 2.5 mg/mL diluted in lidocaine); if unsuccessful, short burst of systemic corticosteroids or clofazimine 100 mg daily for 3–6 months (urine turns red-orange). Once less active, reduction surgery on lip may be required.

30.2 Leukoplakia

► **Definition:** White patch on mucous surface, which will not rub off. (Definition designed to exclude candidiasis, which usually can be rubbed off.) The white color is caused by moist hyperkeratosis.
► **Classification:** There are many different types of leukoplakia:
  • *Inherited:* White sponge nevus is best example.
  • *Acquired:*
    – Infections (Epstein–Barr virus and oral hairy leukoplakia in HIV/AIDS, oral warts).
    – Exogenous agents (tobacco, trauma).
    – Other disorders (lichen planus).
  ◪ **Note:** Confusion can arise from thr use of the term leukoplakia as synonymous with squamous cell carcinoma in situ of the mucosa. This is a more restricted meaning. Selected examples of the different types of leukoplakia are discussed below.
► **Clinical features:** In most instances, the nature of leukoplakia can be established clinically. For example, white linear streaks on the buccal mucosa at the level of the bite line are almost always frictional and reactive. Lesions along the lower labial mucosa where chewing tobacco is held are very often in-situ carcinomas. Verrucous lesions, speckled leukoplakia (mixture of red and white areas), or ulcerated areas are also likely to represent malignant change.
  🗲 *Caution:* In all instances, when the diagnosis of leukoplakia is made, the possibility of a intraepithelial carcinoma should be considered and excluded with a biopsy if clinically needed.
► **Histology:** Microscopic picture can vary from reactive hyperplasia through carcinoma in situ to frankly invasive squamous cell carcinoma. Even when an underlying disorder such as lichen planus is identified, the risk of a secondary squamous cell carcinoma is not completely excluded.
► **Therapy:** Treatment depends on underlying diagnosis.

White Sponge Nevus

► **Definition:** Localized area of marked hyperkeratosis; present since birth and stable.
► **Pathogenesis:** Mutations in keratin type 4 or 13; the major forms expressed in the mucosal basal layer; autosomal dominant inheritance.
► **Clinical features:** Thickened, wave-like or folded plaques on the oral and nasal mucosa; sharply bordered and permanent. Less often vaginal or anal involvement. Rarely symptomatic.
► **Therapy:** No effective therapy available.

Human Papillomavirus (HPV) Infections

▶ **Pathogenesis:** Selected HPV types can thrive on mucosal surfaces; examples include HPV 2 and 4 (warts), HPV 6 and 11 (condylomata acuminata), and HPV 13 and 32 (Heck disease).
▶ **Clinical features:** The clinical distinctions are usually more a matter of degree. Warts may appear more papillomatous or elongated than condylomata. Heck disease usually occurs in Eskimos or Native Americans; patients have 100 s of small oral papillomas.
▶ **Therapy:** Many of the usual wart treatments are difficult to use. Local destruction (electrosurgery, laser) and meticulous hemostasis is the usual approach.

Carcinoma in Situ of the Lip

One must distinguish between carcinoma in situ of the lip, usually caused by sun exposure and a dermatologic problem, and carcinoma in situ of the oral mucosa, usually caused by tobacco exposure and a management responsibility of oral surgeons and otorhinolaryngologists, but often a diagnostic challenge for dermatologists.
▶ **Synonym:** Actinic cheilitis.
▶ **Pathogenesis:** Completely analogous with actinic keratosis; UV-induced carcinogenesis. Nicotine use and immunosuppression may be co-factors. Only difference is that risk of invasive squamous cell carcinoma is greater on lip than skin.
▶ **Clinical features:** Almost exclusively involves lower lip; early lesions may simply feel rough to patient or be slightly white; later lesions can be thickened, erythematous or ulcerated.
▶ **Histology:** Atypical keratinocytes in epithelium, but no evidence of invasion into lamina propria.
▶ **Therapy:** Early lesions can be treated with cryotherapy or laser ablation; any thickened or ulcerated lesions should be biopsied first. More advanced disease usually treated by vermilionectomy (excision of epithelium of lip) with coverage either with a mucosal advancement flap or by secondary intention.

Carcinoma of the Lip

▶ **Definition:** Invasive squamous cell carcinoma of the lip with potential for metastasis.
▶ **Classification:** Shown in Table 30.**1**.

Table 30.1 · Classification of carcinoma of the lip

Stage	Tumor thickness
T1	<5 mm
T2	5–10 mm
T3	10–20 mm
T4a	>20 mm thickness, <20 mm diameter
T4b	>20 mm thickness, >20 mm diameter

▶ **Clinical features:** On lower lip and usually with history of previous treatment of actinic cheilitis. Verrucous, eroded, ulcerated papule or nodule.
▶ **Diagnostic approach:** History, clinical examination; sonographic evaluation of regional lymph nodes; chest radiograph.

- ▶ **Differential diagnosis:** Other causes of leukoplakia; other lip tumors, such as keratoacanthoma and basal cell carcinoma.
- ▶ **Therapy:**
  - Excision with careful control of margins; ideally micrographic surgery.
  - Radiation therapy if inoperable or impossible to completely excise.
  - If lymph nodes are involved, neck dissection.
  - Consideration of chemotherapy depending on status of excision and lymph nodes; mandatory for systemic involvement.
- ▶ **Follow-up:** Every 3 months, with sonography every 6 months and yearly chest radiograph.
- ▶ **Prognosis:** Highly variable; 5-year survival for T1 is 80%; T4, 20%.

30.3 Lesions of Tongue

Furrowed Tongue

- ▶ **Synonyms:** Plicated tongue, scrotal tongue
- ▶ **Pathogenesis:** Unknown; in rare cases associated with Melkersson–Rosenthal syndrome.
- ▶ **Clinical features:** Thickened tongue with deep furrows and splits that look as if they should hurt but are asymptomatic. Appearance often very distressful to patient, as is the name "scrotal tongue," which should be avoided.
- ▶ **Therapy:** Nothing satisfactory.

Geographic Tongue

- ▶ **Synonyms:** Migratory glossitis, exfoliatio linguae areata.
- ▶ **Definition:** Migratory areas of loss of relief of tongue.
- ▶ **Clinical features:** Name comes from resemblance to a map with red smooth areas with white borders; totally asymptomatic but sometimes scares patient; patient changes over hours to days (Fig. 30.1). Usually idiopathic, but occasionally associated with severe psoriasis.

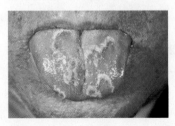

Fig. 30.**1** · Geographic tongue.

- ▶ **Histology:** Atrophic epithelium with exocytosis of neutrophils.
- ▶ **Differential diagnosis:** Candidiasis, other forms of glossitis (as found in deficiency states, for example).
- ▶ **Therapy:** None available.

Black Hairy Tongue

- **Synonym:** Lingua villosa nigra.
- **Definition:** Discoloration of dorsal surface of tongue with elongated papillae.
- **Pathogenesis:** Unknown; smoking and poor oral hygiene may play role, but many patients have no risk factors. May be secondary to pertubation of normal flora during antibiotic therapy. May be more common in HIV/AIDS, but not to be confused with oral hairy leukoplakia.
- **Clinical features:** Dorsal surface of tongue is discolored; long threads are elongated papillae; may bother patient (Fig. 30.**2**).
- **Diagnostic approach:** Clinical examination.
- **Therapy:** Exclude predisposing factors; clean tongue regularly with soft toothbrush. If not helpful, paint with 20% urea solution before brushing, to soften.

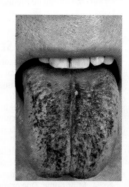

Fig. 30.**2** · Black hairy tongue.

Oral Hairy Leukoplakia

- Almost 100% specific for HIV/AIDS. Result of mixed infection with Epstein–Barr virus most important, but both HPV and *Candida albicans* associated. Fine filaments or "hairs" at lateral edge of tongue. Harmless, but difficult to treat (p. 161).

Glossodynia

- **Definition:** Sensation of burning or discomfort of tongue in the absence of physical findings.
- **Epidemiology:** Most patients are middle-aged women; often they display obsessive-compulsive personality traits.
- **Clinical features:** By definition, the examination is normal. Search for signs of candidiasis, aphthae, blistering diseases.
- **Diagnostic approach:** Culture of mouth and stool for *Candida albicans* frequently recommended; one must be careful since *Candida albicans* can be transiently present in the mouth and stool of almost everyone. Similarly, vitamin and mineral deficiencies may rarely be responsible, but repeated testing often convinces patients that they require special diets and supplements.
- **Therapy:** Short trials of anticandidal agents or vitamin supplements may be indicated in some patients. Antidepressant therapy is also occasionally helpful, but usually resisted by patients.

30.4 Epulis

▶ **Definition:** General name for any gingival tumor.
▶ **Clinical features:** There are many different types:
- *Congenital epulis:* Benign soft tumor, present at birth; usually on maxilla; histologically resembles a granular cell tumor (p. 462).
- *Epulis fissurata:* Also known as fibrous inflammatory hyperplasia; reactive process at edge of ill-fitting denture.
- *Epulis granulomatosa:* Pyogenic granuloma (p. 456) of gingiva; more common in pregnancy or following trauma.
- *Giant cell epulis:* Posttraumatic reaction; tumor rich in giant cells and fibrous stroma; also known as peripheral giant cell reparative granuloma.

▶ **Diagnostic approach:** If the clinical diagnosis is not apparent, biopsy is needed.
▶ **Therapy:** Eliminate predisposing factors; surgical removal.

30.5 Aphthous Stomatitis

▶ **Definition:** Common disorder with small usually painful recurrent oral ulcers with characteristic clinical appearance.
▶ **Synonyms:** Aphthae (singular aphtha), canker sore, recurrent aphthous stomatitis (RAS).
▶ **Pathogenesis:** Cause unknown; stress appears trigger, as does trauma, but variety of autoimmune and vasculitic processes also suggested, with TNFα appearing to be common mediator. Less common in smokers; more common in HIV/AIDS.
Clinical Features:
- Small round or oval ulcers covered with gray exudate and surrounded by erythematous halo. Usually heal over 7–10 days without scarring.
- Several clinical variants:
  - Minor type: One or more aphthae, common recurrences.
  - Herpetiform type: Same as minor, but lesions arranged in herpetiform fashion but no evidence for herpes simplex virus infection.
  - Major type: Larger more severe ulcers which usually cause scarring. Also known as Sutton aphthae or periadenitis mucosa necrotica recurrens.
- Bipolar aphthae: Combination of oral and genital aphthae with no sign of other systemic disease.
- Multiple aphthae also one of diagnostic criteria for Behçet syndrome (p. 256) and associated with cyclic neutropenia where aphthae and drop in WBC occur every few weeks.

▶ **Diagnostic Approach:** Strictly clinical diagnosis; biopsy does not help.
▶ **Differential Diagnosis:** Always exclude Behçet syndrome or bipolar aphthae if multiple lesions are presence or recurrences frequent. Recurrent herpes simplex infections only rarely intraoral and aphthae do not involve lips, but confusion persists.
▶ **Therapy:** No good therapy; try topical anesthetics, corticosteroids or pledgets soaked in tetracycline solution. Rarely systemic corticosteroids necessary; thalidomide highly effective, blocking TNFα but not often used.

31 Diseases of the Hairs and Scalp

A classification of hair disorders is shown in Table 31.1.

Table 31.1 · Classification of hair disorders	
Hypertrichosis	
Localized	*Diffuse*
Faun tail nevus	Hirsutism
Becker nevus	Hypertrichosis lanuginosa acquisita
Hair nevus	Congenital hypertrichosis
Drug-induced hypertrichosis[a]	Drug-induced hypertrichosis
Hypertrichosis associated with metabolic and endocrine disorders[a]	Hypertrichosis associated with metabolic and endocrine disorders
Posttraumatic/postinflammatory hypertrichosis	
Trichomegaly (excessive eye lashes)	
Alopecia	
Localized	*Diffuse*
Nonscarring	
Alopecia areata	Diffuse alopecia areata, alopecia totalis, alopecia universalis
Trichotillomania	Androgenetic alopecia[b]
	Androgen-induced alopecia[b]
Traction alopecia	Hormonal imbalance
Infections (tinea capitis, folliculitis)	Anagen effluvium: toxins (chemotherapy, poisons)
	Telogen effluvium: major illnesses, polytrauma, high fevers, post-partum effluvium, drug-induced, "stress"-induced effluvium
	Loose anagen hair
Scarring	
Lichen planus	Pseudopelade of Brocq
Frontal fibrosing alopecia (Kossard)	Keratosis follicularis spinulosa decalvans
Chronic cutaneous lupus erythematosus	
More severe or advanced infections (deep tinea capitis, massive folliculitis, zoster)	
Physical, chemical or mechanical alopecia	
Aplasia cutis congenita	
Epidermolysis bullosa—junctional, dystrophic or acquired	

Continued Table 31.1 ▶

Table 31.1 · Continued	
Alopecia (Continued)	
Localized	*Diffuse*
Hair shaft abnormalities	
Isolated	*Associated with syndrome*
Monilethrix	Netherton syndrome
Trichorrhexis nodosa	Menkes syndrome
Pili torti	Trichothiodystrophy
	Ectodermal dysplasia syndromes

a Can be either localized (then usually symmetrical) or diffuse.
b Diffuse, but follows a genetically determined pattern (hair loss only in androgen-sensitive scalp hair fol
  licles; hair retained in androgen-insensitive occipital hair follicles).

31.1 Alopecia: Overview

Definitions

▶ **Atrichosis or atrichia:** Congenital complete absence of hairs.
▶ **Hypotrichosis:** Congenital reduction in number of hairs.
▶ **Effluvium:** Sudden loss of hair.
▶ **Anagen effluvium:** Loss of hairs during their growth phase.
▶ **Telogen effluvium:** Loss of resting hairs.
▶ **Alopecia:** Acquired loss of hair; may be partial or complete; scarring or nonscar
  ring.

Diagnostic Approach

▶ Diagnostic methods are summarized in detail on p. 34.
▶ Far and away the most common alopecia is androgenetic alopecia. The only other
  fairly common problems are alopecia areata and telogen effluvium. All other
  alopecias (scarring alopecia, infections, hair shaft anomalies) are uncommon.
▣ *Note:* Every slowly progressive diffuse hair loss in women, as well as every telogen
  effluvium or slow regression of temporal hair line in men, as long as there is no
  suggestion of scarring, should be considered as androgenetic alopecia until proven
  otherwise and so treated. This diagnosis is correct for the vast majority of both
  men and women who complain of losing hair.

Differential Diagnosis

If you are having trouble, always consider these possibilities:
▶ Trichotillomania—easy to overlook.
▶ Diffuse alopecia areata is not so rare; often the patients can remember a solitary
  lesion, perhaps years in the past.
▶ Many patients have both androgenetic alopecia and telogen effluvium (caused by
  abnormal thyroid function, dietary defects, iron deficiency, zinc deficiency, medi
  cations).

➤ Both severe androgenetic alopecia and psoriatic alopecia can rarely show scarring on biopsy.
➤ Always think of unexpected toxin exposure—accidental, suicidal, or homicidal.

Practical Tips for Patient

◼ **Note:** Always take the patient's concerns seriously. Loss of hair is a great problem to many people. They may worry not only about their appearance, but about the possibility of an underlying malignancy or serious disease, as well as poisoning or other environmental hazards.

Always ask about and discuss the following topics:

➤ **Hair washing:** Daily hair washing, using a mild shampoo, is fine. Discrete dandruff and pruritus is often a clue that washing could be more frequent. Lack of care may also increase the telogen rate. It is always appropriate to use conditioners and rinses.

➤ **Cosmetics:**
- Cutting, coloring, and gentle permanent waves without tight curlers scarcely influence hair growth. Hair sprays are also harmless.
- Aggressive permanent waving or frequent blow-drying damages the hair shafts, but does not influence hair growth. When hair dyes (usually paraphenylenediamine) or other products cause allergic contact dermatitis, the telogen rate is increased and hair growth is affected.
- Hairstyles where tension is applied to hairs (corn rows, long pigtails, tightly wound styles) can drive anagen hairs into telogen. If employed for long periods of time they cause traction alopecia, which in rare cases can scar and then became permanent.

➤ **Diet:**
- Almost every patient is convinced that diet plays a great role in hair growth; this issue must be addressd in every case.
- Patients with eating disturbances or on crash diets almost always have telogen effluvium. When a careful history is obtained in young women with diffuse hair loss, dietary factors play a role in at least 25%. Gelatin capsules are popular, but there is no evidence that they offer an advantage over a well-balanced, protein-rich diet.
- At least 20% of young women have an iron deficiency because of blood loss during menses. Low iron levels increase the sensitivity of the follicle to androgens; daily iron replacement is safe and often helps.
- Even in the absence of iron deficiency and associated anemia, low ferritin levels raise an anagen follicle's sensitivity to various hair growth-inhibitory agents (e.g., androgens, thyroid abnormalities, drugs). Therefore, measuring ferritin, and raising it to a level well above the lower normal range by oral iron substitution therapy, is always advisable.
- Biotin and zinc deficiencies are rarer than is often assumed. Zinc deficiency rarely causes isolated hair problems. Biotin also appears to play a minor role. However, supplementation with either material, even in the absence of a manifest deficiency, can be helpful. Any zinc deficiency should be corrected, because zinc is a co-factor of numerous important enzyme systems.

31.2 Congenital Alopecia and Hypotrichosis

Total Congenital Alopecia

▶ **Isolated:** At birth, normal hairs, but later complete loss of all hairs with atrophy o sebaceous glands; autosomal recessive inheritance.
▶ **Associated defects:** Seen with several ectodermal dysplasia syndromes; mos common is hidrotic ectodermal dysplasia (complete alopecia, palmoplantar kera toderma, thickened nails); also seen in progeria.
▶ **Papular atrichia with cysts:** At birth, normal hairs. During puberty, onset of hai loss in face and scalp, later complete alopecia with many tiny papules that are epidermoid cysts. Defect in *hairless* gene at 8p21.2.

Localized Congenital Alopecia

▶ **"Negative" nevus:** Area lacking hair follicles from birth.
  ▣ *Note:* Nevus sebaceus (p. 411) frequently presents at birth as a bald patch on the anterior scalp line. On biopsy, follicles are always seen, and during puberty, the lesion thickens and becomes more clinically apparent.
▶ **Aplasia cutis congenita** (p. 350): Usually isolated finding but can be associated with number of syndromes; typically area on vertex where skin fails to fuse, leav ing atrophic scar.
▶ **Scarring alopecia** can be seen with a variety of other syndromes, including incon tinentia pigmenti.
▶ **Temporal triangular alopecia:** Congenital loss of hair in triangular pattern, usu ally unilateral, nonscarring. Similar lesions may be seen over suture lines or as par of cowlick.

Congenital Hypotrichosis

▶ **Hypotrichosis congenita:**
  • *Autosomal dominant form* (hypotrichosis simplex of the scalp): normal scalp hair at birth and in early childhood, but noticeable hair loss by start of school.
  • *Autosomal recessive form:* Normal hair at birth, but soon thereafter loss of scalp hairs as well as eyebrows and eyelashes.
▶ **Hypotrichosis can be seen with many syndromes, including:**
  • Hidrotic ectodermal dysplasia (p. 351).
  • Anhidrotic ectodermal dysplasia (p. 351).
  • Syndromes with hair shaft anomalies (p. 510).
  • Rothmund–Thomson syndrome (p. 306).
  • Disorders of amino acid metabolism (p. 315).

31.3 Diffuse Nonscarring Alopecia

Telogen Effluvium

▶ **Definition:** Sudden loss of hairs because of altered hair growth cycle, with prema ture shift of hairs into catagen and then telogen phase.
▶ **Pathogenesis:** We do not view telogen effluvium as a disease, but as a symptom almost always reflecting a trigger event.
  • *Androgenetic alopecia:* Most common cause is flare of androgenetic alopecia, i both men and women.

- ▣ *Note:* Telogen effluvium may also be the only sign of a developing androgenetic alopecia where the terminal-to-vellus hair conversion has not yet occurred.
- *Thyroid dysfunction:* Always check thyroid function tests; sometimes normal values in patients on thyroid replacement can still be associated with unexplained hair loss, requiring more detailed endocrinologic studies.
- *Sudden drop in estrogen levels:* Delivery, miscarriage, or discontinuing oral contraceptives.
- *Inadequate diet:* Always ask about eating disturbances, crash diets, or other peculiarities.
- *Iron deficiency:* May be first sign of modest iron deficiency with only abnormal ferritin levels and no laboratory signs of anemia.
- *Scalp diseases:* Seborrheic dermatitis; less often psoriasis, tinea capitis or allergic contact dermatitis.
- ▣ *Note:* Any inflammatory scalp disease increases the shift into telogen phase and thus the rate of hair loss; thus prompt and aggressive treatment required.
- *Medications:* Most common are β-blockers, cimetidine, antithyroid drugs, ACE inhibitors, lipid lowering agents, amphetamines, retinoids, NSAIDs.
- Other possible causes include:
  - Severe acute illnesses, infections, high fever, general anesthesia.
  - Hyperprolactinemia (especially if associated with late-onset acne).
  - Malabsorption and inflammatory bowel disease.
  - Endocrine disorders (Addison disease, Hashimoto thyroiditis).
  - Chronic diseases (connective tissue disorders, chronic infections, malignancies).
  - Psycho-emotional stress.
- **Clinical features:** Typically patient describes markedly increased diffuse hair loss during hair washing and combing, well above the previously observed level. If flare of underlying androgenetic alopecia, often—but not always —the characteristic pattern can be seen.
- **Diagnostic approach:** Examine hairs, trichogram shows >25% telogen hairs (in extreme cases, 80–90%); laboratory screening (complete blood count [CBC], sed rate, liver function tests, renal status, iron, ferritin); more directed testing based on history.
- **Differential diagnosis:**
  - *Anagen effluvium*: Hairs are damaged and lost during growth phase; bayonet hairs without telogen bulb; usual causes chemotherapy, radiation therapy, sepsis; rarely seen with alopecia areata.
  - *Intoxication*: Actual poisoning by thallium or arsenic rarely seen, but many patients convinced they are being poisoned by amalgam, environmental factors, dietary exposure, or (especially problematic) occupational exposures. Careful documentation and discussion required. Usually the underlying disease is ndrogenetic alopecia.
- **Therapy:** Usually no therapy is needed. Most patients accept the message that underlying factors must be corrected and nature given time to restore cycle. In women with androgen-induced telogen effluvium, solutions containing 17-estradiol induce prolongation of anagen phase and are effective.

Androgen-induced Alopecia

- **Definition:** Hair loss because of an endocrine abnormality with increased circulating androgen levels.
- **Epidemiology:** Disease of women.
- **Pathogenesis:** Causes of excesses androgens include ovary (secretory tumors, polycystic ovary disease), adrenal gland (many corticosteroids have androgenetic

function), and pituitary (excess secretion of regulatory hormone). In about 50% of cases, combined ovarian and adrenal hyperfunction. Always exclude adrenogenital syndrome (p. 319).

► **Clinical features:** Diffuse alopecia often starting in centroparietal region, associated with seborrhea; hirsutism (hypertrichosis of beard area, breasts).

► **Diagnostic approach:** General examination; determination of dehydroepiandrosterone sulfate (DHEAS), testosterone, free testosterone, sex hormone binding globulin (SHBG), prolactin levels; trichogram or phototrichogram.

► **Differential diagnosis:** Androgenetic alopecia, diffuse alopecia areata, SAHA syndrome (**s**eborrhea, **a**cne, **h**ypertrichosis, **a**ndrogen-induced alopecia).

► **Therapy:** Treat underlying disease; antiandrogens including cyproterone acetate combined with ethinyl estradiol or chlormadinone acetate.

Androgenetic Alopecia

► **MIM code:** 109200.

► **Definition:** Physiologic process with increased follicle sensitivity to androgens leading to change from terminal to vellus hair follicles with distinct patterns of alopecia, often associated with telogen effluvium.

► **Epidemiology:** At least 80% of men and 60% of women have detectable androgenetic alopecia by 60 years of age.

► **Pathogenesis:** Polygenic inheritance; variable penetrance. The hair follicles have increased numerous of androgen receptors in typical patterns as well as increased activity of 5-α-reductase type II, leading to increased androgen sensitivity. Dihydrotestosterone also causes shift to telogen hairs.

► *Clinical features:* Thinning of hair without scalp disease; two classic pattern schemes used for grading (Figs. 31.**1**, 31.**2**):

• *"Male pattern"* (after Hamilton).

• *"Female pattern"* (after Ludwig).

☐ *Note:* Overlap forms are common in both sexes.

► **Diagnostic approach:** Usually obvious, but many younger patients are skeptical and disappointed in the diagnosis. In men, usually receding frontal hairline; in women, more diffuse thinning and retention of frontal pattern. Vellus hairs usually prominent in areas of loss; hairs are thinner and remain shorter. In women, often associated with telogen effluvium.

• Patients may complain that hairs are finer and grow more slowly, while at other body sites, hair growth may be increased. Often seborrhea more prominent than previously.

• Family history is almost always positive, if one is persistent enough. Many patients initially say that no one in the family was bald, but this typically means only that their father had a relatively full head of hair. Ask about hair loss in grandparents, uncles, aunts.

☐ *Note:* If the clinical diagnosis seems likely but the patient is skeptical, studying old photographs with the patient is often very helpful.

• Trichogram or phototrichogram reveals reduced anagen/telogen ratio, frontal > occipital. Only valuable if rigorously standardized, quality-controlled, and done professionally. In clinical routine, both techniques are dispensable for making correct diagnosis.

• Hormone levels usually normal. Studies only needed when hirsutism, virilization, menstrual problems, infertility, galactorrhea, or other indications of endocrine abnormalities are present. Then DHEAS, free testosterone, SHBG, prolactin, thyroid function; hormone studies should be done on day 3–7 of cycle, ideally after not taking oral contraceptives for 3 months.

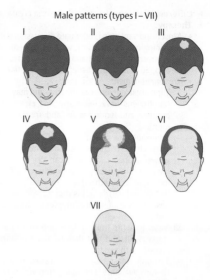

Male patterns (types I – VII)

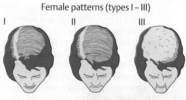

Female patterns (types I – III)

Fig. 31.**1** · Androgenetic alopecia: male pattern (after Hamilton) and female pattern (after Ludwig); men can also develop the Ludwig pattern and women the Hamilton pattern.

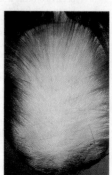

Fig. 31.**2** · Severe androgenetic alopecia in a women.

▶ **Differential diagnosis:** Diffuse alopecia areata, androgen-induced alopecia.
▶ **Therapy:**
• Most important step is adequate discussion with patient. Explain that process is physiologic, normally slow, with occasional bursts. Since the hairs are not lost but converted to vellus hairs, there is good hope that an efficient therapy can be developed to re-convert them. *Be optimistic!.*
• *Treatment of men:*
  – Topical estrogens are ineffective and may lead to gynecomastia. Systemic antiandrogens have too many side effects including testicular atrophy, impotence, and feminization (and are therefore only indicated in transsexual men).
  – *Minoxidil* is a systemic vasodilator, used for severe hypertension, which causes hypertrichosis. Topical minoxidil 2–5% solution is effective in androgenetic alopecia. Minoxidil can also be compounded (p. 697), but considerable care is required as it is poorly soluble. After 4–12 months of usage, hair loss may be stabilized and some regrowth of terminal hair shafts seen in frontal and vertex vellus regions. Side effects include hypertrichosis in undesired locations (face, nipples), allergic contact dermatitis and hypotension.
  ▣ *Note:* Patients must understand that once minoxidil is stopped, hair loss starts again, and that maintaining the status quo, rather than dramatic regrowth, is the goal.
  – Systemic finasteride (5-α-reductase type II inhibitor) is the most effective therapy available. 1 mg/daily "forever" is the dosage. It blocks conversion of testosterone into dihydrotestosterone, the active agent in androgenetic alopecia. Side effects during short-term use (1–3 years) are minimal; the inhibitor is highly specific and even effects on libido are quite rare. The long-term effects over 30 years are still unpredictable. Once stopped, there is rapid progression of hair loss at the pretreatment level.
  – Topical 17-α-estradiol is often employed in Germany; it does not exert estrogen effects, yet may inhibit 5-α-reductase activity and therefore is a safe, but not highly effective, treatment.
  – Combination therapy makes sense and appears more effective, yet has not been rigorously tested; minoxidil and/or 17-α-estradiol solution (men) combined with finasteride.
  – Supportive care includes appropriate grooming, aggressive treatment of seborrheic dermatitis, and avoiding medications that could increase hair loss.
  – Be alert to co-factors such as thyroid disease; appropriate endocrinologic management can help slow progression of hair loss.
  – *Hair transplantation:* Effective technique that depends on donor dominance; plugs or micrografts of hairs taken from an area where androgenetic alopecia does not occur can be transplanted to bald areas and hairs will continue to grow.
  ▣ *Note:* Hair transplants should be done by experienced surgeons, and only in patients in whom the degree and progression of baldness can be assessed. Continued treatment with minoxidil and/or finasteride should also be considered.
• *Treatment of women:*
  – Topical estrogens may be of value. A 17-α-estradiol solution is available commercially in Germany, or appropriate solutions for women and men can be compounded (p. 694). The solutions are applied to scalp and massaged in for 10 minutes daily. Trial of therapy for at least 4 months.
  – Minoxidil also useful; at least 6 months trial, better 12; more risk of facial hypertrichosis in women.

- Systemic antiandrogens can be employed, always in conjunction with oral contraceptives in premenopausal women and usually with monitoring by gynecologist. Various combinations and dosages of cyproterone acetate and chlormadinone are available in Europe but not in the USA.
- Topical antiandrogens are under development. Agents such as spironolactone, ketoconazole, cimetidine or dexamethasone have systemic antiandrogen effects but do little, if anything, topically.
- Hair transplantation usually not indicated in women because of their more diffuse thinning and the impossibility of reliably determining the border between androgen-sensitive and insensitive hair follicles.
- Same supportive measures as in men; also consider iron, zinc, and biotin supplementation.
- Monitor success with hair counts, trichogram or phototrichogram; learning that hair loss is decreasing has immense emotional value for the patient.

31.4 Localized Nonscarring Alopecia

Alopecia Areata

▶ **MIM code:** 104100.

▶ **Definition:** Sudden localized hair loss without clinically visible inflammation; variety of clinical patterns.

▶ **Epidemiology:** Prevalence in the USA is 0.1–0.2%, with an estimated lifetime risk of developing alopecia areata of 1.7%. About 20% of patients with alopecia areata report a positive family history for the disease.

▶ **Pathogenesis:** Alopecia areata is most likely an organ-specific autoimmune disorder, with autoaggressive T cells possibly directed against melanocytes in the anagen follicle. Likely association with other autoimmune diseases such as vitiligo, Hashimoto thyroiditis, and diabetes mellitus; also seen with other thyroid diseases and atopy, as well as with Down syndrome and Turner syndrome, but causal relationship not proven. Despite the severity of the immunologic attack, follicles are only very rarely destroyed and can therefore fully recover. Alopecia areata is so variable that some consider it to be a family of diseases. It occasionally follows severe physical or emotional stress.

▶ **Classification:**
- *Alopecia areata circumscripta:* One or several areas of alopecia on scalp or beard.
- *Alopecia totalis:* Loss of most or all of scalp hair, sometimes with loss of eyebrows and eyelashes.
- *Alopecia universalis:* Loss of all scalp and body hair.

▶ **Clinical features:**
- Round to oval sharply circumscribed areas of hair loss without inflammation (Fig. 31.**3**). Usually starts as single lesion; most often spontaneous resolution. In others, expansion of lesion or development of new patches.
- *Ophiasis:* Band-like loss from ear to ear across the nape; poor prognostic sign.
- Scalp sometimes slightly swollen; doughy or puffy feeling.
- *Exclamation point hairs:* Broken-off 1–2 mm hairs at periphery of patch; when plucked, look like exclamation point with thick bulb.
- *Cadaver hairs:* Hairs broken before they reach surface; also sign of activity and progression.
- Focal areas of *poliosis* (grey hairs) where previous patches have regrown.

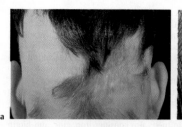
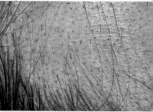

a

Fig. 31.3 · **a** Alopecia areata. **b** Exclamation point hairs.

- *Pitted nails* present in around 20% of adults and up to 50% of children with alopecia areata; association with twenty-nail dystrophy (trachyonychia p. 524); other nail problems less likely. Rare reports of keratitis and hypohidrosis.

► **Histology:** Only indicated for confirmation of suspected diffuse variant of alopecia areata. In early stage, dense lymphocytic infiltrate about lower follicles ("swarm of bees" pattern around anagen hair bulb) and increased number of catagen follicles; later, miniaturization of follicles. If infiltrates present, strong support for diagnosis; their absence does not rule out the possibility of alopecia areata.

► **Diagnostic approach:** History (previous lesions, overlooked lesions in beard area); clinical examination (polished areas with exclamation point or cadaver hairs).

   ▣ *Note:* Use hand lens (dermatoscope) to better visualize exclamation point and cadaver hairs as well as fully maintained follicle orifices (disappear in scarring alopecias); always do pull test at edge of lesion (if positive, high likelihood of progression).

- Biopsy rarely needed. Laboratory examination probably not justified for single lesion, but if disease is progressive or persistent or negative prognostic factors present, then CBS, sed rate, thyroid function (highest yield), search for autoantibodies (ANA, parietal cell, mitochondrial, thyroid); if otherwise sick or lymphadenopathy, or if very many, small, only partially alopecic areas visible, then syphilis serology.

   ▣ *Note:* Check blood pressure. Alopecia areata tends to be more aggressive in young patients from families with high prevalence of hypertension.

► **Differential diagnosis:** Trichotillomania, tinea capitis, syphilitic alopecia, scarring alopecia.

   ▣ *Note:* Combinations of alopecia areata and trichotillomania occur, especially in children.

► **Prognosis:** The outlook is variable; 35–60% experience spontaneous remission in 2 years. Unfavorable signs are:

- Positive personal or family history for atopy, alopecia areata, or autoimmune diseases.
- Onset before puberty.
- Rapid progression.
- Widespread recurrence.
- Persistence for >2 years.
- Ophiasis (alopecia areata involving temporal ands occipital margins of scalp in a continuous band).
- Involvement of eyelids or eyelashes.
- Pitted nails.

▶ **Therapy:**
- Aggressiveness of therapy adjusted to risk factors and prognosis.
- Explain course to patient; initially only vellus hairs (peach fuzz) will be seen; regrowth of terminal hairs takes 6–18 months, depending on hair length.
- Address underlying issues if any have been identified, such as atopy or thyroid disease.
- No curative therapy; two main strategies to alter immune picture around follicles—immunosuppression with corticosteroids or immunomodulation via intentional allergic contact dermatitis.
- Single or few lesions less than 6 months in age:
  - High potency topical corticosteroid solution or gel b.i.d.
  - Triamcinolone acetate 2.5 mg/mL in lidocaine; infiltrate lesion, especially the periphery, and repeat in 4–6 weeks. More than two injections leads to increased risk of atrophy.
  - Add zinc aspartate 50 mg b.i.d. as adjuvant therapy.
  - Consider short burst of systemic corticosteroids in patient with two or more unfavorable prognostic factors. Typical regimen prednisolone for 1 week is 75–75–50–25–25–10–10 mg, then 3 weeks pause. Repeat for three cycles; then re-assess and either offer another three cycles or stop. Carefully consider contraindications and side effects (hypertension, worsening of diabetes mellitus, glaucoma, many others).
▶ Long-term systemic treatment with corticosteroids or cyclosporine can induce hair growth, but it is not stable and the side effects of continued therapy are unacceptable.
▶ Anthralin irritant therapy can be combined with corticosteroid bursts and oral zinc. Use either 1–3% anthralin cream or 2–5% anthralin stick applicator. Apply daily; starting for 5 minutes and increasing in 5 minute increments until irritation is induced or 8 hours is reached. If no irritation, can also increase concentration. Then continue on daily basis, removing the anthralin one burning occurs. Regrowth takes 4–8 weeks to begin after irritation has been induced. Side effects include discoloration and nuchal lymphadenopathy.
▶ If all these approaches have failed despite appropriate usage, then consider inducing contact allergy to diphenylcyclopropenone (*Happle regimen*). Extensive counseling required, as this method is still regarded as experimental:
  - Sensitization with 2% diphenylcyclopropenone applied to scalp with adhesive bandage.
  - Observe positive response; if none occurs, repeat.
  - After 2 weeks, begin treatment starting with 0.0001% solution and slowly working up to 0.5%. Make every effort to maintain a mild allergic contact dermatitis. Explain to patient that occasional severe reactions are hard to avoid; blisters and pigmentary changes can occur.
  - Over months of mild irritation, hair regrowth usually starts.
- Other possibilities include:
  - PUVA or UVB therapy.
  - Minoxidil.
  - Topical immunomodulatory agents (tacrolimus, pimecrolimus).
  ▶ *Note:* In children, the main options are topical corticosteroids, anthralin, and oral zinc.

Trichotillomania

▶ **Definition:** Localized alopecia secondary to plucking, cutting, or rubbing away hairs.

▶ **Clinical features:**
- Poorly circumscribed areas of with broken-off hairs; occasionally follicular hemorrhages. Pull test is negative and trichogram shows few telogen hairs.
- In infants, an almost normal habit of no consequence. May also induce nuchal alopecia simply by rubbing their heads on mattress or pillow. In older children or adults, usually associated with psychiatric disturbances, in the general category of obsessive-compulsive disorder. Clinically tends to be more diffuse than in small children; sometimes entire scalp involved and patient presents with wig.

▶ **Histology:** Biopsy shows perifollicular hemorrhage and damaged follicles; useful to exclude alopecia areata.
  ▣ *Note:* Bear in mind the possibility of trichophagia and the formation of hair ball (trichobezoar) in the gastrointestinal tract, which can cause obstruction and other signs and symptoms.

▶ **Therapy:** Confronting the patient with the diagnosis may help in mild cases. Most teenagers and adults require psychiatric support and therapy. Often manifestation of conflict between child and parents, making management even more difficult.

Self-induced Alopecia

There are several other forms of self-induced alopecia in which there is no underlying psychological problem:

▶ **Traction alopecia:** Hair loss secondary to tight hair styles, such as corn rows in blacks, tight braids, or long, heavy ponytails. If not interrupted, can progress to scarring and permanent hair loss.

▶ **Pressure alopecia:** Hair loss from tightly-fitting helmets, hats, sweat bands, or the like.

▶ **Massage alopecia:** Hair loss following over-aggressive or ritually repeated hair massage.

31.5 Scarring Alopecia

Overview

▶ **Definition:** Irreversible damage to hair follicles leading to scarring and permanent alopecia.

▶ **Pathogenesis:** Many causes including autoimmune diseases (chronic cutaneous lupus erythematosus [discoid], lichen planus, less often morphea or systemic sclerosis), infections (bacterial, fungal, viral), tumors (mycosis fungoides, follicular mucinosis), exogenous factors (ionizing radiation, trauma, overaggressive hair care), embryological defects (aplasia cutis congenita). In some instances, no causative agent is identifiable (*pseudopelade*). In our experience, however, most cases of pseudopelade represent end-stages of lichen planopilaris (most common) or chronic cutaneous lupus erythematosus (less common).

▶ **Diagnostic approach:** The key is not to overlook clinical signs of scarring. Use of the dermatoscope is a priceless, but far too rarely employed, tool for identifying such signs—disappearance of follicular ostia, along with shiny, thin scalp epidermis that has lost its normal surface patterning. Bundles of hairs produced by hair follicles that have become fused by autoaggressive inflammation (*toothbrush sign,* as hairs resemble grouped bristles of toothbrush) are also a frequent sign of scarring alopecia.

► Always look for signs of associated diseases elsewhere on the skin. Sometimes much easier to identify lupus erythematosus or lichen planus on the skin than on the scalp. Also check mouth and nails for discrete signs of lichen planus. Scalp biopsy is always indicated when scarring alopecia is suspected, but quite often is not as helpful as expected. The main reason for that is a wrong biopsy technique (p. 27). Advanced scarring alopecia, no matter how perfect your biopsy is and whatever its cause, looks puzzlingly similar in most cases.

► **Differential diagnosis:** Late disease looks the same, no matter what the cause. Always systematically consider all of the pathogenetic possibilities discussed above, and look for indications to the presence of these problems elsewhere on the skin, mucosa, or nails.

► **Therapy:** If the cause is identified, then it should be treated promptly and aggressively to minimize the amount of scarring. Once scarring has occurred, there is no treatment other than perhaps an attempt at hair transplantation—yet only in the absence of active inflammation and once the alopecia has stopped progressing.

Chronic Cutaneous Lupus Erythematosus (CCLE)

► **Synonym:** Discoid lupus erythematosus.
► **Clinical features:**
  • Scalp involvement is common in CCLE, especially among black women.
  • Early lesions show erythema, follicular plugging, and scale; later hypopigmentation, atrophy, and scarring alopecia (Fig. 31.4).
  ⚠ *Caution:* In rare cases, CCLE can evolve into a squamous cell carcinoma, so always do a biopsy in patients with chronic disease and a changing clinical picture.

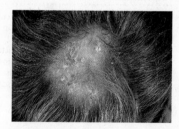

Fig. 31.4 · Scarring alopecia: chronic cutaneous lupus erythematosus.

► **Histology:** Follicular scarring, lymphocytic infiltrates about remaining follicles, epidermal atrophy, telangiectases, mucin deposition, on direct immunofluorescence (DIF) may see lupus erythematosus band.
► **Therapy:**
  • High-potency topical or intralesional corticosteroids (triamcinolone 2.5–5.0 mg/mL in lidocaine). If lesions are hyperkeratotic, then a salicylic acid scalp ointment applied overnight and washed out thoroughly may remove scale and help increase penetration of corticosteroids.
  • If no response, then more rapidly to systemic therapy. Often scalp disease in CCLE is self-limited, so aggressive intervention is warranted. Most useful are

corticosteroid pulse therapy or cyclosporine for a limited time period. Antimalarials are another possibility, but have a slow onset of action and are less suited for the immediate task of arresting scarring.

- Chronic immunosuppressive therapy is not appropriate for scarring alopecia.
- Patients should wear a hat and use high protection factor sunscreens.

Lichen Planus

- ▶ **Synonym:** Lichen planopilaris, lichen follicularis, Graham–Little syndrome.
- ▶ **Epidemiology:** Scalp involvement in 30–60% of patients with lichen planus; usually middle-aged adults. More common in patients with persistent diseases.
- ▶ **Clinical features:** Follicular or perifollicular hyperkeratoses, usually multiple, evolving into atrophic patulous follicles, sometimes with erythematous rim, and then permanent scarring.
- ▶ **Histology:** Dense lymphocytic infiltrate both around residual follicles and sometimes along dermoepidermal junction; epidermis normal with prominent granular layer, no mucin; on direct immunofluorescence, colloid bodies more likely.
- ▶ **Therapy:**
  - High-potency topical or intralesional corticosteroids with salicylic acid ointments.
  - If nonresponsive or rapidly advancing, consider short burst of systemic corticosteroids, perhaps combined with acitretin (0.3–0.5 mg/kg).

Infections

Sometimes the cause of the inflammation leading to scarring is known:
- ▶ Tinea capitis (p. 108).
- ▶ Furuncle, carbuncle (p. 74).
- ▶ Herpes zoster (p. 61).

Folliculitis Decalvans

- ▶ **Definition:** Scarring alopecia with follicular inflammation and usually pustules.
- ▶ **Epidemiology:** In men, usually starts in young adult life; in women, somewhat later.
- ▶ **Pathogenesis:** Divided opinions if bacteria play a primary or secondary role. Possibly a hypersensitivity reaction against persistent bacterial antigens with continued, autoaggressive immune responses.
- ▶ **Clinical features:** Pustules, erythema, scarring and sometimes marked seborrhea (Fig. 31.5).
- ▶ **Histology:** Dense neutrophilic infiltrates with destruction of follicles; often rich in plasma cells.

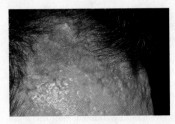

Fig. 31.**5** · Folliculitis decalvans.

Diagnostic approach: Culture often identifies *Staphylococcus aureus*. Biopsy and DIF useful to exclude lupus erythematosus.

Therapy:

- Despite the confusing pathophysiology, empiric antibiotic therapy seems the best approach.
- Rifampicin 300 mg b.i.d., often combined with clindamycin 300 mg b.i.d. for 2 weeks; then rifampicin alone for another 6–8 weeks. Clarithromycin or ciprofloxacin can replace clindamycin.
- Metronidazole 500 mg t.i.d. combined with clindamycin 300–600 mg b.i.d. for 3 weeks.
- If antibiotics are not effective, then consider prednisolone pulse therapy combined with isotretinoin.

Follicular Mucinosis

Synonym: Preferred term is folliculotropic mycosis fungoides; alopecia mucinosa.

Definition: Alopecia associated with lymphocytic infiltrate of hair follicle and intrafollicular mucin deposition.

Pathogenesis: In adults, almost always follicular mycosis fungoides; in children, controversial if perhaps a self-limited form exists. Often mycosis fungoides appears years after the follicular mucinosis (p. 474).

▶ *Note:* If the diagnosis of follicular mucinosis is made, the patient must be examined completely and then followed for development of mycosis fungoides.

Clinical features:

- *Acute form:* 2–5 cm boggy plaques without hairs; usually on face or scalp. Most common in children, young adults. Spontaneous healing may occur over 1–2 years.
- *Chronic form:* In addition, keratotic papules on extensor surfaces or trunk associated with hair loss; often mucinous substance can be expressed.

Histology: Folliculotropic infiltrate of T cells together with mucin deposition in follicles or epidermis. If atypical lymphocytes or clonal rearrangement of T-cell receptor present, then regard as mycosis fungoides.

Therapy:

- If chronic lesion or older adult, treat as mycosis fungoides with PUVA or ionizing radiation (20–30 Gy fractionated over 3–4 weeks) combined with interferon-α-2b.
- If acute lesion in child with no histological evidence for mycosis fungoides, can treat with intralesional steroids. If no response, consider short burst of systemic corticosteroids or dapsone 50–100 mg daily (following hemoglobin level). Follow patient even if remission occurs.

Pseudopelade of Brocq

Definition: Scarring alopecia in absence of identified causative agent.

Pathogenesis: May be the end stage for lichen planus or lupus erythematosus; no convincing evidence available that this really is a specific disease unrelated to other forms of scarring alopecia; possibly an exaggerated form of (physiological) "programmed organ deletion" of hair follicles.

Clinical features: Small confluent atrophic scarred areas (likened to "tracks in the snow"), usually occipital or parietal. Typically bundles of hairs remaining (Fig. 31.**6**). Hair follicles hard to see; affected areas smooth and glistening, sometimes pruritic.

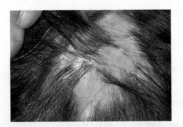

Fig. 31.**6** · Pseudopelade of Brocq.

► **Histology:** Reduced number of follicles with scarring and no evidence for lupus erythematosus or lichen planus.
► **Therapy:**
  • Treat underlying disease.
  • If none seen, empiric use of antibiotics or antimalarials.
  • Symptomatic treatment with wig. Hair transplantation or scalp reduction can be considered if disease is completely quiescent.

31.6 Hair Shaft Anomalies

Definitions

There are a number of structural defects in the hair shaft; some inherited, others acquired. Figure 31.**7** illustrates the most common variants.
► **Trichoptilosis:** Hairs split and feathered.
► **Trichoclasis:** Tranverse split in hair with retained cuticle.
► **Trichoschisis:** Smooth transverse split in hair, associated with trichothiodystrophy.
► **Trichorrhexis nodosa:** Localized longitudinal splitting of shaft; frayed ends pushed upon one another (compared to two paint brushes pushed into one another), causing nodules along shaft.
► **Trichonodosis:** Knots and loops in shaft.
► **Trichorrhexis invaginata:** Distal shaft pushed into bulbus receptacle on proximal shaft (*bamboo hair*); associated with Netherton syndrome (atopy, ichthyosiform skin changes; p. 195).
► **Pili torti:** Hair that is flattened and twisted upon its long axis.
► **Monilethrix:** Shaft has alternate swellings (nodes) and constrictions (lacking medulla), producing beaded effect. Nodal interval 0.7–1.0 cm.
► **Pseudomonilethrix:** Appears similar to monilethrix, but parts of shaft are irregular with nodes while other areas are regular.
► **Pili annulati:** Disturbance in hair color with alternating pigmented and nonpigmented areas. May be confused with pili torti.

Diagnostic Approach

► **Hair shaft anomalies:**
  • *With increased fragility:* Monilethrix, pseudomonilethrix, poli torti, Menke syndrome, Netherton syndrome, trichorrhexis nodosa, trichothiodystrophy.
  • *With normal stability:* Pili annulati, wooly hair, uncombable hair syndrome.

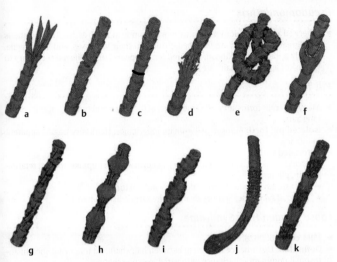

Fig. 31.**7** · **Hair shaft anomalies (after Whiting).** **a** Trichoptilosis. **b** Trichoclasis. **c** Tricho-schisis. **d** Trichorrhexis nodosa. **e** Trichonodosis. **f** Trichorrhexis invaginata. **g** Pilus tortus. **h** Monilethrix. **i** Pseudomonilethrix. **j** Loose anagen hair syndrome. **k** Pilus annulatus.

Therapy

In most instances, no therapy except "tender loving care." Patients should be encouraged to use mild shampoos, with rinses and conditioners to make hairs less likely to tangle or split.

Monilethrix

▶ **MIM code:** 158000.
▶ **Pathogenesis:** Mutations in human hair keratins (HB1 or HB6), both on chromosome 12q13; autosomal dominant inheritance.
▶ **Clinical features:**
- Normal hair at birth, but in the first months hairs begin to break off 1–2 cm above the surface, more prominent on occiput, where small erythematosus follicular keratoses also develop.
- Sometimes spontaneous improvement in puberty or pregnancy.
- Occasionally eyelids, eyelashes, and body hair affected.
- Often associated with keratosis pilaris and nail changes; rarely dental anomalies and juvenile cataracts.
▶ **Diagnostic approach:** Sometimes clinically inapparent, but abnormalities identified with microscopy or scanning electron microscopy.
▶ **Therapy:** No satisfactory therapy; supportive care.

Pseudomonilethrix

▶ Inherited autosomal dominant form, most common in South Africa. The hair shafts vary greatly in caliber, are flattened, turned on their long axes, and very fragile. Usually appears in childhood. Acquired form appears later, believed secondary to trauma or aggressive hair care.

Pili Torti

▶ Many different forms, all with same defect of flattening and twisting of shaft along long axis.
▶ **Isolated pili torti:** Autosomal dominant inheritance. Hairs very fragile, apparent in infancy.
▶ Associated with:.
   • *Menkes kinky hair syndrome* (p. 317): abnormal copper uptake, mental retardation, pili torti.
   • *Bjornstad syndrome:* Sensory deafness and pili torti.
   • *Crandall syndrome:* Sensory deafness, hypogonadism, pili torti.

Loose Anagen Hair Syndrome

▶ **MIM code:** 600628.
▶ **Definition:** Disturbance in binding between hair shaft and inner root sheath; autosomal dominant inheritance with variable expressivity.
▶ **Clinical features:** At birth, hairs are normal. By 4–6 years of age, fine blond hairs that are easily extracted; more common in girls.
▶ **Diagnostic approach:** Light pull test is very positive; on trichogram, almost all the hairs are anagen.
▶ **Therapy:** No effective treatment, but self-limiting disease; in almost every patient, by puberty the hairs are firmly anchored again.

Trichothiodystrophy

▶ **MIM code:** 601675.
▶ **Definition:** Combination of sulfur-deficient hair with complex series of associated defects.
▶ **Pathogenesis:** Mutations in same DNA repair genes responsible for xeroderma pigmentosum (p. 304); in autosomal recessive inheritance. Mutations at some sites in genes cause xeroderma pigmentosum; at others, trichothiodystrophy.
▶ **Clinical features:** The hair findings are the unifying clinical feature.
   • The hairs are easily broken, so patients present with both focal and diffuse alopecia, often involving nonscalp hairs. When examined under polarized light, the hairs are banded (*tiger tail sign*).
   • Associated defects include **p**hotosensitivity, **i**chthyosis, **b**rittle hair, **i**nfertility, **d**evelopmental delay, **s**hort stature. The initial letters are variously combined to create BIDS, IBIDS, PIBIDS; *Tay syndrome* is another name for IBIDS.
   • Despite the relationship to the xeroderma pigmentosum gene, there is no increased incidence of skin cancers.
▶ **Diagnostic approach:** Exact genetic analysis available in specialized centers.
▶ **Therapy:** Multidisciplinary management; no treatment for hair except gentle care.

Other Hair Shaft Anomalies

▶ **Pili multigemini:** Multiple hairs arise from same follicular unit; very common in dogs.

▶ **Trichostasis spinulosa:** Multiple vellus hairs rolled up inside dilated follicle with comedo plug; more common in sebaceous areas, sun-damaged skin; almost normal on nose.

▶ **Woolly hair:** Hairs are excessively curled, fancifully compared to sheep wool, scalp hair of blacks, or even fiberglass; may be inherited (MIM code 194300) or acquired; diffuse or localized (*woolly hair nevus*). Also associated with Naxos syndrome (MIM code 601204: palmoplantar keratoderma, cardiomyopathy, defect in plakoglobin).

▶ **Hair casts:** Small white keratinous sheaths around the hair shaft; may slide; differential diagnostic considerations include nits and trichomycosis axillaris.

31.7 Hypertrichosis

Overview

▶ **Definition:** Growth of hairs that are longer, thicker or more numerous than the location, age, and racial background of the patient would predict. Usually there is a switch from vellus to terminal hairs; in acquired hypertrichosis an anagen shift is usually present.

Hypertrichosis Lanuginosa

▶ Lanugo hairs have a thin depigmented shaft. They are present in utero during months 3–7, but normally shed by birth and replaced by terminal or vellus hairs.

▶ **Hypertrichosis lanuginosa congenital:**
  • MIM code: 145700.
  • Uncommon genodermatosis in which newborn is covered by long lanugo hairs, which are not shed and replaced, but continue to grow. Patient typically winds up with a silvery coat of hairs 10 cm long.

▶ **Hypertrichosis lanuginosa acquisita:** Obligatory paraneoplastic marker (p. 486). Any patient who shows this should be subjected to a rigorous and systematic tumor search.

Generalized Hypertrichosis

▶ There are many causes for diffuse excess numbers of terminal hairs. In all of these disorders, there are still local (regional differences) but the entire body seems affected.

▶ **Hereditary:** Porphyria cutanea tarda and porphyria variegata (primarily facial), mucopolysaccharidoses, chromosome abnormalities (trisomy 18).

▶ **Endocrine:** Pituitary and thyroid disorders.

▶ **Eating disorders** (especially anorexia nervosa), malabsorption, fetal alcohol syndrome.

▶ **Medications:** Cyclosporine, minoxidil, phenytoin are most common; others include diazoxide, streptomycin, corticosteroids, penicillamine, psoralens.

Localized Hypertrichosis

▶ **Nevi** including:
- *Hair nevus:* Uncommon and disputed but sometimes localized area with excess hair follicles and no other abnormalities; if papule in front of ear, search carefully for associated cartilage suggesting accessory tragus with enormous number of vellus hairs.
- *Becker nevus:* Localized mosaic area of increased melanin and increased hair growth. Often relatively hairless until puberty, can be associated with localized acne or underlying smooth muscle hamartoma with cutis anserina (*goose bumps*) as smooth muscles contract (p. 412).
- *Faun tail nevus:* Localized hair growth over sacrum fancifully resembling a fluffy tail, but a most serious marker for potential underlying spinal cord defects or spina bifida. Neurological and radiological work-up mandatory.

31.8 Hirsutism

Overview

▶ **Definition:** Increased growth of terminal hairs in women in androgen-dependent areas, producing male-like hair growth pattern. *Virilization* is the association of hirsutism with other signs of male development, such as voice deepening, clitoral enlargement, increased muscles, loss of breast tissue, acne, and androgenetic alopecia.

▶ **Pathogenesis:** The main causes of hirsutism are summarized in Table 31.2.
- ▶ *Note:* Most cases of hirsutism are physiologic; in many ethnic groups, female body hair does not fit the current Western beauty standard, leading to psychosocial problems as people move between cultures.
- ▶ *Note:* Hirsutism combined with androgenetic alopecia can be a sign of elevated prolactin levels, typically caused by neuroleptic agents, polycystic ovary syndrome, or prolactinoma (usually a small tumor not otherwise symptomatic).

Diagnostic Approach

▶ **History:**
- Onset, course of excessive hairs; family history (hair patterns of other women in family).
- Menstrual history; pregnancies.
- Symptoms of virilization?.
- Medications?.
- History of thromboses (contraindication to estrogen therapy).

▶ **Examination:**
- Signs of virilization, Cushing disease, acromegaly, galactorrhea (Fig. 31.8).
- Complete physical examination; palpate ovaries, Pap smear, breast check.
- *Laboratory:* DHEAS, free testosterone, SHBG, prolactin; others as indicated. Testosterone >2 ng/mL suggests ovarian tumor; DHEAS >9000 ng/mL suggests adrenal tumor.
- ▶ *Note:* If it is not completely clear that the patient has idiopathic hirsutism, refer to endocrinologist or gynecologist for a second opinion.

Table 31.2 · Causes of hirsutism

	Functional	Neoplastic
Endocrine		
Ovarian	Polycystic ovary disease	Variety of functional tumors (hilar cell or Leydig cell, luteoma, arrhenoblastoma
Adrenal gland	Congenital adrenal hyperplasia, idiopathic adrenal hyperandrogenism	Adenomas and carcinomas
Pituitary		Cushing disease, acromegaly, adrenogenital syndrome, prolactinoma
Nonendocrine		
Idiopathic	Most common; genetic-ethnic variation	
Medications	Phenytoin, androgens (danazol, stanozolol, body building pills), corticosteroids, ACTH, oral contraceptives (progesterone has androgen action), metyrapone (used for diagnostic purposes only, so unlikely)	
Achard–Theirs syndrome	Virilization and adult-onset diabetes mellitus in postmenopausal women because of excess adrenocortical androgens	
SAHA syndrome	Seborrhea, acne, hypertrichosis/hirsutism, alopecia; group of disorders with either elevated androgen levels or increased androgen sensitivity	

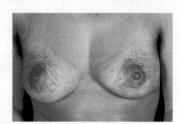

Fig. 31.**8** · Hirsutism.

Therapy

► **Treat underlying disease**.
► **Removal of hairs:**
  • Shaving, wax epilation, chemical epilation (thioglycolate commercial products or compounded, p. 700).
  • Bleaching (6–10% hydrogen peroxide in water).
  • *Electrolysis:* Destruction of individual hair follicles with electrocoagulation or diathermy; time-consuming; frequent re-treatment; works on white or gray hair.
  • *Epilation with lasers* (diode or Nd:YAG) or intense pulsed light source; only works on pigmented hairs but much faster and more effective. Clearly the method of the future.
  • Eflornithine (topical) effective but only as long as used; also expensive.
  • Ionizing radiation **contraindicated**.
  ☒ *Note:* The problem with all attempts at permanent hair removal is that bulge (hair stem) cells are hard to destroy and multiple treatments are often required. Also, complete destruction of these important stem cells ("bone marrow of the skin") does not appear an inherently good idea, since they are needed during wound healing and epidermal regeneration after burn wounds.
► **Hormone therapy:**
  • *Hormones that antagonize androgens:* Corticosteroids or estrogens.
  • *Primary antiandrogens:*
    – Cyproterone acetate.
    – Chlormadinone acetate.
  • *Miscellaneous agents with secondary antiandrogen activity:* Spironolactone, ketoconazole, cimetidine.
  • *5-α-Reductase inhibitor*: Finasteride is not approved for women but effective; must be used with effective contraception because of risk of malformations in male fetuses.
  • *Combination therapy*: Many combinations of estrogens and either cyproterone acetate or chlormadinone acetate are available in Europe.

31.9 Diseases of the Scalp

Dandruff

► **Definition:** Pityriasis capitis.
► **Clinical features:** Familiar fine scale present on scalps of most adults; uncommon in children. Gradual transition with seborrheic dermatitis, in which case erythema or pruritus may be present, as well as involvement of paranasal and retroauricular regions and external ear canal.
► **Therapy:** Medicated "dandruff" shampoos with zinc pyrithione, selenium sulfide, climbazole, octopirox, ketoconazole, and/or tar. Patients should be encouraged to switch between shampoos to reduce tachyphylaxis (product not working after repeated use).

ily Scalp

Synonym: Seborrhoea oleosa.

Clinical features: Likely a variant of seborrheic dermatitis. Patients have very oily skin and hair; often associated with androgenetic alopecia, as androgens stimulate sebum production.

Therapy: Keep hairs cut short, same shampoos as above; if insufficient, use topical estrogens in alcoholic vehicle.

eborrheic Dermatitis

In our view, both of the above conditions are closely related to seborrheic dermatitis, a combination inflammatory condition that overlaps with psoriasis.

▶ *Note:* Treating seemingly minor degrees of scalp inflammation (such as mild seborrheic dermatitis) is essential in managing hair loss, because inflammation causes a telogen shift and thus exacerbates the hair loss.

32 Diseases of the Nails

32.1 Introduction

Anatomy (Fig. 32.1)

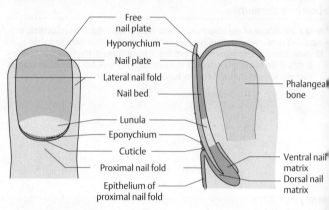

Fig. 32.1 · Anatomy of the nail apparatus.

Components of the Nail

- **Epidermis of dorsal nail fold:** Skin at proximal end of nail; folded upon itself.
- **Cuticle:** Sheet of cells that seals proximal nail fold.
- **Nail matrix:** Epithelium that keratinizes without granular layer (onycholemm keratinization); the lunula is the most distal aspect of the nail matrix, visibl through the nail plate.
- **Nail bed:** Produces a thin sheet of parakeratotic keratinocytes attached to dee surface of nail plate; perhaps helps in attachment, which is also facilitated by a sy: tem of ridges and furrows (zipper effect).
- **Hyponychium:** Skin at point of separation of nail plate from nail bed; lacks de matoglyphics.
  - ▶ *Note:* Nails grow slowly; replacement requires 6–12 months for fingernails an 12–18 months for toenails. Thus any therapeutic effects on the nails are no easily noticed, and treatment requires much patience on the part of physicia and patient alike.

Common nail abnormalities (Fig. 32.2)

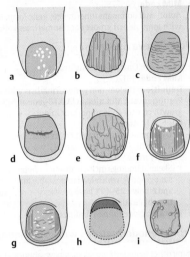

Fig. 32.**2** · **Common nail changes. a** Pits. **b** Longitudinal grooves. **c** Transverse grooves. **d** Beau lines. **e** Trachyonychia. **f** Punctate leukonychia. **g** Longitudinal leukonychia. **h** Onychoschisis. **i** Lichen planus nail. **j** Distal onycholysis.

32.2 Congenital Nail Anomalies

Pachyonychia Congenita

▶ **MIM codes:** 167200; 167210; 260130.
▶ **Definition:** Group of genodermatoses involving keratin mutations with thickened nails and variable associated findings; pachys means thick.
▶ **Pathogenesis:** Two well established types:
  • Jadassohn–Lewandowsky type (PC1): Mutations in keratins 16 and 6A.
  • Jackson–Lawler type (PC2): Mutations in keratins 17 and 6B.
▶ **Clinical features:** Thickened and friable finger and toenails; palmoplantar hyperkeratosis and often hyperhidrosis. PC1 patients have oral leukokeratosis; PC2 patients have steatocystomas, alopecia, and natal teeth. Other clinical forms very rare, poorly established.
▶ **Therapy:** Abrasion of nail with rotary sander; keratolytics, including high-concentration urea ointments; if severe, acitretin may produce temporary improvement.

Isolated Congenital Nail Dystrophy

► **MIM code:** 605779.
► Autosomal dominant inheritance; gene locus 17p13. Patients have thin nail plates with longitudinal grooves and sometimes koilonychia. No associated findings.

Nail–Patella Syndrome

► **Synonym:** Onycho-osteodystrophy.
► **MIM code:** 161200.
► **Definition:** Uncommon genodermatosis with nail and skeletal anomalies.
► **Pathogenesis:** Mutation in *LMX1B* gene at 9q34.1 coding for LIM homeo domain, a growth control gene important in dorsa–ventral patterning of the limbs.
► **Clinical features:**
  • Dystrophic nails; triangular lunulae; longitudinal grooves, splitting and even anonychia (complete or partial); worse on thumbs, which are sometimes exclusively involved.
  • Skeletal findings include absent or hypoplastic patellas (seen on prenatal ultrasonography), which lead to unstable knees; also abnormal iliac horns, scapulas, and elbows. 25–40% have progressive nephropathy and some require dialysis or transplantation.
► **Therapy:** None for nail findings.

Other Genodermatoses with Nail Anomalies

Many other genodermatoses may have abnormal nails. Examples include:
► Non-bullous congenital ichthyosiform erythroderma.
► Darier disease.
► Hailey–Hailey disease.
► Hidrotic ectodermal dysplasia.
► Focal dermal hypoplasia.
► Junctional and dystrophic forms of epidermolysis bullosa.
► Dyskeratosis congenita.

Other Inherited Nail Anomalies

► **Pitted nails**, as well as longitudinal and transverse grooves, can be inherited. Diagnosis made when present early in life and with positive family history, as all are most often acquired.
► Various forms of **anonychia:** Partial or complete absence of nail from birth (In contrast, **onychotrophy** should be reserved for nails that are initially normal and then become thinned or even lost.).
  ☐ *Note:* Anonychia is associated with a wide variety of ectodermal dysplasia syndromes. Always look for associated hair, tooth, and skin findings.

32.3 Nail Apparatus Infections

Acute Paronychia

► **Definition:** Acute infection of nail fold.
► **Pathogenesis:** Most often bacterial infection, facilitated by damage to cuticle; less often herpes simplex; rarely iatrogenic (patients receiving systemic retinoids).

Clinical features:

- Painful swelling of proximal or lateral nail fold region; cuticle usually missing. When staphylococcal, can be bullous (*bulla repens*) and extend under the nail.
- *Herpetic whitlow:* Intensely painful swelling; usually with blisters; if child, often with oral herpetic infection and thumbsucking; in adults, formerly common in dentists, today rare.

▶ **Diagnostic approach:** Culture and sensitivity for bacteria; direct immunofluorescence test for herpes simplex virus.

▶ **Differential diagnosis:** Felon or panaritium refers to a deeper digital infection, often following puncture injury (human or cat bite, trauma). Has potential to spread along fascial planes and tendon sheaths, so requires management by hand surgeon.

▶ **Therapy:** If bacterial, incision and drainage; systemic antibiotics; if viral, no manipulation, systemic antivirals.

Blistering Dactylitis

▶ **Definition:** Streptococcal infection of fingertips.

▶ **Pathogenesis:** No explanation for limited localization of infection.

▶ **Clinical features:** Patients present with asymptomatic distal digits that are swollen and may evolve with blisters. More proximal involvement also possible. Most common in children.

▶ **Differential diagnosis:** Important to distinguish from paronychia or other nail fold infection because of rapid response to antibiotics.

▶ **Therapy:** Oral penicillin or other antistreptococcal antibiotics. Blisters can be drained.

Chronic Paronychia

▶ **Definition:** Chronic infection of the nail fold.

▶ **Epidemiology:** Very common disorder, most often seen in women 30–60 years of age.

▶ **Pathogenesis:** The two most important factors are repeated exposure to water and a damaged cuticle. The usual causative agent is *Candida albicans*; secondary infection with *Staphylococcus aureus* and *Pseudomonas aeruginosa* (dark nail) also occurs.

▶ **Clinical features:** Thumb and index finger are most often involved. Usually starts as slight swelling of proximal nailfold, then loss of cuticle and discharge of pus from under the nailfold. Once the cuticle is damaged, water, irritants, and microorganisms all cause trouble.

▶ **Diagnostic approach:** Smears for culture and sensitivity; search for both bacteria and yeast; secondary contaminants common.

▶ **Therapy:** Treatment of chronic paronychia is difficult, requiring patience on the part of both patient and physician. Important steps include:

- Reducing exposure to moisture and other irritating factors. Elimination is impossible for domestic workers, and difficult in many industrial settings.
- Protection of nail fold:
  - Gloves, ideally washable cotton gloves underneath rubber gloves.
  - Disposable vinyl gloves when working with fruits and vegetables.
  - No direct contact with cleaning fluids, solvents, paints.
  - After exposure, wash hands with mild soap, rinse extensively.
  - Do not manipulate cuticle.
  - In the evenings, apply thick ointment to cuticle area.

- Use topical antimycotic agents q.i.d. and after exposure; ointments adhere better but solutions penetrate better; let patient try both. If bacterial infection identified, then topical antibiotics.
- Bacterial infections may require culture-directed systemic antibiotics; systemic antimycotic agents seldom needed.

Onychomycosis

▶ **Definition:** Fungal infection of the nail apparatus.
▶ **Epidemiology:** 20–30% of adults >40 years of age have onychomycosis, usually involving toenails.
▶ **Pathogenesis:** Dermatophytes are most common cause (>80%) (*tinea unguium*) but also yeasts (8%) and molds (6%).
   ☑ *Caution:* If patient is young and has multiple or severe candidal infections of nail folds and nails, think of chronic mucocutaneous candidiasis or other immune defects.
▶ **Clinical features:** Three common clinical patterns can be seen:
   • *Distal subungual onychomycosis:* Most common form; the fungus penetrates the hyponychium and cross along the ventral nail surface, causing onycholysis and crumbling. Entire nail can become involved (Fig. 32.**3**).

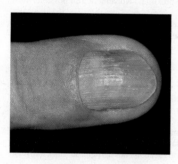

Fig. 32.**3** · Onychomycosis caused by a mold.

   • *Superficial white onychomycosis:* Infection of dorsal surface of nail plate causing scaly white spots.
   • *Proximal subungual onychomycosis:* Penetration occurs at proximal nail fold leading to severe nail dystrophy with diffuse involvement.
▶ **Diagnostic approach:** Clippings from dystrophic nail for microscopic examination; periodic acid–Schiff (PAS) staining of histologic sections both easier and more effective than KOH examination. Culture of nail is gold standard.
▶ **Differential diagnosis:** Psoriasis, trauma.
▶ **Therapy:**
   • Topical therapy (antifungal nail polish) only suitable for superficial, minimal disease.
   • Systemic antifungal agents offer the best chance of cure:
      – Terbinafine for anthrophilic dermatophytes: 250 mg daily for 2 weeks.
      – Fluconazole for yeasts and dermatophytes: 150 mg weekly for 3–6 months.
      – Itraconazole for yeast, molds and mixed infections: 200 mg daily for 3 months or 200 mg b.i.d. for 7 days, then 21 days vacation; repeat for total of three or four courses.

> ▪ *Note:* There are many other regimens and recommendations; the three listed above are clearly the best agents, and we have found these regimens most effective.

- In Germany, shoes are treated with formaldehyde solutions in sealed plastic bags for several days to reduce risk of re-infection.
- Nail removal almost never needed. Surgical removal painful and may damage matrix, leading to permanently dystrophic, susceptible nails. In addition, patients perceive nail removal as a cure, which it is not.
- If a patient cannot tolerate systemic therapy, then the nail can be removed by softening with a 40% urea ointment (p. 697) for a week followed by extraction and treatment with topical antimycotic agents. Once a nail starts to form, topical antifungal agents should be applied.
- Nail polish can be used without problems.

> ▪ *Note:* The biggest problem in treating onychomycosis is recurrence. There are many possible explanations:
>
> - Reinfection from shoes, environment (swimming pools, saunas), or other individuals.
> - Biological predisposing factors (impaired immunity, anatomic disturbances such as overlapping or tightly compressed toes).
> - Persistent microorganisms "hiding" from the systemic agents.
> - In any event, it is wise to warn patient about likelihood of recurrence (at least 50%) and never promise a cure. In addition, the chance of cure drops with age.

32.4 Acquired Nail Changes

Onychodystrophy

Definition: Generic term for any change in color, texture or structure of nails. In addition to distorted growth, other common findings include pits, ridges, and loss of sheen (Fig. 32.**4 a**).

Pathogenesis: Common causes of onychodystrophy include:.

- Trauma.
- Nail biting.
- Nervous tic or other manipulation of nail or cuticle.
- Postinflammatory (chronic dermatitis or paronychia).
- Psoriasis (subungual debris, nail pits, oil spots).
- Lichen planus (atrophy of nail plate, sometimes trachyonychia).
- Ischemic vascular disease.

Leukonychia

Definition: White discoloration of nail caused by alteration of light reflection because of defective keratinization.

Clinical features: Many forms (Fig. 32.**4 b**), including:

- *Leukonychia punctata:* Very common; more often dominant hand; probably microtrauma.
- *Total leukonychia:* Rare, may be genetic; occasionally traumatic (exposure to strong acids).
- *Striate leukonychia:* Longitudinal white bands may reflect disorder of keratinization (Darier or Hailey–Hailey disease) or be traumatic.

Diseases of the Nails

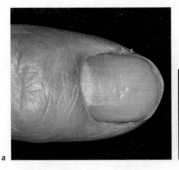
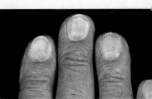

a

Fig. 32.**4** · **a** Pitted nails. **b** Leukonychia.

- *Transverse leukonychia:*
  - Transverse white bands usually from trauma (typist's nails in the past, exce[?]sive manicuring, picking at proximal nail fold).
  - Mees lines: White lines from nail matrix affects of high fever or toxic exp[?]sure (arsenic).
  ◻ *Note:* Isolated longitudinal leukonychia may reflect an underlying nail b[?] tumor.
- *Apparent leukonychia* is the result of nail bed changes in vascularization or on[?]cholysis. The nail itself is not altered:
  - *Terry nail:* White nail seen with cirrhosis.
  - *Muehrcke nail:* White bands in hypoalbuminemia.
  - *Lindsay nail (half and half nail):* Proximal whiteness in uremia.
  - *Distal onycholysis:* Most common cause of distal leukonychia.
▶ **Therapy:** Other than eliminating underlying cause, no treatment is possible.

Trachyonychia

▶ **Synonym:** Twenty-nail dystrophy; trachys means rough.
▶ **MIM code:** 161050.
▶ **Definition:** Uncommon congenital nail dystrophy with autosomal dominant i[?] heritance.
▶ **Clinical features:** All nails have longitudinal grooves, are dull, fragile, and ha[?] adherent scales. Onset in early childhood.
  ◻ *Note:* Involvement of one or several nails can occur in psoriasis, lichen plan[?] alopecia areata, or sporadically.
▶ **Therapy:** No effective therapy; most patients improve with time.

Median Nail Dystrophy

▶ Longitudinal central defect in thumb nail, often bilateral, may be associated w[?] enlarged lunula. Defect may be feathered or branched. Presumed posttrauma[?] No effective therapy.

Beau Lines

- **Definition:** Transverse lines or grooves in nail.
- **Pathogenesis:** Causes include trauma, skin diseases (atopic dermatitis), systemic illnesses (hepatitis, pellagra, acute lupus erythematosus), medications (chemotherapy)—in sum, anything that can disturb nail matrix.
- **Clinical features:** The grooves or lines move distally; the distance from the nail fold lets one assess the time of trauma. In cancer chemotherapy patients, the ridges sometime mirror the multiple courses of chemotherapy.

Onycholysis

- **Definition:** Separation of nail from nailbed.
- **Pathogenesis:** Causes include psoriasis, dermatitis, fungal infections; medications (for example *photo-onycholysis* from tetracyclines or psoralens), thyroid disease, other metabolic disturbances; rarely inherited.
  - *Idiopathic onycholysis* is most common among women; painless separation of nail without apparent cause. Typically, the distal third separates and underlying nail bed becomes darker and thickened.
- **Diagnostic approach:** Fungal culture to exclude distal subungual onycholysis.
- **Therapy:** Cut nail very short to reduce leverage encouraging separation; even in absence of positive studies, apply antifungal solution b.i.d. Usually self-limited process.

Onychogryphosis

- **Definition:** Thickened, distorted, claw-like nail.
- **Pathogenesis:** Usually in elderly; factors include trauma, poorly fitting shoes, neglect, impaired vascular supply, onychomycosis.
- **Clinical features:** Most often great toes; nails dramatically thickened and claw-like (Fig. 32.5 a).
- **Therapy:** Removal of nail using urea paste; if peripheral circulation is intact, surgical removal and matrix destruction is another possibility. Then, roomy footwear and routine clipping.

Ingrown Nail

- **Synonym:** Unguis incarnatus.
- **Definition:** Penetration of nail plate into tissue of lateral nail fold.
- **Pathogenesis:** Almost always involves great toes. Causes include congenital malformation of nail (pincer nail), improper trimming, tightly fitting shoes, and hy-

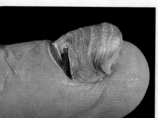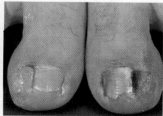

Fig. 32.5 · **a** Onychogryposis. **b** Ingrown toenails.

pertrophy of the lateral lip of the great toe because of pressure from an overlapping second toe.
- ► **Clinical features:** Distorted nail with swelling, pain, and granulation tissue along the lateral nail fold (Fig. 32.**5b**).
- ► **Therapy:**
  - *Mild cases:* Eliminate pressure, trim nail; topical antiseptics as foot soaks or on small piece of cotton wool pushed under affected nail.
  - *Moderate cases:* May benefit from nail brace, shifting pressure away from lateral aspects; applied by podiatrist.
  - *Severe cases:* Emmert procedure, where lateral nail fold is excised and lateral aspect of nail matrix destroyed.

Clubbing

- ► **Synonyms:** Hippocratic nails, drumstick fingers.
- ► **Definition:** Thickened distal digits with rounded nails; first described by Hippocrates.
- ► **Pathogenesis:** Most often associated with chronic pulmonary disease, but can reflect wide variety of underlying disturbances. Acquired clubbing almost always means systemic disease.
  - *Pachydermoperiostosis* (*primary hypertrophic osteoarthropathy, Touraine–Solente–Golé syndrome*): Combination of thickened skin of the scalp (cutis verticis gyrata), hyperhidrosis, periosteitis, enlarged hands and feet, and clubbing.
  - *Hypertrophic pulmonary osteoarthropathy* (*Marie–Bamberger syndrome*): Combination of distal osteitis and clubbing secondary to chronic cardiac or pulmonary disease.
- ► **Clinical features:** The tip of the digit is swollen and the nail is curved over the end. *Lovibond angle* (the angle between the nail and the nail bed) is > 180°.
- ► **Therapy:** Treat underlying disease, sometimes nails also improve.

Koilonychia

- ► **Definition:** Spoon-shaped nails.
- ► **Pathogenesis:** Many causes: normal variant in infants; in adults associated with iron deficiency (Plummer–Vinson syndrome), other deficiencies, occupational trauma, impaired circulation in elderly.
- ► **Clinical features:** Reverse of clubbing; the nail is depressed in its mid-portion and then elevated again distally.
- ► **Therapy:** Treat underlying diseases; biotin 5 mg daily is frequently tried in Germany.

Yellow Nail Syndrome

- ► **MIM code:** 153300.
- ► **Definition:** Triad of primary lymphedema, bronchopulmonary disease, and yellow nails.
- ► **Pathogenesis:** Mutation in forkhead family transcription factor MFH1 (*FOXC2*) autosomal dominant inheritance; overlaps with other forms of lymphedema caused by mutations in same gene.
- ► **Clinical features:** Nails are slow-growing, overly curved and yellow, often with onychodystrophy. Lymphedema and bronchiectasis are associated findings.
- ► **Therapy:** Prompt attention to pulmonary problems, compression for lymphedema; nails are least problem.

ail Tumors

The list of nail tumors is long. They can cause longitudinal discoloration or deformations.

Examples include wart, digital mucous cyst, pyogenic granuloma, glomus tumor, fibroma, subungual exostosis, subungual epidermoid cyst, enchondroma, Bowen disease, keratoacanthoma, squamous cell carcinoma, melanocytic nevus, acral-lentiginous malignant melanoma.

Caution: Subungual malignant melanoma (Fig. 32.6) is often diagnosed too late; always think of the possibility when a longitudinal dark streak appears in an adult nail. It is difficult to distinguish between a streak caused by a nevus and that from a melanoma; often an excisional biopsy is needed in adults. In children who are developing nevi elsewhere, one can usually assume the streak is from another nevus. When the pigment extends to the nail fold or finger tip (*Hutchinson sign*), melanoma is probable. Dermatoscopy is also helpful. The main differential diagnostic consideration is a subungual hematoma, which can almost always be identified with dermatoscopy.

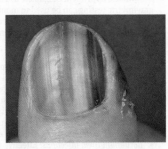

g. 32.**6** · Subungual malignant elanoma.

33 Disorders of Sweat Glands

Hyperhidrosis

▶ **Definition:** Increased eccrine sweating.
▶ **Classification:**
- *Emotional (cortical) hyperhidrosis:* Usually localized to axillae, groin, palms, a soles.
- *Thermoregulatory (hypothalamic) hyperhidrosis:* Usually diffuse, such as swea ing when hot or active, or with variety of metabolic triggers, infections, vascul or neurological diseases.
- *Gustatory hyperhidrosis:* Reflex hyperhidrosis following eating or other senso stimulation; can be generalized but most often localized to distribution auriculotemporal nerve following injury or parotid gland surgery.
▶ **Clinical features:** Hyperhidrosis causes a variety of problems. "Sweaters" are u able to work with metals and often avoid social contacts.
▶ **Diagnostic approach:** Diagnostic usually made easily on history; starch iodide gravimetric testing can be used to monitor therapy.
▶ **Differential diagnosis:** Exclude underlying diseases (diabetes mellitus, hype thyroidism, pheochromocytoma, and many others) that can cause hyperhidrosi
▶ **Therapy:**
- *Aluminum salts:*
  - Extra-strength ordinary antiperspirants.
  - 15–20% aluminum chloride solution or compounded mixture (15.0C $AlCl_3.6H_2O$, 2.50% hydroxyethyl cellulose to thicken, 82.5% distilled water
  - Apply to axillae each evening for 5 nights; rinse in morning; then u 1–2×weekly. Main problem is irritation; can discolor fabrics. Do not use ir mediately after shaving. For palms and soles, can use 30%.
- *Tap water iontophoresis:* 10–15 mA; easier for palms and soles.
- *Botulinum toxin injections:* Effective for axillae, as well as palms and soles, b far less painful in axillae.
- *Surgery (only for axillae):* Subcutaneous curettage of sweat glands, suction r moval or excision; sympathectomy is last resort.

Miliaria

▶ **Definition:** Erythematous papules associated with sweat duct occlusion follow ing heat exposure.
▶ **Epidemiology:** Miliaria are most common in first week of life as infant adjusts environment; also occur in any age with excessive heat, sweating, occlusion, combinations thereof.
▶ **Pathogenesis:** The eccrine sweat pore become macerated and then occludes t duct. This leads to superficial clear vesicles (*miliaria crystallina*) or deep, mc painful red papules or nodules (*miliaria rubra*). Most common sites trunk, neck; occluded areas (sporting equipment).
▶ **Differential diagnosis:** Usually mistaken for folliculitis or one of its varian *Neutrophilic eccrine hidradenitis* is closely related, occurs with chemotherapy episodically in children; extreme miliaria with inflammatory response.
▶ **Therapy:** Cooling measures, zinc oxide lotion.

Bromhidrosis

▶ Unpleasant odor usually caused by axillary sweat. Interaction of apocrine and eccrine sweat probably responsible. Factors such as medications (DMSO), garlic, or amino acid disorders affect only eccrine sweat. Co-factors include improper hygiene, secondary bacterial and fungal infections, as well as nonabsorbent clothing. Mainstay of treatment is to reduce sweating, as for hypohidrosis.

Pseudobromhidrosis

▶ Delusion of unpleasant body odor, when none is present. A monosymptomatic delusion, similar to acarophobia. Very difficult to manage; approach only in cooperation with psychiatry.

Chromhidrosis

▶ Discoloration of eccrine or apocrine sweat. Normal eccrine sweat is always colorless; discoloration is the result of colored salts on the skin (copper miners), infections with chromogenic microorganisms (*Corynebacterium*), or other subtle exposure to dyes. Apocrine sweat, on the other hand, is rich in lipofuscin and can be discolored intrinsically, or secondary to metabolic diseases (ochronosis) or medications (clofazimine).

Fox–Fordyce Disease

▶ **Definition:** Pruritic papules in axillae and anogenital region.
▶ **Pathogenesis:** Uncommon disease, almost limited to women; probably apocrine miliaria with plugging of follicle and secondary inflammation.
▶ **Clinical features:** Intensely pruritic papules in axillae and inguinal region.
▶ **Differential diagnosis:** Folliculitis.
▶ **Therapy:** No good treatment; some patients improve with oral contraceptives; high-potency topical corticosteroids may suppress itch. If small area affected, excision can be tried.

34 Diseases of Sebaceous Glands

34.1 Acne

► **Definition:** Multifactorial disease primarily of teenagers with follicular plugging and inflammation.

► **Epidemiology:** Most common skin disease; affects almost every individual. Most commonly in puberty, but special forms seen in other age ranges.

► **Pathogenesis:** Many different factors play a role:
- Altered hormonal status with increased androgens in men and increased androgenic properties of progesterone and other hormones in women.
- Follicular keratinization: Hyperkeratotic plugs form in follicle opening.
- Hyperplasia of sebaceous glands with increased sebum production, secondary to hormonal changes.
- Colonization of follicles by *Propionibacterium acnes*, which produces lipase splitting free fatty acids and releasing inflammatory mediators.

► **Clinical features:**
- *Acne vulgaris:* Traditionally divided into two overlapping subcategories:
  - *Acne comedonica:* Primarily open comedones (whiteheads) and closed comedones (blackheads). Comedones develop only in sebaceous follicles concentrated on face, chest, and mid-back, which have small hairs and large sebaceous glands. Black color is melanin from follicle, not dirt. Most common sites for comedones are forehead, cheeks, perioral region (Fig. 34.1 **a, b**).

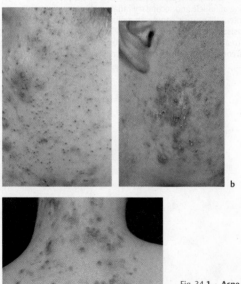

Fig. 34.**1** · **Acne vulgaris. a** Primarily comedones. **b** Comedones and pustules **c** Papulopustular stage.

- *Acne papulopustulosa:* Follicular pustules or inflammatory papules; comedones rupture, neutrophils are attracted, and process accelerated (Fig. 34.1 c).

▸ *Acne variants with marked inflammation:*
  - *Acne conglobata:* Features inflammatory nodules and pseudocysts with marked scarring; typical sites are face, sternum, and back in young men (Fig. 34.2 a).
  - *SAPHO syndrome:* **S**ynovitis, **a**cne conglobata, **p**almoplantar pustulosis, **h**yperostosis, and **o**steitis; sternoclavicular joints most common bony sites.
  - *Acne inversa:* Furunculoid lesions in axilla, groin, perianal region, and submammary area with sinus tracts and fistulas.

☐ *Note:* Almost all "chronic furunculosis" of these sites is acne, not recurrent bacterial infections. The old name of *hidradenitis suppurativa* is no longer appropriate.
  - *Acne tetrad:* Combination of acne conglobata, acne inversa, perifolliculitis capitis abscedens et suffodiens (sterile dissecting folliculitis of scalp), and pilonidal sinus; more common in men.
  - *Acne fulminans:* Sudden severe acne with systemic signs and symptoms (fever, leukocytosis, osteomyelitis, pericarditis); patients present with severe acne conglobata with necrosis of lesions leaving gelatinous debris (Fig. 34.2 b); often tender sternoclavicular joints; treated initially with high-dose corticosteroids to control inflammation; then retinoids.

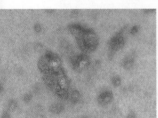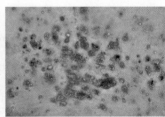

b

Fig. 34.2 · **a** Acne conglobata with cysts. **b** Acne fulminans.

- *Other special forms of acne:*
  - *Mallorca acne (acne aestivalis):* Acne flare of acne following sun intense sun exposure; often winter vacations among Europeans; comedones produced by combination of heat, sweating, and occlusive sun screens; probably variant of polymorphous light eruption (p. 300).
  - *Contact acne:* Caused by comedogenic makeup and other skin care products, as well as tars and other industrial contacts.
  - *Chloracne:* Systemic or topical exposure to halogenated hydrocarbons causes severe comedonal acne, often permanent, as well as liver disease; mass industrial exposure (Seveso accident), military use (Agent Orange in Vietnam war), or intentional poisoning (Ukrainian presidential election in 2005).
  - *Acne neonatorum:* Acne as a result of elevated hormone levels in utero with sebaceous gland hyperplasia; resolves spontaneously.
  - *Acne infantum:* Onset age 3–6 months; caused by elevated levels of luteinizing hormone (LH), follicle-stimulating hormone (FSH), and testosterone; always rule out endocrine disorder; check free and total testosterone, DHEA, DHEAS, LH, FSH.

- *Acne excoriée des jeunes filles:* Mild acne in young women with overaggressive self-manipulation leading to excoriations and erosions.
- *Mechanical acne:* Head bands, shoulder pads, and many other items causing occlusion and pressure can induce comedones.
- *Late-onset acne (acne tarda):* Onset of acne in women well past puberty; always exclude hyperprolactinemia and polycystic ovary syndrome.
- *Localized acne:* Two situations where acne can be limited to patch of nonfacial skin as variant of epidermal nevus (p. 412):
  Munro nevus: Mosaic defect in FGFR2 with localized acne
  Becker nevus: Androgen-sensitive epidermal mosaic, often with hypertrichosis and localized acne.
- *Medication-induced acne:* Details are given in Table 34.1. In almost all instances the reaction is acneiform, with follicular papules or pustules but not comedones.

Table 34.1 · **Medications causing acne**

Category	Examples
Hormones	Corticosteroids, androgens, oral contraceptives (progesterone dominant), body-building steroids
Antiepileptic medications	Trimethadione, phenytoin, and related compounds
Halogens	Compounds with bromides, iodides
Antabuse	Disulfiram
Anti-TB drugs	Isoniazid, ethionamide, rifampicin
Psychopharmaceuticals	Lithium, amitriptyline, barbiturates
Immunosuppressive agents	Cyclosporine
Monoclonal antibodies	Cetuximab (EGFR inhibitor)
Thyroid-suppressive agents	Thiouracil
Antibiotics	Tetracyclines (rarely, but then a clinical problem)

- ▣ *Note:* Not all diseases with comedones are acne. *Favre–Racouchot disease* (nodular elastosis with cysts and comedones) is caused by chronic UV exposure but always has comedones without inflammation. *Nevus comedonicus* is a form of epidermal nevus with comedones but no inflammation. In addition, not all diseases with acne in their name belong in the acne family. *Acne urticata* is facial excoriations without acne, while *acne varioliformis* is a form of folliculitis limited to the frontal hairline.
- ▶ **Prognosis:** The course and prognosis of acne is highly variable. It is impossible to look at a patient and say "You will have trouble for only a few months." All acne causes scars, but the more promptly the disease is treated, the less severe the scarring is likely to be. It is a very emotionally distressing disease, especially for teenagers already at a difficult stage of life. Few groups of patients are more grateful than acne patients, who usually respond promptly to a variety of measures but then require long-term treatment and support.
- ▶ **Therapy:** The main principle of acne therapy is that there are many options; the treatment plan should be adjusted to the severity and course of the acne. Combination therapy is usually required. Our therapeutic approach is summarized in Table 34.2 and Fig. 34.3.

Table 34.2 · Choice of acne treatment based on clinical features

	Substance	Comedones	Seborrhea	Pustules	Inflammation
topical	Azelaic acid	++	–	++	+
	Benzoyl peroxide	(+)	–	+++	(+)
	Adapalene	+++	–	(+)	++
	Tretinoin	+++	–	(+)	–
	Antibiotics	(+)	–	+++	+
systemic	Tetracycline	(++)	–	+++	+
	Isotretinoin	+++	+++	(+++)	++
	Antiandrogens	++	+	(+)	?

– = no effect; + = effective; ++ = very effective; +++ = extremely effective; (+) = indirect effect;?= unclear effect.

	Lesion type / Medication	Comedones	Papules, pustules	Papules, pustules, nodules	Nodules, cysts
Topical	Topical retinoids		a	b	
	Benzoyl peroxide (BPO)			b	
	Azelaic acid		a	d	
	Topical antibiotics		c	b	
Systemic	Systemic antibiotics		c	d	
	Systemic isotretinoin				
	Antiandrogens			a	e

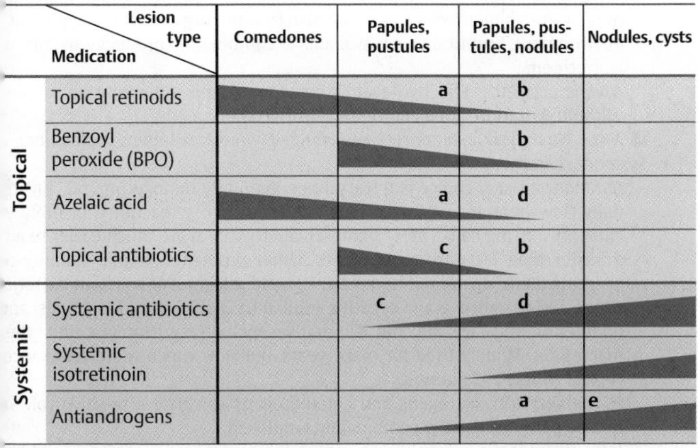

a = Combine with BPO or topical antibiotics
b = Combine with systemic antibiotics or antiandrogens
c = Combine with topical retinoids
d = Combine with antiandrogens
e = Combine with systemic antibiotics and isotretinoin

Fig. 34.**3** · Strategies for acne therapy (after Orfanos and Garbe).

- *General measures:* Always discuss the following points with patients and parents (if patient agrees):
  - Diet is not a major factor. Patients should eat what they enjoy.
  - Lack of cleanliness is not the crucial issue. Gentle mild cleansing twice daily is completely adequate. There is no reason to buy expensive cleansers. Abrasive cleansers can be too irritating.

- *Topical therapy:*
  - *Topical retinoids:* Far and away the best treatment for comedones. Since all acne lesions develop from comedones, almost every acne patient benefits from topical retinoids. Several forms are available; the most widely used is tretinoin, but isotretinoin and adapalene are also available and less irritating. Tretinoin comes in various concentrations as a cream and gel. It must cause a bit of irritation to be effective. It should be used in the evening because it is slightly photosensitizing. Easily combined with other products for morning use.

  🗹 *Caution:* Acne almost always flares as topical retinoid therapy is started. Always warn the patient.
  - Benzoyl peroxide 5–10%: Also comes as wash, cream, water-based gel, or alcoholic gel; can be used as monotherapy b.i.d. or mornings in combination with topical retinoids; bleaches hair and clothes, slightly irritating; no resistance of microorganisms.
  - *Topical antibiotics:* Antibiotics are used to inhibit *Propionibacterium acnes* and reduce the lipolytic acne, decreasing follicular irritation. The most widely used topical antibiotics are erythromycin and clindamycin. Topical usage avoids systemic side effects, but antibiotic resistance does develop, not only by *Propionibacterium acnes* but also by other organisms in the patient's environment. Erythromycin is available as combination product with zinc or ·isotretinoin.
  - *Azelaic acid 20%:* Effective against comedones and inflammation; almost without irritation; good choice for sensitive skin.

  ▷ *Note:* No topical agent or regimen effectively reduces sebum production.
- *Systemic therapy:*
  - *Antibiotics:* Usual choice is tetracyclines, generally minocycline 50–100 mg daily (low phototoxicity, occasional hypersensitivity reactions) or doxycycline 50–100 mg daily (more photosensitivity). Both are much easier to administer than ordinary tetracyclines. Other problems include staining of erupting teeth (do not use under age 12), and selection of resistant bacteria strains. May cause gram-negative folliculitis with painful pustules and nodules on mid-face and chin. Alternatives include erythromycin and other macrolides. Widely used for many years, but now much more reluctance typical course 2–3 months.
  - *Hormones:* Both estrogens and antiandrogens can play a positive role in female patients. Usually combination employed.
  - *Isotretinoin* is the only sebostasis agent, inhibits comedo formation and has immunomodulatory actions. It is indicated for severe acne, but highly effective in all forms. Usual dosage 0.5–1.0 mg/kg for 3–6 months. Detailed recommendations (p. 622).

  🗹 *Caution:* Isotretinoin is teratogenic. Female patients must employ effective contraception under the guidance of a gynecologist, with pregnancy testing before initiation of therapy. Do not bend the rule; assume the worst.
  - Other cautions include:
    Do not combine with tetracyclines because of risk of pseudotumor cerebri
    Watch for elevated cholesterol, triglycerides, and liver function tests
    Be aware of likelihood of skeletal pain in physically active patients; always question patients about sporting activities; if competitive athletes, treat in off-season.

- *Supplementary measures:*
  - Light chemical peels with α-hydroxy acids (AHA) or other mild agents are sebostatic and help with superficial scars.
  - Surgical management of scars requires individual adjustment; can include laser ablation, dermabrasion, cryotherapy, collagen injections.
  - Acne inversa usually requires surgery.

34.2 Rosacea

▶ **Definition:** Chronic inflammatory facial dermatosis in adults.

▶ **Epidemiology:** Common disorder, more often seen in fair-skinned individuals (skin types I–II, "curse of the Celts").

▶ **Pathogenesis:** Unclear; not related to acne despite superficial similarities as no comedones are present. Key factors include flushing (vascular reactivity) and inflammation. Genetic predisposition; other factors may include *Demodex folliculorum*.

▶ **Clinical features:**
  - *Stage I:*
    - Flushing; vascular dilation; triggered by alcohol, spicy foods, caffeine, nicotine, hormonal change, UV light, heat and cold. In early stages, reversible.
    - Persistent erythema; telangiectases but no comedones or pustules.
  - *Stage II:*
    - Persistent erythema, papules and pustules (Fig. 34.**4a**). Does not respect the hairline (as does acne). Usually mid-facial; only rarely involves chest or trunk.
  - *Stage III:*
    - May develop independent of earlier stages; perhaps mediated by TGF-β.
    - Rhinophyma: swollen nose with sebaceous gland hyperplasia and fibrosis, usually red because of telangiectases (Fig. 34.**4b**).
  - *Special variants:*
    - *Ocular rosacea:* Patients may have blepharitis, conjunctivitis, iridocyclitis, or keratoconjunctivitis without obvious rosacea; usual scenario is lid rosacea plus ocular problems (Fig. 34.**4c**). Complain of foreign body sensation or photophobia.
    - ⚠ *Caution:* Untreated, ocular rosacea can advance to severe keratitis with corneal scarring.
    - *Rosacea fulminans* (*pyoderma faciale*): Severe inflammatory reaction, analogous to acne fulminans. Young women with sudden severe conglobate disease with necrosis but without comedones.
    - *Lupus miliaris disseminatus faciei:* Tiny brown papules periorbital region; granulomatous histology.
    - *Steroid rosacea:* Topical corticosteroids may induce a rosacea-like picture; more often they are responsible for perioral dermatitis.

▶ **Histology:** Biopsy rarely needed, but may show granulomatous changes including caseation; thus often confusion over relationship of rosacea and tuberculosis.

▶ **Diagnostic approach:** History, clinical examination.

▶ **Differential diagnosis:**
  - Acne is always mentioned first, but easy to tell them apart; different age groups, and rosacea has no comedones.
  - *Perioral dermatitis:* Different clinical picture but exact relationship to rosacea still unclear.

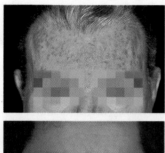
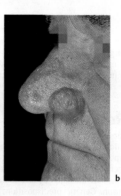
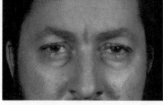

Fig. 34.**4** · **a** Rosacea. **b** Rhinophyma. **c** Ocular rosacea.

- Rosacea and seborrheic dermatitis frequently present in same patient.
- In past, relationship to tuberculids was confusing. Today granulomatous rosacea is an accepted histologic variant; lupus miliaris disseminatus faciei is regarded as periocular granulomatous rosacea and not a form of tuberculosis.
- Demodicosis often complicates rosacea; pustules may be full of mites. More controversial is primary inflammatory condition caused by *Demodex folliculorum* mimicking rosacea; if it exists, then pustules on normal skin without the underlying erythema.
- ◩ *Note:* Always ask and ask again about the use of topical corticosteroids, a frequently overlooked trigger.
▶ **Therapy:**
  - *Stage I:* Topical metronidazole gel; commercially available in most countries or can be compounded (p. 695). Apply b.i.d. Alternatives include topical erythromycin, which is less effective. Use sun screens; avoid triggers if any seem clinically relevant.
  - ◪ *Caution:* Topical corticosteroids are absolutely contraindicated in rosacea. They are responsible for worsening in many cases.
  - *Stage II:*
    – Systemic antibiotics, usually minocycline 50 mg daily or b.i.d for 3 months. Tetracycline 250 mg q.i.d. on empty stomach for 3 months. In either case, can gradually taper dose.
    – Isotretinoin 0.2–1.0 mg/kg for 6 months; not with tetracycline.
    – Short burst of systemic corticosteroids plus isotretinoin for rosacea fulminans.
  - *Stage III:* Surgical invention; debulking with scalpel, dermabrasion, or laser ablation.

34.3 *Perioral Dermatitis*

▶ **Definition:** Papular dermatitis primarily involving perioral region, with distinctive pattern.

▶ **Epidemiology:** Most common in young women.

▶ **Pathogenesis:** Controversial. Most patients present having used topical corticosteroids, which are agreed to be a causative factor. But for what condition did the patient receive the corticosteroids, and how does one explain the occasional patient who has never used corticosteroids? Two likely lines of evidence: overuse of moisturizers leads to follicular occlusion and reaction; problem worse in those with atopic diathesis.

▶ **Clinical features:**
- Tiny 1–3 mm erythematous papules and pustules without comedones Fig. 34.**5**); grouped around mouth with distinctive grenz zone between vermilion and first lesions; true name *peri-perioral dermatitis*.
- May also be periorbital or perinasal.

▶ **Diagnostic approach:** Clinical examination, history of corticosteroid use.

▶ **Differential diagnosis:** Rosacea, demodicosis, folliculitis.

▶ **Therapy:**
- Absolute prohibition of topical corticosteroids.
- ◪ *Note:* Explain to patient that her disease will flare initially because of "steroid withdrawal," but that she must resist the temptation to restart topical corticosteroids. This is the classic nightmare in treating perioral dermatitis—the patient has an ample supply of corticosteroids and re-employs them, with the expected flare.
- Short course of systemic antibiotics; tetracycline or erythromycin for 6 weeks.
- Topical immunomodulatory agents may also be helpful in early weeks.
- Choose just one, bland moisturizer.

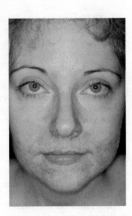

Fig. 34.**5** · Perioral dermatitis.

35 Diseases of Subcutaneous Fat

35.1 Lipodystrophy and Lipoatrophy

Overview

Definition: Group of disorders with localized or generalized changes in fat. Frequent overlaps between dystrophy and atrophy:

- *Lipodystrophy:* Includes both increase in fatty tissue, abnormal distribution of fat, or disappearance of fat.
- *Lipoatrophy:* Refers exclusively to loss or disappearance of fatty tissue.

Congenital Lipodystrophy

▶ **Congenital generalized lipodystrophy (CGL)** (Berardinelli–Seip syndrome); rare disorder; autosomal recessive inheritance, with two different mutations:
  - *CGL1* (MIM code 608594): mutation in *AGPAT2* at 9q34.3.
  - *CGL2* (MIM code 269700): mutation in seipin at 11q13.
  - Widespread loss of fat, extensive acanthosis nigricans, hirsutism, acromegaly, insulin resistance with extremely high insulin levels and hypertriglyceridemia.

▶ **Familial partial lipodystrophy (FPLD):** Three types recognized in OMIM, although not all agree with splitting. All feature localized loss of fat with some degree of excess fat at other sites:
  - *FPLD1 (Köbberling type, MIM code 608600):* Mutation unknown. Loss of adipose tissue on extremities with normal or increased amounts on face, neck, and trunk.
  - *FPLD2 (Dunnigan type, MIM code 151660):* Mutation in lamin A/C; autosomal dominant inheritance. Patients lose fat over their limbs and trunk, developing a pseudomuscular appearance, but at same time have increased deposits on the neck and sometimes labia. They are insulin-resistant and usually develop diabetes mellitus and elevated triglycerides; acanthosis nigricans and hirsutism may also occur.
  - *FPLD3:* Similar to type 2, but with mutations in *PPARG* gene.

▶ **Partial progressive lipodystrophy (MIM code 608709, Barraquer–Simons syndrome):** Genetic basis unclear. Loss of fat on face, trunk, and arms, producing starved appearance, with normal distribution on buttocks and legs; have associated IgG antibody against C3 (C3 nephritogenic factor) leading to renal disease in about 50%.

Acquired Lipodystrophy

▶ Most common cause today is truncal and nuchal lipodystrophy in HIV/AIDS patients; etiology unclear, but in many·instances secondary to highly active antiretroviral therapy (HAART).

▶ Buffalo hump and moon facies of Cushing syndrome are classified by some as lipodystrophy.

▶ Acquired generalized lipoatrophy (Lawrence syndrome) resembles Berardinelli–Seip syndrome but starts in adult life, following severe systemic illness. Very rare.

▶ **Localized disease:**
  - Following injections of corticosteroids; rarely other medications.
  - Secondary to panniculitis (inflammatory lipoatrophy).

- *Lipoatrophia semicircularis*: linear depressed bands on thighs of women; in most instances posttraumatic (tight pants, water-skiing tow ropes).
- *Lipodystrophia centrifugalis abdominalis infantilis*: Idiopathic disorder in Japanese infants with loss of subcutaneous fat starting in groin or axilla and spreading to trunk.

▸ **Differential diagnosis:** Sometimes it is difficult to tell which layers of skin are deficient; for example:
- Atrophoderma of Pasini–Pierini: atrophic morphea.
- Hemifacial atrophy (Parry–Romberg): extensive loss of tissue on one side of face including skin and muscle, as well as fat; also probably extreme morphea variant.

35.2 Panniculitis

Overview

▸ **Definition:** Inflammation of the subcutaneous fat.
▸ **Classification:** There are many different ways to classify panniculitis:
- *In order of frequency:*
  - Erythema nodosum is common.
  - All the others are extremely rare.
- *Clinically:*
  - On the shin: usually erythema nodosum.
  - On calf, above knee, or not on legs: Consider other possibilities.
- *Histologically:*
  - Septal versus lobular.
  - With or without vasculitis.

A working classification is shown in Table 35.1.

Table 35.1 · Classification of panniculitis		
Septal	Without vasculitis	Erythema nodosum
		Connective tissue panniculitis
	With vasculitis	Superficial thrombophlebitis
		Polyarteritis nodosa
Lobular	Without vasculitis	Pancreatic
		Lymphoma
		Traumatic (cold, injections, injuries)
		Neonatal fat necrosis
		α_1-Antitrypsin deficiency
		Infectious
		Lipoatrophic panniculitis (Rothman–Makai lipogranulomatosis, other variants)
		Lupus erythematosus (lupus profundus)
		Sarcoidosis
		Weber–Christian disease (idiopathic)
	With vasculitis	Erythema induratum/nodular vasculitis

► **Diagnostic approach:**

- If not erythema nodosum, do biopsy. Take a long thin ellipse through the subcutaneous fat, not a punch biopsy, and label the specimen clearly as "rule out panniculitis." Otherwise, many dermatopathology laboratories routinely trim the fat from specimens.
- If the lesion drains oily liquid when incised, suspect liquefying panniculitis, which almost always means α_1-antitrypsin deficiency or artifact.
- Many special clues from the histology:
  - Lobular vs. septal; vasculitis or not.
  - Plasma cells: lupus erythematosus.
  - Saponification: pancreatic disease.
  - Foreign bodies: factitious disease.
  - Organisms: infections.
  - Atypical lymphocytes: lymphoma.
  - ▷ *Note:* Always consider the possible triggers and underlying diseases when confronted with panniculitis. Few disorders display more interplay between the skin and systemic disease.

Erythema Nodosum

► **Definition:** Self-limited panniculitis with sudden onset of red-brown, bruise-like patches and nodules on shins; usually reactive.

► **Epidemiology:** Female:male ratio 3–5:1; typically young adults.

► **Pathogenesis:** Triggers include:

- *Medications:* Oral contraceptives, penicillin, other antibiotics, salicylates, bromides, iodides, immunotherapy agents (vaccines, hyposensitization regimens).
- *Infections:*
  - *Bacteria:* Most common are streptococcal and mycobacterial infections, as well as brucellosis, yersiniosis, and chlamydial infections (psittacosis), but almost every bacterial infection has been associated with erythema nodosum. *Erythema nodosum leprosum* is a late reactive stage and not true erythema nodosum.
  - *Deep fungal:* Most patients with coccidioidomycosis or histoplasmosis have erythema nodosum; also with blastomycosis and sporotrichosis.
  - ⚠ *Caution:* Always take travel history. If a young adult returns from holidays in southwestern desert areas of the USA (California, Arizona, New Mexico) and has erythema nodosum, the risk of acute coccidioidomycosis is considerable. If the patient is pregnant and not treated, the risk to the child is also significant.
  - *Viral:* Hepatitis B, hepatitis C.
- *Malignant diseases:* Rare marker for Hodgkin lymphoma, other lymphomas, leukemias, and following radiation therapy.
- *Chronic inflammatory diseases:* Inflammatory bowel disease, Behçet syndrome, and Reiter syndrome can all present with erythema nodosum.
- *Sarcoidosis,* especially *Löfgren syndrome:* Sarcoidosis with hilar lymphadenopathy, arthritis, and erythema nodosum.
- *Pregnancy.*

► **Clinical features:**

- *Prodrome:* Fever, chills, perhaps joint pain; varies with trigger.
- *Skin findings:* Usually multiple, bilateral bruise-like tender or painful nodules and plaques covered by a smooth epidermis (Fig 35.1). Almost always on shins, rarely thighs, arms. May be associated with continuing fever, malaise, or arthritis. Resolve after weeks.

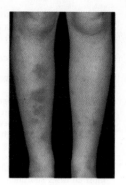

Fig. 35.**1** · Erythema nodosum.

➤ *Special variants:*
- *Erythema nodosum migrans:* Multiple smaller nodules, evolve into rapidly spreading plaques with central healing. *Subacute nodular migratory panniculitis* (Vilanova–Piñol-Aquadé) is the same or similar.
- *Erythema nodosum chronicum:* Otherwise typical lesions but persistent.
- *Nodose erythema:* Refers to clinically atypical lesions such as those located on calves and not shins.
➤ **Histology:** Thickened septae, granulomas, giant cells, fat lobules relatively spared.
➤ **Diagnostic approach:** Examination, detailed history, screening laboratory work (streptococcal screen, pregnancy test, chest radiograph, tuberculosis skin test) and others as directed by history.
➤ **Differential diagnosis:** Other forms of panniculitis, Sweet syndrome, necrobiosis lipoidica, granuloma annulare, pernio (usually on feet).
➤ **Therapy:**
- Compression stockings, NSAIDs; if severe, bed rest if possible (most young mothers cannot get bed rest).
- High-potency corticosteroids under occlusion.
- No systemic steroids, as they may mask underlying signs and symptoms; exception is acute sarcoidosis.

Erythema Induratum

➤ **Synonyms:** Bazin disease, nodular vasculitis.
➤ **Definition:** Panniculitis associated with granulomatous vasculitis involving mid-sized vessels.
➤ **Epidemiology:** Almost limited to adult women.
➤ **Pathogenesis:** Controversial; relationship to tuberculosis not firmly established. *Mycobacterium tuberculosis* DNA is rarely identified in lesions. The issue is nodular vasculitis—same clinical appearance but no evidence for tuberculosis.
➤ **Clinical features:** Firm nodules almost always on back of legs. Tend to ulcerate and heal with scars.
➤ **Histology:** Granulomatous vasculitis.
➤ **Differential diagnosis:** Other forms of panniculitis; erythema nodosum never ulcerates.

► **Therapy:** Compression stockings, NSAIDs; wound care if ulcerated.
  • If evidence in history or examination for tuberculosis, then consider tuberculo-static therapy.

Other Forms of Panniculitis

Most of these diseases are very rare, and many are covered elewhere in this book. Here are just a few tips:

► Both **pancreatitis** and **pancreatic neoplasms** can cause panniculitis. The pancreatic enzymes cause saponification.

► **α_1-Antitrypsin deficiency:** Consider with liquefying panniculitis, when several members of same family have panniculitis; responds to dapsone; patients should be warned about smoking and pulmonary disease.

► **Lymphoma:** Subcutaneous lymphomas are usually T-cell in origin (p. 479). Erythrophagocytosis is not uncommon. Histiocytic cytophagic panniculitis is in almost all cases subcutaneous panniculitis-like T-cell lymphoma. Rare disorders exist with virally triggered hemophagocytosis and fat involvement.

► **Trauma:** Cold panniculitis is common, ranging from popsicle panniculitis (children sucking icy desserts) of the cheeks to neonatal fat necrosis, a benign condition. Fat is a favored site for injection of materials, ranging from silicone for cosmetic enhancement to feces, urine, and even more bizarre materials to induce artifactual disease.

► True infectious panniculitis is uncommon; in most instances infections trigger erythema nodosum.

► **Lupus profundus** (p. 206): Usually signs of lupus erythematosus elsewhere, but sometimes isolated. Panniculitis plus overlying mucin or epidermal atrophy, or rich in plasma cells, should suggest lupus erythematosus.

► **Weber–Christian disease** (relapsing febrile nodular nonsuppurative panniculitis) is controversial; probably most cases reflect α_1-antitrypsin deficiency, pancreatic disease, or lymphoma. Before making this diagnosis, investigate the patient extensively and observe for at least 6 months.

36 Anogenital Diseases

36.1 Anal and Perianal Diseases

Hemorrhoids

- **Definition:** Hyperplasia of the physiologic hemorrhoidal vascular complex, which is an erectile tissue essential in maintaining rectal continence. In the USA, such hemorrhoids are referred to as internal hemorrhoids.
- **Epidemiology:** Every adult has some degree of hyperplasia of these normal structures.
- **Pathogenesis:** Factors leading to signs and symptoms of disease include chronic constipation with straining for bowel movements, genetic predisposition, low-fibre diets, and abuse of laxatives.
- **Clinical features:** Hemorrhoids are divided into four grades:
  - *Grade I:* Enlarged cushions of hemorrhoidal complex, visible on proctoscopic examination.
  - *Grade II:* Hemorrhoids can prolapse through anal canal, but retract spontaneously.
  - *Grade III:* Hemorrhoids frequently prolapse but can be repositioned.
  - *Grade IV:* Permanent anal prolapse.
- **Diagnostic approach:**
  - Careful inspection, ideally after bowel movement, and with pressing.
  - *Palpation:* Grade II can be palpated, as can thrombosed lesions.
  - Proctoscopic examination, ideally with Blond proctoscope, which has side opening into which hemorrhoids may prolapse. Routine proctoscopy can overlook hemorrhoids.
  - ▶ *Note:* Never be content to blame rectal pain or bleeding on hemorrhoids. A complete examination is necessary to exclude other conditions, such as a carcinoma of the rectum.
- **Therapy:**
  - High-fibre diet.
  - Anal exercises; tightening anal sphincter for 10–20 seconds repeatedly several times a day, perhaps tightening against anal dilator.
  - Destruction with rubber band ligature, sclerosing solution, infrared coagulation or operation, depending on severity.
  - ⚠ *Caution:* Hemorrhoidal ointments and suppositories cannot address the underlying problem. They may provide temporary relief from pain and pruritus, but have a high risk of causing allergic contact dermatitis.

Anal Vein Thrombosis

- **Synonym:** Pile, external hemorrhoid.
- **Definition:** Sudden painful thrombosis of external anal vein.
- **Clinical features:** Blue-purple nodule, often eroded, very tender; on anal ring; often appears after defecation.
- **Therapy:** Incision and expression of clot, NSAIDs, sitz baths.

Anal Tags

▶ **Clinical features:** Lax, fibrotic skin folds, usually the long-term sequelae of thrombosed anal veins. They may become inflamed or irritated, as well interfering with continence.
▶ **Therapy:** Symptomatic lesions easily excised.

Anal Fissure

▶ **Definition:** Extremely painful fissure or ulcer in anal canal.
▶ **Pathogenesis:** Controversial; increased sphincter tone plays a role, but other factors unclear.
▶ **Clinical features:**
  • Fibrinous fissure or ulcer with callused border; almost always at 6 o'clock position with patient in dorsal lithotomy position.
  • Extremely tender; pain after completion of bowel movement almost unbearable; patients tend to resist bowel movements and become constipated, worsening problem.
  • Increased sphincter tone, sentinel pile (proximal hypertrophic anal papilla).
▶ **Therapy:**
  • Apply local anesthetic before attempting examination; sometimes injection is required.
  • Acute fissures can be painted with 1% aqueous silver nitrate solution.
  • 2% nitroglycerine ointment is sometimes helpful; can cause headaches. Apply t.i.d.–q.i.d. In theory, sphincter is relaxed and dilated.
  • Injection of botulinum toxin also appears to relax sphincter tone.
  • Chronic or unresponsive fissures must be excised; wide variety of surgical approaches available.

Perianal Dermatitis

▶ **Definition:** Dermatitis in perianal region; usually extremely pruritic.
▶ **Epidemiology:** Common; many patients do not present to physician.
▶ **Pathogenesis:** Many causes, including:
  • Anal incontinence with irritation of perianal skin by anal discharge.
  • Inadequate anal hygiene.
  • Allergic contact dermatitis to cleansing tissues, hemorrhoidal preparations other medications.
▶ **Clinical features:** Few clues to cause on clinical examination; erythema, maceration, fine fissures. Often excoriations; some patients complain of considerable interference with work, social life, or sleep.
▶ **Diagnostic approach:** Look for skin disease elsewhere, complete proctologic examination, patch testing, stool examination for ova and parasites, cultures of stool and perianal skin for yeasts and dermatophytes; if disease persists, biopsy.
▶ **Differential diagnosis:** See summary in Table 36.1.
▶ **Therapy:** Improve hygiene, eliminate triggers, short course of mid-potency corticosteroid ointment; use zinc oxide paste for long-term protection.
  ◪ *Note:* Important to discourage the patient from overenthusiastic cleansing which can often worsen the problem and develop into a neurosis.

Table 36.1 · Differential diagnosis of perianal disease

Disease	Clinical features
Candidiasis	Macerated patches with erosions and peripheral pustules
Tinea inguinalis	Involves medial thigh, not scrotum or labia; scaly patch with prominent erythematous border
Psoriasis	Red macerated plaques without characteristic silvery scale; very difficult to diagnose without other signs of psoriasis
Seborrheic dermatitis	Look for clues elsewhere; sometimes worst in perianal region
Lichen planus	Often eroded and intensely pruritic
Lichen sclerosus	Both girls and women may have genital and perianal involvement; often hemorrhagic; in children mistaken for child abuse
Atopic dermatitis	Search for other stigmata; sometimes primarily here in adults
Contact dermatitis (allergic, toxic)	Erythema, scale, papulovesicles; appropriate history (usually hemorrhoid creams)
Other causes of anal dermatitis	Hemorrhoids, anal tags, worms, anal polyp, anal fissure, anal fistula—because of the risk of rectal carcinoma, every patient with an unclear perianal dermatitis deserves a proctologic examination
Condyloma acuminata	White papillomatous papules which can coalesce or become macerated
Extramammary Paget disease	Weeping eroded plaques, perianal or inguinal, associated with underlying adenocarcinoma in some cases
Bowen disease	Erythematous plaques; formerly common in patients who had received ionizing radiation for psoriasis
Condylomata lata	Eroded weeping broad-based plaques; perianal and intertriginous; lesion of secondary syphilis
Crohn disease	Draining sinus tracts and fistulas

Perianal Lesions

▶ Many of the same diseases affecting the genitalia also involve the perianal region. Always think of the possibility of rectal disease with secondary perianal problems.

Pruritus Ani

▶ **Definition:** Perianal pruritus without visible skin changes.
▶ **Pathogenesis:**
  • Most common causes are eating spicy foods and improper anal hygiene.
  • All of the conditions that cause anal dermatitis can also cause pruritus ani.
  • Other factors include pinworms, candidiasis, food allergies, emotional factors.
▶ **Clinical features:** In true pruritus ani, nothing is to be seen.

▶ **Diagnostic approach:** Careful examination to exclude anal and rectal diseases, especially those causing stool incontinence; search for condyloma; culture stool and skin for *Candida albicans*; patch testing.

▶ **Therapy:**
- Few diseases are as burdened with emotional overtones as pruritus ani. Patients are hesitant to discuss the problem. Often there are hidden guilt factors, such as anal intercourse or other forms of penetration.
- **⚠ Caution:** Always consider child abuse in children who complain of pruritus ani or anal pain.
- Bland, high-fibre diet.
- Some individuals develop severe pruritus from the tiny residual amounts of stool left behind after cleansing with toilet paper, and must plan their activities so that they can clean the area adequately.
- Topical antipruritic agents, such as polidocanol ointment in nonsensitizing base.
- Systemic sedating antihistamines in the evening.

36.2 Diseases of Male Genitalia

There are many diseases that may involve the male genitalia. We will only touch upon some of the most common.

Balanitis

▶ **Definition:** Inflammation of the glans penis. *Balanoposthitis* refers to inflammation of the glans and prepuce, which is the more likely clinical setting.

▶ **Pathogenesis:** The main risk factor is the presence of an occlusive foreskin. Other factors include infections, diabetes mellitus (with glycosuria), immunosuppression, lack of cleanliness (with irritation from smegma), excessive trauma, and underlying skin diseases such as atopic dermatitis or psoriasis. The most common infectious organism causing balanitis is *Candida albicans*, but trichomonas, herpes simplex, *Chlamydia*, and many others can play a role. Another factor is allergic contact dermatitis to hygiene items, topical medications, or latex.

▶ **Clinical features:** Acute balanitis features erythema, pain, and often a weeping discharge. In many instances it may be accompanied by phimosis. Always search for lymphadenopathy or ulcerations as clues to infections. Chronic balanitis is usually candidal and often occurs in diabetics.

▶ **Diagnostic approach:** Culture for bacteria (often mixed infections) and yeasts. If any question, syphilis serology. If urethral discharge, culture for gonorrhea.

▶ **Differential diagnosis:** The differential diagnostic considerations are shown in Table 36.2.

▶ **Therapy:**
- Treat underlying disease.
- Always use lotions or thin creams; heavy pastes or ointments cause additional "debris" to accumulate beneath the foreskin and exacerbate the problem.
- Wicking is essential in uncircumcised men. A strip of moistened gauze 1–2 cm wide is placed in coronal sulcus and the foreskin is pulled over it. Tap water suffices; high concentrations of disinfectants under occlusion (from the foreskin) can lead to necrosis.
- If no diagnosis is apparent, then assume *Candida albicans* is involved and use imidazole lotion or cream b.i.d.
- Chronic persistent balanoposthitis may require circumcision.

Table 36.2 · Differential diagnosis of balanitis

Disease	Clinical features
Chronic irritative balanitis	Erythema, maceration, painful; more common in uncircumcised; more common when partner has discharge
Candidal balanitis	Pustules are peripheral; partner history? diabetes mellitus?
Contact dermatitis	Erythema, pruritus, appropriate history; condoms, hygiene products
Herpes genitalis	Grouped blisters on erythematous base, rapidly pustular, painful, history of recurrences
Psoriasis	Red macerated plaque; look for psoriasis elsewhere; can be solitary or just associated with arthritis
Lichen planus	Eroded plaque; look for lichen planus elsewhere; can be solitary
Lichen simplex chronicus	Area of persistent rubbing, exaggerated skin markings; occasionally on penis
Plasma cell balanitis (Zoon)	Circumscribed smooth red plaque; almost always in uncircumcised; biopsy diagnosis
Erythroplasia of Queyrat	Circumscribed velvety red plaque; variant of squamous cell carcinoma in situ; biopsy diagnosis
Erythema multiforme	Target lesions on extremities, palms and soles; sometimes on glans penis; blue-violet center with white intermediate zone and erythematous rim
Lichen sclerosus	White sclerotic area on glans or inner prepuce; common cause of phimosis; also known as balanitis xerotica obliterans
Circinate balanitis	Erythematous erosions with white periphery; associated with Reiter syndrome (reactive arthritis, keratoderma blennorrhagicum, signs of psoriasis)
Fixed drug eruption	Red-brown patch or plaque; history of recurrence in exactly the same site with ingestion of same drug

Human Papillomavirus (HPV) Infections (p. 70)

▶ **Clinical features:** In the anogenital lesion, HPV on mucosal or transitional surfaces or in occluded or macerated areas are white and thus often not instantly recognized as warts; they are also generally designated condylomata acuminata. Intrameatal warts are not uncommon; they may cause dysuria or even mild obstruction with a distorted stream of urine. Similar lesions on the shaft of the penis are usually darker.

▶ **Histology:** Some lesions may show squamous cell carcinoma in situ; they are known as *bowenoid papulosis* (p. 71). Despite the worrisome histologic appearance, many of these lesions resolve spontaneously. Biopsy of genital warts is usually not needed, but should be considered in recalcitrant lesions.

► **Differential diagnosis:** HPV infections of the genitalia are common, but they are also often misdiagnosed. Table 36.**3** shows just some of the conditions that are erroneously diagnosed as "warts" in the anogenital region.

► **Therapy:** Mucosal warts respond more readily to topical agents such as podophyllotoxin or imiquimod.

Table 36.3 · Differential diagnosis of genital warts

Disease	Clinical features
Bowenoid papulosis	Variant of condylomata acuminata, larger lesions, often on shaft of penis or labia minora; histologically squamous cell carcinoma in situ; some regress, others become squamous cell carcinoma
Molluscum contagiosum	Skin-colored 1 – 5 mm delled papules, often grouped
Free sebaceous glands	Tiny yellow papules on prepuce or labia minora
Pearly penile papules	Tiny angiofibromas in sulcus of glands; often mistaken for warts; harmless; female equivalent is hirsuties vulvae
Lichen planus	Polygonal violet flat-toped papules, lacy white network often seen on glans or labia minora; pruritic
Lichen nitidus	Miniscule white papules; favor penis shaft
Condylomata lata	Eroded weeping broad-based plaques; perianal and intertriginous; lesion of secondary syphilis

Penile Ulcers

► **Pathogenesis:** Genital ulcers are a major problem because they are often transmissible, painful, interfere with sexual intercourse, and may reflect a serious underlying disease (syphilis, chancroid).

  ◪ *Note:* Genital ulcers are often overlooked in women. This is reflected in the transmission of herpes simplex by asymptomatic women and in the lower incidence of chancres in female syphilis patients.

► The causes of penile ulcers include infections, trauma, aphthous diseases (both idiopathic genital ulcers and Behçet syndrome), squamous cell carcinoma, and especially artifact.

► **Clinical features:** Classically the distinction is made between the relatively painless firm, punched-out chancre of syphilis (hard ulcer) and the soft, jagged, painful ulcer of chancroid. The most common genital ulcers are caused by herpes simplex virus; they are typically small, grouped erosions, as the vesicular stage is often overlooked.

► **Diagnostic approach:** Always take a careful history, check other mucosal sites (mouth, rectum, conjunctiva), and consider trauma and artifact. If the diagnosis is not 100% clear, do syphilis serology and bacterial culture.

► **Differential diagnosis:** The same infections and other problems create genital ulcers in women, but the risk of their being overlooked is greater. Thus, we discuss penile ulcers as prototypical of all genital ulcers. The differential diagnostic considerations are shown in Table 36.**4**.

► **Therapy:** Treat underlying disease. Genital ulcers heal rapidly; avoid occlusive medications, which are messy and so often not employed by patient.

Table 36.4 · Differential diagnosis of penile ulcers

Disease	Clinical features
Herpes genitalis	Grouped blisters on erythematous base, rapidly pustular, painful, history of recurrences; most common cause of small penile blisters
Chancre	Firm hard, button-like lesion with superficial erosion; usually painless
Chancroid	Painful, dirty, genital ulcer with ragged edges
Lymphogranuloma venereum	Small solitary soft erosion; often overlooked; main finding lymphadenopathy
Pyoderma	Painful dirty ulcer; often arises after traumatic sexual intercourse, zipper injury
Squamous cell carcinoma	Irregular tumor, often ulcerated, almost invariably in uncircumcised individuals
Behçet syndrome	Recurrent aphthae, genital ulcers; more common in Asia and Middle East; genital lesions often large and persistent
Artifact	Bizarre morphology; penis is favored site for injections, chemical burns, other self-induced changes
Fournier gangrene	Sudden aggressive ulcer; necrotizing fasciitis of the genitalia; mixed bacterial infection; associated with trauma, surgery, systemic infections

Sclerosing Lymphangiitis

A peculiar condition in which the lymphatics (or on occasion veins) of the penile shaft become irritated or inflamed. Not infectious, but often follows sexual intercourse, presumably because of trauma. Presents as painful cord, easily felt because of lack of subcutaneous tissue. No treatment required; NSAIDs are sometimes helpful.

36.3 Diseases of Female Genitalia

Vaginitis

Vaginal infections rarely present to the dermatologist. Nonetheless, it is important to inquire about vaginal discharge whenever confronted with a vulval dermatitis, as the drainage may be irritating. Similarly, partners of women with vaginitis are likely to develop balanitis. The most common infectious causes of vaginitis are *Candida albicans*, *Trichomonas vaginalis*, and *Gardnerella vaginalis*, which causes bacterial vaginosis with its characteristic fishy smell. *Chlamydia* are more likely to cause cervicitis, while *Neisseria gonorrhoeae* can lead to a purulent discharge, especially in children whose vaginal epithelium better supports the infection.

Chronic vulvovaginitis has many overlaps with chronic balanitis; diabetes mellitus and obesity are particular risk factors, while *Candida albicans* is frequently present and should be treated. Allergic contact vaginitis also occurs, triggered primarily by feminine hygiene products and latex, but most such reactions are irritant in nature.

Foreign bodies are another consideration, especially in children, who are also occasionally irritated by bubble baths.

Atrophic vaginitis is a problem that may involve dermatologists. Every women experiences some degree of vaginal atrophy after the menopause, with thinning of the epithelium and a rise in pH favoring Gram-negative, anaerobic bacteria. If a discharge is present, it is watery. Topical estrogens or estrogen vaginal suppositories are the usual treatment. Some of these patients have lichen sclerosus, as discussed below.

Vulvar Dermatitis

When confronted with a patient with vulvar dermatitis, the two most important issues are:

► Presence of vaginal discharge with irritation.
► Evidence of underlying skin disease such as:
  • *Atopic dermatitis:* Many women with chronic vulvar dermatitis have other stigmata of atopic dermatitis.
  • *Psoriasis:* Classic intertriginous disease, may involve vulva almost exclusively; look for other clues (nails, scalp).
► Some rare diseases also regularly involve the vulva. Examples include necrolytic migratory erythema as a marker for glucagonoma and acrodermatitis enteropathica as a sign of zinc deficiency.
  ▣ *Note:* Always consider nutritional deficiencies and eating disorders when confronted with vulvar dermatitis.
► **Therapy:** Treatment is based on identifying and correcting the underlying disorder. To control pruritus, topical corticosteroid and anesthetics (polidocanol) lotions or creams are useful.

Lichen Sclerosus

This common inflammatory dermatosis often involves the vulva in both small girls and older women. The clinical picture is distinctive, with an ivory-white plaque usually with a violaceous ring. In the genital area, a "figure 8" pattern occasionally occurs as the disease involves both the anus and the vaginal orifice (p. 217).

A careful search for clues to lichen sclerosus is indicated in several clinical settings:

► **Potential child abuse:** Because of the abnormal connective tissue in papillary dermis, patches of lichen sclerosus frequently show hemorrhage. When periorificial, the findings can be confused with sexual abuse.
► **Vulvar pruritus and pain:** The affected skin is more fragile and easily damaged by irritants or physical trauma. In addition, late lesions are sclerotic and atrophic producing a restricted vaginal orifice and pain on intercourse.
► **Vaginal atrophy** often reflects overlooked lichen sclerosus.
► **Vulvar lichen sclerosus** is rarely a site for the development of squamous cell carcinoma. Keratotic or ulcerated lesions in this setting must always be biopsied.
► **Therapy:** Surprisingly, topical corticosteroids (usually high potency) and topical calcineurin inhibitors are more effective than topical estrogens.

Pruritus Vulvae and Vulvodynia

► **Definitions:** Although there are overlaps and cases that are hard to define, it is clinically helpful to separate two conditions:
  • *Pruritus vulvae:* Intense vulvar itching, with almost invariably secondary excoriations or lichenification.
  • *Vulvodynia:* Vulvar burning or pain, usually associated with pain on intercourse (*dyspareunia*).

Pruritus vulvae: Most often reflects underlying pruritic dermatosis (atopic dermatitis, contact dermatitis, lichen sclerosus), vaginal discharge, infestation (scabies), or underlying cause of pruritus (renal disease, diabetes mellitus). Always check for what is being applied topically, taking detailed and persistent history. Physical examination should include perianal region, as rectal discharge can also lead to vulvar irritation. Sometimes biopsies are useful to identify clinically subtle lichen sclerosus or even bullous pemphigoid in the elderly. Search for any erosions, ulcerations, or scars, as they might point to herpes genitalis or aphthae. In some instances, one finds no cause.

▶ *Note:* Pruritus vulvae can simplistically be viewed as lichen simplex chronicus of the female external genitalia. No matter what the cause, a chronic itch–scratch cycle develops and lichenification is the result.

● *Therapy:* Topical corticosteroids or anesthetics are most useful; they can be combined with systemic antihistamines or even antidepressants, depending on the severity.

Vulvodynia: A much more difficult problem. Generally no positive physical findings. Classic symptom is pain or burning.

▶ *Note:* A patient with vulvodynia generally corrects a physician who asks "How long have you been *itching?*" They feel pain, not itching.

● One must search for any signs of dermatologic disease that could explain the pain. Sometimes when the vulvar vestibule (area between labia minora where urethra and vagina open) is exquisitely sensitive, the diagnosis of vulvar vestibulitis is made. Some then treat for HPV infection of the vestibule, but results have been clinically less than impressive.

Therapy: Try to work together with a gynecologist and psychotherapist interested in this extremely challenging and time-consuming clinical problem. Most patients do not benefit from topical therapy, and require antidepressants or other psychotropic medications.

37 Phlebology

37.1 Anatomy and Function of Leg Veins

Anatomy of the Leg Vein System (Fig. 37.1)

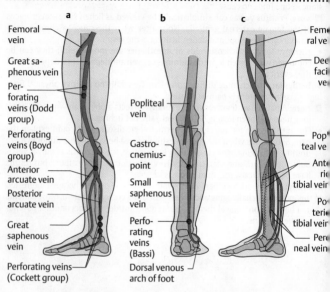

Fig. 37.1 · **Anatomy of the leg veins. a** Epifascial greater saphenous vein with most important perforating veins. **b** Epifascial lesser saphenous vein with most important perforating veins. **c** Deep subfascial veins.

There are two systems of leg veins, both containing unidirectional valves directing the blood flow upward:

▶ **Superficial epifascial veins:**

- Two major veins, great saphenous vein and small saphenous vein, as well as their branches.
- The *great saphenous vein* runs into front of the medial malleolus and along the medial aspect of the leg to the groin where it joins the femoral vein at the *saphenofemoral junction*; it is the longest vein in the body.
- The *small saphenous vein* runs from above the lateral malleolus over the calf to join with the popliteal vein at the sapheno-popliteal junction in the popliteal fossa.
- The *posterior arcuate vein* (posterior saphenous vein) is the most important smaller vein; it runs from behind the medial malleolus up the calf and joins the great saphenous vein. It has connections to the *subfascial posterior tibial vein*

(Cockett perforating veins); incompetent valves in this system are a major cause of venous leg ulcers.

▶ **Deep subfascial veins:**
- The deep veins of the lower leg are paired with the corresponding arteries; they include the *anterior tibial, posterior tibial,* and *peroneal veins.*
- Above the knee, the deep veins are the *popliteal, superficial femoral,* and *deep femoral veins.*
- Anatomic variants are common in this system.

▶ **Perforating veins** connect the two systems; their valves direct the blood flow to the deep system.

Function of Leg Veins

▶ **Muscle pump:** The energy for venous return is provided primarily by the pumping action of the leg muscles combined with the unidirectional valve system. Each time the muscles contract, venous blood is directed upward and inward. Adequate contraction of the muscle pump depends on a fully flexible ankle joint.

▶ **Other factors:** The arterial pressure plays little part. Each step empties the venous pads of the soles.

37.2 Varicose Veins

Overview

▶ **Definition:** Varicosities are dilated superficial veins. They are divided into primary and secondary forms.

Primary Varicose Veins

▶ **Definition:** Varicose veins that develop without an apparent cause.

▶ **Epidemiology:**
- Female:male ratio 2:1; onset usually 20–30 years of age.
- Strong family predisposition.
- By age 70, 70% of women and 60% of men are affected; in 70%, both legs are involved.
- Co-factors include number of pregnancies, occupation requiring prolonged standing, and obesity.

▶ **Pathogenesis:** The wall is dilated to an extent that the valves are no longer competent. This starts a vicious cycle of reflux, further dilation, and impaired return.

▶ **Clinical features (Figs. 37.2, 37.3):**
- *Starburst or spider varicosities:* Fine microvaricosities usually located on inner aspect of calf and outer aspect of thigh. When arranged along edge of foot, known as *corona phlebectatica paraplantaris* (venous crown).
- *Reticular varicosities:* Netlike dilated superficial veins without hemodynamic consequences.
- *Accessory varicosities:* Involve branches of the main veins; often asymptomatic but hemodynamically significant.
- *Truncal varicosities (saphenous vein varicosities):* Involve the major veins of the leg; in 70% of cases associated with incompetent perforating veins; hemodynamically significant.
- The classification of varicosities devised by Hach is shown in Table 37.1 and Fig. 37.4.

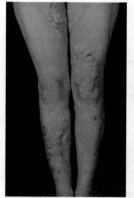

Fig. 37.2 · Prominent varicosities involving major veins.

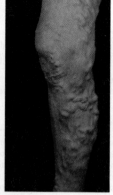

Fig. 37.3 · Closer view of marked varicosities.

Table 37.1 · Level of insufficiency of major veins

Reflux	Grade
Great saphenous vein	
One handsbreadth below junction	I
Above the knee	II
Below the knee	III
To the ankle	IV
Small saphenous vein	
Below the knee	I
Mid-calf	II
To the ankle	III

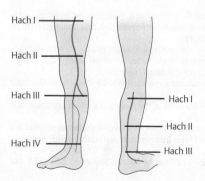

Hach I

Hach II

Hach III

Hach IV

Hach I

Hach II

Hach III

Fig. 37.4 · Level of venous insufficiency (after Hach).

Secondary Varicose Veins

- **Definition:** Varicose veins secondary to a known cause.
- **Pathogenesis:** The most common cause of secondary varicosities is the *post-thrombotic syndrome.* Uncommon causes are angiodysplasias (vascular malformation syndromes) and other underlying diseases, such as connective tissue defects. In the postthrombotic syndrome, a deep venous thrombosis leads to damage to the valves and reflux, which then places excess demands on the perforating and collateral veins. Over years the perforating and then epifascial veins become dilated and incompetent. In both primary and secondary varicosities, the number of incompetent perforating veins is the best correlate for the degree of hemodynamic compromise.
  - ▶ *Note:* Suprapubic varicosities are almost always a sign of a pelvic vein thrombosis. They are occasionally confused with an inguinal hernia.
- **Chronic venous insufficiency:** The reduced venous return is hemodynamically significant and causes clinical disease, divided into three stages (after Widmer):
  - *Stage I:* Corona phlebectatica paraplantaris.
  - *Stage II:* I + atrophie blanche, hemosiderin deposits, dermatosclerosis, stasis dermatitis.
  - *Stage III:* II + ulceration.

Complications

- Thrombophlebitis, varicophlebitis.
- Rupture of varicose veins with minor trauma.
- **Arthrogenic stasis syndrome:** Thickening of skin and pain restrict motion of ankle joint, starting a vicious circle of inadequate pumping and then worsening problems. The impaired mobility of the ankle joint later becomes the most important obstacle to ulcer healing.
- Venous leg ulcer (ulcus cruris venosum, stasis ulcer).
- Muscle atrophy, subcutaneous bone dysplasia.

Diagnostic Approach

Detailed information on the phlebologic diagnostic process is given on p. 39. The most useful approach for chronic venous insufficiency is Doppler and duplex sonography. Other approaches such as light reflection rheography (LRR), digital photoplethysmography (DPPG), and venous plethysmography (resting and dynamic) can be used as indicated. When deciding on the possibility of surgery for the postthrombotic syndrome with secondary varicosities, invasive phlebodynametry (actual measurement of venous pressure with intravascular needle) is often required. Phlebography is usually not necessary when the above approaches are employed.

Therapy

- **Basic principles:**
  - Regular compression therapy is the mainstay of treating varicosities.
  - Varicosities in the great and small saphenous vein require surgical correction.
  - Accessory vein varicosities can be treated surgically or sclerosed.
  - Reticular and starburst veins can be treated with sclerotherapy, or in the case of starburst veins, with laser ablation.
  - Incompetent perforating veins should be interrupted surgically.
  - Vein stripping (Babcock procedure) can produce long-term improvement.

venous leg ulcers heal with compression therapy. When accompanyin
cose veins are treated, most ulcers heal more rapidly.

.edure depending on phlebologic evaluation:

No deep reflux but varicosities: LRR or DPPG indicate improvement possible
then:

- Remove incompetent vein segments surgically.
- Strip the main vein and then either excise or sclerose the accessory veins.
- General, regional or tumescent local anesthesia can be employed.
- If varicosities recur, repeat operation possible.

2 *Deep reflux and varicosities:* LRR or DPPG indicate improvement possible, then
- Completely remove varicosities as above.
- If the reflux in the deep veins stops, then life-long compression not required

3 *Deep reflux and varicosities:* LRR or DPPG indicates no improvement possible
then:
- Life-long compression therapy required.

☐ **Note:** Patients with compensated varicose veins *can* be treated; those wit
chronic venous insufficiency *must* be treated.

▶ **Operative approach to venous leg ulcers:** The entire surgical palette discusse
above can be employed when leg ulcers are present. Prompt therapy of chroni
venous insufficiency should hopefully prevent advancement to stage III disease. I
addition, early surgery reduces the likelihood of deep vein insufficiency. If
complete stripping is not possible or has already been accomplished, then option
include:

- Sclerosis of veins about the ulcer.
- Ligature of isolated perforating veins, especially those in Cockett group.
- Endoscopic subfascial resection of perforating veins is another alternativ
  when severe dermatosclerosis or a leg ulcer is present; recurrences are not un
  common.
- Radical excision of ulcus to fascia and paratibial fasciotomy are seldom used.
- Shaving excision of ulcer followed by mesh grafting offers the chance of long
  term relief.
- If all other procedures have failed, split-skin grafting and compulsive compres
  sion therapy will shorten the healing time.

▶ **Alternative surgical methods:** There are a number of new promising approache
that have not been clinically validated and must still be regarded as experimenta
- *CHIVA* (**c**onservative and **h**emodynamic method for **v**enous **i**nsufficiency on a
  ambulatory basis): After duplex sonographic mapping, all perforating veins ar
  tied off under local anesthesia but no attempt is made to remove the varicosi
  ties, which regress somewhat on their own.
- *Endoluminal laser therapy:* The great saphenous vein is exposed or entered per
  cutaneously just below the knee. A glass fiber is advanced to the junction. Then
  with tumescent local anesthesia, the vein is coagulated with a diode laser whil
  the glass fiber is slowly retracted.
- *Radiowave sclerosis:* Similar to the endoluminal laser therapy, but the vein is de
  stroyed with a disposable catheter attached to a high-frequency electrosurgica
  unit.
- *Valvuloplasty:* The junction is exposed and the great saphenous vein wrappe
  with a Gore-Tex cuff or partially ligated so that its valve system functions onc
  again.

37.3 Inflammation of Veins

Superficial Thrombophlebitis

Note: When speaking with patients, always emphasis the difference between *thrombophlebitis* (inflammation of vein) and *phlebothrombosis* (primary thrombosis, far more serious).

Pathogenesis: The elements of the *Virchow triad* (vessel wall damage, increased coagulability, delayed blood flow) remain the crucial factors for thrombosis.

Clinical features: Erythematous warm and tender cord without generalized signs and symptoms. Most common on calf in area of varicosities; uncommon without accompanying varicose disease. Also may develop on arm following long-term intravenous therapy.

Diagnostic approach: History, clinical examination.

Differential diagnosis: Erythema nodosum, erysipelas, phlebothrombosis.

Therapy: Compression therapy with class II stockings or relatively firm elastic wraps. No bedrest. NSAIDs. If ascending, prophylactic heparinization. If the junction is involved, emergency surgery; if the thrombosis enters into the deep venous system, then treatment as below.

Varicophlebitis

Definition: Localized phlebitis in a varicose vein.

Clinical features: Tender, long, firm thrombosis in a varicosity of one of the major veins. May be localized or widespread. When the great saphenous vein is involved on the thigh, both deep vein involvement and pulmonary emboli may occur.

Therapy: Standard therapy as above; also consider operative removal of primary varicosity or incision with expression of thrombus.

Thrombophlebitis Saltans

Definition: Recurrent thrombophlebitis in nonvaricose veins; involves both arms and legs.

Epidemiology: Most common in young men.

Clinical features: Involvement of both arms and legs should always suggest trouble when dealing with thrombophlebitis.

Diagnostic approach: Check for underlying vasculitis (Bürger syndrome).

Caution: Thrombophlebitis saltans can be a paraneoplastic marker, especially for lung and pancreas carcinomas.

Therapy: NSAIDS; if Bürger disease is present, consider systemic corticosteroids or immunosuppressive agents.

Mondor Disease

Definition: Thrombophlebitis of the thoracoepigastric vein.

Pathogenesis: Unknown.

Clinical features: Sudden onset of firm, tender cord up to 40 cm long on the lateral thoracic wall.

Diagnostic approach: Pathognomonic clinical picture.

Therapy: Nothing or NSAIDS. Lesion resolves spontaneously over weeks.

37.4 Deep Venous Thromboses

Arm Vein Thrombosis

▶ **Classification:**
  - Subclavian-axillary vein thrombosis (Paget–Schroetter syndrome).
  - Thrombosis as complication of venous catheterization.
  - Thrombosis secondary to predisposing conditions.

▶ **Clinical features:** Subclavian–axillary vein thrombosis typically affects you men; the most common cause is thoracic inlet syndrome. The onset is usually slo with pain, swelling, and a sense of heaviness, as well as loss of strength. The vei in the shoulder region may be more prominent and cyanosis of the limb c develop.

▶ **Complications:** Pulmonary emboli develop in 10%; rarely life-threatening. Pos thrombotic features very uncommon.

▶ **Diagnostic approach:** Compression sonography or duplex sonography; if n clear, phlebography. D-dimer test.

▶ **Differential diagnosis:** External of axillary vein by tumors, metastases, scars, fe lowing radical mastectomy, callus formation after clavicular facture, substerr thyroid tissue, and cervical rib.

▶ **Therapy:**
  - Low molecular weight heparin and coumarin; once the INR is in the range 2 for 2 days, then heparin can be discontinued (see below).
  - Thrombolysis or surgery in early phase in young patients.
  - In thoracic inlet syndrome, surgical correction usually possible.

Deep Vein Thrombosis (DVT)

▶ **Synonyms:** Phlebothrombosis, deep leg vein thrombosis.

▶ **Pathogenesis:** Risk factors include trauma, lack of physical activity (especially a solute bedrest), aberrant coagulability (following surgery, miscarriage, or pre nancy), use of oral contraceptives, underlying malignancy, smoking, long airpla flights, and excessive physical activity in poorly trained individuals (Sund mountain climbers).

▶ **Clinical features:**
  - In nonhospitalized patients, onset usually dramatic. In hospitalized patien often slow and easily overlooked.
  - Sense of heaviness and tension, tugging pains, pain in the groin or flank, fatig anxiety, increased pulse.
  - Leg may be livid or show prominent veins.
  - ⚠ *Caution:* May present as pulmonary embolus.
  - *More severe forms:*
    – *Phlegmasia cerulea dolens:* Acute fulminating DVT with reactive arter spasm, cyanosis and edema; multiple veins may be involved.
    – *Phlegmasia alba dolens:* Femoral vein phlebitis leading to limb swelling a pallor.
  - ▶ *Note:* If a patient has unexplained calf pain, leg edema, tense muscles or tende ness, always think of DVT.

▶ **Diagnostic approach:**
  - Clinical diagnosis extremely difficult and unreliable; must always be co firmed.
  - *D-dimer test:*
    – Fibrin split products, which always appear when clotting occurs.

- Always positive after surgery, infections (erysipelas); return to normal after 2–3 days.
  - Available as rapid screening test or can be quantitatively determined.
  - Only for screening test to exclude diagnosis.
- *Compression sonography:*
  - Method of choice.
  - If diagnosis unclear, repeat after short period of time or do phlebography. Doppler sonography and vein compression plethysmography are only sensitive for pelvic vein thrombosis.
- **Differential diagnosis:** Sport injuries, hematomas, thrombophlebitis.
- **Therapy:** (p. 676).
  - Subcutaneous heparinization with a low molecular weight heparin (for example, fraxiparin 0.1 mL/0 kg b.i.d. subq.). On first or second day, also start coumarin with a goal of INR 2–3. Once the INR level has been obtained for 2 days, heparin can be stopped.
  - ⚠ *Caution:* Check platelets before starting heparin therapy and then weekly, because of risk of heparin-induced thrombocytopenia (HIT).
  - Duration of therapy 6 months for thrombosis below pelvis; 12 months for pelvic vein thrombosis or recurrence.
  - Compression therapy with compression bandages and then once edema has resolved, compression stockings class II.
  - Bed rest for 5 days in the case of pelvic vein thrombosis.
  - In younger patients, thrombolysis or operative thrombectomy should be considered. If an operation is planned, then nonfractionated heparin should be administered by continuous i.v. infusion, as it is more easily counteracted with protamine sulfate.
  - ◨ *Note:* Calf vein thrombosis may require less aggressive therapy (p. 676).
- **Complications:**
  - *Pulmonary embolus:*
    - Clinical signs and symptoms include tachycardia, dyspnea, right-sided cardiac overload, oxygen saturation < 92%, pain. About 10% of untreated DVT patients develop clinically apparent pulmonary emboli.
    - Diagnostic procedures include EKG, scintigraphy, sonography, chest radiograph, and pulmonary artery angiography.
  - Later complications include development of secondary varicosities or postthrombotic syndrome.

Postthrombotic Syndrome

- **Definition:** Chronic venous insufficiency of leg following phlebothrombosis.
- **Pathogenesis:** Following postthrombotic recanalization with valve defects, there is usually a period of years without problems, then development of incompetent perforating veins and secondary varicosities. The chronic venous insufficiency leads to disturbances in microcirculation with tissue damage including ulceration, obliterating lymphangiopathy, and arteriolar occlusion.
- **Clinical features:** Initially pitting edema, later induration. Small varicosities and blowout veins as first signs of incompetent perforating veins. Other signs of stasis are *atrophie blanche* (white atrophic scars) and *purpura jaune d'ocre* (yellow-brown chronic purpura about ankles) (Fig. 37.**5**).
- **Therapy:** Life-long use of compression stockings (Table 37.**2**) or compression bandages. Usually a below-the-knee stocking is sufficient.

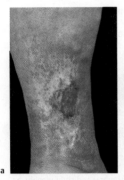
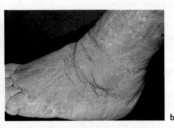

a   **b**

Fig. 37.**5** · **a** Atrophie blanche with ulceration. **b** Dermatosclerosis and verrucous edema i postthrombotic syndrome.

Table 37.2 · **Classes of compression stockings**

Class	Features
I	Light compression, pressure 15 – 20 mmHg, mild superficial effect
II	Medium compression, pressure 23 – 32 mmHg, moderate superficial effect
III	Strong compression, pressure 34 – 36 mmHg, superficial and deep effects
IV	Very strong compression, pressure > 49 mmHg, marked deep effects

37.5 Stasis Dermatitis and Venous Leg Ulcers

Overview

► **Pathogenesis:** Crucial factor is reduced tissue oxygen levels caused by venous hy pertension and stasis.
► **Clinical Features:** Venous ulcers are usually on medial side of ankle; they can var greatly in size and clinical appearance (Fig. 37.**6**).
► **Diagnostic approach:** Evaluation to rule out arterial and neuropathic ulcers, a well as ulcerated tumors and trauma. Differential diagnostic considerations for le ulcers are listed on p. 728.
◘ *Note:* The biggest mistake is to overlook an ulcerated tumor (basal cell carcinom squamous cell carcinoma, amelanotic malignant melanoma, lymphoma); if i doubt or if ulcer fails to respond, always biopsy.

Therapy

► **Overview:**
  • Compression therapy, mobilization, and consideration of surgical measures t eliminate varicosities.
  • Stage-adjusted management of venous ulcer with moist wound therapy wit goals of cleaning, encouraging granulation, and facilitating re-epithelializatio

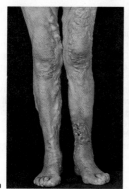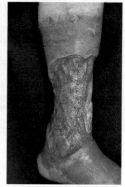

a **b**

Fig. 37.**6** · **a** Bilateral varicosities with venous leg ulcer. **b** Extensive venous leg ulcer.

⚠ *Caution:* Avoid use of topical agents with potential for contact sensitization; rare use of topical antibiotics; systemic antibiotics only for clinically apparent infection, then short-term and culture-directed.

Compression and mobilization:
- Firm compression bandages; maximal variant is Unna boot (zinc paste bandages).
- Variety of stockings available for ulcer care.
- Mobilization; physical therapy to retain mobility of ankle joint because of its crucial role in pumping.
- Consider manual or instrumental lymphatic drainage.

▶ *Note:* Meticulous attention to compression and mobilization is the cornerstone of all effective venous leg ulcer treatment.

Topical therapy around ulcer.
- *Goals:* Clean and protect nonulcerated periphery, treat underlying dermatitis.
- *Cleansing:* Daily washing in tub or shower; moist compresses with physiologic saline (0.9%). Compresses with 5.0% saline are more effective but may be irritating or painful. Olive oil is useful for removing crusts and residual creams or ointments.
- *Superinfection with exudation:* Antiseptic solutions with moist compresses.

▶ *Note:* Moist compresses left on until almost dry are much more effective for debridement than soaking.
- *Resistant infections:* Culture and sensitivity; then consider fusidic acid ointment or mupirocin ointment. In most instances, systemic antibiotics are preferable.
- *Dermatitis therapy:*

▶ *Note:* Always exclude allergic contact dermatitis caused by topical agent or preservative. Common allergens include balsam of Peru, wool wax alcohols, cetyl sterol alcohol, emulgators, preservatives (parabens), antibiotics (especially neomycin, gentamicin, chloramphenicol). Use of any of these agents should be considered carefully.
  – If the dermatitis is dry, use a corticosteroid ointment or emollient cream. A useful compound is betamethasone valerate 0.1% in white petrolatum (p. 692).
  – If the dermatitis is moist or weeping, then clioquinol lotion or cream (p. 691) is helpful.

- *Skin protection:* Zinc oxide paste or white petrolatum can be applied to norm
  skin around the ulcer.
- ⚠ *Caution:* White petrolatum has an occlusive effect, which encourages th
  growth of bacteria. It must always be combined with appropriate cleansing.

▶ **Topical therapy of ulcer:** Goals are pain relief, cleansing, encouragement o
  granulation, encouragement of reepithelialization, protection.

- *Pain relief:*
  - Topical anesthetics before cleansing (EMLA under occlusion for 45 minutes
    alternatively, local anesthetic solution injected beneath ulcer.
- ⚠ *Caution:* Lidocaine creates an alkaline environment, favoring bacterial grow
  and inhibiting keratinocyte proliferation.
  - Analgesics (usually NSAIDs suffice).
  - Choose dressings that are easy to remove. If dressing is adherent, soak wit
    tap water or physiologic saline for 5–10 minutes.
- *Cleansing:*
  - *Physiologic-osmotic:* NaCl solution in increasing concentration
    (0.9%–2%–5%–10%) or crystalline sugar.
  - *Antiseptic solutions:* H_2O_2:H_2O 50:50, 0.1–0.5% methylrosaniline chloric
    aqueous solution (p. 697); always rinse with physiologic saline.
  - *Mechanical debridement:* Curettage after adequate anesthesia.
  - *Autolytic debridement:* Alginate or hydrocolloid dressings.
  - *Enzymatic debridement:* Many available, none clearly superior; possibiliti
    include streptokinase/streptodornase, collagenase, and papain-ure
    chlorophyll.
  - *Absorption:* Activated charcoal granules, also available with additional silv
    other compounds.
- ▣ *Note:* Most of the cleansing measures also stimulate granulation tissue.
- *Encouragement of granulation:*
  - *Physiologic-osmotic:* 5–10% saline solution, sugar or sugar:sand mixtures.
  - *Mechanical debridement:* scarification of periphery with scalpel and the
    airtight occlusion.
  - *Increase perfusion:* Infrared light, Nd:YAG laser, or physical activity.
  - *Moist wound care:* Polyurethane foams, alginate pads.
  - *Vacuum closure technique:* Polyurethane foam is applied, covered with occl
    sive membrane and then placed under suction pressure with pump
    vacuum bottle. Often painful at start.
- *Encouragement of epithelialization:*
  - *Moist wound care:* Hydroactive gel or hydrocolloid dressing.
  - *Impregnated gauze nonadhering dressings.*
  - *Autologous keratinocyte cultures,* if technically possible.
  - *Protargol zinc paste:* 0.1% silver nitrate, 30.0% zinc oxide, 69.9% whi
    petrolatum.
- *Protection:* Zinc oxide paste or ointment, panthenol ointment.

▶ **Rheologic therapy:** If there is an arterial component, consider low-dose aspir
  low-dose heparin, pentoxifylline; prostacyclin infusions possible but value n
  proven. Foot of bed should be lower than head, and no compression therapy if art
  rial systolic pressure at ankle < 80 mm Hg. Check for hyperviscosity syndrome a
  treat.

- ▣ *Note:* Always maximize treatment of accompanying varicosities, venous i
  sufficiency, or arterial disease; otherwise an ulcer will take much longer to he
  Be alert to accompanying neuropathies. If response is slow, check again to
  sure you have identified the cause correctly.

37.6 Phlebologic Surgery

▶ **Preoperative planning:**
- Exact diagnosis incorporating Doppler and duplex ultrasonography, as well as phlebography. To document function of deep and pelvic veins, ascending press phlebography is best.
- Identify all incompetent veins, including perforating veins and accessory, collateral, or atypical main veins.
- To reduce complications, usually best to operate on just one leg; the other one can then be addressed in 6–8 weeks. This approach minimizes the postoperative restriction of motion,

▶ **Operative approach for varicosities:**
- **Procedure:** Recommended procedures are shown in Table 37.**3**.

Table 37.3 · **Operative approach to varicosities**

Stage (after Hach)	Procedures
I	Crossectomy of the great saphenous vein/small saphenous vein
II	Crossectomy of the great saphenous vein/small saphenous vein and stripping with Babcock method to knee
III	Crossectomy of great saphenous vein and stripping to mid-calf Crossectomy of small saphenous vein and stripping of the complete posterior calf
IV	Crossectomy of great saphenous vein and stripping of entire calf

▶ **Technique:**
- On the evening before the operation, mark the junctions and the course of the major veins, as well as the perforating veins and other varicosities; shave the groin and thighs.
- After sterile preparation and draping, incision to expose the oval fossa of the thigh. Exposure of the junction of the great saphenous vein and the femoral vein. Tie off all contributing branches; then suture ligation of great saphenous vein with additional safety ligature.

  🔲 *Caution:* Place ligatures carefully so as not to reduce lumen of femoral vein.
- If possible, insert stripper into the distal great or small saphenous vein and then advance it in direction of venous valves. Retrograde insertion increases risk of damaging vein wall. Always advance stripper slowly and control its progress with palpation.

  🔲 *Caution:* Do not introduce stripper via perforating veins.
- Once the stripper has been passed and its head attached, dissect out and ligate the perforating and accessory veins. Then extract the stripper, removing the vein, and immediately applying compression dressings. This minimizes blood loss.

▶ **Postoperative care:** Compression therapy with custom-fitted class II stockings for 8–10 weeks. Thereafter consider sclerotherapy of accessory varicosities.

  🔲 *Caution:* Recurrent varicosities should always be treated on an inpatient basis because of the risk of excessive bleeding.

Venous Leg Ulcer

▶ **Chronic venous ulcer:**
- Conservative antiseptic therapy, closing the skin defect.
- Simultaneous attention to incompetent main, accessory, or perforating veins will speed heeling.

▶ **Marked dermatolipofascial sclerosis:**
- Radical fasciectomy to relieve pressure.

▶ **Less severe changes:**
- Endoscopic subfascial dissection of perforating veins is often just one.
- Sufficient to allow healing of ulcer.

▶ **Large infected ulcers:** *Vacuum sealing method* offers excellent approach following radical excision of ulcer to condition base. Its use can greatly reduce the time a patient is immobilized.

38 *Occupational Dermatoses*

38.1 *Overview*

▶ Skin disorders are the second most common cause of occupational disability in most developed countries accounting for around 25% of days lost. (The most common is musculoskeletal problems, accounting for around 50%.).
▶ Scandinavian studies suggest an incidence of 5–15:10000. The vast bulk of this is occupational allergic-irritant dermatitis of the hands.

38.2 *Occupational Hand Dermatitis*

▶ **Epidemiology:** About 1% of the population has hand dermatitis. In working populations, the prevalence may exceed 10%. Some professions at very high risk include:
- Beauticians/hairdressers and barbers.
- Bakers.
- Gardeners and florists.
- Machinists.
- Construction workers.
- Dental technicians.
- Other health care personnel.
▶ **Pathogenesis:** The vast bulk of occupational hand dermatitis is irritant in nature. Typical irritants include soaps, cutting oils, and other petroleum products. Prolonged immersion of hands in water is also a factor, by greatly damaging the barrier and facilitating entry by other agents. Strong irritants cause chemical burns and are usually recognized and avoided. Frequent exposure to minor irritants is the usual scenario.
- Allergic contact dermatitis may rise on the background of irritant dermatitis or independently. Typical allergens include:
  - Rubber components.
  - Epoxy resins.
  - Chromate.
  - Aromatic amines (parabens, hair dyes).
  - Fragrances.
  - Preservatives.
▶ **Clinical features:** The diagnosis and treatment of hand dermatitis is covered in detail (p. 200).
  - ☐ *Note:* Assume every case of hand dermatitis is potentially occupational, and detail the information in your history. This will both allow you to intervene early and institute preventive measures, perhaps even for other employees, and save you much anguish later when contacted by the employer or workmen's compensation bureau.
▶ **Diagnostic approach:**
- Search for preexisting or aggravated skin diseases. Both atopic dermatitis and psoriasis can cause problems. The issue is always whether the disease was already present but made worse by the occupational exposure, or was "caused" by the job. Understandably, the distinction is difficult and the financial impact on the employee, employer, and insurer is immense.

- Document what happens to the dermatitis on nonworking days, weekends, and during vacation.
- Is there distant spread to sites beyond the hands? This hints at allergic contact dermatitis.
- Do patch testing. This information will be required in almost every case. Obtain detailed instructions on how to test for the specific materials with which the patient has contact. Two common errors are:
  - Blind reliance on standard patch test series (p. 43).
  - Failure to properly dilute suspected substances, thus causing irritant reactions instead of testing for allergic ones.

▶ **Differential diagnosis:** The initial diagnosis is easy. One should exclude tinea and psoriasis.

▶ **Therapy:** The treatment is standard, including emollients, topical corticosteroids and in severe cases systemic corticosteroids or other immunosuppressive agents. In addition, in almost all cases, the patient must be temporarily excused from work.

▶ **Prophylaxis:** The ideal approach is avoidance or prophylaxis. This can take many forms:
- *Primary prevention:*
  - Advise patients with atopic dermatitis not to enter high-risk professions.
  - Screen individuals entering high-risk professions for preexisting skin diseases and teach them about skin protection and avoidance maneuvers.
  - Be sure appropriate protective measures are available in the workplace, including protective gloves and skin barrier creams. Using a fluorescent marker in the hand cream and a Wood's light, patients can be shown how to apply their protective creams correctly.
  ◨ *Note:* The three-step approach to skin protection involves protection, cleansing and maintenance care.
- *Secondary prevention:*
  - Prompt attention to early irritant hand dermatitis, with increased emphasis on protection and maintenance to avoid severe disease.
  - In Germany, all physicians are required to refer patients in whom an occupational hand dermatitis is suspected to a qualified dermatologist for expert assessment and management.
  - Working with trades unions and employers, it is often possible to remove potential allergens or irritants from the workplace and find suitable replacements.
- *Tertiary prevention:*
  - Once the disease is severe, patients can be taught how to deal with it better or retrained in other professions.

38.3 Occupational Contact Urticaria

▶ Contact urticaria (p. 172) is a common problem among bakers, veterinarians, food handlers, and health care workers.

▶ Nonimmune contact urticaria is more common and represents a reaction to chemicals such as sorbic acid. Immune contact dermatitis involves a reaction to protein constituents, such as those in meats, foods, animal dander, or especially latex.

▶ Latex has an interesting history. In the 1980s, with increased interest in preventing hepatitis B and the advent of HIV/AIDS, the demand for natural rubber latex (NRL) gloves rose dramatically. With the introduction of cheaper manufacturing methods in Asia, producing NRL gloves with a high protein content, latex allergy dramatically increased in the 1990s, with sensitization rates up to 20% in hospital personnel. New regulations limiting the amount of protein in NRL gloves to $< 200\,\mu g/g$ (low-protein gloves) and the provision of powder-free NRL gloves have reversed the trend, with sensitization rates dropping in most series.

► In most instances, the patients suffer from contact urticaria initially. Later, latex allergy may lead to life-threatening reactions as some patients develop anaphylaxis.

► The diagnostic approach includes specific IgE testing and then prick testing with a latex extract. The sensitivity of the specific IgE testing has been greatly increased to around 70% by using recombinant Hev b 5 and Hev b 13 (Hev refers to *Hevea brasiliensis*, the rubber tree), which are the major latex allergens. The sensitivity and specificity of prick testing depends on the allergen extract used, and may vary depending on its origin.

38.4 *Other Occupational Dermatoses*

Infections

► **Bacterial infections:**
  • *Staphylococcal and streptococcal infections:* Any profession exposed to minor trauma, such as butchers, farmers, construction workers; more serious problem in health care workers because of risk of resistant strains and possibility of further transmission.
  • *Anthrax:* Contact with infected animals or hides contaminated with spores can cause local inoculation or pulmonary disease.
  • *Erysipeloid: Erysipelothrix rhusiopathiae* is present in many animals; inoculation injury for hunters, butchers.

► **Viral infections:**
  • *Warts:* Human papillomavirus 7 and occasionally other strains cause butchers' warts.
  • *Orf:* Parapox virus common in sheep and goats can be transmitted to farmers, shepherds, and veterinarians.
  • *Milker's nodule:* Closely related to orf, but infects udders of cows and is transferred to dairy farmers and veterinarians.

► **Fungal diseases:**
  • *Candidiasis:* Candidal paronychia are common in bakers and food handlers.
  • *Sporotrichosis:* Inoculation of plant material can transfer *Sporothrix schenckii* to gardeners, forestry workers.
  • *Dermatophyte infections:* Those around cattle often acquire severe but self-limited infection with *Trichophyton verrucosum* during first period of exposure.

Acne (p. 530)

► **Chloracne:** Caused by exposure to halogenated hydrocarbons, such as dioxin, chloracne features closed comedones and cysts, as well as hyperpigmentation. Exposure may be via military service (Agent Orange pesticide exposure in Viet Nam), contaminated foods, industrial accidents (Seveso accident), or even poisoning as occurred in a prominent Ukrainian politician in 2005.

► **Tar acne:** Pitch, tar, and oils can cause comedonal or pustular acne. Today cutting oils are most common; be suspicious when acneiform lesions are seen on anterior thighs or abdomen where oils can be splashed.

Skin Cancers

▶ **UV exposure** is the most common cause, playing a role in skin cancers across the range of occupations including pilots, farmers, military personal, athletes, welders, and many others.

▶ **Hydrocarbons**, such as pitch, tar, and other compounds, may also cause skin cancers. The first known report of occupational cancer was scrotal cancer in chimney sweeps. Today risk groups include road construction workers, roofers, and refinery workers.

▶ **Arsenic** exposure in mining activites in areas such as Taiwan and Argentina, as well as in industrial processes, can cause skin cancers. Today most exposure worldwide is through contaminated ground water in Bangladesh.

Vibration Syndrome

▶ The use of tools with marked vibration such as jackhammers, stamping machines, or chain saws may lead to vasospasm or white fingers. Smoking and cold weather are co-factors. The spasm is different from Raynaud syndome in that it is asymmetrical. Raynaud syndrome and acro-osteolysis can be induced by exposure to vinyl chlorides, while systemic sclerosis with Raynaud syndrome can be caused by exposure to silica.

39 *Skin Diseases in Different Age Groups*

39.1 *Skin Diseases in Pregnancy*

Overview

▶ Many skin changes occur during pregnancy. They can be grouped into physiologic variations, changes in preexisting dermatoses, and pregnancy-specific dermatoses.

◪ *Note:* Remember that what is common in nonpregnant patients is also common in pregnancy. Always think of common diseases first—atopic dermatitis, acne, and scabies are all commonly misdiagnosed as other, more exotic conditions.

▶ **Physiologic changes:** Most are likely caused by hormonal changes:
- Striae distensae.
- Hyperpigmentation of nipples, genitalia, and perianal region. Linea alba (midline of abdomen) darkens and is known as *linea nigra*. Facial hyperpigmentation known as *melasma* or "*mask of pregnancy*" (p. 379).
- Seborrhea, hyperhidrosis, hypertrichosis.
- Androgenic alopecia may improve with increased levels of estrogens.
- Postpartum telogen effluvium.
- Eruptive vascular lesions (nevus araneous or vascular spiders) and palmar erythema.

▶ **Changes in pre-existing or latent dermatoses:**
- Darkening, growth and perhaps increase in number of melanocytic nevi.
- Growth of neurofibromas.
- *Tend to improve:* Acne, acne inversa, psoriasis and sarcoidosis.
- *May improve or worsen:* Atopic dermatitis, pustular psoriasis.
- *Tend to worsen:* Autoimmune collagen-vascular disorders (lupus erythematosus, dermatomyositis, systemic sclerosis), autoimmune bullous diseases (fetal involvement possible via transplacental transfer of antibodies), invasive or metastatic melanoma, porphyria cutanea tarda, Ehlers–Danlos syndrome, pseudoxanthoma elasticum, viral and fungal infections.

▶ **Pregnancy-specific dermatoses**.

Cholestasis of Pregnancy

▶ **Synonym:** Pruritus of pregnancy.
▶ **Pathogenesis:** Common disorder occurring in up to 2% of pregnancies; idiosyncratic hormonally driven reduction in bile transport.
▶ **Clinical features:** Presents with intense pruritus in second or third trimester; rarely accompanied by dark urine or jaundice. No problems in mother, but slight increase in fetal mortality and prematurity. Likely to recur in subsequent pregnancies and perhaps with oral contraceptives.

◪ *Note:* The most common cause of jaundice in pregnancy is viral hepatitis.
▶ **Diagnostic approach:** Elevated bilirubin with possible mild elevations in AST, ALT; any other changes should mandate search for other liver disease.
▶ **Differential diagnosis:**
- *Pruritus:* Look for other signs of pruritic diseases, such as scabies or atopic dermatitis.

- *Jaundice:* Hyperemesis gravidarum, viral hepatitis, acute fatty liver of pregnancy.
- *Jaundice + thrombocytopenia:* HELLP syndrome (**h**emolysis, **e**levated liver enzymes, **l**ow **p**latelets).
▶ **Therapy:** Cholestyramine 8–12 g daily in 2–3 divided doses for itch. Vitamin K if hypoprothrombinemia develops. Consider induction of labor.

Erythema Nodosum Gravidarum

▶ Just as erythema nodosum occasionally appears correlated with menses or oral contraceptives, sometimes it appears in the first trimester or early second trimester without apparent cause. Patient must be investigated just as any other patient with erythema nodosum (p. 540). If secondary to pregnancy, usually resolves by third trimester but may recur with subsequent pregnancies or hormone exposure.
🗷 *Caution:* NSAIDs should not be used in the third trimester; they may cause premature closure of the ductus arteriosus.

Pemphoidus Gestationis

This is the most specific dermatosis of pregnancy, an autoimmune bullous disease that may also transiently affect the newborn (p. 238).

Pruritic Urticarial Papules and Plaques of Pregnancy

▶ **Synonym:** PUPPP (acronym), polymorphic eruption of pregnancy.
▶ **Definition:** Intensely pruritic eruption, usually occurring in last trimester.
▶ **Clinical features:** The distended abdomen is the most common site; sometimes the urticarial papules and plaques preferentially involve the striae. May also involve trunk, thighs, and upper arms. No other signs and symptoms and no complications. Resolves after delivery. No risk to child.
▶ **Histology:** Not diagnostic. Superficial and deep perivascular lymphocytic and eosinophilic infiltrates. Sometimes spongiosis or acanthosis.
▶ **Therapy:** Topical corticosteroids; in rare cases, systemic corticosteroids needed.

Prurigo Gestationis

▶ **Definition:** Association of intense pruritus in third trimester with excoriations and prurigo papules.
▶ **Pathogenesis:** Many of these patients have atopic diathesis, and their skin diseases flares in pregnancy.
▶ **Clinical features:** Marked pruritus, excoriations, erosions, prurigo nodules.
▶ **Diagnostic approach:** No specific clinical or histologic criteria.
▶ **Differential diagnosis:** Exclude hepatic disease (cholestasis of pregnancy occurs early but hyperemesis, HELPP occur late), folliculitis and other pruritic dermatoses (scabies). Search for stigmata of atopy.
▶ **Therapy:** Symptomatic topical antipruritic measures.

Impetigo Herpetiformis

▶ **Definition:** Severe annular pustular psoriasis (p. 265) in pregnancy.
▶ **Pathogenesis:** Unknown, but may be associated with or lead to hypoparathyroidism.
▶ **Clinical features:** Erythematous patches with peripheral pustules and central scales favoring abdomen or upper inner thighs. Systemic signs and symptoms in

cluding fever, chills, nausea and vomiting; in some cases hypocalcemia with tetany. Potentially fatal, and increased fetal mortality.

▶ **Histology:** Intraepidermal accumulations of neutrophils without evidence for infectious agents.

▶ **Diagnostic approach:** Clinical examination, history of psoriasis, leukocytosis, elevated sed rate, calcium level, exclude hypoparathyroidism.

▶ **Differential diagnosis:** Occasionally described in nonpregnant patients; then we prefer diagnosis of pustular psoriasis. IgA pemphigus may appear similar; consider immunofluorescence studies.

▶ **Therapy:** Multidisciplinary management with obstetrician and pediatrician. Systemic corticosteroids and meticulous supportive care, usually in hospital, are required.

39.2 Dermatoses in Childhood

The differential diagnostic considerations for the classic childhood exanthems are shown in Table 39.1.

Table 39.1 · Classic exanthems

Diagnosis	Clues
Measles	Fever, sniffles, cough, skin changes start behind ears, Koplik spots
German measles (rubella)	Resembles common cold, skin changes start on face, lymphadenopathy
Scarlet fever (scarlatina)	Starts on neck, favors flexures, pharynx dark red, tonsils enlarged/inflamed, white strawberry tongue
Dukes disease	No longer diagnosed
Erythema infectiosum (fifth disease)	Begins on trunk, later face ("slapped cheeks"), sometimes lacy pattern on arms, pharyngitis, fever, malaise
Roseola infantum (exanthem subitum, sixth disease)	Infants, sudden high fever, as the fever resolves, pale red macules on trunk which last about 1 day, no lymphadenopathy
Varicella (chickenpox)	1–2 cm oval erythematous macules with central blister, lesions in various stages, scalp and oral mucosa affected, palms and soles spared, pruritic

Classic Childhood Exanthems

Traditionally, there were six childhood exanthems. Many have become rare today because of immunization or the wider use of antibiotics, and nowdays most childhood exanthems are caused by Cocksackie and enteroviruses. The left-hand column indicates the numbers attached to the classic exanthems over 100 years ago. The terms "fifth disease" and "sixth disease" are still occasionally used.

Most of these have fortunately become uncommon because of effective immunizations. The ill-advised trend of avoiding immunizations in many developed countries has led to increasing numbers of all the exanthems in recent years.

Measles

▶ **Synonym:** Morbilli.
  ☐ *Note:* The name rubeola means measles in German and English, but rubella in French and Spanish—thus best avoided.
▶ **Definition:** Acute viral infection of childhood with typical exanthem and severe general signs and symptoms.
▶ **Pathogenesis:** Measles virus is a paramyxovirus, spread by droplets. Highly infectious; over 90% of infected individuals are clinically ill.
▶ **Clinical features:** Three stages:
  • *Incubation period:* 9–12 days.
  • *Prodrome:* 3–4 days.
    – Fever, runny nose, cough, conjunctivitis (worse on lids, making eyes appeared circled), photophobia.
    – Tiny white spots on buccal mucosa (Koplik spots) persist into exanthem phase. Patchy erythema of palate (3–4 days).
  • *Exanthematous phase:* 3–4 days.
    – Initially fever disappears, but then recurs.
    – Maculopapular exanthem starts behind ears and on forehead; later spreads to neck and trunk and finally to extremities including palms and soles. Initially pale, but becomes deep red and may scale.
    – Complications include encephalitis, pneumonia, otitis media, and as delayed effect, subacute sclerosing panencephalitis.
▶ **Diagnostic approach:** Clinical features, exposure, lack of immunization; increase in titer of IgG antibodies.
▶ **Differential diagnosis:** Rubella, other viral infections, scarlet fever.
▶ **Therapy:** Supportive care, bedrest, antipyretics; in severe cases or with complications, antibiotics or immunoglobulins.
▶ **Prophylaxis:** Immunization is part of MMR (measles, mumps, rubella) administered at 12–15 months. This provides long-term immunity, as does primary infection.

Rubella

▶ **Synonyms:** German measles, 3-day measles.
▶ **Definition:** Common relatively mild viral infection of children and young adults; causes severe fetal damage if contracted in early pregnancy.
▶ **Pathogenesis:** Rubella virus is a togavirus, spread by droplet infection with high infection rate, but more asymptomatic cases than measles.
▶ **Clinical features:**
  • *Incubation period:* 14–21 days.
  • *Prodrome:* Minimal complaints, mild common cold; 3–4 days.
  • *Exanthematous phase:* 2–3 days.
    – Starts on face; erythematous macules and papules with pale periphery spread rapidly to neck, trunk, and extremities; disappear over 3 days (much more transient than measles).
    – Prominent retroauricular, occipital, and cervical lymphadenopathy; sometimes tender.
    – Complications include fetal defects in first 16 weeks of pregnancy (*Gregg syndrome:* ocular, hearing, and cardiac problems), as well as purpura, encephalitis, and in adults arthritis.
▶ **Diagnostic approach:** Clinical features, lack of immunization, increase in IgG or IgM titers; prenatal diagnosis of viral RNA in amniotic fluid or later fetal blood antibodies possible.

► **Differential diagnosis:** Measles, other viral exanthems, scarlet fever.
► **Therapy:** None needed; with complications, immunoglobulin available. Isolation from pregnant or potentially pregnant women. If pregnant patient is exposed, multidisciplinary consideration for immunoglobulin; only helps if given before exanthem develops.
► **Prophylaxis:** Immunization with MMR. All girls who do not have titers by puberty must be immunized to reduce risk of fetal malformations.

Scarlet Fever

► **Definition:** Generalized exanthem caused by erythrogenic toxins from group A streptococci.
► **Epidemiology:** Most patients are children < 10 years of age.
► **Clinical features:**
  • The cutaneous and mucosal features in scarlet fever appear 1–2 days after the pharyngitis and tonsillitis. Patients are ill with fever, chills, and malaise.
  • *Enanthem*: The pharynx is usually dusky red, when enlarged, inflamed tonsils. The tongue initially has a white cover, then the red papillae become apparent (*white strawberry tongue*), and then later the coating is shed, revealing a red swollen tongue (*strawberry tongue*).
  • *Exanthem*: The rash usually starts on neck and spreads to trunk and extremities. After 2 days, spread is complete. The flexures are most prominently affected (*Pastia lines*), while the palms and soles are spared. Running one's hand over the skin is described as the "*sandpaper sign.*" The erythema resolves after 3–5 days, followed by widespread shedding, most noticeable on the palms and soles.
► **Complications:** Glomerulonephritis, rheumatic fever, otitis, sinusitis.
► **Diagnostic approach:** Throat culture.
► **Therapy:** Penicillin V–K 250 mg t.i.d. for 10 days; acutely ill children may benefit from initial intramuscular dose.

Erythema Infectiosum

► **Synonym:** Fifth disease.
► **Definition:** Infection with parvovirus B19 causing fever and distinctive skin reaction pattern.
► **Epidemiology:** Occurs between 5 and 10 years of age; moderately contagious, occurs in epidemics; 50% of teenagers have immunity.
► **Pathogenesis:** B19 has affinity for bone marrow erythropoietic cells via P antigen. Causes considerable problems in pregnancy, as well as in patients with chronic anemia and immunosuppression, especially bone marrow transplantation patients.
► **Clinical features:**
  • Two classic skin findings:
    – *Slapped cheek sign:* Erythema of cheeks, sometimes figurate.
    – *Garland sign:* Reticulate erythema of extensor surfaces of arms.
    – Both may be missing, and patient may have pruritus and a maculopapular exanthem
  • Associated findings include fever, lymphadenopathy, pharyngitis.
  • Infection in children with chronic anemia, bone marrow transplantation patients, and other immunosuppressed patients can lead to *aplastic crisis*.
  • Infection in pregnancy may lead to fetal death (first trimester), hydrops (second trimester), or transient aplastic anemia (third trimester).

▶ **Diagnostic approach:** In child or adult, if any clinical question, check IgM antibodies or PCR for viral DNA, especially if contact with pregnant individual. In pregnancy, multidisciplinary approach with fetal ultrasound monitoring, search for antibodies and viral DNA.

▶ **Differential diagnosis:** Other viral exanthems, especially when classic findings not present.

▶ **Therapy:** Symptomatic.

Exanthema Subitum

▶ **Synonyms:** Exanthem subitum, roseola infantum, sixth disease.

▶ **Definition:** Viral infection of small children with high fever and transient rash.

▶ **Epidemiology:** Usually affects children 6 months–3 years of age; caused by human herpesvirus 6 (HHV-6) (and less often HHV-7). Runs in epidemics.

▶ **Clinical features:**
- Sudden high fever (40°C) lasting 3–5 days, with child surprisingly asymptomatic. Enanthem possible.
- As fever breaks, pale pink-red macules on trunk lasting 1 day.
- No lymphadenopathy or other associated findings.

▶ **Diagnostic approach:** Usually clinical diagnosis, but leukopenia, IgM antibodies and HHV can be identified.

▶ **Differential diagnosis:** Many other viral exanthems.

▶ **Therapy:** Symptomatic.

Other Childhood Exanthems

Erythema Toxicum Neonatorum

▶ **Definition:** Common erythemato-squamous eruption of first week of life.

▶ **Epidemiology:** Present in up to 50% of infants; usually starts 1–2 days after birth.

▶ **Clinical features:** Erythematous macules on trunk and extremities; associated with wheals and pustules; harmless and not toxic.

▶ **Diagnostic approach:** Smear from pustule rich in eosinophils.

▶ **Differential diagnosis:**
- *Neonatal pustular melanosis*: Possible variant of erythema neonatorum, more common in dark-skinned infants; pustules plus scaly hyperpigmented macules representing older lesions.
- *Impetigo:* Child sick, smear contains neutrophils.
- *Miliaria:* Usually occurs later, often intertriginous or on trunk.
- If purely pustular, consider neonatal *herpes simplex* and *Candida* infections.
- If child is older, consider *infantile acropustulosis*.

▶ **Therapy:** None required.

Gianotti–Crosti Syndrome

▶ **Synonyms:** Infantile acrodermatitis, papular acrodermatitis of childhood, acrodermatitis papulosa infantum.

▶ **Definition:** Acral viral exanthem caused by many different agents.

▶ **Epidemiology:** 90% of patients are < 4 years of age.

▶ **Pathogenesis:** Initially associated with hepatitis B, but now clear that many different viruses can cause same clinical picture. Most common cause in countries where hepatitis B immunizations are used is Epstein–Barr virus. Some form of aberrant immune response, seen only in small percentage of infected patients.

▶ **Clinical features:**
- Lichenoid red-brown papules on cheeks, extensor surfaces of extremities and buttocks. Resolve spontaneous over a few days; in rare cases, more persistent. Usually nonpruritic.
- Associated signs and symptoms vary with causative virus.

▶ **Diagnostic approach:** Clinical diagnosis; search for HBsAg, but not necessary to do extensive viral epidemiology.

▶ **Differential diagnosis:** Easy clinical diagnosis in young children; in older children and adults, consider lichen planus, lichen nitidus and lichenoid drug eruption.

▶ **Therapy:** Symptomatic.

Papular Purpuric Gloves and Socks Syndrome

▶ Caused by many different viruses; most commonly B19, HHV-6. Patients present with edema and purpura of the palms and soles; occasional spread to dorsal surfaces of hands and feet or onto limbs. Many have enanthem and about 10% have lymphadenopathy. Self-limited, clearing in 1–2 weeks; only supportive care is needed.

Unilateral Laterothoracic Exanthem

▶ **Synonym:** Asymmetric periflexural exanthem of childhood.

▶ Peculiar eruption usually starting in one axilla and spreading centrifugally. Cause unknown. Features macules, papules and lacy spreading rings. Eventually thorax is then involved and then dissemination may occur to other half of body. Other signs and symptoms minimal. Resolves over 1–2 weeks. Symptomatic treatment.

Child Abuse

▶ Dermatologists have a responsibility not to overlook signs of possible child abuse, and at the same time not to misdiagnosis dermatologic conditions as child abuse. Neither task is easy.

▶ In many health systems, specially trained nurses and physicians are available to help evaluate such cases in order to insure that no abused child is overlooked, but that at the same time the rights and feelings of parents are respected. In most instances physicians are legally required to report suspected child abuse.

⚠ *Caution:* Every dermatologist must be informed about the local legal and social aspects of referral for potential child abuse.

▶ It is usually wisest to say to the parents something like, "This seems to be a difficult type of case, not responding as we had expected; we would like to have one of our special nurses examine your child." Confrontation during the physical examination is almost always a social disaster and sometimes a legal one.

▶ **Clinical features:** Any difficult-to-explain clinical finding in a child raises the question of abuse. Examples include:
- Bruises or hematomas that seem excessive or recurrent, or follow lines that suggest use of a belt for whipping.
- Anogenital warts, tears, fissures, or bruises, gaping anus.
- Blisters and ulcers not fitting pattern for childhood bullous diseases.
- Uniform skin lesions about the diameter of a cigarette.
- Burns with peculiar patterns, suggesting body part was dipped or held in hot water.

⚠ *Caution:* Recurrent appearances in the emergency room with bruises, trauma, or unexplained findings are an absolute danger sign.

- The reverse side of the coin is conditions that can mimic child abuse (Table 39.2). Accusing parents of child abuse when they are innocent may also have catastrophic effects. There are several reports in the medical literature of "epidemics " of child abuse in communities caused by overzealous physicians or nurses misinterpreting harmless findings.

Table 39.2 · **Diseases that can mimic child abuse**

Clinical finding	Possible abuse
Hematomas following accident, especially in children with hematologic disorders	Beating
Dermatitis artefacta	Beating, burning, cutting
Ehlers–Danlos syndrome (hematomas, scars, fragile skin)	Beating
Epidermolysis bullosa (fragile skin)	Burns, scalds
Lichen sclerosus (perianal subtle hemorrhage)	Sexual abuse
Epidermal nevus in anogenital region	Viral warts following sexual abuse
Localized pemphigoid in anogenital region (ulcers, erosions)	Sexual abuse
Mongolian spot (blue-gray dermal pigmentation)	Trauma
Phytophotodermatitis	Burns, scalds, whipping
Bleomycin hyperpigmentation (hyperpigmented bizarre streaks)	Whipping
Staphylococcal scalded skin syndrome	Burns, scalds
Pityriasis lichenoides et varioliformis acuta	Cigarette trauma
Genital psoriasis	Sexual abuse
Striae distensae	Whipping
Diaper dermatitis	Inadequate care, sexual abuse
Crohn disease (gaping anus)	Sexual abuse

39.3 *Geriatric Dermatology*

Overview

▶ There are two major types of cutaneous aging:
  - *Instrinsic aging:* Natural changes: "ticking of biological clock".
  - *Extrinsic aging:* Major extrinsic factor is UV irradiation; effects of chronic UV exposure include increased risk of cutaneous malignancy, as well as many other changes.
    ◻ *Note:* The easiest way to form visual image of extrinsic versus intrinsic aging is to compare the skin of the forearm to the skin of the buttocks in an elderly individual.
  - As both life expectancy and UV exposure increase, the number of aging-related cutaneous disorders has increased and will continue to do so.

▶ **Intrinsic aging (functional changes):** Epidermal atrophy, decreased cell turnover leading to reduced wound repair, fewer Langerhans cells and generally impaired immune response, decreased sensation, drier skin (less sebum and epidermal lipids), decreased hairs, less vitamin D production, less sweating (impaired thermoregulation) and less vascular reactivity.

▶ **Extrinsic aging (UV-induced changes):** DNA and mitochondrial damage leading to basal cell carcinomas, actinic keratoses squamous cell carcinomas and malignant melanomas; induction of matrix metalloproteinases (solar elastosis); accelerated cell death; vascular changes.

▶ **Clinical features**
- Skin is generally drier, less turgid, often with fine scaling.
- Excessive washing or inadequate lubrication leads to increased scaling, dryness and pruritus; main factors are altered epidermal lipids and sebum, as well as changes in sweating.
- *Changes in hair:*
  - *Both sexes:* Graying of hair (canities) and reduced density of genital and axillary hairs.
  - ▶ *Note:* The temporal bone acquired its name because it typically underlies the first site where gray hairs appear (tempora is the plural of the Latin tempus = time).
  - *Women:* Increased moustache or beard hairs, as well as androgenic alopecia.
  - *Men:* Most have some degree of androgenic alopecia; increased hair growth in ears, nostrils, eyebrows.
- *Nails* grow more slowly, become dry and brittle, often develop longitudinal ridges and on the feet may become thickened and dystrophic, either with or without accompanying onychomycosis.
- *Light-exposed skin* features wrinkles, deep furrows (especially on nape), focal hyper- and hypopigmentation, telangiectases, senile purpura (hemorrhages on forearms secondary to weakened vessels), stellate pseudoscars (white irregular patches on forearms). Likelihood of malignancies depends on skin type and amount of UV exposure; almost every patient in Western countries has a few actinic keratoses. A peculiar finding is periorbital comedones (Favre–Racouchot disease).
- Seborrheic keratoses are an almost normal finding, most commonly on the trunk.

▶ **Skin care:**
- Nondrying soaps or synthetic detergents should be used; skin should be promptly lubricated after bath or shower. Many older patients require help to do this.
- Extremely dry skin benefits from use of lotions or creams containing urea or lactic acid. Just as in children, the greater sensitivity of elderly skin may lead to burning after application.
- Topical retinoids and hydroxy acids seem to be the most effective simple approaches to arresting or partially reversing photodamage. They should be combined with adequate sun protection.

▶ **Common dermatoses in elderly people:**
- *Scalp:* Seborrheic dermatitis; in those with bald heads—actinic keratoses, basal cell carcinoma, squamous cell carcinoma.
- *Face:* Angular stomatitis (perlèche) from improperly fitting dentures or drooling, actinic cheilitis, rosacea, rhinophyma, xanthelasma, seborrheic keratoses, keratoacanthoma, basal cell carcinoma, squamous cell carcinoma, lentigo maligna melanoma.

- *Trunk:* Seborrheic keratoses, candidiasis, tinea corporis, senile angiomas, basal cell carcinoma (superficial type), Bowen disease, Paget disease, superficial spreading melanoma, nodular melanoma, lymphoma.
- *Extremities:* Squamous cell carcinoma, basal cell carcinoma, Bowen disease, extramammary Paget disease, superficial spreading melanoma, acral-lentiginous melanoma, nodular melanoma, lymphoma.
- *Anogenital region:* Candidiasis, erythroplasia (mucosal squamous cell carcinoma in situ), lichen sclerosus, extramammary Paget disease, Bowen disease, plasma cell balanitis or mucositis.
- *Entire body:* Erythroderma, large-patch parapsoriasis, lymphoma, zoster, paraneoplastic markers.
- Treatment is covered in the respective chapters.

40 Psychodermatology

Overview

Definition: Psychodermatology concerns itself with the psychological causes of skin diseases and the patient's psychological adjustments to having skin diseases. Skin diseases can be completely somatic (seborrheic keratosis), somatic but with marked effect on psyche (malignant melanoma), somatic but with apparent emotional triggers (atopic dermatitis), or completely psychological (delusions of parasitosis).

The skin has long been considered a "mirror of the soul". We become red with anger or pale with fear. Our language also supports this connection; someone who annoys you "gets under your skin."

The skin, and especially the skin appendages, are richly innervated. Melanocytes, Merkel cells, and cutaneous nerves all arise from the neuroectoderm. Modern advances in psychoneuroimmunology have shed light on the fascinating interactions between the psyche, nervous system, endocrine organs, and immune system. For example:

- The immune system is innervated.
- Hematopoietic cells and neurons share certain receptors for neuropeptides and neurotransmitters.
- Lymphocytes can secrete many neuropeptides and other neuroendocrine factors.
- Cells of the immune system and nervous system can produce and react to the same cytokines.

There are two classic ways in which the nervous system and immune system communicate:

- Neuroendocrine peptides (growth hormone, prolactin, ACTH, β-endorphin, others) are secreted by the pituitary gland, which is controlled by factors secreted by the hypothalamus.
- The autonomic and sensory nervous systems interact directly with the immune system.

Many cutaneous cells (keratinocytes, melanocytes, fibroblasts, sebocytes) produce a variety of neurohormones, neurotransmitters, neuropeptides, and neurotrophins (nerve growth factor and others). In addition, they may express the corresponding receptors, a feature formerly considered to be limited to endocrine and neural cells.

The organs of the lymphoid system have sympathetic and cholinergic innervation. Sympathetic nerve endings are in close contact with antigen-presenting cells, T cells, and even B cells. Direct connections between cutaneous nerve endings and Langerhans cells or mast cells have also been shown. One can therefore postulate mechanisms for the neural and thus psychic control of the immune response in disorders such as atopic dermatitis. The old designation of neurodermatitis becomes modern once more, although we do not advocate switching names again.

Every pruritic dermatitis can become worse with stress. There are numerous possible mechanisms, including the central release of endorphins, which have analgesic and euphoric actions but also cause pruritus. Peripheral nerve endings may be triggered by stress to release various neuropeptides that cause mast cell degranulation and the release of histamine and other mediators as well as inflammatory infiltrates. The interactions between pruritus and stress can thus evolve into a vicious cycle.

Psychosomatic Dermatoses

Examples of dermatoses in which it is extremely difficult to separate the physical and emotional comments include atopic dermatitis, chronic urticaria, psoriasis, idiopathic pruritus, prurigo simplex, lichen simplex chronicus, acne excoriée, and stress-induced telogen effluvium. The exact neurophysiologic mechanisms influencing these disorders remain a subject of discussion and research.

The mainstay of therapy should be appropriate topical and systemic treatment. Without question, psychotropic medications, psychological therapy (behavior therapy, relaxation therapy) and even psychodynamic approaches (group therapy, individual therapy) can be useful supplements, as can training of patients and parents in how to best cope with the disease.

Body Dysmorphic Disorder

▶ **Synonym:** Dysmorphophobia.
▶ **Definition:** Mental disorder in which a person of normal appearance is preoccupied with an imagined defect in appearance, or overconcerned about a minor abnormality.
▶ **Epidemiology:** Estimated that 1% of population and 10% of dermatologic practice suffer from this disorder; typical patients are young, unhappy, worried women.
▶ **Pathogenesis:** These patients display features both of obsessive-compulsive behavior (frequently checking mirror) and of delusional thinking (firmly convinced of an abnormality).
▶ **Clinical features:** Typical complaints include:
   • Facial burning, unclean skin, too many vessels, burning, other defects that are not visible to anyone else.
   • Scalp or tongue burning.
   • Anogenital problems (pruritus, discharge, fear of venereal diseases or HIV).
▶ **Diagnostic approach:** Absolutely essential to exclude underlying diseases, but at the same time not reinforce disease perception by endless testing. Requires tremendous skill as physician to walk this line.
▶ **Therapy:**
   • Establish confidence, assure patient that you take the problem seriously.
   • Consider referral to psychologist or psychiatrist; this is almost always refused.
   • Neurotropic agents can be helpful:
      – Selective serotonin re-uptake inhibitors (SSRI) are preferred for obsessive-compulsive problems.
      – Antipsychotic agents are required for those with delusional behavior.
   ⚠ *Caution:* We deliberately avoid recommending medications or dosages. Any physician who feels they want to employ psychotropic medications for dermatologic patients is ethically obliged to obtain special training and expertise in the use of these agents.

Delusions of Parasitosis

▶ **Synonyms:** Monosymptomatic hypochondrial psychosis, delusional disorder—somatic type.
▶ **Definition:** Psychiatric disorder in which patients are firmly convinced they have a parasitic infestation.
▶ **Epidemiology:** Uncommon disease, usually involves middle-aged or older women, often from higher socio-economic groups. In younger patients, male:female ratio is equal and there is often history of substance abuse.

Pathogenesis: These patients are not psychotic, because their psychosis centers around just one point; other mental functions are surprisingly normal. Some speak of an *encapsulated psychosis*.

Clinical features:

- The patients typically present with widespread excoriations, a long history, and often carrying a small bottle or box. In the box they have meticulously saved all the "parasites" harvested from their skin, but microscopic examination of the contents reveals only threads, scales, and dirt. They may complain of *formication* (sensation of arthropods crawling on their skin, biting and stinging them). Most have been diagnosed several times as having scabies and treated with scabicides.
- Two other monosymptomatic hypochondrial psychoses may occasionally be seen by dermatologists:
  - *Delusions of bromhidrosis (unpleasant body odor):* Patients exude a normal body odor but they are convinced they smell so bad that no one can bear to be in their presence.
  - *Delusions of facial asymmetry:* Patients are convinced their face is distorted, usually presenting with a mirror to demonstrate the asymmetry explicitly. Careful morphometric studies actually show that every face is asymmetrical, but this is no consolation to the patient.
- A final fascinating aspect is the frequency with which family members come to share the delusion—known as *folie à deux*. The "deux" is not always accurate, as sometimes many individuals are involved.

Diagnostic approach:

- Exclude all causes of pruritus that have not been already investigated.
- Force yourself to examine the contents of the box or bottle again.

Therapy:

- Unless scabies is identified, resist the temptation to try a scabicide one more time, just in case.
- Topical antipruritics.
- Antipsychotic medication is the only thing that helps. The most effective agent is pimozide, approved for Tourette syndrome. We have found it useful to explain to the patient that we know they do not have Tourette syndrome (thank goodness) but for a peculiar reason unknown to all, they seem to require the same medication. Pimozide is not easy to use and newer antipsychotics will likely replace it. Once again, training and experience in using psychotropic medications is required.

Dermatitis Artefacta

Definition: Psychocutaneous disorder in which the patient inflicts cutaneous damage to satisfy underlying need.

Epidemiology: Rare disease, almost limited to women, and often those with connection to health care field.

Pathogenesis: Most patients have borderline personality disorder and there is no clear social explanation for their behavior. In some instances, the skin damage is a reaction to stress that they cannot otherwise manage.

Clinical features:

- Lesions are highly variable, but typically difficult to assign to an established dermatosis, absent from areas patient cannot reach (mid-back), common on forearms, face, and breasts, and more likely to be on contralateral side from dominant hand. They may appear as erosions, ulcers, burns, hemorrhagic lesions, or abscesses.

- Typical measures include applying irritating chemicals, injecting urine, feces, milk, or the like, or excessive painful manipulation. Cigarette burns are favorite trick; always be suspicious of lesions roughly the diameter of a cigarette. Self induced ulcers are typically highly irregular. Another classic feature is a failure to respond to therapy.

▶ **Diagnostic approach:** Once again, one must may every effort to exclude nonartifactual disease, such as vasculitis, pyoderma gangrenosum, hematologic disorders or immune defects. Cultures from abscesses revealing mixed pathogenic organisms often suggests artifactual disease.

▶ **Differential diagnosis:** There are several other psychodermatological considerations:

- *Malingering:* Patient induces lesions intentionally for a conscious benefit, such as creating the suspicion of an occupational injury.
- *Munchausen syndrome:* An extreme example of a factious disorder in which the patient intentionally simulates signs and symptoms of disease for the purpose of obtaining treatment, but without any apparent motive.
- *Munchausen syndrome by proxy:* Occurs when someone else induces lesions in another so that the second party receives unnecessary diagnostic and therapeutic attention. In Munchausen by proxy, skin lesions are more common because it is easier to show the physician something on the other person.

▶ **Therapy:**

- Occlusive bandages or dressing will give the lesions a chance to heal and help confirm the working diagnosis.
- It is not usually helpful to confront the patient at first.
- If underlying psychiatric disorder is present (depression, generalized anxiety), treatment may help. Antipsychotic drugs are occasionally helpful.

Other Artifactual Diseases

There are a number of other diseases in which self-manipulation is clearly responsible, but where there is little evidence of accompanying emotional problems and the disease is usually controllable with antipruritic measures. Examples discussed elsewhere in this book include:

▶ Prurigo simplex subacuta (p. 329).
▶ Prurigo nodularis (p. 330).
▶ Lichen simplex chronicus (p. 330).
▶ Lip dermatitis from repeated biting, licking (p. 489).
▶ Trichotillomania; other forms of hair and nail manipulation (p. 506).

1 *Topical Therapy*

1.1 *Overview*

e skilled use of topical agents is what distinguishes a dermatologist from other ysicians. An old truism is that a dermatologist can usually achieve more by choos- the best vehicle than can a non-dermatologist by using active ingredients in the ong vehicle. Most of the advances in modern topical agents have been achieved by rmatologists working with industrial partners.

pical Pharmacokinetics

Diffusion: The movement of molecules along concentration gradient via random motion. For a topically applied agent to enter the skin, it must diffuse between the vehicle and the stratum corneum.

Adsorption: The attachment of topically applied substances to the skin.

Absorption: The uptake and storage of topically applied substances in the skin. Both adsorption and absorption are dependent on many factors, including:

- *Location* (for example, number of hair follicles present).
- *Age of patient:* Absorption much greater in neonates.
- *Condition of skin:* Intact stratum corneum has maximum barrier function; as stratum corneum is abnormal or damaged, uptake of lipophilic agents is dramatically increased.
- *Environmental factors:* Humidity, temperature.
- *Choice of vehicle.*

Resorption: The uptake of topically applied substances with transfer to blood vessels or lymphatics. In the case of most dermatologic agents, resorption is not desirable. For example, the less systemic uptake of corticosteroids, the better. On the other hand, in transdermal delivery systems (usually patches, sometimes ointments), resorption is the goal (estrogen, clonidine, nitroglycerin, scopolamine, and analgesic patches; nitroglycerin ointment).

Metabolism: Cutaneous agents can be metabolized in the skin or resorbed and then metabolized in the liver. The skin contains all the relevant enzymes needed to metabolize foreign materials including oxygenases, hydrolases, transferases, and esterases; their activity is 1–5% of the corresponding liver enzymes. For example, benzoyl peroxide is almost 100% converted to benzoic acid in the skin.

pical Agents

topical medication consist of one or more active ingredients combined with a ve- cle. The vehicle contains a base to which have been added preservatives, emulsi- rs, fragrances, and other products. Water is present in almost every product.

Note: Ideally, a product should contain only one active ingredient. Occasionally two or three are present, but such products should be considered exceptions.

Vehicle:

- The vehicle is very important in determining the pharmacokinetics. For example, the active ingredient must be more soluble in the outer layer of the stratum corneum than in the vehicle, or diffusion will not start. Many tricks are used to insure maximum penetration, including adding agents that alter the stratum corneum (urea), or creating carrier structures (microsomes).
- The following vehicles are recognized in the European prescribing regulations:
  - Hydrophobic (lipophilic) ointments.

- Absorption ointments: Water-in-oil (W/O) or oil-in-water (O/W) mixture capable of taking up water.
- Hydrophilic ointments: Polyethylene glycol (macrogol) ointments.
- Hydrophobic creams (W/O creams).
- Hydrophilic creams (O/W creams).
  ▪ *Note:* An aqueous liniment is an O/W emulsion with a high water content and is easily washed off. This is in sharp contrast to the older lay definition of a liniment as an almost oily liquid applied to the skin.
- Ambiphilic creams: Features of both O/W and W/O creams.
- O/W lotions.
- Hydrophobic gels.
- Hydrophilic gels.
- Shake lotions.
- Hard pastes.
- Soft pastes.
- Liquid pastes.
  ▪ *Note:* In lay terms, an ointment is greasy, a cream rubs in, a gel is clear or translucent, and a paste or shake lotion contains a nondissolved powder.
- The most widely used ointment and cream bases in Germany are listed in Table 41.1. They are based on the *Neues Rezeptur Formularium* (NRF), the *Deutsche Arzneibuch* (DAB) 2004 edition and the *Deutscher Arzneimittel Codex* (DAC) 2004 edition.

Table 41.1 · Common ointment vehicles

	% Composition
Wool wax alcohol ointment DAB (Unguentum alcoholum lanae) (W/O absorption ointment with wool wax alcohol)	
Wool wax alcohol	6.0
Cetearyl alcohol	0.5
White petrolatum	93.5
Aqueous wool wax alcohol ointment DAB (Unguentum alcoholum lanae aquosum) (Hydrophobic or W/O cream)	
Wool wax alcohol ointment	50.0
Water	50.0
Hydrophobic Basiscreme DAC (NRF 11.104.) (Hydrophobic cream, W/O cream without wool wax)	
Triglycerol diisostearate	3.0
Isopropyl palmitate	2.4
Hydrophobic Basisgel DAC	24.6
Potassium sorbate	0.14
Water-free citric acid	0.07
Magnesium sulfate heptahydrate	0.5
Glycerol 85%	5.0
Water	64.29

Table 41.1 · Continued

	% Composition

Cooling ointment DAB (Unguentum leniens)
(W/O cream without emulsifiers)

Yellow wax	7.0
Cetyl palmitate	8.0
Peanut oil	60.0
Water	25.0

Basiscreme DAC
(Ambiphilic cream)

Glycerol monostearate	4.0
Cetyl alcohol	6.0
Mid-chain triglyceride	7.5
White petrolatum	22.5
Macrogol-1000 glycerol monostearate	7.0
Propylene glycol	10.0
Water	40.0

Hydrophilic ointment (Unguentum emulsificans) DAB
(O/W absorption ointment, capable of taking up water)

Emulsifying cetearyl alcohol (Type A)*	30.0
Thick paraffin	35.0
White petrolatum	35.0

Aqueous hydrophilic ointment (Unguentum emulsificans aquosum) DAB (Hydrophilic O/W cream—anionic)

Hydrophilic ointment DAB	30.0
Water	70.0

Nonionic hydrophilic cream DAB (Unguentum emulsificans nonionicum aquosum) (Hydrophilic, O/W cream—nonionic)

Polysorbate 60	5.0
Cetearyl alcohol	10.0
Glycerol 85%	10.0
White petrolatum	25.0
Water	50.0

* Mixture of cetearyl alcohol and godium cetearylsulfate

► **Preservatives and emulsifiers:**
  • *Preservatives* are essential to prolong shelf life and to reduce the rate with which products decay when used. Common preservatives include sorbic acid potassium sorbate, parabens, propylene glycol, and occasionally benzoic acid o sodium benzoate.
  • *Emulsifiers* are used creative mixtures containing two immiscible substances One substance is distributed in small globules throughout the other. The emul sifiers currently approved in Germany are shown in Table 41.2.

Table 41.2 · Common emulsifiers

Oil/water	Emulsifying cetearyl alcohol (type A)*
	Macrogol** sorbitan monostearate
	Macrogol** cetearyl ether 100
	Macrogol**-8-stearate
	Macrogol**-1000 monocetylether (Cetomacrogol 1000)
Water/oil	Wool wax and wool wax alcohols
	Triglycerol diisostearate
	Glycerol monostearate
	Sorbitan monostearate

* Mixture of cetearyl alcohol and sodium cetearylsulfate
** Macrogol is also known as polyethylene glycol

► An overview of the use of topical agents is presented in Table 41.3. It is based on the German formularies, but will still be useful to those working in other systems as a rough guideline.
◨ *Note:* As one moves down chart, the cooling, drying and anti-inflammatory action decreases, while the lubrication and water retention increases!

Table 41.3 · Use of dermatologic vehicles in different stages of diseases

Vehicle	Examples	Stage of disease	Effect
Wet dressing		Acute	Cooling, debridement
Powder		Acute	Cooling, absorption
Shake lotion		Acute	Cooling, drying, anti-inflammatory
Non-stabilized	Lotio alba aquosa DAC or skin-colored (NRF 11.22.)		
	Lotio alba spirituosa (NRF 11.3.) or skin-colored		
Stabilized	Emulsified zinc oxide shake lotion (NRF 11.49.)		
	Aqueous zinc oxide paste FH Z.3		

Table 41.3 · Continued

Vehicle	Examples	Stage of disease	Effect
Hydrophilic paste	Hydrophilic zinc oxide paste 40% with ammonium bituminosulfonate 5% (NRF 11.108.)	Acute	Cooling, drying, anti-inflammatory
	Zinc oxide shake lotion 25% (NRF 11.109.)		
	Emulsified zinc oxide shake lotion (NRF 11.49.)		
Solutions	Aqueous	Acute	Cooling, drying, anti-inflammatory
	Alcoholic		
Hydrogels		Acute	Anti-inflammatory
Non-ionic	Hydroxyethyl cellulose gel DAB		
Anionic	Sodium carmellose gel DAB		
	Aqueous carbomer gel DAB		
	2-propanol carbomer gel DAB		
O/W lotion		Subacute	Anti-inflammatory
Non-ionic	Hydrophilic emulsion base (NRF S. 25.)		
	Cetomacrogol lotion FN		
Anionic	Tegin lotion		
O/W cream			
Nonionic	Aqueous liniment SR DAC (NRF 11.93.)	Subacute	Anti-inflammatory
	Nonionic hydrophilic cream DAB		
	Nonionic hydrophilic cream SR DAC (NRF S. 26.)		
	Nonionic aqueous liniment DAC (NRF 11.92.)		
Anionic	Unguentum emulsificans aquosum DAB		
	Anionic hydrophilic cream SR DAC (NRF S. 27.)		
Ambiphilic cream	Basiscreme DAC		Anti-inflammatory
Pseudo W/O cream	Cooling ointment DAB		Anti-inflammatory
O/W absorbent ointment			
Nonionic	Unguentum Cordes		
Anionic	Unguentum emulsificans DAB		

Continued Table 41.3 ▶

Vehicle	Examples	Stage of disease	Effect
Table 41.3 · Continued			
W/O creams			
With wool wax	Unguentum alcoholum lanae aquosum DAB	Subacute	Anti-inflammator
	Eucerin cum aqua		
	Lanolin DAB		
Without wool wax	Hydrophobic Basiscreme DAC (NRF 11.104.)		
	Cremor sorbitansequioleati		
	Cremor vaselini MB 59		
W/O absorbent ointments		Chronic	Lubrication, retains moisture
With wool wax	Unguentum alcoholum lanae DAB		
Without wool wax	Unguentum sorbitansequioleati		
	Emulsifying ophthalmic ointment (NRF 15.20.)		
Lipophilic pastes			Lubrication, retains moisture
Hard	Zinc paste DAB (2 phase paste)		
	Zinc oxide-starch absorption ointment ZL (2 phase paste)		
Soft	Soft zinc oxide paste DAB (2 phase paste)		
Liquid	Oleum zinci (NRF 11.20.)		
Carbohydrate and lipo gels	White petrolatum Ph. Eur.		Lubrication, retains moisture
	Simple ophthalmic ointment DAC		
	Hydrophobic basis gel DAC (Oleo gel)		
	Lard DAB (Lipo gel)		
Plaster			Activation
Occlusion			

From Wolf G, Süverkrüp R *Rezepturen: Probleme erkennen, lösen, vermeiden*. Deutscher Apotheker Verlag 2002, pp. 117–172.

Urea

Urea is a very useful addition. It is hygroscopic (water-binding) and keratolytic, as well as antiproliferative. Furthermore, it almost never causes allergic contact dermatitis. It is irritating and burns upon application, especially with higher concentrations, damaged skin, or in children.

Indications: Urea can be used as a primary active ingredient for dry skin or hyperkeratotic lesions. It is useful for hyperkeratotic atopic dermatitis and psoriasis. In addition, it increases the penetration of corticosteroids and dithranol. In higher concentrations (40%), it can be used to remove dystrophic or onychomycotic nails (p. 697). Because it is nonsensitizing, it is ideal for long-term therapy.

Caution: Use cautiously in acute dermatitis; once healing has started, increase gradually 3% → 5% → 10%. In children, be sure they understand it will burn for a few minutes; if they are too young to understand, use 1–3%.

Salicylic Acid

Excellent keratolytic agent; used at 2–10% concentration to remove scales in psoriasis and at higher (10–20%) concentrations for palmoplantar keratodermas and other markedly hyperkeratotic lesions. Like urea, it is irritating in acute stages.

Often combined with dithranol, not only to increase penetration but also to stabilize the product.

Caution: Use with great care in children; absorption can rapidly lead to salicylism.

41.2 Topical Antiviral Therapy

Wart Therapy

Although there are a number of therapeutic approaches, none achieves more than a 70% cure rate. Flexibility is the key.

Keratolytics: Salicylic or lactic acid (in concentrations from 5% to 20%) can be used in plasters, flexible collodion, or solutions:
- The key to use is regular debridement (sanding, trimming, visits to office) coupled with daily application, ideally with some form of occlusion.
- Many different mixtures with a variety of other ingredients including trichloracetic acid, oxalic acid, and even 5-fluorouracil are available.

Caution: Many stronger formulations are designed to be applied 1–2 × weekly by physician or nurse. Be sure you know the requirements for solutions you use.

Podophyllotoxin: Antimitotic effect on microtubules; effective for mucosal warts but not cutaneous lesions. The specific commercial product containing purified podophyllotoxin is preferable to the older mixtures of podophyllin resin, which varied highly in contents and efficacy.

Topical immunotherapy: Imiquimod is effective on genital warts but not cutaneous warts because the vehicle does not provide sufficient penetration (see below).

Cryotherapy:
- Liquid nitrogen is sprayed on the wart or applied with a special sound. If a cotton applicator is used, it must be large (such as a vaginal swab); an ordinary cotton bud does not transfer enough cold.
- The cold kills the adjacent tissue and induces a blister; it does not kill the virus particles. Usual regimen is freeze for 10 seconds, allow to thaw, and repeat twice.

▪ *Note:* Initially observe patients frequently after freezing until you develop a fe for how hard you must freeze to induce a blister.
- Freezing can be repeated 1–2 × weekly; once every 2 weeks is not adequate, too much healing occurs in the interval.
- *Side-effects* include pain on application, painful blisters and erosions, slow hea ing. Difficult to use around the nails, or in children with multiple lesions.

► **Surgical measures:**
- Patients often assume that when a wart is surgically removed, the cure rate much higher than with other methods. This is not the case, leading to disa pointed patients and recurrent warts in surgical scars.
- Many approaches, all under local anesthesia, include curettage and cauter electrosurgery alone, or scalpel excision.

► **Laser therapy:**
- Ablation with CO_2 laser.
- Destruction of feeder vessels with tunable dye laser.

► **Suggestion:** Placebo treatment is rarely indicated in dermatology, but in th special case, it can be endorsed. Warts have a relatively high spontaneous cure ra in children, so the approach has a scientific background. One can employ pure sug gestive therapy, painting with fluorescent material and irradiating with Wood light, or sham radiotherapy. Another possibility is to use a laser at doses so low th there is no tissue effect.

► **Other measures:**
- Intralesional bleomycin (0.1 mg every 1–4 weeks); best avoided on acral area
- Interferon (IFN)-α-2a or interferon-α-2b: 3 million IU weekly, along with de structive measures.

Imiquimod

► **Mechanism of action:** Stimulation of Toll-like receptor 7 on plasmacytoid den dritic cells and induction of cytokines essential to innate immune response, e pecially IFN-α, interleukin (IL)-6, IL-8, and tumor necrosis factor (TNF).
► Major indication is condylomata acuminata and other mucosal warts; also prom ising for actinic keratoses and superficial basal cell carcinomas.
► Condylomata are treated 3 × weekly; medication applied and washed off afte 6–10 hours. Erythema of treated areas indicates inflammatory response is bein elicited. Treatment should last until lesions have healed, with maximum use fo 16 weeks.
► For nonmucosal surfaces, prior handling with keratolytics, occlusion, or mo frequent application may be needed.
► Suggested regimens for actinic keratoses and superficial basal cell carcinomas ar 3 × weekly for 6 weeks, and then if inflammatory response is good, 2 × weekly fo the next 6 weeks.
► Side effects include local irritation, varying depending on tissue and method of ap plication.
► Proprietary products containing imiquimod are relatively expensive.

Acyclovir

► **Mechanism of action:** Inhibition of viral DNA polymerase by insertion of foreig base analogue.
► Topical acyclovir is widely available and frequently employed, but not very effec tive. It can be tried 5 × daily for 5 days, *starting immediately with first sign of tin gling or pain,* in mild cases of recurrent herpes simplex virus infection.

- Side effects include burning, erythema, and rarely allergic contact dermatitis.
- *Note:* Systemic therapy is cheaper, more effective, and without serious side effects.

41.3 Topical Antibiotics

Overview
....

Topical antibiotics are controversial. At first glance, they appear a wise choice as one achieves effective control of bacteria without systemic risks. There are two excellent reasons *not* to use them:

- Induction of allergic reaction, which then makes systemic use of entire classes of antibiotics impossible.
- Increasing use is one possible factor in development of community-based resistant strains of bacteria.

In addition, there are many other antibacterial agents that can be employed (see next section).

Available Agents
....

- **Gentamicin:**
  - Optimum effect at pH 7.8; thus, does not combine with other products, especially those with acidic base.
  - Available as 0.1% creams and ointments.
  - Effective against staphylococci, *Proteus*, and *Klebsiella*.
  - *Side effects* include sensitization, ototoxicity, and even nephrotoxicity.
  - If chosen, only for short-term use on small wounds or superficial pyodermas.
- **Oxytetracycline:**
  - Available in 1–3% concentration as ointment, cream, solution, or ophthalmic ointment.
  - Effective against staphylococci, *Propionibacterium acnes.* When combined with polymyxin B, also against Gram-negative species such as *Pseudomonas aeruginosa*, *Proteus*, and *Klebsiella*.
  - Solutions used in acne vulgaris; problems with discoloration of skin.
  - Should not be used on wide areas during pregnancy nor around the nipple in nursing women because of effects on fetal teeth.
  - Terramycin ointment is a mixture of oxytetracycline and polymyxin B.
- **Erythromycin:**
  - Available as 0.5–4% cream, ointment or gel; also can be compounded using erythromycin base.
  - Effective against staphylococci, streptococci, and *Propionibacterium acnes*.
  - Widely used in acne.
  - Use with care during pregnancy or nursing.
  - Zineryt contains both erythromycin and zinc acetate, designed for acne.
- **Fusidic acid:**
  - Available in many forms including cream, ointment, gel, powder, impregnated gauze.
  - Effective against staphylococci, enterococci.
  - Widely used in Europe for wound care, pyoderma, secondarily infected dermatitis, and ulcers.
  - Very low rate of sensitization; rarely employed systemically.
  - *Note:* Probably the antibiotic best suited for topical use, with no apparent disadvantages for short-term use.

► **Metronidazole:**
  • Azole with unique nitro group; long used orally for trichomonas and rosace.
    also effective against Gram-negative bacteria (such as in Gram-negative to
    web infections and Gram-negative folliculitis).
  • Available as 0.5–1.0% creams and gels, or can be mixed (p. 695) for rosacea.
► **Chloramphenicol:**
  • Widely used for acne in Europe as alcoholic solution.
  • Controversial because of development of allergic contact dermatitis and, in ra
    but well documented cases, of bone marrow failure and aplastic anemia.
  ▣ *Note:* No longer recommended.

41.4 Dyes and Antiseptics

Overview

Dye solutions have long been a mainstay of dermatologic therapy in Europe, but the
never received widespread acceptance in the USA. They have now been remove
from some European formularies because of a (largely theoretical) risk of carcino
genesis.
► **Mechanism of action:** Antimycotic, antibacterial, drying, and in some instance
  anti-inflammatory.
► **Advantages:** Inexpensive, low incidence of allergic contact dermatitis, almost n
  resistance.
► **Disadvantages:** Stain everything, may inhibit keratinocyte and fibroblast pro
  liferation in ulcers, theoretical risk of carcinogenesis. None has excellent evidenc
  for effectiveness, although many have been used for almost a century.

Available Agents

► **Arning tincture:**
  • Active ingredients are anthrarobin and ammonium bituminosulfonate.
  ⚠ *Caution:* Anthrarobin is often not available in pharmaceutical quality.
  • Weakly antimicrobial effect; very drying and somewhat anti-inflammatory.
  • Burns on use but does not stain.
► **Methylrosaniline chloride:**
  • Known in USA as methyl violet; main component of gentian violet, which it ha
    replaced in Europe.
  • Used as 0.5–1.0% solution for candidiasis and intertrigo.
► **Gentian violet:**
  • No longer allowed in Europe; replaced by methylrosaniline chloride.
  • Available in USA; usually employed as 0.5–1.0% aqueous solution for candidia
    sis and intertrigo.
  • In higher concentrations, under occlusion (such as under foreskin) or in infant
    can be irritating and cause necrosis.
► **Eosin:**
  • Available as both alcoholic and aqueous solutions for superficial infections.
► **Castellani paint:**
  • Long favorite for dermatophytosis in intertriginous sites, especially betwee
    toes; antimycotic, antibacterial, and drying.

- Also known as *carbolfuchsin topical solution* (USP). Contains basic fuchsin, phenol, resorcinol, acetone, alcohol, and water, as well as chlorocresol in some formularies. Resorcinol and chlorocresol no longer recommended in Europe.
- Replaced by 0.5% fuchsin solution in ethanol (NRF 11.26).

Brilliant green:
- Difficult to manufacture without extensive heavy metal contamination.
- No longer employed in Europe.

Other Antimicrobial Agents

Clioquinol (iodochlorhydroxyquin):
- Best known in USA under its trade name of Vioform.
- Available as 0.5–3.0% cream, ointment, or pastes. Also combined with low-potency corticosteroids (Vioform–HC).
- Popular for secondarily infected atopic dermatitis.
- Can also be compounded (p. 692).
- Inactivated by zinc and other cations; avoid using simultaneously in aqueous vehicle systems.

Chinolinol (8-hydroxy chinolin):
- Close relative of clioquinol.
- Bacteriostatic and fungicidal.
- Widely used as 0.1% solution (NRF 11.127.) for wet dressings in pyoderma. If mixed as cream, care needed as it is inactivated by anionic hydrophilic creams or O/W creams.

Octenisept:
- Combination of octenidine HCl 0.1 g and phenoxyethanol 2.0 g in 100 mL aqueous solution.
- Useful for skin and mucous membrane disinfection.
- Effective against broad range of bacteria, fungi, and viruses.

Povidone-iodine:
- Combination of iodine and the complex polymer povidone (polyvinylpyrrolidone); slowly releases iodine.
- Antibacterial.
- Available in every imaginable form, usually at 10% concentration, including soaps, impregnated sponges for preoperative use, gels, creams, suppositories, and impregnated gauzes.
- Best known in USA as Betadine.
- Used for wound and ulcer care, pyoderma.
- Best avoided in all conditions where iodine is contraindicated (hyperthyroidism, dermatitis herpetiformis); avoid in pregnancy.

Silver sulfadiazine:
- Silver derivative of sulfadiazine, a sulfonamide.
- Broad spectrum of antibacterial action; also effective against yeasts.
- Widely used for burn patients, known colloquially as "burn butter".
- Probably best reserved for acute use, as chronic use may increase risk of sensitization.
- ◪ *Note:* Silver sulfadiazine is a sulfonamide, capable of causing reactions in individuals sensitized to topical or systemic sulfonamides.
- Proprietary products have an excellent moisturizing base, which enhances their efficacy.

Potassium permanganate:
- Dark-violet crystals; dissolves in water have weak antiseptic effect but very strong staining effect—can permanently stain towels and even bathtubs.

- Warn patient that skin and nails will have brown discoloration.
- Irritating if patient exposed to higher concentrations or especially nondissolve crystals.
- Use 1.0% stock solution (NRF 11.82) and dilute to provide concentrations in th range of 1:1000–1:5000.

► **Triclosan:**
- Organochloride compound with wide spectrum of action against Gram-neg tive and Gram-positive bacteria; also somewhat effective against yeasts an fungi. Can be compounded: hydrophobic triclosan cream 2% (NRF 11.122).
- Used as preservative; also for surgical soaps, in deodorants, and as surface di infectant in 0.1–0.2% concentration.

  ⚠ *Caution:* If compounded, the triclosan must be pharmaceutical grade an certified free of dioxins, which can be contaminants in the manufacturin process.

41.5 Topical Antifungal Agents

There is a wide variety of topical antifungal agents, summarized in Table 41.**4**. Th biggest family is the imidazoles, with over 20 representatives. Differences betwee members of the same class are minimal, despite manufacturers' claims to the cor trary. Daily application suffices in most instances. There is no truly effective topic agent for onychomycosis, although nail varnishes are now available.

Table 41.4 · Topical antifungal agents

Agent	Spectrum		
	Dermatophytes	Yeasts	Molds
Polyenes			
Amphotericin B		+	
Nystatin		+	
Imidazoles			
Many	+	+	+
Allylamines			
Naftifine	+		
Terbinafine	+		
Hydroxypyridones			
Ciclopirox	+	+	+
Morpholines			
Amorolfin	+		

41.6 Topical Antiparasitic Agents

Permethrin

▶ **Mechanism of action:** Synthetic pyrethroid; mimics arthropod growth hormone and also interferes with sodium transport.

▶ **Indications:** Scabies, pediculosis; around the world, varying degrees of resistance; check with local public health authorities for recommended approach if unsure. Usual first-line agent.

▶ **Contraindications:** Can be used in pregnancy; nursing should be stopped for 3 days application; avoid in infants < 2 months.

▶ **Use:**
  • *Pediculosis capitis:* Use 1% lotion; apply to washed scalp for 30–45 minutes; rinse. Repeat in 1 week if live lice are found.
  • *Scabies:* Use 5% cream or lotion (2.5% for infants < 12 months); apply to entire body; leave on 12 hours; wash off. One application usually suffices.

▶ **Side effects:** Can be irritating; rare difficulty breathing or asthma.

Lindane

▶ **Synonym:** Gamma benzene hexachloride.

▶ **Mechanism of action:** Penetrates chitin exoskeleton; potent neurotoxin.

▶ **Indications:** Scabies, pediculosis; around the world, varying degrees of resistance; check with local public health authorities for recommended approach if unsure.

▶ **Contraindications:** Best avoided in pregnancy, nursing and infants < 2 years of age.

▶ **Use in scabies:**
  • Available as lotions and shampoos. Tend to be irritating and drying, especially if overused. Absorption (infants, damaged skin) can lead to neurotoxicity.
  • *Adults:* Apply lindane lotion each evening for three consecutive evenings (or for two consecutive evenings and then again in 1 week); wash off in morning. Wash bedding, clothes; treat all close contacts (sexual partners, children).
  • *Children 3–10 years:* Apply lotion to entire body for two consecutive days for 2 hours; wash off.
  • *Children < 3 years:*
    – Consider alternative agent.
    – Apply lotion to half of body for 2 hours; wash off; repeat on each side twice (total of 4 days of treatment).

▶ **Use in pediculosis:**
  • Use shampoo for 5 minutes or lotion for 12 hours. Wash off. Repeat in 1 week if viable organisms seen. Problems with resistance.

Malathion

▶ **Mechanism of action:** Organophosphorus insecticide; inhibits cholinesterase, blocking nerve transmission.

▶ **Indications:** Pediculosis; only agent without significant resistance; *not effective in scabies.*

▶ **Contraindications:** Occasional contact dermatitis; quite toxic if ingested.

▶ **Available** as 0.5% lotion.

▶ **Use:** Apply for 8–12 hours; rinse; repeat in 1 week if live lice are still present.

Benzyl benzoate

▶ **Mechanism of action:** One of the active substances in balsam of Peru; damages chitin exoskeleton.
▶ **Indications:** Second line treatment for scabies, pediculosis. Approved for careful use in pregnancy.
▶ **Available** as 25% solution or lotion in Europe; in USA has to be compounded as 25% lotion.
▶ **Use:** Apply nightly for three nights in scabies; apply $1-2 \times$ for pediculosis.

Other Agents

▶ **Crotamiton:** Relatively ineffective agent against scabies and lice. Can be used during pregnancy or nursing. Apply daily for 3–5 days; leave on for 24 hours; wash and re-apply. Has some intrinsic antipruritic effect.
▶ **6–10% precipitated sulfur in petrolatum:** Old, messy, relatively ineffective treatment for scabies; advantage is that it is 100% safe in pregnancy and infancy; apply b.i.d. for 7–14 days.
▶ Many **natural pyrethrins** are available for the treatment of pediculosis. They tend to be irritating..

41.7 Topical Corticosteroids

Pharmacology

Corticosteroids are 21-C steroids synthesized by the adrenal cortex gland in response to ACTH, or less often angiotensin II. They are divided into *glucocorticoids*, which influence carbohydrate, fat and protein metabolism, and *mineralocorticoids*, which regulate electrolyte and water balance. Glucocorticoids are used almost exclusively in dermatology.

▶ The *resorption* of topical corticosteroids is very dependent on the site of application. Resorption is 1% on the forearm, 4% on the scalp, 7% on the forehead, and 36% on the scrotum. Resorption is also greater in infants and children. Both urea and DMSO can enhance resorption up to 4-fold. The influence of salicylic acid is controversial. Occlusion clearly enhances resorption.
▶ If corticosteroids are applied over a long period of time, *tachyphylaxis* develops; in this instance, the effectiveness of the corticosteroid drops considerably. Thus application once or at most twice daily is recommended.
▶ Corticosteroids accelerate *gluconeogenesis* (synthesis of glucose from amino acids) and thus have proteolytic and anti-insulin effects. Their main effects have a delayed onset, as they primarily depend on altered protein synthesis, but direct membrane effects also occur.
▶ They are used in dermatology for their *anti-inflammatory*, *immunosuppressive* and *antiproliferative* actions.
☐ *Note:* Therapy with topical corticosteroids is always symptomatic, never curative

Indications and Contraindications

▶ **Indications:**
  • *Topical:* Allergic and irritant contact dermatitis, atopic dermatitis, other forms of dermatitis, psoriasis, cutaneous lupus erythematosus, lichen planus, sarcoidosis.

- *Intralesional:* Granuloma annulare, alopecia areata, hypertrophic scars and keloids, less often psoriasis and discoid or hypertrophic lupus erythematosus.
- *Systemic:* Wide range of uses including bullous autoimmune diseases, collagen-vascular disorders, severe forms of dermatitis and others.

▶ **Contraindications:** Bacterial, viral, or fungal infections, wounds, ulcers, atrophy. Many relative contraindications depending on strength of corticosteroid, site of application, and age of patient; for example, high-potency corticosteroids are never applied to the scrotum of boys.

▶ **Side effects:**
- Sufficient high-potency topical corticosteroids can be absorbed to cause Cushing syndrome. This is especially true in infants. Conversely, if high-potency agents are abruptly stopped, there may be sufficient suppression of the pituitary–adrenal axis to cause an Addisonian crisis.
- Local effects include atrophy, striae, telangiectases, purpura (vessel fragility), hypertrichosis, infections, and perioral dermatitis.

Use
....

In Europe corticosteroids are divided into four classes, on the basis of increasing potency from I (least potent) to IV (most potent). The standard American classification is into seven groups ranging from 1 (most potent) to 7 (least potent). Representative members of the European group are shown in Table 41.**5**. Most are available from more than one pharmaceutical firm, and many have become generic. Many class I agents are available over the counter.

▶ **Available agents:**
- It is impossible to remember all the available agents. Pick one to two agents in each group and use them.
- Choose an agent available in multiple forms, such as ointment, emollient cream, and gel. In Europe, many manufacturers make the nonmedicated vehicle available for maintenance therapy. Such products have a high degree of patient acceptance.
- Some agents can be compounded, as indicated in Table 41.**5**. Assuming a reliable pharmacy is available, considerable cost savings can be achieved by compounding 500 mg or 1 kg jars. Since preservatives are less effective in compounded products, patients should be instructed to work out of a smaller container and remove material from the large jar only with a sterile instrument.
- Choice of vehicle is incredibly important. In most instances, potency ranges are as follows: ointment > gel > cream > lotion.
- Do not follow the percentages. Notice that the highest percentage concentration (2 %) is used in the weakest agent, hydrocortisone. Patients invariably read the label and may be annoyed when they receive a lower concentration. Always explain this point.
- The fourth-generation or soft corticosteroids are group II agents, indicated in italics in Table 41.**5**, which are prodrugs. The 21-ester bond is split in the skin, so the drugs are inactivated before entering the circulation. They have extremely favorable risk:benefit ratios and are widely used in pediatric dermatology.
- Maximum effect can be achieved by intralesional injection (usually triamcinolone acetonide (1–5 mg/mL). Although problems with particle size have been resolved, injection around the eye is usually avoided because of fear of retinal artery embolization.
- Another effective approach is to use a corticosteroid-impregnated tape, containing flurandrenolide 4 μg/cm^2.

Topical Therapy

Table 41.5 · Classes of topical corticosteroids

Class	Agent	Concentration (%)
I (weak)	Dexamethasone	0.1
	Fluocortinbutylester	0.75
	Hydrocortisone[a]	0.5–2.0
	Hydrocortisone acetate[a]	1.0
	Prednisolone[a]	0.4
II (medium)	Betamethasone valerate	0.05
	Clobetasone butyrate	0.5
	Flumethasone pivalate	0.2
	Fluocinolone acetonide	0.25
	Fluprednidene acetate	0.1–0.5
	Hydrocortisone aceponate[b]	0.1
	Hydrocortisone buteprate[b]	0.1
	Hydrocortisone butyrate[b]	0.1
	Methylprednisolone aceponate[b]	0.1
	Prednicarbate[b]	0.25
	Triamcinolone acetonide[a]	0.25–0.5
III (strong)	Betamethasone diproprionate	0.05
	Betamethasone valerate	0.5
	Amcinonide	0.1
	Desoximetasone	0.25
	Diflucortolone valerate	0.1
	Fluocinolone acetonide	0.2
	Fluocinonide	0.5
	Halcinonide	0.1
IV (very strong)	Clobetasol propionate[a]	0.05
	Diflucortolone valerate	0.3

a Can be compounded.
b Fourth-generation corticosteroids.

- Many compound products are available, containing corticosteroids combine with antibiotics or antifungal agents. They may be helpful in very acutely in flamed dermatitis or tinea, but in general it is wiser to use two separate agent at different times, separated by at least 2 hours, to achieve maximum benefit from both the corticosteroid and the antimicrobial agent.
► **Helpful hints:**
  - Choose strength of corticosteroid based on pathogenesis of disease; hyper proliferative disorders require class III or IV agents.
  - Watch for tachyphylaxis; application more than b.i.d. is almost never correct.

- Use with care on face and in intertriginous areas; exceed class II only with definite indications (localized bullous pemphigoid, nonresponsive chronic cutaneous lupus erythematosus).
- Never go above class II in children.
- Avoid using corticosteroids in infectious processes (pyoderma, tinea) unless the underlying disease is being simultaneously treated.
- Always think about steroid-sparing approaches (phototherapy, tar, retinoids, vitamin D analogues, calcineurin inhibitors, dithranol, urea).

41.8 Calcineurin Inhibitors

Overview

Definition: Immunomodulatory substances (*tacrolimus* and *pimecrolimus*) that have been used for years in transplantation medicine but are also available as topical agents for atopic dermatitis and other inflammatory dermatoses.

Mechanism of action:
- Preferential immunosuppressive action on T cells, Langerhans cells, and mast cells; potent and prolonged antipruritic effect.
- Both substances bind to a cytosol receptor (macrophilin-12) forming complexes that inhibit calcineurin. Calcineurin dephosphorylates NFAT (**n**uclear **f**actor of **a**ctivated **T** cells), a cytosol transcription factor. If the dephosphorylation is blocked, NFAT cannot reach the nucleus and the transcription of inflammatory cytokines is blocked.
- Tacrolimus and pimecrolimus both also cause mast cell degranulation, perhaps via release of neuropeptides from cutaneous nerves. Consequently there is burning on application at onset of therapy but with rapid accommodation; this is more of a problem for tacrolimus than for pimecrolimus.
- They also interact directly with cutaneous nerve fibers to have additional antipruritic effects.

Side effects:
- Initial burning on application; resolves rapidly.
- In contrast to corticosteroids, no cutaneous atrophy.
- Theoretical risk of reduced immunosurveillance and increased cutaneous tumors; long-term studies in progress to test hypothesis.
- A warning in 2005 from the FDA regarding increased risk of UV-induced cutaneous neoplasms and lymphomas is not supported by data and has been denounced in Europe.

▣ *Note:* Both agents are very expensive, which has been the main limiting factor in their acceptance and use.

Tacrolimus

Synonym: FK506.

Isolated from the bacterium *Streptomyces tsukubaensis*.

Indications:
- Moderate to severe atopic dermatitis; officially approved for adults and children > 2 years of age but can be used in infants.
- Also employed in other dermatoses such as lichen planus, lichen sclerosus, graft-versus-host disease, scrotal dermatitis, chronic hand dermatitis, renal pruritus, different forms of prurigo, inverse psoriasis, rosacea.

► **Contraindications:**
  • Sensitivity to tacrolimus.
  • Do not use in florid viral infections; can make disorders such as eczema herpe-
    catum persist.
  • Avoid in Netherton syndrome (p. 195); abnormal barrier leads to excess absor-
    tion and toxicity.
  • Do not use in pregnancy or during nursing.
  • Do not combine with UV light because of theoretical increased tumor risk.
► **Cross-reactions:** None known. Theoretical problem with immunizations, whi
  should be delayed for 14–28 days after discontinuation of tacrolimus.
► **Use:** Apply b.i.d. to involved areas as long as inflamed or pruritic. Long-term inte
  mittent use up to 12 months is unproblematic. If no response after 6 weeks, re-e
  amine indications and options.
► **Side effects:** Initially burning on application in > 10%; less often erythema, prur
  tus, folliculitis. Rarely bacterial and viral infections. Disulfiram effect: adu
  patients who use tacrolimus on face and drink alcohol may experience pain
  flushing and erythema.

Pimecrolimus
► Semi-synthetic ascomycin derivative.
► **Indications:**
  • Mild to moderate atopic dermatitis. Officially approved for children > 2 years
    age but can be used safely in infancy.
  • Other uses as under tacrolimus.
► **Contraindications:**
  • Sensitivity to pimecrolimus.
  • Other contraindications as for tacrolimus.
► **Cross-reactions:** Same as tacrolimus.
► **Use:** Apply b.i.d. to involved areas as long as inflamed or pruritic. Long-term inte
  mittent use up to 12 months is unproblematic. If no response after 6 weeks, re-e
  amine indications and options.
► **Side effects:** Initially burning on application but less common than wi
  tacrolimus, thus making pimecrolimus a better choice in infants and sma
  children who cannot be warned about burning. Other problems as wi
  tacrolimus.

41.9 Vitamin D Analogues

Overview
....

Cholecalciferol (vitamin D_3) is synthesized from 7-dehydrocholesterol in the sk
under the influence of UV light and then converted in the liver to 25-hydrox
cholecalciferol. The most potent form is the renal product 1,25-dihydroxycholeca
ciferol (calcitriol). In some settings, this potent molecule is also synthesized in th
skin.
► **Mechanism of action:**
  • Mobilizes calcium from bone and increases reabsorption of calcium and pho
    phorus in kidney.
  • In the skin, blocks proliferation and enhances differentiation. Also increases e
    pression of corticosteroid receptors, and has immunomodulatory role.

Available agents: All three have similar spectrum of action; the analogues are used more than calcitriol itself:

- *Calcitriol:* Chemical structure 1,25-dihydroxycholecalciferol (1,25-dihydroxy vitamin D_3).
- *Calcipotriol:* Analog of vitamin D_3.
- *Tacalcitol:* Analog of vitamin D_3.

Indications:

- Mild to moderate psoriasis, including facial psoriasis.
- HIV/AIDS-associated psoriasis.
- Under investigation for some disorders of keratinization.

Contraindications:

- Pustular psoriasis.
- Severe renal or hepatic disease; abnormal calcium metabolism.
- Pregnancy or nursing.
- Not officially approved for children.

Use:

- *Calcipotriol:*
  - Apply to maximum of 30% of body surface.
  - Use $< 15\,g$ daily.
- *Tacalcitol:*
  - Apply to maximum of 10% of body surface.
  - Use $< 5\,g$ daily.
- *Both:*
  - Apply daily or b.i.d.; as long as totals observed, can be used long-term.
  - Can be combined with UVB, PUVA, or dithranol.
  - Less than 1% of single dose is absorbed.
  - Monitor serum calcium levels prior to and during treatment; likelihood of abnormalities minimal with analogues.

Side effects: Irritating on application; limits use in flexures, intertriginous areas.

1.10 Retinoids

etinoin

Synonym: Vitamin A acid, all-trans retinoic acid.

Mechanism of action: Binds to nuclear vitamin A receptors and modifies gene expression. Direct effects including altering keratinization, especially in follicle, reducing sebum production, and antiproliferative action.

Indications: Acne vulgaris—since the primary lesion in all types of acne is a comedo, and tretinoin is the most effective agent against comedones, it is useful for almost all acne patients. Also effective for prophylaxis and treatment of sun-damaged skin. Less dramatic effects in disorders of keratinization including some forms of ichthyosis, Darier disease.

Contraindications: Although absorption is minimal, best avoided during pregnancy to avoid potential medico-legal problems.

⚠ *Caution:* All retinoids are potent teratogens and should be avoided in pregnancy.

Many different forms available.

▶ *Note:* The vehicle plays a very important role in determining the strength and thus imitating effect of tretinoin. For example, 0.025% gel tends to be stronger than 0.5% cream.

- Special formulations include:
  - Oily base for photo-aged skin.
  - Delayed-release system to reduce irritation.
► **Use:**
- Apply sparingly and avoid periorbital region; use only in evening (because photosensitizing effect).
- Explain to patient that tretinoin is irritating, and that they will look worse aft 1–2 weeks as comedones are highlighted.
  - ◨ *Note:* The therapeutic goal is best achieved when mild irritation of the skin induced.
- Start with low concentration and apply every other night. As tolerance creases, apply nightly and then increase concentration if minimal erythema not obtained.
- If treated sun-damaged skin, use very low concentration, do not attempt to i crease. Many patients do well on twice weekly application.
- Either benzoyl peroxide or a topical antibiotic (usually erythromycin) can used in the morning.
- Insist patients use sunscreen regularly.
► **Side effects:** Initial irritation, drying, photosensitivity. If too irritating, post flammatory hypo- and hyperpigmentation.

Other Topical Retinoids

► **Adapalene:**
- Less irritating than tretinoin; used in same way.
► **Isotretinoin:**
- 13-cis retinoic acid.
- Less irritating than tretinoin; used in same way.
► **Tazarotene:**
- Retinoid prodrug with affinity for multiple retinoid receptors.
- Primarily indicated for mild to moderate psoriasis; often chosen for palmopla tar psoriasis and then by analogy for palmoplantar keratoderma and chro hyperkeratotic hand dermatitis.
- Also effective in treating photodamage.

41.11 Other Topical Agents

Coal Tars

► **Overview:** Coal tar has a long history of use in dermatology. Today it has unfo tunately fallen into disrepute because of theoretical concerns about carcinoge sis, which are not supported by 100 years of clinical experience.
► **Mechanism of action:** Tars are antipruritic, anti-inflammatory, antiproliferati and photosensitizing.
► **Available agents:** There is no uniform single "coal tar." Each batch is obtained the destructive distillation of bituminous coals, so there are striking variations composition, which includes oils of varying weights as well as residues (pitch). compounding, two products are available:
- Pix lithanthracis (DAB6).
- Liquor carbonis detergens (LCD), an alcoholic extract of coal tar.

Many finished products are also available, including tar gels, creams, ointments, shampoos, and bath additives. The compounded products have two advantages: they are less expensive, and it is easy to gradually increase the concentration of tar. The list of possible compounding instructions is endless; use the local standard or consult with an experienced pharmacist.

Indications: Psoriasis (usually in combination with UV light—Goeckerman regimen—or dithranol), seborrheic dermatitis, any chronic dermatitis.

Contraindications: Acute dermatitis, exudative or pustular psoriasis.

Use: Apply $1-2 \times$ daily; when combined with phototherapy, be alert to phototoxicity. Remissions induced by tar therapy tend to be longer-lasting than those with corticosteroids. Thus, in general, start with corticosteroids and then simultaneously taper corticosteroids and introduce tars in increasing concentrations.

▶ *Note:* Tars are very messy and difficult for patients to use at home. Thus, with the shift away from inpatient care of psoriasis, a very effective agent has fallen into relative neglect.

ther Tars

Shale tar: Two major products:

- Ammonium bituminosulfonate is sulfur-rich.
- Ammonium sulfobitol is sulfur-poor.

Less irritating than coal tar; used in 2–5% concentration for chronic dermatoses. Best known form is ichthyol.

Wood tars: Many different wood tars are available. They are not photosensitizing, but more allergenic. Examples include:

- Oil of cade (juniper tar, pix juniperi).
- Pine tar (pix liquida).
- Beech (pix fagi).
- Birch (pix betulina).

All have modest anti-inflammatory activity and can be used in mild chronic dermatitis. Many have become more popular in recent years as interest natural medicine has increased in Europe; main effect has been increase in allergic contact dermatitis.

thranol

Synonyms: Anthralin, cignolin.

Mechanism of action: Dithranol is antiproliferative, but the exact mechanisms are unknown. Radical form is responsible both for effect and discoloration. Maximum concentration in skin achieved 60–300 minutes after application. Metabolized in the skin and excreted in inactive form by kidneys.

Indications: Psoriasis; irritant in alopecia areata.

Contraindications: Exudative or pustular psoriasis; use sparingly in intertriginous areas.

Available agents: Standard compounding recipes available for dithranol in washable or nonwashable ointments, usually combined with salicylic acid; most useful because concentration can be best manipulated (p. 693). Commercial ointments and creams available in a wide range of concentrations. Once again, the standard product is very messy and difficult to use at home.

Use:

- *Long-term therapy:* Start with 0.1–0.25% dithranol ointment, increasing through the concentrations 0.5–1.0–2.0–3.0–5.0%, each time waiting until the irritant reaction (dithranol dermatitis) has resolved. The dithranol is applied once daily.

- *Ingram regimen:* Combination of dithranol, coal tar, and UV light.
- *Minute therapy:* Higher concentrations of dithranol (1–5%) applied for short pe
  riods of time (10–60 minutes); then washed off. Applied once daily. Can be use
  at home; the commercial cream form is especially useful. More often employe
  for alopecia areata or very localized psoriasis.
► **Side effects:**
- *Dithranol dermatitis:* Almost invariable; not controlled by corticosteroids o
  NSAIDs; must be used as "intrinsic monitor".
- *Dithranol pigmentation:* The skin, bedding, and clothes all acquire a purple
  brown color. Commercial prewash stain removers are usually effective.
- *Dithranol pseudoleukoderma:* When surrounding skin turns brown and psori
  atic lesions resolve, they appear hypopigmented.
- Allergic contact dermatitis rare.

Benzoyl Peroxide

► **Mechanism of action:** Releases H_2O_2; has marked antibacterial effect, lesser ef
  fects on comedones and sebum production.
► **Indications:** Acne, especially inflammatory forms.
► **Contraindications:** Should not be combined with phototherapy.
► **Available agents:** Hundreds of commercial products available, ranging from 2.5
  to 10% concentration in gel (alcohol or water-based), cream, emulsion, and wash
  forms.
► **Use:** Apply 1–2 × daily; easily combined with topical retinoids; topical or systemic
  antibiotics. On face 2.5–5.0% is sufficient; on back, can try 10% or wash. Pay atten
  tion to vehicle; patients with acne and dry skin do better with water-based prod
  ucts.
► **Side effects:** Often irritating, rarely (<2%) causes allergic contact dermatiti
  bleaches hairs and may cause hypopigmentation in dark-skinned patients.

41.12 Sunscreens

Overview

► **Endogenous UV protection:** Melanin, hairs, reactive thickening of stratum cor
  neum (light-induced callus), antioxidants, DNA repair mechanisms.
► **Broad spectrum filters:**
- Many new organic filter or blocking molecules have been recently approved
  and will reach the market soon.
- Two agents—*drometrizole trisiloxane* and *bis-ethylhexyloxyphenol methoxy
  phenyl triazine*—are widely effective against UVA and UVB; others have
  markedly improved UVA coverage.
► **UVB filters:**
- Para-aminobenzoic acid (PABA): First widely used agent, but today not often
  found because of allergic contact dermatitis and burning around eyes.
- PABA esters (pentyl-*p*-dimethyl aminobenzoate [Padimate] or *p*-dimethyl
  aminobenzoate.
- ⚠ *Caution:* Patients sensitive to para-compounds (sulfonamides, parabens) can
  have marked photoallergic reactions.
- Cinnamates.
- Salicylates.
- Phenylbenzimidazole sulfonic acid.

UVA filters:
- Benzophenones.
- Avobenzone, which is widely used and undergoes photodegradation to form potent allergens.

Blockers:
- Titanium dioxide.
- Zinc oxide.
- Micronized or silicone-coated particles are equally effective; popular because they do not appear as white pastes on the skin.

Other protection: Special UV-protective clothing is available and is a very good choice for children or those requiring maximum protection.

un Protection Factor

Describes the degree of protection offered by a sunscreen.

In simple terms, if someone can stay in noonday sun for 20 minutes without sunscreen before getting red and 300 minutes with a sunscreen, then the SPF is 15. The real world is more complicated:
- European, Australian and American standards for UVB SPF.
- No accepted in-vivo UVA SPF method.
- Water resistance and persistence of sunscreen also must be assessed.
- Measurements are made with a defined fairly generous application of sunscreen/cm². Many studies have shown that the average patient applies far less.
- Much skepticism over incredibly high ratings; SPF 60 is not 4 × as effective as SPF 15. Some movement to stop at SPF 30.

se

Indications: Protection from sunburn, reduction of chronic UV exposure with photoaging and carcinogenesis; maximum protection for those with photoallergic, phototoxic, or intrinsic photosensitivity disorders.

Note: Although the effectiveness of long-term sunscreens in ameliorating chronic photodamage and carcinogenesis has not been proven (because of the long time and many patients required), there is no reason to think that it will not be helpful. Arguments of opponents center around:
- *Reduced vitamin D production:* Elderly people should perhaps not use maximum sun protection or take vitamin D supplements.
- *Increased risk because individuals then increase their sun exposure:* Can only be corrected by public education campaigns.

Side effects: Many patients become sensitized to sunscreen components; thus PABA is rarely used any more; such patients can use blocking agents.

1.13 Phototherapy

heck before Starting Phototherapy

Rule out dermatoses caused or worsened by light.

Be sure patient is not taking photosensitizing or immunosuppressive medications.

Obtain written informed consent.

Require protective eye covers and genital shielding.

Apply topical agents following phototherapy; some enhance effects (tars, ointments); others decrease them (vitamin D analogues).

UVB Phototherapy

▶ **Overview:**
- Available sources includes:
  - *Broad spectrum:* 280–320 nm.
  - *Selective UVB phototherapy (SUP):* 305–325 nm.
  - *Narrow band:* 311 nm (TL 01).
  - *Excimer laser:* 308 nm.
- Narrow band has replaced regular UVB in most settings because of increased effectiveness and decreased amount of erythema-inducing irradiation.

▶ **Indications:**
- Major indication is psoriasis; most effective wavelengths center around 311 nm (304–314 nm).
- Atopic dermatitis, pruritus (especially renal pruritus), pityriasis lichenoides et varioliformis acuta, pityriasis lichenoides chronica.
- Hardening in polymorphous light eruption.
- Simulation of repigmentation in vitiligo.

▶ **Contraindications:** Photosensitivity, reduced minimal erythema dose (MED) for UVB.

▶ **Use:**
- Determine MED (p. 49); if not determined, then based on skin test and previous experience with specific light source.
- *Psoriasis:* Start with 70% of MED; increase each time by 10–30%. Administer 3–5 × weekly; maximum reaction at 24 hours so easy to observe. Usually complete remission achieved in 4–6 weeks.
- *Atopic dermatitis:* Use as adjunct in patients who tolerate light well; start with 70% of MED.
- *Polymorphous light eruption:* Start 4–6 weeks before spring or planned vacation; start with 70% of MED, increase by 10–20% until mild erythema is induced; then drop back slightly and slowly increase again.
- *Vitiligo:* Narrow band UVB; start with very low dose (0.1–0–2 J/cm²) and increase up to 1 J/cm² over months.

▶ **Combinations:**
- With UVA for hardening in polymorphous light eruption or in pruritus.
- With salt water baths (27% table salt solution or equivalent in tub for 15 minutes); excoriated lesions may burn.
- With psoralens (PUVB): sometimes tried in vitiligo, but no well-controlled studies.

UVA Phototherapy

▶ **Overview:**
- Available sources include:.
  - Broad spectrum conventional: 320–400 nm.
  - UVA1: 340–400 nm.
- UVA light is often touted as noncarcinogenic, but this is not true. It does not cause the erythema and sunburn associated with UVB, but instead penetrates more deeply and elicits a different sort of tan. UVA requires much longer exposure periods to have a biologic effect. Most sources also produce visible and infrared light; cold UVA uses filters to eliminate the infrared component.

▶ **Indications:** Acute atopic dermatitis, morphea, pruritus, perhaps urticaria pigmentosa.

▶ **Contraindications:** Photosensitivity; most drug-induced photosensitivity occurs with UVA.

► **Use:**
- *Broad spectrum:* 2–12 J/cm^2.
- *UVA1:* Low dose 10–30 J/cm^2; medium, 40–70 J/cm^2; high 80–139 J/cm^2.

41.14 Photochemotherapy

Overview

....

► The elegant combination of psoralens and UVA (PUVA), as developed in the mid-1970s by the Harvard group of Parrish, Fitzpatrick, and Pathak, is one of the greatest success stories in dermatologic therapy.

► The psoralen molecules intercalate between strands of DNA and are then activated by UVA light. They have a broad spectrum of action, interfering with DNA synthesis but also altering many aspects of immune response. Neither the psoralens nor the UVA alone has any effects (in the doses used).

► The small long-term risk of carcinogenesis is probably related to both DNA damage and immunosuppression.

Oral PUVA Therapy

....

► **Indications:** Psoriasis, pustular psoriasis, lichen planus (especially exanthematous forms), mycosis fungoides, other low-grade cutaneous T-cell lymphomas, urticaria pigmentosa, graft-versus-host disease, severe hand and foot dermatitis, vitiligo, polymorphous light eruption (hardening), solar urticaria (hardening), chronic actinic dermatitis (hardening).

► **Contraindications:** Severe renal or hepatic disease, pregnancy, nursing, lupus erythematosus, DNA repair defects (such as xeroderma pigmentosum).

► **Pretreatment evaluation:**
- *History:*
  - Photosensitivity, excessive solar damage, photodermatoses (lupus erythematosus, porphyria cutanea tarda); ingestion of photosensitizing medications.
  - Epilepsy (medications, risk of seizure during treatment).
  - In case of psoriasis, previous treatment with methotrexate, radiation therapy or arsenic; all increase risk of carcinogenesis.
  - Renal or hepatic disease.
  - Pregnancy, nursing; desire for future children.
- *Laboratory:*
  - Complete blood count.
  - Renal and hepatic function.
  - Ophthalmologic examination; prescription of sunglasses with maximum UV protection.
- Determination of minimal phototoxicity dose (MPD) (p. 51).
- ⚠ *Caution:* Never start therapy before you have all of the above documented and a signed informed consent.

► **Use:**
- Administer 0.6 mg/kg of 8-methoxsalen (8-methoxypsoralen) (in USA usually 0.4 mg/kg of Oxsoralen ultra); round off using the standard 10 mg tablets.
- After 2 hours, administer broad spectrum UVA light. Treat 4 × weekly (M–T–Th–F).
- Start with 70% of MPD; increase the dose gradually assessing erythema on non-involved skin. Never increase dose 2 days in a row.

⚠ *Caution:* PUVA erythema first develops after 72 hours.
- If MPD is not available, then:
  - *Skin type I/II:* 0.5 J/cm² ; increase by 0.3 J/cm² every 3 days until erythema appears.
  - *Skin type III/IV:* 1.0 J/cm² ; increase by 0.5 J/cm² every 3 days until erythema appears.
- Patient remains photosensitive for 12 hours; must wear special sunglasses, sunscreen, and avoid exposure.
- Psoralens were initially combined with natural sun exposure, first as "suntan pills" and later to treat vitiligo. This approach may be an option in areas where easy access to UVA phototherapy units is limited, but it is very difficult to control because of the variability in sun exposure.

► **Side effects:**
- *Acute:* Sunburn, gastrointestinal distress.
- *Chronic:* Photodamaged skin, PUVA lentigines, actinic keratoses, squamous cell carcinomas, basal cell carcinomas and malignant melanomas.
  ⚠ *Caution:* The increase in the already high background risk of developing a malignant melanoma is minimal, but every PUVA patient must be monitored lifelong to insure early identification.

Topical PUVA Therapy

► **Overview:** Many "tricks" have been developed to avoid the systemic ingestion of psoralens with resultant ocular risk and photosensitivity. Possibilities include limited degree of UVA exposure (hand and foot PUVA) and applying the psoralens topically (bath, shower, or cream PUVA). Topically applied psoralens lose their effects after 2–3 hours. Can be used in pregnancy. No need for sunglasses after treatment.
  ⚠ *Caution:* Extremely low concentrations of topical psoralens are required. In the USA, the initial commercial product was far too concentrated and difficult to use. It is no longer available.

► **Indications:** Same as for oral PUVA.
► **Contraindications:** Many fewer, as process is limited to lesional skin.
► **Cream PUVA:**
- Methoxsalen 0.006% cream in unguentum cordes or other bases.
- Store at 4°C.
- Apply for 1 hour before irradiation; some use with plastic foil occlusion.

► **Bath PUVA:**
- Require special facilities with bath or shower for PUVA; special plastic sheeting in tub can reduce amount of psoralens required.
- Final concentration is around 1 mg methoxsalen to 1 liter water.
- After 15 minutes, immediate irradiation.
  - Dosage: Treat 4 × weekly; onset of erythema is goal. Start with 30% of MPD and increase rapidly to reach erythema threshold. If MPD is not available, then:
    - *Skin type I/II:* 0.3 J/cm² ; increase by 0.2 J/cm² every 3 days until erythema appears.
    - *Skin type III/IV:* 0.5 J/cm² ; increase by 0.3 J/cm² every 3 days until erythema appears.
    - When erythema appears, no increase in dosage.

Topical Therapy

41.15 *Photodynamic Therapy*

Overview

▶ Photodynamic therapy (PDT) is a special form of photochemotherapy. Special photosensitizers are employed which concentrate in tumors or inflamed tissue and then can be activated with concentrated light sources whose emission spectrum corresponds to the activation spectrum of the sensitizer.

▶ The usual sensitizer is α-aminolevulinic acid (ALA), one of the intermediates in porphyrin metabolism. A form of "local iatrogenic porphyria" is induced in the target tissue.

▶ More ALA is taken up by tumor cells than by normal surrounding skin. Irradiation with 630 nm bright red light (LEDs) leads to destruction of tumor cells and endothelial damage in feeder vessels.

Method

▶ **Indications:** Actinic keratosis, supercoil basal cell carcinoma, superficial squamous cell carcinoma, Bowen disease, isolated superficial cutaneous lymphoma; perhaps condylomata acuminata and psoriasis. Only effective for superficial lesions.

⚠ *Caution:* Diagnosis must be confirmed histologically before commencing PDT.

▶ **Light source:**
  • *Monochromatic source:* Pumped rhodamine dye laser (628 nm) or gold vapor laser (628 nm).
  • *Polychromatic source:* Slide projector with 250–500 watt lamp and filter; xenon lamp with filter.

▶ **Use:**
  • Apply 10–20% ALA cream or methylaminolevulinate for 4 hours under occlusion and protected from light.
  • Apply light for 15–20 minutes.
  • Repeat in 2–3 months.
  • When dealing with multiple actinic keratoses, the ALA can be used to highlight the lesions, which are then treated.
  • Painful: Systemic analgesics and lidocaine/prilocaine (EMLA) may be needed for irradiation. Heals with necrosis and crusting.

41.16 *Balneotherapy*

▶ **Overview:** Baths are a very effective way of treating a large area quickly. They are expensive, because of requirements for personal facilities. Bathing or balneotherapy has long occupied a major role in German dermatology, driven primarily by the emphasis on inpatient care and spa visits paid for by health insurance.

▶ **Cleansing baths:** Baths are incorporated into therapy plans to remove crusts, scales, and residual medications. A variety of tensides can be added. Additionally, 3–5% sodium chloride or sodium bicarbonate may be useful for loosening scales in psoriasis or ichthyosis.

Anti-inflammatory Baths

▶ **Acute exudative or infected dermatitis:**
  • Adding bolus alba (white clay powder) 250 g/tub has a soothing effect.

- Tannins or synthetic equivalents are useful for their astringent properties. Useful for local baths or wet dressings for intertrigo, as well as hand and foot dermatitis. Tannosynt is best known product in Europe; difficult to find in USA.
► **Chronic skin disorders:**
  - Useful for chronic dermatitis, psoriasis, lichen planus, prurigo simplex chronica.
  - Most useful choice is coal tar baths; photosensitizing can be used for advantage in psoriasis.
  - Polidocanol can be added for antipruritic effect.

Disinfectant Baths

► Chinolinol 0.1 % in bath water is antibacterial and antifungal. Low sensitizing potential. Binds to emulsifiers and metal salts with resultant inactivation.
► Potassium permanganate baths have a similar effect but permanently discolor bathtubs. Usual concentration 1:5000 (several crystals completely dissolved in full tub). Should be used alone, as inactivated by many substances.

Oil Baths

► Oil baths are the most effective to re-lubricate dry skin in atopic dermatitis or psoriasis.
► Three approaches:
  - Miscible oils are spread through the bath and leave some residues on skin.
  - Nonmiscible oils remain on the bath surface and coat the body on exit.
  - Both can also be applied to wet skin immediately after bathing.
► Many different oils employed.
► **Cleopatra's bath:** 1 glass of milk with 1 teaspoon each of olive oil and honey; shaken thoroughly; added to bath.
▣ *Note:* All baths are drying if the skin is not lubricated at the end. Many people with dry skin enjoy soaking in the tub or taking long hot showers, but fail to re-lubricate their skin and end up with more dryness and pruritus.

41.17 Aesthetic Dermatology

Overview

Dermatologic therapy has always sought to produce both medicinal and aesthetic results. Today there are so many options that a subspecialty of aesthetic dermatology is in the process of establishing itself. It includes the use of appropriate tested cosmetics, instruction in maintenance approaches following therapy, and correction of skin conditions that are primarily aesthetic in nature but may also have medical or psychological aspects.

Botulinum A Toxin

► **Mechanism of action:**
  - Botulinum toxin is made by *Clostridium botulinum* as an exotoxin, which blocks the release of acetylcholine and thus inhibits neuromuscular transmission and causes muscle paralysis. There are seven types; type A is the most effective and has the longest duration of action.
  - The molecule is relatively unstable, with two subunits bound by a disulfide bond that is easily split.

- Effects first appear after 1–3 days with maximum effect reached at 2 weeks. Average duration of effect 3–6 months. Muscles then become re-innervated.
- The strength of botulinum A toxin is given in biological units based on the effect in mice.

▶ **Indications:** Botulinum A toxin was initially developing for strabismus; paralyzing the ocular muscles was far more effective and safer than corrective surgery. It also is effective for hyperhidrosis, providing several months of relief for axillary or palmar excessive sweating. The main dermatologic indication is correction of facial wrinkles. The following features must be considered:

- *Type of wrinkle:* Only those caused by muscles of facial expression (mimic wrinkles) are amenable to correction.
- *Consider expectations of patient:* Those with reasonable expectations will be happiest; those with few wrinkles, or perception disorders, will be disappointed.

▶ **Informed consent:**

- Some products such as Dysport and Botox (now widely used as generic name) are not at present approved for cosmetic usage. Patient must be aware of this.
- Inform patients about other ways to treat wrinkles.
- Counsel regarding the side effects discussed below.
- Patient must agree to pay; insurance plans do not cover cosmetic procedures.
- Take photographs before treatment, and then as needed.

▶ **Contraindications:**

- *Absolute:* Rare diseases with decreased muscle activity such as myasthenia gravis or Eaton–Lambert syndrome; simultaneous use of macrolide or aminoglycoside antibiotics; pregnancy or nursing; infection in area of injection, psychiatric problems.
- *Relative:* Coagulopathy or therapeutic anticoagulation.

▶ **Use:**

- Define injection points.
- Draw up botulinum A toxin.
- ⚠ *Caution:* The commercially available products have different concentrations, different degrees of activity, and different methods of dilution. They are not interchangeable.
- Disinfect area and let dry completely, to avoid denaturing botulinum A toxin.
- Inject target muscle with 30 or 32 gauge needle.
- Cool.

▶ **Side effects:** Hematoma, pain on injection, burning, pressure sensation, headache, numbness, swelling, undesired muscle paralysis, ptosis of the eyelid when treating the glabellar area, ptosis of the eyebrows when treating the forehead, allergic reaction to individual components.

▶ **Specific sites:**

- *Glabellar wrinkles:*
  - Very suitable.
  - Always inject 1 cm from orbital rim.
  - 3–5 injection points.
  - *Specific side effects:* Hematomas, headache, paralysis of levator muscle; if ptosis occurs, can use apraclonidine eye drops; 1–3 drops daily stimulates Müller muscle and elevates upper lid.
- *Forehead wrinkles:*
  - Suitable.
  - Always inject in the middle of the forehead.
  - 4–6 injection points.
  - *Specific side effects:* Drooping or elevation of eyebrows.

- *Periorbital wrinkles:*
  - Suitable.
  - Always inject 1 cm lateral to orbital rim.
  - 2–3 injection points.
  - *Specific side effects:* If the lateral rectus muscle is paralyzed, then diplopia (very rare).
- *Perioral and neck wrinkles:* Only for experienced operators.

Soft Tissue Augmentation

▶ **Overview:** Wrinkles can also be corrected by injection permanent or nonpermanent fillers. Permanent fillers, such as silicone or polymethyl acrylates, have the great disadvantage that not only the effect but also the side effects, such as a foreign body reaction, are persistent. In addition, some filler material may shift in the skin. For this reason, nonpermanent fillers have assumed a predominant role. All fillers should be used with the same precautions and documentation as botulinum A toxin.

▶ **Hyaluronic acid:**
- Hyaluronic acid (HA) is a polysaccharide of *N*-acetyl glucosamine and glucuronic acid. It is present in many tissues and accounts for about 50% of the ground substance of normal skin.
- Both linked and unlinked HA preparations are available. The linked products have larger molecules and persist longer. Both glutaraldehyde and butanediol diglycide ether (BDDE) are using for linking. HA is broken down to H_2O and CO_2 over 3–8 months.
- *Indications:* Wrinkles, lip augmentation, scars.
- *Contraindications:* Pregnancy, nursing, active autoimmune diseases, use of aspirin; some forms derived from rooster combs cannot be used in patients with eggwhite allergy.
- **Use:**
  - Topical anesthesia.
  - Inject with 27–30 gauge needle with either drop technique or tunnel technique. Larger areas such as cheeks are most easily enhanced using tunnel technique.
  - *Side effects:* Hematoma, erythema, edema, pain, granuloma formation, infection.

▶ **Poly–L-lactic acid:**
- Combination of polylactate microspheres, mannitol, and carboxymethylcellulose.
- Suited for larger defects such as deeper wrinkles and lipoatrophy.
- Use similar to HA. Granuloma formation more common.

▶ **Bovine collagen:**
- Several collagens are available. Cross-linked collagen will persist longer. All are derived from cattle in an isolated herd to eliminate risk of prion disease.
- Test injection 0.1 mL intradermal on arm recommended because some patients have allergic reactions to animal proteins. Positive reaction consists of erythema or swelling that persists 6 hours after injection. About 1–3 % of those not reacting to skin test will react to collagen.
- Uses similar to HA.
- Several forms of human-derived collagen are now available in various stages of development. See specialized texts.

Chemical Peeling

▶ **Definition:** Use of toxic exfoliative substances to remove skin. Depth of removal depends on agent, concentration, body location, length of exposure, and degree of occlusion, as well as status of skin and previous treatments.

▶ **Available agents:**

- α-*Hydroxy acids (AHA)* and derivatives (glycolic acid, lactic acid, citric acid):
    - Most originally obtained from fruits and thus known as fruit acids.
    - Multiple effects, primarily reduce keratinocyte adhesion and induce fibroblast activity.
- β-*Hydroxy acids*; *salicylic acid:* Very superficial peel, removing stratum corneum.
- *Trichloracetic acid (TCA):* Mainstay of peeling; denatures tissue; not absorbed.
- *Retinoids* (p. 601).

▶ **Levels of peeling:** Three levels usually considered:

- *Superficial peel:*
    - Removal of outer part of epidermis.
    - Mild procedure; sometimes called soft peel or lunch peel. Little toxicity; rapid, but short-term improvement. Can be used anywhere on body.
    - Agents include AHA 20–40%, and TCA 10%.
    - Can be done by nurses or other auxiliary personnel.
    - Indications include dry skin, superficial keratoses, photoaging, mild acne, hyperpigmentation, melasma.
    - Side effects minimal but include erythema, pigmentary disturbances, triggering of recurrent herpes simplex virus infections.
- *Medium peel:*
    - Removes entire epidermis and impinges on papillary dermis.
    - Agents include AHA 50–70% and TCA 35%.
    - Usually done by physician.
    - Indications include acne scars, actinic keratoses, plane warts, melasma, tiny wrinkles, photoaging. Should not be used in Type IV–V skin.
    - Side effects include persistent erythema, pigmentary disturbances and scarring.
- *Deep peel:*
    - Reaches to reticular dermis.
    - Agents include TCA 50% (or pretreatment plus 30%) and phenol.
    - Usually done under general anesthesia, always by physician.
    - Indications include deeper wrinkles, photoaging, thicker keratoses or lentigines.
    - Same problems as with medium peel but scarring more liking; when phenol is used, risk of cardiac arrhythmias.

▶ **Procedure:**

- Explanation, informed consent, photos, as for botulinum A toxin.
- Pretreatment for 2–4 weeks with AHA 8–15%.
- Clean skin, then apply peeling agent either with brush or sponge or with gloved hand. Apply with constant pressure.
- Start with lowest usual concentration, leave on for 2 minutes, neutralize if applicable and cool.
- Re-emphasize need for sunscreens.

Bleaching

▶ **Available agents:**
- *Azelaic acid:* Blocks tyrosinase to cause depigmentation (also keratolytic and antibacterial). Usual concentration 15%.
- *Hydroquinone:* Most widely used bleach; blocks oxidation from tyrosine to dopa. Used in 2–4% concentration in variety of "lightening creams." Higher concentrations, available especially in Africa and Asia, carry risk of exogenous ochronosis and hyperpigmentation.
- *Monobenzyl ether of hydroquinone:* Highly effective, causing irreversible pigmentation, also at sites distant to application. Only used to complete depigmentation in widespread vitiligo.
- *Kojic acid:* Tyrosinase inhibitor obtained from malted rice; used at around 2% concentration.
- ▣ *Note:* All attempts at bleaching must be combined with regular use of a sunscreen.

Cosmetic Care

In Germany many dermatology clinics have a cosmetician who is involved in treatment of acne and rosacea patients. In some instances, the health insurance pays for the treatment.

▶ **Acne treatment:**
- *Superficial treatment:* Mild debridement with abrasive soaps or scrubs; similar to what patient can accomplish at home.
- ▣ *Note:* Not everyone is convinced that abrasive scrubs or treatments are helpful. They feel good, but cause follicular irritation and may worsen acne in some patients. In addition, they reinforce the erroneous connection between unclean skin and acne.
- *Acne surgery:* Comedones are incised and expressed; produces short-term improvement but studies have shown that lesions refill over 1–2 weeks.

▶ **Rosacea:** Sobye suggested a pattern of massage to move lymphatic fluid in parts of the face that move relatively little with facial expression. Effectiveness minimal, but may be useful adjunct. Massage is directed centrally, involving forehead, temples, nose, and lateral cheeks. Patients best taught to do procedure themselves at home (up to 3 × daily).

Camouflage

Special make-up is one of the most overlooked tools in the dermatologic trade. In Europe, advice is often given in the clinic or practice. In the USA, patients are referred to the cosmetic company. Diseases such as vitiligo and vascular malformations can often be covered more effectively than treated. In addition, skilful use of make-up, such as using a green base to reduce erythema, helps many erythematous and vascular processes.

Fine Needle Electrosurgery

Fine needles at a low (1–3 A) setting can be used to selectively destroy telangiectases or carry out epilation. In recent years, both tasks have been replaced to a large extent by lasers, which are more effective and far quicker.

Sclerotherapy

Small telangiectases, especially starburst telangiectases, can be treated by injection with variety of sclerosing agents, as discussed under phlebology (p. 555).

42 Systemic Therapy

42.1 Antiviral Therapy

Acyclovir

▶ **Mechanism of action:** Blocks viral DNA polymerase. Herpes virus thymidine kinase selectively phosphorylates acyclovir (a guanosine analog), which is then incorporated into viral DNA and blocks synthesis.
▶ **Indications:** Infections with herpes simplex virus (HSV) 1 and 2, acute varicella infection; herpes zoster; cytomegalovirus prophylaxis following solid organ and bone marrow transplantation; widely used for prophylaxis for recurrent herpes simplex virus infections.
▶ **Contraindications:** Carefully chosen during pregnancy and nursing; small risk of fetal malformations outweighed by risks from maternal varicella and perhaps maternal primary herpes simplex virus with viremia.
▶ **Dosage:**
  • *Immunocompetent patients:* 200–800 mg p.o. 5 × daily or 5 mg/kg i.v. t.i.d. (200 mg for herpes simplex, 800 mg for herpes zoster).
  • *Immunosuppressed patients:* 10 mg/kg t.i.d.
  • Adjust dosage in patients with renal insufficiency.
  • Prophylaxis for herpes simplex: 200 mg p.o. b.i.d.–t.i.d.
  ⚠ *Caution:* Cimetidine and probenecid slow the excretion of acyclovir.
▶ **Side effects*:** **Seizures, headache, dizziness,** glomerulonephritis, acute renal failure.

Valacyclovir

▶ **Mechanism of action:** Prodrug of acyclovir; converted in first pass through gastrointestinal tract and liver to acyclovir.
▶ **Indications:** Infections with HSV-1 and -2; herpes zoster; prophylaxis for recurrent HSV infections. Probably better for zoster than acyclovir. Not approved in immunosuppressed patients.
▶ **Contraindications:** Pregnancy and nursing; wiser to use acyclovir, which has more safety data.
▶ **Dosage:**
  • *Infections:* 1000 mg p.o t.i.d. for 7–10 days for zoster, acute HSV.
  • *Prophylaxis:* 1000 mg p.o. b.i.d.
▶ **Side effects:** See acyclovir.

Brivudin

▶ **Mechanism of action:** Blocks viral DNA synthesis by interacting with deoxythymidine kinase and DNA polymerase.
▶ **Indications:** Infections with varicella-zoster virus and HSV-1, especially severe mucocutaneous forms.
▶ **Contraindications:** Pregnancy and nursing; cannot be used with systemic 5-fluorouracil or other analogues.
▶ **Dosage:** Adults: 125 mg p.o. q.i.d.

---

* Side effects printed in boldface are potentially fatal.

► **Side effects:** Gastrointestinal distress, headache, elevated liver enzymes, rare cutaneous drug reactions.

Famciclovir
....

► **Mechanism of action:** Prodrug of penciclovir; good gastrointestinal absorption, converted in first pass through gastrointestinal tract and liver to active form, which also interferes with DNA polymerase.
► **Indications:** Herpes zoster—as effective as valacyclovir but considerably more expensive; also approved for acute HSV infections.
► **Contraindications:** Pregnancy and nursing.
► **Dosage:**
  • *Zoster:* 250 mg p.o. t.i.d.
  • *Recurrent herpes genitalis:* 125 mg p.o. b.i.d.
► **Side effects:** Headaches, diarrhea, nausea; sometimes confusion in elderly patients.

42.2 Dapsone

► **Synonym:** Diaminodiphenylsulfone, DDS, DADPS.
► **Mechanism of action:** Unclear; competitive antagonist of PABA interfering with normal synthesis of folic acid by bacteria; also seems to have antineutrophil action; metabolizes to aminohydroxyldiphenylsulfone, which is responsible for methemoglobulinemia and hemolysis. Excreted via kidneys (90%) with a half-life of 2–4 days.
► **Indications:**
  • Leprosy, dermatitis herpetiformis, prophylaxis for *Pneumocystis carinii.*
  • Employed for many other dermatologic disorders including pyoderma gangrenosum, autoimmune bullous diseases, bullous LE, granuloma faciale, erythema elevatum et diutinum and leukocytoclastic vasculitis.
► **Contraindications:** Severe cardiovascular disease, marked renal insufficiency, pregnancy, sulfonamide allergy.
► **Drug interactions:** See Table 42.**9**.
► **Precautions:**
  • *Before therapy:*
    – Complete blood count (CBC) and hemoglobin (Hgb).
    – Determine glucose-6-phosphate dehydrogenase (G6PD). Patients with relative deficiency have more hemolysis; common among blacks, Asians.
  • *During first 3 months of therapy:*
    – Weekly, then biweekly, CBC, Hgb, and methemoglobin.
  • *Later:*
    – CBC, Hgb and methemoglobin every 2–3 months; liver functions and renal status every 6 months.
► **Dosage:** Start with 50–100 mg daily and observe response; can increase to 150 or maximal 200 mg daily; many patients with dermatitis herpetiformis do fine on 50 mg daily or q.o.d.
🚩 *Caution:* With impaired renal function, divide dose by two. If creatine clearance is < 15 mL/minute, do not use.
► **Side effects:**
  • *Methemoglobinemia:* Everyone gets it, but few have problems. Cyanosis can appear with values as low as 3%. Symptoms usually appear with levels > 10%.
  • *Hemolysis:* Usually starts with 50 mg daily, dose-dependent. At 150 mg daily, a drop in Hgb of 2 g/dl is expected. Usually reversed to some degree by increased

production. Patients with limited cardiovascular or marrow reserve may not tolerate this stress.

- Agranulocytosis, aplastic anemia.
- Nephrotic syndrome, renal papillary necrosis.
- *Peripheral motor neuropathy:* Occurs after long-term use; more common in those with G6PD defects.
- *Sulfone syndrome:* Flu-like illness with malaise, exanthem, hepatitis, lymphadenopathy and eosinophilia. Usually resolves when dapsone stopped.

▶ **Alternatives:** Sulfapyridine 1.5–2.0 g daily is reasonable substitute in dermatitis herpetiformis.

42.3 Antifungal Agents

Griseofulvin

▶ **Mechanism of action:** Griseofulvin is incorporated into newly synthesized keratin, so it must be taken for a long time—up to 18 months in the case of toe nails. Its half-life is around 24 hours; micronized forms are better absorbed and distributed. It interferes with microtubule formation.

▶ **Indications:** Dermatophyte infections; griseofulvin is not effective against yeasts and molds. Organism should be cultured before starting therapy.

▶ **Contraindications:** Liver disease, porphyria, LE, pregnancy.

▶ **Drug interactions:** Griseofulvin is metabolized in the liver and interacts with many agents (Table 42.**9**) including:
- Impairs action of coumarin.
- Reduces effectiveness of oral contraceptives.
- Cross-reactions with penicillin possible.

▶ **Dosage:** Griseofulvin is still the only agent approved for tinea capitis in children; it has been replaced in most of its other uses by the more effective imidazoles.
- Children 10 mg/kg daily; adults 500–100 mg p.o. daily.
- If no response, dose can be doubled after 2 weeks.

▶ **Side effects:**
- Hepatic toxicity, gastrointestinal bleeding, leukopenia, granulocytopenia.
- Check CBC before therapy and after 2–3 weeks.
- Exanthems, urticaria, photosensitivity.
- May trigger acute intermittent porphyria or systemic lupus erythematosus.

Itraconazole

▶ **Mechanism of action:** Inhibits cytochrome P450-dependent synthesis of ergosterol, a key component of fungal cell walls.

▶ **Indications:** Effective against dermatophytes, molds, and many yeasts. Excellent against *Candida albicans* and *Candida krusei*; moderately effective against other *Candida* species.
- Cutaneous mycoses, including onychomycoses.
- Mycoses in HIV/AIDS.
- Mucocutaneous and systemic candidiasis.
- Recurrent vaginal candidiasis.
- Aspergillosis.
- Soft tissue mycotic infections.

▶ **Contraindications:** Pregnancy; contraception until 4 weeks after end of therapy.

▶ **Drug interactions:** Inhibits cytochrome P450; many interactions (Table 42.**9**); enhances coumarin, oral hypoglycemic agents, theophylline, and phenytoin.

▶ **Dosage:**
  • *Cutaneous mycoses:* 100–200 mg p.o. daily for 2–4 weeks.
  • *Onychomycosis:* Interval therapy; 200 mg p.o. b.i.d. for 7 days; repeat in weeks 4 and 7.
  • *Vaginal candidiasis:* 200 mg p.o. twice in one day.
  • Longer-term, higher-dose therapy in HIV, soft tissue, and systemic mycoses.
▶ **Side effects:** Only common effect is nausea.

Fluconazole

▶ **Mechanism of action:** Inhibits cytochrome P450-dependent synthesis of ergosterol, a key component of fungal cell walls.
▶ **Indications:** Effective against dermatophytes and yeasts; not molds. Effectiveness reduced against *Trichophyton mentagrophytes*, *Candida glabrata*, and *Candida guilliermondii*.
  • Useful for candidiasis in almost all settings from acute vaginal to HIV/AIDS to chronic mucocutaneous candidiasis.
  • Dermatophyte infections, including onychomycoses.
▶ **Contraindications:** Severe liver disease, pregnancy and nursing; contraception until 7 days after completing therapy.
▶ **Drug interactions:** Inhibits cytochrome P450; many interactions (Table 42.**9**). Enhances coumarin, midazolam, oral hypoglycemic agents, phenytoin, tacrolimus, theophylline.
▶ **Dosage:**
  • *Vaginal candidiasis:* Single dose of 150 mg.
  • *Systemic candidiasis:* 200–800 mg p.o. daily (depending on organism) in adults; can be used in children if no suitable alternative: 3–6 mg/kg p.o. daily.
  • *Dermatophytes:*
    – Adults: 50 mg p.o. daily.
    – Children: 1–2 mg/kg p.o. daily; higher dose for zoophilic fungi.
  • *Onychomycosis:* 150 mg weekly in single dose, for 3–6 months (fingernails) or 6–12 months (toenails).
▶ **Side effects:**
  • Seizures, leukopenia, thrombocytopenia.
  • **Hepatic injury**—monitor liver enzymes.
  • **Toxic epidermal necrolysis;** be very cautious about continuing in patients developing an exanthema.

Terbinafine

▶ **Mechanism of action:** Inhibits sterol biosynthesis by blocking squalene peroxidase causing accumulation of squalene and cell death.
▶ **Indications:** Primarily dermatophytes.
▶ **Contraindications:** Renal or hepatic disease.
▶ **Dosage:** Cutaneous disease 250 mg daily p.o. for 2–4 weeks; onychomycosis 250 mg daily p.o. for 6–12 weeks or interval therapy.
▶ **Side effects:** No common serious side effects; elevated liver enzymes, disturbed taste; rare toxic epidermal necrolysis.

42.4 Antihistamines

▶ **Mechanism of action:** Antihistamines share structural similarities with histamine and block its actions by competing for receptor sites. There are two main types of histamine receptors, H1 and H2. Both are found in the skin, and H2 receptors are also found in the gut. H2 blockers decrease gastric section and are used for peptic ulcer disease. H3 receptors are limited to the CNS. In most instances, classic H1 antihistamines are adequate for cutaneous disease; in some instances combined H1–H2 blockage is more effective.

▶ **Indications:** Urticaria, anaphylaxis, allergic rhinitis, allergic conjunctivitis. Antihistamines are not as effective in atopic dermatitis as in other manifestations of atopy. They are also frequently employed for other forms of dermatitis, pruritus, and prurigo, but when itch is not histamine-mediated their effectiveness is comparable to that of a sedating placebo.

Table 42.1 · **Classification and use of antihistamines**

Class	Agent[a]	Dose	Sedating	Comments
Ethanolamine	Diphenhydramine	25–50 mg q4–6 h	+++	
	Clemastine	1–2 mg b.i.d.	+	
Ethylenediamine	Tripelennamine	25–50 mg q4–6 h	++	
Piperazine	Hydroxyzine	10–50 mg q6–8 h; 50 mg HS	++	Physical urticarias, nighttime use
Alkylamine	Chlorpheniramine	2–4 mg q4–6 h	+	
Phenothiazine	Promethazine	12.5 mg t.i.d.–q.i.d.; 25 mg HS	+++	Nighttime use
Piperidine	Cyproheptadine	4 mg q4–6 h	+	Cold urticaria, nighttime use; antiserotonin activity
Nonsedating H1	Azelastine	2 mg b.i.d.	–	
	Cetirizine	10 mg daily or b.i.d.	–	
	Levocetirizine	5 mg daily or b.i.d.	–	
	Ebastine	10 mg daily or b.i.d.	–	
	Fexofenadine	60 mg b.i.d. or 60–180 mg daily	–	Not metabolized in liver
	Loratadine	10 mg daily	–	Long half-life
	Desloratadine	5 mg daily	–	Long half-life; not metabolized in liver
	Mizolastine	10 mg daily	–	
Thioguanidine	Cimetidine	300 mg q.i.d.	–	For skin diseases, used with H1 blocker; also immunomodulatory and antiandrogenic
Tricyclic antidepressant	Doxepin	10–20 mg q.i.d.	++	H1, H2 blocker: cardiac side effects

a For the older classes, only a single well-known example is cited

▶ **Contraindications:** Generally best avoided during pregnancy; more information on older antihistamines. Clemastine generally recommended in Germany. Few are approved for children < 2 years of age; dimethindene is available in Germany for infants > 1 month.

▶ **Dosage:** It is best to start at a low dose of antihistamines and gradually increase. It may also be wise to use two different antihistamines from different chemical classes to maximize effect. The nonsedating H1 antihistamines, which poorly cross the blood–brain barrier, have been a tremendous advance and have replaced many of the older sedating H1 blockers. On the other hand, in some instances the sedating action is desirable and an older agent serves better. There are also phenothiazines (promethazine) and tricyclic antidepressants (doxepin) with significant antihistamine effects. The antihistamines are summarized in Table 42.**1**.

▶ **Side effects:**
  ▢ *Note:* Acquaint yourself with the specific side effects and their likelihood in the antihistamines you routinely prescribe.
  • Sedation is only a problem with the older agents. However, one is legally mandated to warn the patient about driving, operating heavy equipment, or doing anything requiring alertness when an antihistamine is prescribed, even a nonsedating one.
  • Terfenadine, one of the first nonsedating antihistamines, is no longer available in the USA because of its propensity to cause **life-threatening cardiac arrhythmias.** This problem was made worse by its interaction with macrolide antibiotics and imidazole antifungals.
  • None of the other nonsedating antihistamines has the same high risk, but patients with preexisting cardiac disease, especially rhythm disturbances, should be evaluated carefully.
  • Many are metabolized by the cytochrome P450 enzymes, so that multiple drug interactions are possible (Table 42.**9**).
  • Anticholinergic effects, including urinary retention, dry mouth, even predisposition to heat stroke (decreased sweating).
  ▢ *Note:* Many of the antihistamines, especially doxepin and diphenhydramine, are effective topically. Unfortunately they are potent sensitizers and thus probably best avoided, as sensitized patients may then be allergic to systemic antihistamines, which are often administered in an emergency setting.

Other Antiallergic Agents

▶ **Cromolyn:**
  • Mast cell stabilizer; poorly absorbed; primarily used for asthma, allergic rhinitis, and allergic conjunctivitis in the form of inhalers, nose drops, and eye drops.
  • Available as pill with indication for use in systemic mastocytosis; absorption minimal, but helps stabilize gastrointestinal mast cells.
▶ **Ketotifen:**
  • H1 receptor antagonist and mast cell stabilizer.
  • Useful in allergic asthma and as eye drops in allergic conjunctivitis.
  • Treatment of choice for pruritus associated with neurofibromatosis.

42.5 Antimalarials

▶ **Mechanism of action:** Stabilize membranes, especially lysosomes; downregulate expression of MHC molecules; hinder neutrophil and eosinophil migration and function; interact with complement system; inhibit prostaglandin synthesis; many other undoubtedly important immunological interactions.

▶ **Indications:** The antimalarials were discovered to be effective against lupus erythematosus, as American soldiers receiving malaria prophylaxis during World War II noted improvement in their disease. They are now used for this indication as well as rheumatoid arthritis, polymorphous light eruption, and sarcoidosis. In much lower dosages, they are employed in porphyria cutanea tarda. Our comments apply only to their use in dermatology, not to their worldwide use against *Plasmodium*.

▶ **Contraindications:** Pregnancy, nursing, G6PD deficiency, simultaneous use of hepatotoxic agents or monoamine oxidase (MAO) inhibitors, myasthenia gravis, hematopoietic diseases.

▶ **Drug interactions:** Increase levels of digoxin.

▶ **Precautions:**
- Ophthalmologic examination before starting therapy and then every 6–12 months.
- CBC, liver, and kidney parameters before starting therapy; check CBC after 1 month and all parameters at 6 months.

▶ **Available agents:**
- Chloroquine (CQ) 250 mg.
- Hydroxychloroquine (HCQ) 200 mg.
- ◫ *Note:* 250 mg CQ is roughly equal to 400 mg HCQ. Each agent has found favor in different countries.

▶ **Dosage:** Usually either 200–400 mg HCQ or 250 mg CQ as required. When treating porphyria cutanea tarda, the usual dosage is 125 mg CQ 2–3 × weekly.
- ◫ *Note:* Full dosages of CQ or HCQ can be fatal in porphyria cutanea tarda (p. 312).

▶ **Side effects:**
- Agranulocytosis, blood dyscrasia, hemolytic anemia.
- Irreversible retinal damage: The risk of retinopathy is generally accepted to be less with HCQ than with CQ, but the key is careful monitoring, not choice of agent. One study suggested safe ranges of < 4.0 mg/kg daily of CQ or < 6.5 mg/kg daily of HCQ. Conflicting data on total cumulative dose. Similar retinal changes can be seen in systemic LE and macular atrophy.
- ◫ *Note:* Deposits can be seen in the retina with a split lamp. They are reversible, but the visible damage is not.
- Seizures, EKG abnormalities.
- Anorexia, nausea, vomiting (common).
- Pigmentary changes including blue-gray discoloration of hairs especially in redheads; blue discoloration of tibia, palate, face, nail bed.
- Lichenoid and urticarial exanthems; rarely toxic epidermal necrolysis.
- General wisdom is that antimalarials make psoriasis worse, but this was not supported by experience during the Viet Nam War, and there are studies showing effectiveness of HCQ in psoriatic arthritis.

Quinacrine

Quinacrine (Atabrine) 100 mg has been used in the past as a back-up agent when CQ and HCQ are not tolerated. It is no longer easily obtained and it used primarily as a local irritant injection for pneumothorax or nonsurgical female sterilization. It causes a yellow skin discoloration but not a retinopathy.

Systemic Therapy

42.6 Retinoids

Mechanism of Action

Retinoids modulation the differentiation and keratinization of keratinocytes, alter fibroblast activity and modulate the T-cell response. They lead to desquamation and epidermal thinning, and can block tumor promotion in epithelial tumors.

Indications and Contradictions

► **Indications:**
  • *Isotretinoin:*
    – Acne and rosacea; far and away most important indication for systemic retinoids.
    – Chemopreventive agent in xeroderma pigmentosum and nevoid basal cell carcinoma syndrome to reduce number of new tumors, not to treat existing lesions.
  • *Acitretin:* Psoriasis (especially erythrodermic, pustular and arthritic forms), Darier disease, pityriasis rubra pilaris, lichen planus, disorders or keratinization, chronic cutaneous lupus erythematosus, epidermodysplasia verruciformis, and multiple keratoacanthomas.
  • *Bexarotene:* Used for cutaneous T-cell lymphomas.
  • *Tretinoin:* Used topically in acne but systemically only for acute promyelocytic leukemia to induce differentiation of neoplastic cells; not further discussed here.
► **Contraindications:**
  • Women of childbearing age.
  🛈 *Caution:* The retinoids are potent teratogens. They can be taken by women of childbearing age only with effective contraception, ideally employing two methods. Female patients must sign informed written consent; in many countries, manufacturer offers pretreatment gynecologic consultation and assistance in follow-up. Patient should have negative pregnancy test and normal period before starting therapy.
  • Patient should have severe disease, not responsive to other measures.
  • Pregnancy and nursing.
  • Abnormal liver function, disorders of lipid metabolism, severe diabetes mellitus.
► **Precautions:**
  • Pregnancy test before starting treatment.
  • Baseline liver function tests, cholesterol and triglycerides; monitor monthly for 3–4 months and then every 3 months.
► **Drug interactions:**
  • Vitamin A (exaggerates effect).
  • Tetracycline (pseudotumor cerebri).
  • Methotrexate (hepatotoxicity).
  • Alcohol (hepatotoxicity, cumulative effect on triglycerides).
  • See also Table 42.**9**.

Dosage

► **Isotretinoin:**
  • Severe acne including acne conglobata.
    – 0.2–0.5 mg/kg daily for 4–10 months with a desired total dose of 120 mg/kg.
    – May start with 0.7–1.0 mg/kg daily for first 2–3 months.

- Therapy-resistant less severe acne: 0.2 mg/kg daily for 4–6 months.
- Rosacea, Gram-negative folliculitis, severe sebaceous hyperplasia: No firm guidelines, but usually 0.2–0.5 mg/kg daily for 2–6 months; effects less dramatic and less permanent than with acne.

► **Acitretin:**

- Psoriasis: 0.3–1.0 mg/kg daily for 2–4 months; often combined with phototherapy.
- Other inflammatory dermatoses (pityriasis rubra pilaris, lichen planus, hyperkeratotic hand dermatitis, Reiter syndrome, pustular disorders); dosages similar to psoriasis.
- Genodermatoses: Generally lower doses, 0.2–0.4 mg/kg daily.
- ☒ *Note:* When treating disorders of keratinization, treatment must be continued for months to years. Whenever it is stopped, the disease can be expected to recur. Tricks include higher initial dosages to gain control, then lower maintenance dosages, and therapy-free intervals.

► **Bexarotene:**

- Dosage: 300 mg/m² daily; adjusted to 200 mg/m² and then 100 mg/m² depending on tolerability and effectiveness.
- Used for advanced stages of cutaneous T-cell lymphoma.
- Response rate 50%; exact indications remain to be determined.

Side Effects

► **Teratogenicity:** Single most troublesome side effect. Responsible for numerous medico-legal problems in USA. Well-defined embryopathy. Women must not only practice meticulous contraception while taking medication but must continue for at least 1 month after stopping isotretinoin and 2 years after stopping acitretin.

► **Mucosal disease:** The problem is dryness, which effects every patient—cheilitis, conjunctivitis, dry eyes, dry nose with nosebleeds, dry mouth. The effects are reversible and can usually be controlled with lubrication, artificial tears, and artificial saliva.

► **Skin:** Dry skin, alopecia, and brittle nails are all common. The dry skin is desirable in acne patients, but less so in those with papulo-squamous or keratinization disorders.

► **Depression:** Ongoing controversy over the role of isotretinoin in depression and suicidal ideation in teenagers.

► **Liver function:** Abnormal liver function tests common but rarely clinically significant in teenagers. In adults, careful monitoring required.

► **Lipid metabolism:** Elevated triglycerides and cholesterol are the rule, not the exception. Once again, in teenagers, rarely necessary to stop or alter therapy. In adults or those requiring long-term therapy, major problem with risk of pancreatitis and acerbated cardiovascular disease.

► **Skeletal problems:**

- *Arthralgias* and *myalgias* are common.
- ☒ *Note:* Do not treat teenage athletes during their active season. The effects are sufficient to interfere with performance.
- *Hyperostosis:* Children treated for longer periods of time, as is the case in disorders of keratinization, are at risk to develop **d**iffuse **i**diopathetic **s**keletal **h**yperostosis (DISH syndrome) involving the spine.
- *Calcification:* Tendons and ligaments, especially of distal legs, may be calcified.

► **Others:**

- Pseudotumor cerebri.
- Impaired night vision.
- Hyperthyroidism (bexarotene).

42.7 Corticosteroids

Mechanism of action: Corticosteroids are secreted in a circadian fashion with maximum production in the early morning. For this reason, they should be prescribed in a single morning dose to minimize adrenal suppression or in divided doses to maximize immunosuppressive effects in emergency situations.

► A relatively low dose (prednisolone 10 mg daily) over a period of weeks is sufficient to induce adrenal suppression, so systemic corticosteroids must always be tapered. There is no clear benefit to administering ACTH instead of corticosteroids.

► The physiologic and pharmacologic actions of corticosteroids help explain the side effects and include:

- *Gluconeogenesis*, leading to diabetes mellitus and a catabolic state with osteoporosis (hip fractures) and muscle atrophy.
- *Fat mobilization*, leading to redistribution of body fat (moon facies, buffalo hump).
- Increased numbers of neutrophils, decreased numbers of lymphocytes with suppression of T and B cell activity, leading to increased risk of infections, but providing the *profound immunosuppressive effects*.
- Increased numbers of erythrocytes and thrombocytes leading to *thrombotic state*.
- Multiple *anti-inflammatory mechanisms* with reduced wound healing, striae as side effects.
- *Hypocalcemia* worsening osteoporosis.
- *Mineralocorticoid effects* of sodium retention and potassium excretion leading to fluid retention, weight gain, and hypertension. Glucocorticoids are about 1:1000 as potent as aldosterone, but at higher dose, clinically significant.

► **Available agents:** Only a limited number of agents is needed; almost every dermatologic condition that requires systemic corticosteroids can be managed with prednisolone. a selected list of glucocorticoids, referred to throughout this book as corticosteroids, is shown in Table 42.**2**.

► **Indications:** The indications for systemic corticosteroids are lengthy. They are summarized, along with the dosage and administration guidelines, in Table 42.**3**.

*Table 42.2 · **Systemic corticosteroids***

Agent	Relative potency	Cushing dosage (mg/day)	Comments
Hydrocortisone	1	30	Used for replacement therapy
Prednisolone	4	8	Standard agent
Prednisone	4	8	Converted to prednisolone; interchangeable
Methylprednisolone	5	6	Available i.v. form pulse therapy
Triamcinolone	5	6	Often used intralesionally; in past also i.m. for prolonged effect but no longer so employed. No mineralocorticoid effect
Dexamethasone	30	1	More rapid action; used in shock, cerebral edema, brain metastases

Table 42.3 · Indications for systemic corticosteroids

Regimen	Indications	Comments
Short-term, medium dose	Severe allergic contact dermatitis (poison ivy)	More effective than topical corticosteroids
	Drug reactions	Often used; little data
	Erythema nodosum	Rule out infections first
	Erythema multiforme	Works fine even if HSV present
	Hemangioma	
	Lichen planus (exanthematous form)	Treat for 6–8 weeks
	Leukocytoclastic vasculitis	Often responds to short course
	Sweet syndrome	May require 3–4 weeks
High dose or pulse	Alopecia areata	Pulse
	Angioedema	Single dose
	Jarisch–Herxheimer reaction	Single dose
	Lupus erythematosus	Pulse therapy for CNS disease, severe renal disease, vasculitis
	Pressure urticaria	Sometimes hard to control without bursts
	Pyoderma gangrenosum	May require long-term low dose until healed
Long-term	Autoimmune bullous diseases	May require treatment for months–years
	Connective tissue diseases	May require treatment for months–years
	Sézary syndrome	Modest doses, but long-term
	Vasculitis	Depends on type; usually long-term

- **Contraindications:** Severe infections, osteoporosis, gastrointestinal ulcers, myopathies, psychosis, glaucoma, recurrent thrombosis. In every case, the contraindications are relative and must be weighed against the possible benefits, but also documented and discussed with patient.
- **Drug interactions:** Long list of interactions, including:
  - *Antidiabetics:* Increased blood sugars.
  - *Barbiturates, carbamazepine:* Increased corticosteroid levels.
  - *Estrogens:* Enhanced corticosteroid effects.
  - *Isoniazid:* Reduced levels of isoniazid.
  - *Phenytoin:* Reduced levels of corticosteroids.
  - *Rifampin:* Reduced levels of corticosteroids.
  - See also Table 42.**9**.

▶ **Dosage:** There are a number of general principles to follow in using systemic corticosteroids:

- In dermatologic diseases, corticosteroids are never curative; they only provide symptomatic relief.
- The longer they are used and the higher the dose, the greater the certainty of side effects.

▶ *Note:* It is wise to have a treatment strategy before starting corticosteroids, as their use is a slippery slope. It is often quite difficult to discontinue therapy, and then one is overwhelmed by the negative effects.

- *Short-term medium-dose regimens:*
- Prednisolone 40–60 mg p.o daily for 1–2 weeks as needed.

▶ *Note:* Develop your favorite regimen and always use the same one: this makes answering questions easier. One possibility is 60 mg daily for 4 days, 40 mg daily for 4 days, 20 mg daily for 4 days, and stop.

- *Short-term high-dose and pulse regimens:*
  - Prednisolone 80–120 mg p.o daily.
  - Methylprednisolone 500 mg i.v. q12 h for 3–5 days.
- *Long-term therapy:*
  - Prednisolone, starting at dosages of 80–120 mg to obtain disease control and then tapering as soon as possible, switching to q.o.d. regimens and using steroid-sparing agents to minimize size effects.
  - Goal is prednisolone 10 mg p.o. in morning; even at this level, both osteoporosis and Cushing syndrome possible.
  - If embarking on long-term therapy, document bone density and institute osteoporosis prophylaxis. Typical regimen includes calcium (1.0–1.5 g daily, depending on diet, vitamin D (400 IU daily), and often bisphosphonate (alendronate 5 mg daily), as well as weight-bearing exercise.
  - Exclude inactive tuberculosis.

▮ *Caution:* Three common dermatologic diseases require special mention:

- *Atopic dermatitis:* Rapid response to corticosteroids, but equally rapid flare when stopped. Better never to use.
- *Lupus erythematosus:* There are no cutaneous indications for systemic corticosteroids; save this agent for severe systemic problems.
- *Psoriasis:* Best to avoid because of limited effectiveness and inevitable flare when corticosteroids are tapered. Withdrawal may lead to pustular psoriasis in patients who have previously not had this form.

▶ **Side effects:** Most of the side effects have been alluded to under the mechanism of action. They include:

- *Osteoporosis:* After 6 months, 50% have osteoporosis; incidence of hip fracture varies from 4–25% depending on duration and patient group.
- *Hypertension:* Careful monitoring, routine care.
- *Diabetes mellitus:* Monitor those at risk for diabetes mellitus and carefully control those with the disease.
- Be alert for accompanying *infections*.
- Most other side effects fall under *Cushing syndrome* (p. 318).

42.8 Immunosuppressive Agents

Because of the many side effects of long-term corticosteroid therapy, and because of the failure of some conditions to respond to corticosteroids, a wide number of other immunosuppressive agents are employed.

Azathioprine
....

- **Mechanism of action:** Purine antagonist that interferes with NK, T, and B cells.
- **Indications:** The steroid-sparing agent of choice in LE, dermatomyositis, and overlap syndromes, as well as in transplantation medicine. Also useful in many forms of vasculitis, Behçet syndrome, pyoderma gangrenosum, and chronic actinic dermatitis.
- **Contraindications:** Pregnancy, liver disease, bone marrow damage, active infections.
- **Drug interactions:** Allopurinol increases toxicity of azathioprine.
- **Precautions:** Thiopurine methyltransferase (TPMT) levels should be measured before starting therapy; individuals with low activity (genetic polymorphism) will experience greater immunosuppression.
- Monitor CBC, hemoglobin, platelets; if neutrophils drop below 3000/µL.
- **Dosage:** 1–3 mg/kg p.o. daily (3–5 mg/kg in transplantation medicine). If no response, increase dose cautiously but remember that response to azathioprine is slow. Some patients once under control do amazingly well on q.o.d. doses.
- **Side effects:**
  - Leukopenia, thrombocytopenia, pancytopenia.
  - Pancreatitis.
  - Nausea, vomiting, toxic hepatitis, arthralgias, stomatitis.
  - Long-term risk of increased cutaneous malignancies.

Chlorambucil
....

- **Mechanism of action:** Alkylating agent that interferes with DNA synthesis.
- **Indications:** Best established combined with corticosteroids in pemphigus vulgaris, mycosis fungoides, and Sézary syndrome; widely used in hematologic oncology.
- **Contraindications:** Pregnancy, bone marrow damage, acute infections.
- **Drug interactions:** Phenylbutazone, phenobarbital, vitamin A increase toxicity.
- **Precautions:** Men should avoid fathering a child for 6 months after conclusion of therapy; sperm storage recommended in oncology patients.
- **Dosage:** No established dose in dermatologic disease; in Winkelmann regimen for Sézary syndrome usual dosage is 4 mg daily, increase to 6 or 8 mg possible, with close monitoring of CBC and platelets.
- **Side effects:**
  - Bone marrow suppression.
  - Gastrointestinal toxicity rare.
  - Mucositis, peripheral neuropathy.
  - Rare but serious toxic hepatitis and pulmonary fibrosis.
  - Reproductive side effects (azoospermia with > 400 mg).

Cyclophosphamide
....

- **Mechanism of action:** Alkylating agent, blocks DNA and RNA.
- **Indications:** Steroid-sparing agent in pemphigus vulgaris; also used in LE, vasculitis, Wegener granulomatosis, pyoderma gangrenosum, Behçet syndrome. Widely used in oncologic therapy, especially for hematologic malignancies.
- **Contraindications:** Pregnancy, reduced bone marrow function.
- **Drug interactions:**
  - *Allopurinol:* Increases cyclophosphamide toxicity.
  - *Digoxin:* Reduced absorption of digoxin tablets.
  - *Succinylcholine:* Neuromuscular blockade prolonged.
  - *Warfarin:* Decreased effectiveness.

► **Dosage:**
- *Routine therapy:* 1–3 mg/kg p.o. daily.
- *Pulse therapy:*
  - *Oral:* 15 mg/kg in single dose; once monthly.
  - *Intravenous:* 500 mg 1.0 g/m^2 once monthly; hydrate aggressively before hand to reduce bladder toxicity and administer mesna.

► **Side effects:**
- Cardiotoxicity, hepatotoxicity.
- Myelosuppression, thrombocytopenia, leukopenia, pancytopenia.
- Nausea, vomiting, diarrhea.
- Hemorrhagic cystitis (<5% except with pulse therapy).
- Sterility, azoospermia, amenorrhea.
- Alopecia.

Cyclosporine

► **Mechanism of action:** Cyclosporine inhibits helper T-cell function by blocking interleukin (IL)-2 function; also blocks other lymphokine release including IL-1, IL-3, IL-8, tumor necrosis factor (TNF) α and INF-γ.

► **Indications:** Standard for many years in transplantation medicine. In dermatology used in severe therapy-resistant psoriasis, severe or erythrodermic atopic dermatitis, severe hand dermatitis, pyoderma gangrenosum, and autoimmune diseases.

► **Contraindications:** Underlying malignancy, hypertension, renal disease; pregnancy; active infection.

► **Drug interactions:** Many interactions that require close attention:
- *Methotrexate:* Increases toxicity of both agents.
- *Aminoglycosides, amphotericin B, co-trimoxazole, NSAIDS, sulfonamides:* Increase nephrotoxicity.
- *Amiodarone, anabolic steroids, chloroquine, imidazoles, macrolides, oral contraceptives, retinoids:* Increase cyclosporine levels.
- *Calcium channel blockers:* Diltiazem and verapamil increase cyclosporine levels; others do not.
- *Carbamazepine, co-trimoxazole, phenytoin, rifampicin, sulfonamides:* Reduce cyclosporine levels.
- *Digitalis:* Cyclosporine raises levels.
- *HMG-CoA reductase inhibitors:* Risk of myopathy.

► **Precautions:**
- Before starting therapy, obtain CBC, creatinine, BUN, uric acid, bilirubin, liver function tests, potassium and lipids; check urine.
- Every 2 weeks, check blood pressure, renal status, uric acid, and potassium.
- Prompt attention to infections.

► **Dosage:**
- 2.5–5.0 mg/kg p.o. daily. Usually start at 2.5 mg/kg; work up if no response within 2 weeks; be prepared to taper down.
- Dosage reductions required:
  - If *creatinine* exceeds pretreatment or normal value by 30%.
  - If *potassium* exceeds normal values.
  - If *bilirubin or liver enzymes* exceed pretreatment or normal values by 200%.
  - *and* the increase persists for 2 weeks, then reduce cyclosporine dose by 25%. If not normalized within 2 weeks, must stop drug.
  - If diastolic blood pressure >95 mm Hg, reduce dose or stop. Treat hypertension with nifedipine, which does not interact with cyclosporine.

▶ **Side effects:**
- Renal failure.
- Leukopenia.
- Hypertension (50–90%).
- Headache, tremors.
- Gingival hyperplasia, oral candidiasis.
- Hirsutism.
- ⚠ *Caution:* Patients should avoid UV radiation because of increased risk of cutaneous malignancies. Cyclosporine should not be combined with phototherapy.

Methotrexate

▶ **Mechanism of action:** Folic acid antagonist.

▶ **Indications:** Severe psoriasis, psoriatic arthritis, bullous pemphigoid.

▶ **Contraindications:**
- *Absolute:* Pregnancy, gastrointestinal ulcer, hepatic cirrhosis.
- *Relative:*
  - Renal or hepatic dysfunction, hepatitis, alcoholism.
  - Anemia, leukopenia, thrombocytopenia.
  - Desire for children.
  - Severe infections.
- ⚠ *Caution:* Both men and women should practice contraception for 12 months after taking methotrexate.

▶ **Drug interactions:**
- *Binding resins:* Reduce methotrexate levels.
- *Co-trimoxazole, NSAIDS, omeprazole, penicillin, probenecid, salicylates:* Increase methotrexate levels.
- *Cyclosporine:* Increase toxicity of both agents.
- *Phenytoin:* Reduce levels of phenytoin.

▶ **Precautions:**
- Avoid alcohol and salicylates when on methotrexate; use NSAIDS with caution.
- Increase fluid intake.
- Monitor liver status; risk of hepatic fibrosis.
- ☐ *Note:* Changes in routine liver function tests are a poor predictor of the development of hepatic fibrosis.
  - Serum procollagen III aminopeptide (PIIINP) levels are the most sensitive indicator of hepatic fibrosis; if they remain normal, liver biopsy is not needed.
  - Other centers employ sonographic evaluation of liver every 6 months.
- ⚠ *Caution:* Consult with hepatologist regarding liver biopsy if PIIINP increases, sonographic picture changes or once total dose > 1.5 g. Adjust strategy to national guidelines.
- *Other laboratory tests.*
  - *Before treatment:* CBC, hemoglobin, leukocytes, thrombocytes; renal function; chest radiograph.
  - *During treatment:*
  - CBC, leukocytes, thrombocytes weekly at first, then monthly. If leukocyte count < 3000/μL or platelet count < 100 000/μL, withhold therapy.
  - Renal function every 3 months.

▶ **Dosage:**
- *Oral:*
  - 7.5–25 mg p.o. once weekly.
  - *Weinstein regimen:* 2.5–7.5 mg q12 h × 3; repeat weekly.
- *Parenteral:* 10–25 mg i.m. or i.v. once weekly.

■ *Note:* The dermatologic dosages should never be confused with the considerably higher dosages employed in oncology. The lessons learned from rheumatology using low-dose methotrexate for rheumatoid arthritis are valuable; most dermatologists employ < 15 mg weekly of methotrexate and encounter few problems.

▶ **Side effects:**
  • Bone marrow suppression with leukopenia, thrombocytopenia, pancytopenia and hemorrhage: Despite the concerns over liver disease, the greatest risk to patients on methotrexate is profound hematologic problems. An antidote is available—leukovorin 12 mg i. m. q6h for 4–6 doses.
  • Hepatotoxicity: See precautions for discussion of monitoring. The duration (> 3 years) and total dose (> 1.5–2.0 g) are key risk factors for hepatic fibrosis. After long-term use, about 10% have hepatic fibrosis and 3% cirrhosis.
  • Pulmonary fibrosis.
  • Gastrointestinal bleeding, anorexia, nausea, vomiting.
  • Renal failure.
  • Seizures.
  • Defective spermatogenesis.
  • Stomatitis, alopecia, reactivation of phototoxic disorders.
  • *Cutaneous ulcerations:*
    – *Superficial:* Erosions and ulcers of psoriatic plaques; heal rapidly when dose is lowered.
    – *Deep:* Develop in damaged skin (stasis dermatitis); very persistent.
  ■ *Note:* Remember, most of these catastrophic side effects occur during oncologic therapy. Nonetheless, the dermatologist cannot afford to ignore them.

Mycophenolate mofetil

▶ **Mechanism of action:** Inhibits inosine monophosphate dehydrogenase, an essential enzyme in guanidine nucleotide synthesis, in lymphocytes. The enzyme is scarcely influenced in other cells and tissues. Also influences mast cell degranulation and lipoxygenase activity.

▶ **Indications:**
  • Psoriasis vulgaris, as monotherapy or combined with topical medications.
  • Severe cases of atopic dermatitis, dyshidrotic dermatitis.
  • Widely used in transplantation medicine as steroid-sparing agent; now used in same way in pemphigus vulgaris, bullous pemphigoid, vasculitis, pyoderma gangrenosum, and other corticosteroid-responsive disorders.

▶ **Contraindications:** Pregnancy, nursing; caution with history of gastrointestinal ulcer or renal disease.

▶ **Drug interactions:**
  • *Acyclovir, ganciclovir:* Levels of both antivirals and mycophenolate mofetil increased.
  • *Antacids:* Reduced absorption.
  • *Probenecid:* Increases levels of mycophenolate mofetil.
  • *Resins:* Decreased absorption.
  • *Retinoids:* Decreased levels of both agents.
  ■ *Note:* Routinely combined with cyclosporine in transplant patients; has less bone marrow toxicity than azathioprine and is replacing it in many settings; latter two should not be combined with azathioprine.

▶ **Precautions:**
  • CBC weekly for 1 month, then tapered to every 2 weeks and then monthly.
  • Hepatic and renal function pretreatment, after 1 month and then every 2–3 months.

▶ **Dosage:** 500 mg 2–4 × daily.
▶ **Side effects:**
  • Bone marrow suppression with leukopenia, thrombocytopenia, anemia.
  • Pain, headache.
  • Hypertension.
  • Nausea, vomiting, diarrhea.
  • Increased risk of infections.

42.9 *Biologicals*

▶ **Definition:** Biologicals or immunobiologicals are molecules capable of altering the normal cellular immune response; they are usually molecules designed to interrupt pathways of cell signaling, activation and cytokine production.
▶ **Nomenclature:** The naming of biologicals is initially confusing, but in fact easily understandable. The following terms are used:
  • *mab:* Monoclonal antibody.
  • *cept:* Fusion protein with receptor effect.
  • *mu:* Human antibody.
  • *xi:* Chimeric (mouse-human) antibody.
  • *zu:* Humanized mouse antibody.
  • *li:* Anti-inflammatory.
▶ For example, Inf-li-xi-mab is an anti-inflammatory, chimeric, monoclonal antibody.
▣ *Note:* At this time (January 2006), many biologicals are approved and under review for a perplexing range of indications, varying from one regulatory agency to the next. Consult Internet sources for latest information in your country. The biologicals used for psoriasis are considered in detail elsewhere (p. 271).

42.10 *Antiemetic Therapy*

Overview
....
Dermatologists in Germany administer chemotherapy for malignant melanoma and other tumors. A crucial part of cancer chemotherapy is antiemetic therapy, as anorexia, nausea, and vomiting are the most common side effects. Drugs such as DTIC and cisplatin induce vomiting in > 90% of patients. Vomiting is triggered by 5-hydroxytryptamine (5-HT3) and dopamine receptors in the gastrointestinal tract and CNS (zona postrema).

Antiemetic Agents
....
▶ **Antihistamines:** Several categories minimally effective.
▶ **Dopamine receptor antagonists:** Metoclopramide 10–20 mg q4 h.
▶ **Serotonin receptor antagonists (5-HT3-RA):** Ondansetron 16–32 mg i.v.; then 8 mg q12 h i.v. or tropisetron 5 mg i.v., then 5 mg i.v. or p.o.
▶ **Corticosteroids:** Dexamethasone 10–20 mg i.v. before chemotherapy.
▶ **Phenothiazine:** Triflupromazine 10–30 mg q4 h.
▶ **Benzodiazepine:** Diazepam 10 mg before starting chemotherapy, then 5 mg daily.
  • *Highly emetogenic regimens:* 5-HT3-RA + antihistamines + dexamethasone + diazepam.

- *Delayed vomiting (often from cisplatin):* 5-HT3-RA + dexamethasone.
- *Anticipatory vomiting:* 5-HT3-RA + diazepam.
- ⚠ *Caution:* Combinations are preferred to maximum dosages. 5-HT3-RA can cause extrapyramidal signs and symptoms. Dexamethasone should not be used in patients receiving immunotherapy.

42.11 Pain Therapy

Overview

The other mainstay of care for tumor patients is adequate pain relief, which is the single greatest factor in increasing qualify of life for these unfortunate people. Basic principles of pain therapy include:

▶ Always work together with pain center or pain therapy specialists.
▶ Try to manage with oral agents. Infusion of i. v. agents should be reserved for those who are still uncomfortable with oral therapy.
▶ Continuous infusion or on-demand infusion are preferred to bolus injection of pain medications.
▶ Do not be afraid to use the agents in their maximum therapeutic range.
▶ Adjuvants are effective in increasing the effect of pain drugs (Table 42.4).
▶ Be alert to side effects; opiates always cause constipation, so provide laxatives or stool softeners.
▶ Pay close attention to potential drug interactions.
▶ **Dosage:** A modified stepwise therapy scheme is shown in Table 42.5.
  ⚠ *Caution:* The agents and adjuvants used for pain relief have a vast number of drug interactions. Discussion of these exceeds the limits of a dermatology text, but if you are treating pain patients you must inform yourself about this aspect.

Table 42.4 · Adjuvant pain therapy

Indication	Agent	Dose
Depression	Tricyclic antidepressant (clomipramine)	25 mg HS, may increase to 25 mg t.i.d. or 75 mg in time release dose
Burning dysesthesia (neuropathy)	Haloperidol	3 × 0.5 – 1.0 mg
Nerve compression, increased CNS pressure	Dexamethasone	4 mg i.v.; can repeat 3–6 × daily
Intermittent, lancinating pain	Carbamazepine	2 × 200 mg daily; maximum 800 mg daily
	Valproic acid	3 × 300 mg daily; maximum 4 × 600 mg
Muscle spasms	Muscle relaxants (Baclofen)	3 × 5 mg; maximum 3 × 25 mg

Table 42.5 · Stepwise approach to pain therapy

Agent	Duration (hours)	Dose (24 hours)
1st stage + adjuvants		
Paracetamol	4	4–6 × 0.5–1.0 g
Ibuprofen	3–4	4–6 × 400–600 mg
Diclofenac	4–8	2–3 × 100 mg
Metamizole	4–6	4–6 × 0.5–1.0 g
2nd stage (+ above and adjuvants)		
Tramadol	4–8	4–6 × 50–100 mg
Codeine	2–3	4–6 × 20–100 mg
Tilidine–naloxone	8–10	2–3 × 100–200 mg
3rd stage (+ above and adjuvants)		
Morphine sulfate drops or suppository	2–4	4–8 × 10–30 mg
Morphine sulfate time-release	12	2–3 × 30–80 mg
Buprenorphine	>30	2–3 × 0.2–0.4 mg
Fentanyl TTS (transdermal)	48–72	0.6–6.0 mg daily
4th stage		
Peridural or subcutaneous opiates; regional anesthesia		

Modified from WHO guidelines; see also www.painweb.de

42.12 Miscellaneous Agents

Clofazimine

◪ **Note:** Not readily available in most countries; check with public health authorities.
► **Mechanism of action:** Phenazine dye used in leprosy therapy; has antineutrophil effect, but mechanisms unknown.
► **Indications:** Approved for leprosy and erythema nodosum leprosum; incorporated into some regimens against *Mycobacterium avium-intracellulare*; often tried for Melkersson–Rosenthal syndrome, pyoderma gangrenosum, necrobiosis lipoidica, granuloma annulare, and granuloma facile. Formerly recommended for pustular psoriasis but not effective.
► **Contraindications:** Pregnancy.
► **Dosage:** 100 mg daily–t.i.d.; reduce with clinical response; long-term therapy possible.
► **Side effects:**
  • Nausea and vomiting.
  • *Long-term use:* Eosinophilic enteritis, crystal deposition enteropathy.

- Pink to brown discoloration of skin, tears, urine, sweat, and other bodily fluids may persist long after therapy is stopped.

Colchicine

▶ **Mechanism of action:** Inhibits microtubular system, thus interfering with cell division, migration, other neutrophil functions, collagen synthesis, and deposition of amyloid.
▶ **Indications:** Mainstay of gout therapy. In dermatology used for Behçet syndrome, vasculitis, and amyloid deposition primarily in familial Mediterranean fever.
▶ **Contraindications:** Pregnancy; established teratogen.
▶ **Drug interactions:**
  • *Cyclosporine:* Increased levels of cyclosporine.
▶ **Precautions:** Check CBC, platelets before therapy and then every 2 weeks, later every 1–2 months.
▶ **Dosage:** Start with 0.5–1.0 mg daily; maximum tolerated dose is 1.5–2.0 mg daily. Try to reduce as soon as possible.
▶ **Side effects:**
  • Thrombocytopenia, pancytopenia, agranulocytosis, aplastic anemia: Rare and idiosyncratic.
  • Nausea, vomiting, diarrhea: Inevitable, almost everyone at 1.5 mg daily has problems.
  • Azoospermia, myopathy, alopecia.

Cyproterone

▶ **Mechanism of action:** Antiandrogen.
▶ **Indications:**
  • *Low-dose with estrogens:* Acne, hirsutism, androgenic alopecia.
  • *Mid-dose:* Severe hyperandrogenism.
  • *High-dose:* Prostate carcinoma; reduction of sexual drive in sexual offenders.
▶ **Contraindications:** Pregnancy, severe hepatic dysfunction, thromboembolic disease, estrogen-dependent tumors.
▶ **Dosage:**
  • *Low-dose:* 2 mg cyproterone and 0.035 mg ethinyl estradiol on days 5–25 of menstrual cycle.
  • *Mid-dose:* 2 mg cyproterone and 0.035 mg ethinyl estradiol + 10 mg additional cyproterone on days 5–19.
  • Treatment must be continued for months to years. The mid-dose should be reserved for severe hirsutism.
▶ **Side effects:** Headache, nausea, vomiting, weight gain, breast tenderness, irregular menses, mood changes, loss of libido.
▣ *Note:* Not available in USA.

Fumaric Acid Ester

Fumaric acid is the trans isomer of maleic acid. The natural product contains a variety of esters complexed with different salts; a standardized product is available in Germany.
▶ **Mechanism of action:** Blocks NFκB signaling and thus many aspects of inflammatory reaction; also effects on apoptosis, cytokine production and dendritic cell function.
▶ **Indications:** Moderate to severe psoriasis.
▶ **Contraindications:** Pregnancy, severe or chronic gastrointestinal disease.

▶ **Dosage:** Fumaric acid is available as.
- *Fumaderm initial:* 30 mg dimethyl fumarate, 67 mg ethyl hydrogen calcium fumarate, and small amounts of the zinc and magnesium salts.
- *Fumaderm:* 120 mg dimethyl fumarate, 87 mg ethyl hydrogen calcium fumarate, and small amounts of the zinc and magnesium salts.
- The recommended mode of administration is shown in Table 42.**6**.

Table 42.6 · Dosage scheme for Fumaderm

Day	Morning	Noon	Night	Form
1–3	0	0	1	Fumaderm Initial
4–6	1	0	1	Fumaderm Initial
7–9	1	1	1	Fumaderm Initial
10–12	1	1	2	Fumaderm Initial
13–15	2	1	2	Fumaderm Initial
16–18	2	2	2	Fumaderm Initial
19–21	0	0	1	Fumaderm
22–24	1	0	1	Fumaderm
35–27	1	1	1	Fumaderm
28–30	1	1	2	Fumaderm
31–33	2	1	2	Fumaderm
34–36	2	2	2	Fumaderm

Then continue with 2–2–2

Precautions: Follow laboratory parameters as shown in Table 42.7.

▶ **Dosage reduction:** Follow laboratory parameters as shown in Table 42.**7**. If the following parameters are obtained, then the dosage should be reduced to previously tolerated level; if problems persist, medication should be stopped.
- WBC < 4000/μL.
- Lymphocytes < 500/μL.
- Creatinine > 30% of initial value.
- Proteinuria.
- Persistent eosinophilia (> 25% for > 6 weeks).

Table 42.7 · Laboratory testing in patients receiving fumaric acid esters

Time	CBC	Liver enzymes	Renal function, urine status
Before therapy	Yes	Yes	Yes
1st month	Every 14 days	Once	Once
2nd month	Every 14 days	Once	Once
3rd month	Every 14 days	Once	Once
4th month (if no problems)	Once	Once	Once

▶ **Side effects:**
- To begin with, diarrhea and flushing are common, but they usually resolve with continued therapy.
- Lymphopenia, leukopenia.
- Nephrotoxicity with proteinuria.

Thalidomide

▶ **Mechanism of action:** Another antineutrophil medication with unclear mechanisms; may have anti-TNF effect. Originally used as mild sedative, but turned out to be potent teratogen, producing characteristic limb defects.
▶ **Indications:** Agent of choice for erythema nodosum leprosum; effective in Behçet syndrome, severe aphthosis, pyoderma gangrenosum, LE (especially hyperkeratotic variants), and prurigo nodularis.
▶ **Contraindications:** Women of childbearing age must use double contraception; signed, witnessed informed consent. In most countries, not available as prescription drug but through public health officials or the manufacturer.
▶ **Dosage:** In acute disease, usually start with 300–400 mg daily, but taper rapidly; usual maintenance dosage is 25–100 mg.
  ◨ *Note:* Usually obtained from manufacturer or leprosy treatment centers.
▶ **Side effects:**
- Teratogenic, causing limb defects.
- Peripheral neuropathy (dose-dependent; not always reversible).
- Nausea, vomiting, dizziness, constipation.

42.13 Drug Interactions

Overview

The more systemic medications one employs, the greater the likelihood of an interaction between the two drugs, increasing or decreasing the effectiveness of one or both. It has been estimated that if a patient is taking more than five medications, the likelihood of a drug interaction is 50%; with more than 10 medications, it approaches 100%.

Alert pharmacists, with computerized records of all medications a patient is receiving, can help greatly to alert the physicians to possible problems. For this reason, every outpatient should be encouraged to use a single pharmacy. As of 2005, patients in Germany receive a slight financial benefit if they do so.

Causes

The major causes of drug interactions are:
▶ **Cytochrome P-450 (CYP):** A group of enzymes involves in the metabolism of many drugs. When increased amount of CYP are induced, increased active metabolites are available and the drug potency increased. Conversely, when production of CYP is impaired, then the potency is reduced. The most important enzyme is CYP3A; its main interactions are shown in Table 42.**8**.
- *Inducers* are medications that increase levels of CYP3A, thus leading to increased metabolism and loss of effectiveness of other drugs.
- *Inhibitors* block CYP3A and thus lead to decreased metabolism and gain in effectiveness.

- The *substrate drugs* are those metabolized primarily by CYP3A, which are thus most influenced. Note that several drugs are both inhibitors and substrates, thus when used they inhibit their own metabolism.
▶ **Renal resorption:** When several agents compete for renal resorption, variations in amount excreted and thus variations in potency are possible.
▶ **Impaired gastrointestinal absorption** because of antacids leads to loss in effectiveness, as does competition for bile acids by resins or different agents.

Table 42.8 · **CYP3A substrates, inhibitors, and inducers**
▫ *Caution:* This table is designed to demonstrate the broad spectrum of CYP3A interactions. Consult more detailed sources when prescribing.

Substrates	Inhibitors	Inducers
Benzodiazepines	*Calcium channel blockers*	*Anticonvulsants*
Calcium channel blockers	Diltiazem	Carbamazepine
Diltiazem	Verapamil	Phenobarbital
Felodipine	*Imidazoles*	Phenytoin
Nifedipine	Itraconazole	*Anti-HIV agents*
Verapamil	Ketoconazole	Some NNRTIs
Immunosuppressive agents	*Macrolides*	*Rifampin (and other*
Cyclosporine	Erythromycin	*rifamycins)*
Tacrolimus	Clarithromycin	*Others*
Macrolides	*Not azithromycin;*	St. John's wort
Erythromycin	*thus few interactions*	
Clarithromycin	*Protease inhibitors*	
Protease inhibitors	*Others*	
Statins (not all)	Grapefruit juice	
Others	Mifepristone	
Losartan		
Sildenafil		

Based on Table 2 in Wilkinson GR. Drug metabolism and variability among patients in drug response. N Engl J Med 2005; 352:2211–21.

Table 42.9 · Drug interactions for systemic dermatologic agents

⚠ Caution: This table summarizes the most important drug interactions for the systemic agents discussed in the chapter. It is not intended to be exhaustive, but rather designed to highlight severe or common reactions. The multiple interactions associated with antiemetic and pain therapeutic agents are not listed; they should be sought in specialized books. Always check latest prescribing information for information on drug interactions.

Interaction with	Effect
Antibiotics	
Macrolides (erythromycin, clarithromycin)	Potent inhibitor of CYP3A (Table 42.**8**); always check for all possible interactions before prescribing
Astemizole, terfenadine (**both no longer available**)	Levels ↑ with cardiotoxicity
Carbamazepine	Effectiveness ↑
Coumarin	Effectiveness ↑ ↑
Cyclosporine	Levels ↑
Indinavir, other protease inhibitors	Effectiveness of both ↑
Itraconazole	Effectiveness ↑
Penicillin	Effectiveness ↓ ▶ *Note:* Azithromycin only interacts with penicillin
Prednisolone	Effectiveness ↑
Tetracyclines	M = minocycline, D = doxycycline Many agents (antacids, calcium, food, iron, zinc) block absorption with effectiveness ↓
Oral contraceptives	Controversial slight loss of effectiveness
Carbamazepine (D,M)	Antiobiotic ↓
Coumarin (D, m)	Effectiveness ↑
Phenobarbital (D,M)	Antibiotic ↓
Antifungals	
Griseofulvin	
Coumarin	Anticoagulant effect ↓
Oral contraceptives	Menstrual irregularities, increased risk of pregnancy
Penicillin	Cross-reactions possible
Phenobarbital	Griseofulvin ↓
Imidazoles	F = fluconazole, I = itraconazole
Antacids	Absorption ↓; imidazoles down ↓
Astemizole	QT prolongation, arrhythmias (no longer available)
Benzodiazepines	Sedation ↑

Table 42.9 · Continued

Interaction with:	Effect
Antifungals (Continued)	
Calcium channel blockers (I)	Effectiveness ↑
Carbamazepine	Imidazoles ↓
Cimetidine (F)	Fluconazole ↓
Cisapride	Levels of cisapride ↑ , dysrhythmias
Corticosteroids	Effectiveness ↑
Coumarin	Anticoagulant effect ↑
Cyclosporine	Effectiveness ↑
Digoxin	Effectiveness ↑
Estradiol (F)	Effectiveness ↓
Food	Absorption ↑ ; imidazoles ↑
HMG-CoA reductase inhibitors (I)	Effectiveness ↑ ; myopathy, rhabdomyolysis
H2-blockers	Itraconazole absorption ↓ but metabolism also ↓ ; effect variable
Isoniazid (I)	Itraconazole ↓
Omeprazole	Effectiveness ↓
Oral hypoglycemic agents	Antidiabetic effect ↑
Phenobarbital	Itraconazole ↓
Phenytoin	Itraconazole level ↓
Rifampicin	Itraconazole level ↓
Tacrolimus	Effectiveness ↑
Terfenadine	QT prolongation, arrhythmias (no longer available)
Theophylline	Effectiveness ↑
Terbinafine	
Rifampicin	Terbinafine ↓
Tricyclic antidepressants	Terbinafine ↑
Antihistamines	
Most sedating H1	
CNS depressants	Sedation ↑
Astemizole, terfenadine	(No longer available)
Imidazoles	QT prolongation, arrhythmias
Macrolides	QT prolongation, arrhythmias

Continued Table 42.9 ▶

Systemic Therapy

Table 42.9 · Continued

Interaction with:	Effect
Cyproheptadine	
Serotonin antagonists	Effectiveness ↓ with increased suicide risk
Fexofenadine	
Macrolides	Fexofenadine ↑
Loratadine	
Imidazoles	Levels ↑ but not clinically manifest
Macrolides	Levels ↑ but not clinically manifest
Promethazine	
CNS depressants	Effectiveness ↑
Antiviral agents	
Acyclovir	
Cimetidine	Acyclovir ↑
Probenecid	Acyclovir ↑
Theophylline	Effectiveness ↑
Brivudin	
5-fluorouracil, other fluoropyrimidine	Effectiveness ↑
Azathioprine	
Allopurinol	Azathioprine ↑
Tubocurarine	Effectiveness ↓
Clofazimine	
Cyclosporine	Effectiveness ↑
Chlorambucil	
Phenobarbital	Chlorambucil toxicity ↑
Phenylbutazone	Chlorambucil toxicity ↑
Vitamin A	Chlorambucil toxicity ↑
Chloroquine or hydroxychloroquine	
Ampicillin	Effectiveness ↓
Cimetidine	Chloroquine ↑

Table 42.9 · Continued

Interaction with:	Effect
Chloroquine or hydroxychloroquine (Continued)	
Cyclophosphamide	Cyclophosphamide ↑
Cyclosporine	Effectiveness ↑
Digoxin	Effectiveness ↑
Magnesium salts	Absorption ↓, effectiveness ↓; antacids ↓
Metronidazole	Toxicity (dystonia) ↑
Phenylbutazone	Risk of toxic epidermal necrolysis ↑
Colchicine	
Cyclosporine	Effectiveness ↑
Corticosteroids	
Aminoglutethimide	Corticosteroids ↓
Carbamazepine	Corticosteroids ↓
Cholestyramine	Absorption down, corticosteroids ↓
Estrogens	Corticosteroids ↑
Isoniazid	Effectiveness ↓
Ketoconazole	Corticosteroids ↑
Macrolides	Corticosteroids ↑
Oral hypoglycemic agents	Blood sugar ↑
Phenobarbital	Corticosteroids ↓
Phenytoin	Corticosteroids ↓
Rifampin	Corticosteroids ↓
Salicylates	Excretion ↑, effectiveness ↓
Cyclophosphamide	
Allopurinol	Cyclophosphamide ↑
Coumadin	Effectiveness ↓
Digoxin	absorption ↓, effectiveness ↓
Succinylcholine	Neuromuscular blockade ↑
Cyclosporine	Caution: Long list—monitor carefully.
Aminoglycosides	Nephrotoxicity ↑
Amiodarone	Cyclosporine ↑
Amphotericin B	Nephrotoxicity ↑
Anabolic steroids	Cyclosporine ↑

Continued Table 42.9 ▶

Table 42.9 · Continued

Interaction with:	Effect
Calcium channel blockers	
Diltiazem, verapamil	Cyclosporine ↑
Nifedipine	No interaction
Carbamazepine	Cyclosporine ↓
Chloroquine	Cyclosporine ↑
Co-trimoxazole	Nephrotoxicity ↑, cyclosporine ↓
Digoxin	Effectiveness ↑
HMG-CoA reductase inhibitors	Effectiveness ↑, myopathy, rhabdomyolysis
Imidazoles (all)	Cyclosporine ↑
Macrolides	Cyclosporine ↑
Methotrexate	Both agents ↑, enhanced toxicity
Metoclopramide	Cyclosporine ↑
NSAIDS	Nephrotoxicity ↑
Oral contraceptives	Cyclosporine ↑
Phenytoin	Cyclosporine ↓
Rifampin	Cyclosporine ↓
Sulfonamides	Nephrotoxicity ↑, cyclosporine ↓
Dapsone	
Didanosine	Dapsone ↓
Probenecid	Dapsone ↑
Trimethoprim (co-trimoxazole)	Blocked excretion, both ↑
Methotrexate	
Charcoal, binding resins	Methotrexate ↓
Co-trimoxazole	Methotrexate ↑
Cyclosporine	Both agents ↑, enhanced toxicity
NSAIDs	Methotrexate ↑
Omeprazole	Methotrexate ↑
Penicillin	Methotrexate ↑
Phenytoin	Methotrexate ↑
Probenecid	Methotrexate ↑
Retinoids	Hepatotoxicity ↑ (especially acitretin)
Salicylates	Methotrexate ↑
Sulfonamides	Methotrexate ↑; also folate deficiency ↑

Interaction with:	Effect

Table 42.9 · Continued

Mycophenolate mofetil

Acyclovir, ganciclovir	Both ↑
Antacids	Mycophenolate mofetil ↓
Binding resins	Mycophenolate mofetil ↓
Probenecid	Mycophenolate mofetil ↑
Retinoids	Both ↓

Retinoids

Cyclosporine	Retinoids ↑
Methotrexate	Hepatotoxicity ↑ (especially acitretin)
NSAIDs	Retinoids ↑
Phenobarbital	Effectiveness ↑
Phenytoin	Effectiveness ↑
Tetracycline	Also causes pseudotumor cerebri
Vitamin A	Toxicity ↑

43 *Radiation Therapy*

Overview

Ionizing radiation has long been known to have effects on the skin. The early pioneers, including Pierre Curie, experienced erythema and ulceration after exposure. Many of the advances in radiation therapy were made by dermatologists. Today, a combination of surgical advances, public fear of X-rays, and simple office economics threaten the existence of cutaneous radiation therapy.

Definitions

▶ **Radiation:** Energy transmitted through space or medium by waves.
▶ **Ionizing radiation:** High-energy radiation.
▶ **Dose:** Energy administered to a volume.
▶ **Rad** (radiation absorbed dose): The absorbed dose of ionizing radiation, resulting from the transfer of 0.01 J of energy to 1 kg kilogram of tissue. Now superseded by Gray.
▶ **Gray (Gy):** Standard unit; 1 Gy = 100 rad.
▶ **Dose rate:** Dose per unit time or intensity. The dose rate varies inversely with the square of the source-skin distance (target-skin distance); known as inverse square law.
▶ **Half-value layer (HVL):** The thickness of a given substance that reduces the intensity of a beam of radiation to $1/2$ of its original value (half-value thickness).
 • Both the nature of the absorbing material and the energy of the radiation determine how much diminution occurs.
▶ **Half-value depth (HVD):** The depth in a given tissue at which $1/2$ of the surface dose is administered.

Sources

▶ **Soft or superficial radiation:** Uses high-energy photons produced by traditional dermatologic X-ray machines with combination of filters; capable of producing HVD of 2.0–5.0 mm.
▶ **Electron beam:** Uses electrons produce by linear accelerator; electrons lose energy rapidly when penetrating skin; can be applied to entire skin surface.

Indications

Malignant tumors
▶ The ideal tumor for radiation treatment is a relatively superficial basal cell carcinoma, perhaps in a difficult surgical site in a patient who requires anticoagulation. Common indications include basal cell carcinoma, squamous cell carcinoma, lymphoma, and Kaposi sarcoma.
▶ Malignant melanoma is not usually irradiated, except for lentigo maligna melanoma in situ.
▶ Merkel cell carcinoma is best treated with excision and radiation therapy.
▶ A histological diagnosis should be available before radiation therapy is planned. Often the dermatopathologist can measure the depth of tumor, making more precise treatment possible.
▶ Radiation therapy may be used for palliative treatment of inoperable tumors.
▶ Electron beam therapy can be tailored for treated cutaneous malignancies, usually using a surface gel bolus to concentrate the dosage more superficially.

➤ The main indication for electron beam is total skin electron beam therapy (TSEBT) for mycosis fungoides. In specialized centers, this is an effective first line treatment, which induces relatively long remissions but apparently few cures. Electron beam can also be used in more advanced cutaneous lymphomas, as well as in larger or deep basal cell carcinomas, as a higher dose at depth can be achieved.

Benign conditions

➤ In the past a wide variety of conditions were treated with radiation therapy, including plantar warts, psoriasis, acne, and hirsutism. In each instance, the treatment was temporarily effective but in most cases overused, leading to radiation dermatitis and secondary tumors.

➤ Keloids are perhaps the only benign condition that can be considered for radiation therapy today.

Treatment Regimens

➤ Exact treatment plans should be determined by physicians experienced in radiation therapy. Today the trend is to use fractionated dosages, which provide better sparing of normal tissue.

➤ Basal cell carcinoma and squamous cell carcinoma are usually treated with around 50 Gy—either 6 Gy × 8 sessions or 12 Gy × 4, or variations in between.

➤ Lentigo maligna melanoma in situ requires a higher dose, around 100 Gy, often fractioned over 20 sessions.

➤ Kaposi sarcoma and most lymphomas are much more radiation sensitive; dosage ranges are 20–30 Gy for Kaposi sarcoma and 5–15 Gy for lymphoma, sometimes given in only 1–2 sessions.

Radiation Reactions

➤ **Skin:** Around 4 Gy is sufficient to cause erythema after 1–2 days. The erythema peaks after a week, then resolves, usually with hyperpigmentation. The clinical picture is often more complex as the patient is being repeatedly exposed. As a general rule, up to 8 Gy are tolerated with complete healing. Above this dose, some degree of chronic radiation dermatitis is expected.

➤ **Appendages:**
- 3–4 Gy are sufficient for temporary epilation; 8 Gy can cause permanent loss of hair.
- Sweat and sebaceous glands are also temporarily inhibited by 4 Gy and may suffer permanent damage at 8 Gy.
- ◪ *Note:* These effects explain why ionizing radiation was so popular for acne and hirsutism.

➤ **Radiation dermatitis:**
- *Acute radiation reactions* following therapy or accidental exposure (as in Chernobyl) can be classified as follows:
  - *Grade I:* Erythema.
  - *Grade II:* Vesicles, blisters.
  - *Grade III:* Erosions, ulcers, necrosis.
- *Chronic radiation dermatitis* is the prototype of poikiloderma with telangiectases, hypo- and hyperpigmentation, and atrophy. The tissue also becomes sclerotic and has a tendency to ulcerate and then heal extremely poorly.

➤ **Secondary tumors:** The latency period is 20–30 years, but then the risk of basal cell carcinoma and squamous cell carcinoma is considerable. The tumors are more difficult to treat in the background of radiation dermatitis, and may be intrinsically more aggressive. There is a linear correlation between dose and risk of tumors; no absolutely safe dose has been established.

▶ **Treatment:** There is no effective prophylaxis for radiation dermatitis, other than careful selective of exposure parameters to minimize effects. The surrounding skin must be protected with shielding, usually with lead sheeting. The erythematous phase may be helped by topical corticosteroids or a bland ointment. Once chronic radiation dermatitis has developed, the patient should be instructed in how to best protect the area from subsequent trauma and monitored frequently for the development of radiation keratoses (analogous to actinic keratoses) and more aggressive tumors. If radiation keratoses develop, best to excise entire area of radiation damage if feasible; otherwise treat individual lesions as squamous cell carcinoma in situ.

44 *Therapy During Pregnancy and Nursing*

Overview

▣ *Note:* The basic rules are simple:
► Prescribe as few medications as possible during pregnancy.
► Always have firm indications.
► Use single agents; not mixtures.
► Check every drug prescribed during pregnancy in a reference source.
► Always try topical agents first; absorption is possible, but guaranteed to be less than systemic.
► Oral administration is preferred to intravenous or intramuscular because then the medication is easier to remove from the body.
► Document carefully.

It is relatively simple to follow these rules because every pregnant women shares the concerns of her physicians. The real problem is before a pregnancy has been identified, which can sometimes take months. The most critical period is 15–60 days after conception, as this is the time frame for organogenesis.

Drug Ratings

The categories used to rate drugs for use in pregnancy are shown in Table 44.1.
▨ *Caution:* The dermatologic agents listed in Table 44.2 are either D or X and should not be used. There are other D and X agents; this list is not exhaustive.

Table 44.1 · Rating of drugs for use in pregnancy

Category	Explanation
X	Contraindicated. Never use in pregnancy
D	Evidence of risk for fetus; only use in rare circumstances
C	Possible risk; human studies lacking
B	No risk to humans, or no risk in animals and human studies not performed
A	Controlled studies have shown no risk

Table 44.2 · Contraindicated medications

Category D	Category X
Azathioprine	Acitretin
Colchicine	Estrogens
Cyclophosphamide	Danazol
Hydroxyurea	Finasteride
NSAIDs	Flutamide
Potassium iodide	Isotretinoin
Tetracyclines	Methotrexate
	Stanozolol
	Thalidomide

⚠ Caution: No medication is 100% safe during pregnancy. No common dermatologic agents are category A. Remember that even without medications, pregnancy is fraught with dangers:

- Spontaneous abortion rate is around 3%, but less than 1% if fetal heart beats are identified in weeks 10–12.
- Spontaneous malformation rate is 2–4%.

Antibiotics

▶ **Pregnancy:**
- *First choice:*
  - Penicillins, cephalosporins, erythromycin.
  - Cephalosporins are excreted more rapidly and more widely distributed, so dose must be increased.
  - Spiramycin (another macrolide) is treatment of choice for toxoplasmosis during pregnancy.
- *Alternatives:* Clindamycin, lincomycin; sulfonamides (not in third trimester because of risk of jaundice).
- *Relative contraindications:* Metronidazole is best administered as a suppository for trichomoniasis, and not used systemically. Toxic in animal studies and controversial in humans.
- *Absolute contraindications:*
  - Tetracyclines: Increased risk of hepatotoxicity in mother; dental and bony defects in fetus after 15th week.
  - Aminoglycosides: Ototoxic.
  - Chloramphenicol: Gray syndrome (potentially fatal toxic reaction in fetus).
  - Gyrase inhibitors: No enough data.
- *Topical agents:* Neomycin, bacitracin, and fusidic acid have minimal absorption and are safe. In acne therapy, topical erythromycin is safest. Aminoglycosides, chloramphenicol, and tetracyclines are systemically absorbed and should be avoided.

▶ **Nursing:**
- *First choice:* Penicillins, cephalosporins, erythromycin.
- *Alternatives:* Aminoglycosides and tetracycline with appropriate indications; minimal transfer to fetus.
- *Relative contraindications:* Stop nursing when metronidazole is administered.
- *Absolute contraindications:* Gyrase inhibitors cause irreversible cartilage damage.

Antifungal Agents

▶ **Pregnancy:** No agent can be recommended.
- *First choice:* Terbinafine is rated B but still should only be used when absolutely necessary.
- *Relative contraindications:* Amphotericin B can be used for life-threatening infections (such as coccidiomycosis).
- *Absolute contraindications:* Griseofulvin and the imidazoles are category C and best avoided.
- *Topical agents:* Imidazoles and nystatin are generally safe.
- *⚠ Caution:* Avoid intravaginal use in first trimester and use on other mucosal surfaces, especially if eroded.

> **Nursing:**
> - Avoid imidazoles on breast while nursing.
> - Imidazoles appear in milk, but risk unclear; if appropriate, use oral nystatin instead.

Antihistamines

> **Pregnancy:**
> - All can be used topically, but other reasons to avoid (e.g. allergic contact dermatitis).
> - For systemic use, those with B ratings include clemastine, dimethindene, and chlorpheniramine. All should be avoided close to delivery.

> **Nursing:**
> - Triprolidine, meclizine often recommended; clemastine probably best avoided.

Local Anesthetics

> **Pregnancy:** Local anesthetics enter the circulation and are transferred to the fetus where they can have systemic effects.
> - *First choice:*
>   - Esters are preferred to amides, as fetuses have higher esterase activity.
>   - Those esters with marked protein binding such as bupivacaine cross the placenta with greater difficulty.
> ☐ *Note:* A small excision need not be deferred in pregnancy; the need for procedures where large amounts of local anesthetics are required should be considered carefully.

> **Nursing:** Prilocaine can cause methemoglobinemia and is best avoided; otherwise no problems for routine use.

Analgesics

> **Pregnancy:**
> - Opiates should only be used with strict indications. Codeine and hydrocodone preferred to morphine. Contraindicated just prior to delivery or if miscarriage is threatened.
> - NSAIDs must be avoided in third trimester because of risk of premature closure of ductus arteriosus; should be used only for strict indications in the first and second trimesters.

> **Nursing:** Transfer to fetus possible; only with strict indications.

Immunosuppressive/Chemotherapy Agents

> **Pregnancy:**
> - Chemotherapy agents should only be used for life-threatening processes, in consultation with obstetricians and oncologists.
> - Cyclosporine is category C; the other common agents are all D or X.

> **Nursing:** Careful indications; cyclosporine is also to be used with care, as it can cause immunosuppression, growth retardation, and perhaps carcinogenesis in infants.

Other Agents

> **Acyclovir:** Very complex; limited studies but widely used in pregnancy despite definite small risks to fetus, because risk of fetal varicella or neonatal herpes considered greater.

► **Benzoyl peroxide:** Safe.
► **Corticosteroids:** Can be used safely both topically and systemically. Possible systemic effect is adrenal suppression, so pediatrician should be alerted at delivery as treatment may be required. No evidence of teratogenicity in humans. During nursing, if dosage is >40 mg prednisolone daily, then pause for 4 hours after administration.
► **Dithranol:** Category C; used without problems.
► **Lindane:** Best avoided in pregnancy because of recurrent medico-legal controversies; official category B.
► **Permethrin:** First choice during pregnancy for scabies and pediculosis; alternatives include benzyl benzoate (scabies) and pyrethrins (pediculosis).
► **Podophyllin:** Contraindicated; no reliable data.
► **Povidone-iodine:** Contraindicated; risk of fetal hypothyroidism.
► **PUVA:** Contraindicated; insufficient data; bath PUVA assumed safer than systemic PUVA.
► **Retinoids:** Systemic retinoids absolutely contraindicated. Topical retinoids best avoided although used for years in acne without incident; category C, but once again medico-legal status is cloudy.
► **Salicylic acid:** Avoid widespread use in pregnancy because of absorption and transfer to fetus; do not use on breast during nursing.
► **Vitamin D analogues:** Limited data, but appear safe.

45 *Operative Dermatology*

45.1 *Principles of Dermatologic Surgery*

Informed Consent

▣ *Note:* Except for emergencies and very minor procedures, both verbal and written preoperative information should be provided at least 24 hours before surgery. In the case of minors, the discussion must always include a parent or legal guardian.

Information that should be provided includes:

▶ **General risks:** Anesthesia; wound infection; scarring; nerve, vessel or lymphatic injury.
▶ **Operation-specific risks:**
  • Structures likely to be damaged.
  • Need for multiple procedures (especially in micrographic surgery).
  • Possible need for skin graft if primary closure is anticipated to be difficult.
  • Grafts or flaps should be diagrammed, showing where donor tissue will be taken or how tissue will be moved.
  • Likelihood of impaired healing and necrosis (especially with flaps and grafts).
  • Risk of recurrence in the case of tumor surgery.
  • Likelihood of scarring, especially if history of keloids or surgery in high-risk location.
  • Risk of thrombosis if immobilization is anticipated.

▣ *Note:* Although forms are essential and save a great deal of time, it is best to also write a note documenting that everything has been explained. The patient (or parent) should be given a chance to ask questions, given a 24 hour waiting period, and allowed to sign the consent form without pressure. In some countries, a witness is required.

Preoperative Diagnosis

▣ *Note:* The need for preoperative diagnostic evaluation depends greatly on the extent of the procedure and the general health of the patient. Routine physical examination and laboratory studies are of little benefit, as documented in a study of 20000 patients scheduled for elective hemorrhoidectomy.

▶ **Always consider:**
  • *Risk of bleeding:* Always ask about use of aspirin, heparin, or coumarin. If the history suggests a disorder of coagulation, then detailed laboratory investigation including von Willebrand factor, factor Xa, platelets, and hemoglobin. If platelet count is normal, but history suspicious, also do bleeding time as functional test.
  • *Problems with wound healing:* Ask about previous problems; consider role of systemic corticosteroids, diabetes mellitus, polyneuropathy, chronic venous insufficiency, peripheral arterial disease.
  • *Allergies:* Local anesthetics (usually an overdosage or hyperventilation, but always ask); analgesics, antibiotics; others.
  • *Associated diseases;* HIV/AIDS, hepatitis, cardiovascular disease.

Preoperative Disinfection

▶ Risk of infection varies greatly, depending on vascularity of tissue; rare on scalp and face, common on feet.
▶ Periorificial operations are always confronted with only a semisterile field, as the mouth or anus always has residual microorganisms.
▶ Risks of infection increase greatly with extent and duration of procedure. Also influenced by individual factors, especially diabetes mellitus and immunosuppression.
▶ Usually use Octenisept or 3% peracetic acid ester solution. In special cases:
  • When a flap is be developed, it is best to use a clear solution (such as peracetic acid) so that vascularity of flap can be assessed.
  • Mucosal surfaces can be sterilized with 0.1% benzalkonium chloride solution or Octenisept solution.
▶ Disinfectant always applied from center to periphery in circular strokes of increasing size.

Preoperative Sedation and Anesthesia

▶ **Preoperative sedation:**
  ◨ *Note:* This can be very useful in anxious patients or children, to expand the range of operations that can be accomplished without intubation anesthesia.
  • In children, midazolam is preferred.
  • In adults: usual choice is benzodiazepines (diazepam or oxazepam); 5–10 mg 30–50 minutes before surgery.
  ⚠ *Caution:* Both midazolam and benzodiazepines are respiratory depressants.
  • In high-risk patients or when a long operation is anticipated:
    – Insert venous access line.
    – Have oxygen and suction available.
▶ **Topical anesthetics:**
  • EMLA, a commercial mixture of lidocaine and prilocaine, is the most effective topical anesthetic.
  • Indications include venipuncture sites in children, spinal puncture, preparing a site for injection of local anesthetic, or as sole agent for minor procedures such as removing molluscum contagiosum or skin tags.
  • The ointment is applied 45–60 minutes before the procedure and covered with occlusive foil; self-adhering products are simplest to employ.
  ⚠ *Caution:* EMLA is a vasoconstrictor, so small vascular lesions may disappear.
▶ **Cryoanesthesia:**
  • Highly overrated technique; not suitable for digits or areas where poor wound healing is expected.
  • Suitable for very minor procedures and for preparing for an injection.
  • Use ethyl chloride spray at a distance of 20–30 cm, spraying until skin just turns white. Then proceed immediately.
  ⚠ *Caution:* Never use liquid nitrogen cryospray for anesthesia. The risk of necrosis is too great.
▶ **Infiltration anesthesia:**
  • Almost every example of skin surgery can be done with local infiltration anesthesia, including biopsies, simple excisions, flaps, and grafts.
  • Choice of agents is important (Table 45.**1**), as is attention to maximum volume and addition of epinephrine.
  • Prefer lidocaine 1–2% in combination with epinephrine. Maximum dose is 55 mg/kg.

Table 45.1 · Local anesthetic agents

Agent	Onset (m)	Dura-tion (h)	Max dose (with epi)	Max dose (without epi)	Comments
Articaine	1–3	1	600	400	Rapidly metabolized
Lidocaine	1–2	1–2	500	300	Most often used; marked vasodilation
Mepivi-caine	1–2	1.5–3	500	300	Long lasting; minimal vaso-dilation
Prilo-caine	1–2	1–3	600	600	Can cause methemoglobine-mia; careful in children
Ropiva-caine	1–5	2–6	–	200	Long postoperative pain con-trol; used in nerve blocks

From Table 1.1 in Kaufmann R, Podda M, Landes E. *Dermatologische Operationen*. Thieme, Stuttgart, 2005, p. 7. (epi = epinephrine)

- ◨ *Note:* Standard wisdom is not to use epinephrine when administering local anesthetics to digits, penis, nose or ears, or for nerve blocks. Recent studies indicate that when the circulation to the distal part is normal, epinephrine is a safe useful adjunct.
- Use an 18–21 gauge needle, insert once along line of incision, and inject while withdrawing along course.
- ► **Nerve block:** Can be used for large procedures, areas that are hard to inject (digits, penis, nose, ear, lips), and supplemented with additional infiltration.
  - ◨ *Caution:* Nerve blocks are always done using a local anesthetic without epinephrine.
  - **Finger block:** Point of injection just distal to metacarpal-phalangeal joint. With continuous back aspiration, inject 1–2 mL of anesthetic on each side of finger while advancing toward the palm. Also inject the dorsal aspect of the finger with 1–2 mL. Numbness within 5–10 minutes.
  - **Supraorbital nerve (forehead and nose):** Infiltrate above the eyebrow just medial to the supraorbital notch or foramen.
  - **Infraorbital nerve (lower lid and medial cheek):** Infiltrate within the mouth above and posterior to the second upper premolar.
  - **Mental nerve:** Infiltrate within mouth just distal to second lower premolar and mental foramen.
  - **Penis block:** Inject 2–4 mL lateral to dorsal penis vein bilaterally, with infiltration of both dorsal and ventral sides; the latter must sometimes be extended to frenulum.

Postoperative Dressing

- ◨ *Note:*
  - The initial wound dressing should be left in place for 48 hours. The risk of contamination is greatest during this period. Later the wound is relatively closed, although without tensile strength.
  - For complex flaps, use a transparent dressing so the vitality of the transplanted tissue can be observed without removing the entire dressing.
- ► **Dry sterile dressing:** Uncomplicated primarily closed wounds without exposed bone, cartilage, or fascia can be closed with a traditional dry dressing. Adhesive wound closures such as Steri-Strips can be used to better approximate the wound

Operative Dermatology

edges if needed. They should be left in place until the wound is stable and removed carefully (or allowed to fall off).

► **Moist sterile dressing:**
  • Preferred for superinfected and moist wounds, especially if a wound contains exposed bone, cartilage, or fascia, requires conditioning or following skin transplantation.
  • Sterile dressings are moistened with Octenisept solution, which does not interfere with granulation tissue. Ideal for use with pinch grafts and split skin grafts on infected wounds.
  • Either physiologic saline or lactated Ringer solution can be used to moisten dressings over exposed bone and cartilage.
► **Dressing materials**: Usually combination of antiseptic ointment (povidone iodine or fusidic acid), mesh dressing, and sterile bandages or hydrocolloid dressing.

Wound Infections

► **Clinical features:** Pain, erythema and heat—the classic signs.
► **Therapy:**
  • In most instances, suture material must be at least partially removed and wound re-explored. Systemic antibiotics and topical disinfectants are important but not sufficient measures.
  • If the wound contains pus, rinse with 1% H_2O_2 solution or povidone-iodine solution.
  • Carry out culture and sensitivity so that antibiotic therapy can be as specific as possible. Start with locally accepted broad-spectrum coverage.

45.2 Basic Techniques

Scissor Excision, Curettage, Biopsy

► **Anesthesia:**
  • Cryoanesthesia.
  • Lidocaine/prilocaine (EMLA).
  • Infiltration anesthesia.
► **Scissor excision:**
  • *Indications:* Skin tags.
  • *Technique:* Rapid excision using tip, not throat, of scissors.
► **Curettage:**
  • *Indications*: Benign epidermal lesions including seborrheic keratosis, actinic keratosis, wart, molluscum contagiosum.
  • *Technique:*
    – Disinfect; then local anesthetic. Place skin under tension between thumb and forefinger; grasp curette like a pencil and move across the surface of the lesion.
    – With experience, one can feel the difference between lesional tissue and the firmer normal dermis.
    – Curettes are sharp (or should be kept sharp), so be careful and do not exert undo pressure.
    – Bleeding can be controlled with ferric subsulfate (Monsel's) solution (which may discolor), 35% aluminum chloride solution, or 5–10% trichloracetic acid. Some prefer to use mild electrocautery.

– Warts are best treated with curettage combined with electrocautery or laser destruction of base.

► **Punch biopsy (p. 26):**
- *Indications*: Diagnostic biopsy.
- *Technique:*
  – Punches available in 2, 3, 4 and 6 mm sizes; 3 and 4 mm are most practical for routine purposes.
  – Disinfection and local anesthesia.
  – Despite the name "punch," the trick is to place the skin under tension in a direction perpendicular to skin tension lines and then to gently turn the instrument with mild downward pressure until a "pop" is felt, indicating the subcutaneous fat has been reached.
  – Extensive pressure is not needed if the punch is properly sharpened.
- ▣ *Note:*
- Punch biopsies are not suited for sampling subcutaneous fat, for which a long thin ellipse is preferred.
- Most punch biopsies can be removed for the skin by pressing down on both sides of the defect so the plug is elevated, cutting the base with a curved iris scissors, and lifting the biopsy out and placing it is formalin solution with the scissors. Forceps are almost never needed.
  - ▣ *Note:* A crushed biopsy with forceps marks makes interpretation difficult and is a sign of sloppy work.

► **Excisional biopsy:**
- *Indications*: This type of biopsy is designed to sample subcutaneous fat, or sample transition from normal to abnormal skin (needed primarily when defects in collagen or elastin are suspected).
- *Technique:* Disinfection and local anesthesia; long thin ellipse to minimize tension; close with simple sutures.

Excision with Primary Closure

► **Indications:** Almost all benign and malignant lesions.
► **Technique:**
- Disinfection and local anesthesia.
- Excision of ellipse with scalpel, usually # 15 blade. Angle at tip of spindle should be <30° to avoid the development of dog ears, which then require additional attention.
- Plan the ellipse around the long axis of the lesion. On the face, and in most instances elsewhere, try to place parallel to skin tension lines (Fig. 45.**1**). On the face, pay attention to the aesthetic units (forehead, periorbital region, nasal region, perioral region).
- Benign lesions should be excised with the excision placed just beyond the visible border of the lesion.
- The excision should always extend into subcutaneous fat, making undermining and closure much simpler. Closure is usually with a few dermal stitches to approximate and reduce tension, followed by simple skin closure with single stitches. Larger lesions or those under tension require more extensive subcutaneous or even epifascial undermining.
- Simple deeper lesions, primarily cysts and lipomas, can often be extruded through a small incision in the overlying epidermis. The ellipse should include the central pore in the case of a cyst. The lesion can be carefully mobilized with a blunt curved dissecting scissors. With lipomas, the risk of bleeding at the base is significant, especially with larger lesions or angiolipomas. Electrocautery may be needed if pressure is ineffective.

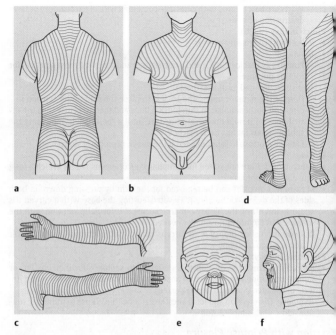

Fig. 45.**1** · Relaxed skin tension lines (modified from Borges and Konz).

Micrographic Surgery

▶ Indications: Basal cell carcinoma, especially if large, recurrent, or located in prob lem zone (perinasal, periorbital, periauricular); squamous cell carcinoma, derma tofibrosarcoma protuberans, other sarcomas, lentigo maligna melanoma.

    ▣ *Note:* The indications for micrographic surgery remain controversial. Practi tioners of the method tend to employ it for all cutaneous malignancies, al though evidence-based medicine is just starting to accumulate data to de lineate the appropriate usage.

▶ **Technique:** There are two basic approaches (Figs. 45.**2**, 45.**3**):

- Tübinger Torte (in Germany) and Mohs' technique (in USA).
- Both are based on meticulous histologic control of the entire margin of the exci sion; the Torte accomplishes this by an ingenious sectioning plan taking a sma peripheral ring, while Mohs depends on flattening the excision and cutting sec tions from the entire base.
- Each requires extensive marking and detailed sketches.
- In most instances, the dermatologic surgeon also does the microscopic exami nation. If permanent sections are used, the wound is temporarily covered unt the final results are available. If the margin is involved, the procedure is re peated in just that area.

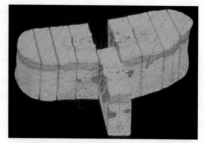

Fig. 45.**2** · Bread loaf technique, showing how easily this standard approach can miss a positive margin.

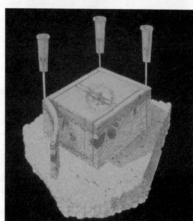

Fig. 45.**3** · Microscopic control of margins.

- Once the entire tumor has been removed and this has been confirmed microscopically, then closure is accomplished, sometimes primarily, but often with a flap or graft.
- ☐ *Note:* Micrographic surgery offers the highest cure rates (95–99%) coupled with the maximum sparing of normal tissue.

Suture Technique

▶ **Sutures:**
- As general rule, atraumatic nonabsorbable sutures are used for skin closure and absorbable sutures for dermal and subcutaneous work.
- *Exceptions:*
  - On the scalp, coarse polyfilament sutures are used to allow rapid closure and tight knots.
  - In the mouth and perianal region, rapidly absorbed polyfilament sutures are used; they dissolve within 14 days, eliminating the need for suture removal.
- Recommendations for various body regions are shown in detail in Table 45.**2**.

Table 45.2 · Recommended suture material for different body regions

Region	Suture material
Face and neck	Subcutaneous: Slowly absorbable monofilament sutures (PDS 4/0 or Serrasynth 4/0) or rapidly absorbable braided sutures (Vicryl 4/0) Skin: Nonabsorbable monofilament sutures (Ethilon 5/0, 6/0)
Scalp	Nonabsorbable braided sutures 2/0, 3/0
Mouth, tongue	Rapidly absorbable braided sutures (Vicryl rapid 3/0, 4/0)
Trunk	Subcutaneous: Slowly absorbable sutures (PDS 2/0 or Serasynth 2/0, 3/0) Skin: Nonabsorbable Prolene 3/0, 4/0
Extremities	Subcutaneous: Slowly absorbable monofilament sutures (PDS 3/0, 4/0 or Serasynth 3/0, 4/0) Skin: Nonabsorbable monofilament sutures (Ethilon 3/0, 4/0)
Hands and feet	Nonabsorbable monofilament sutures (Ethilon 4/0, 5/0)
Anogenital region (mucosa)	Rapidly absorbable braided suture (Vicryl rapid 3/0, 4/0)

▶ **Suture placement:** General guidelines include:
- Generous undermining for mobilization to allow placement of subcutaneous sutures under relatively little tension.
- The subcutaneous knots should point downward, so an inverted suture is required.
- Low-tension skin sutures are essential for best cosmetic results.
- On the scalp, more tension is acceptable as necrosis does not occur and the stitches must also produce hemostasis.
- On the hands and feet, as well as the periorbital region, the approximation should be somewhat less tight.
- ◨ *Note:* Resist the temptation to pull a wound together. It should move easily together and your stitches simply hold it in the new position.

▶ **Knots:**
- *Single simple knot:*
  - Easiest knot; gives excellent cosmetic result if under low tension and removed promptly.
  - Should be combined with subcutaneous sutures to ease closure.
- *Vertical mattress:*
  - The advantage of either the Allgöwer (intracutaneous on one side) or Donati (penetrates skin on both sides) stitches is excellent wound edge approximation. Pressure is better distributed.
  - In difficult areas such as inguinal or axillary regions or when infection is likely, we prefer the Allgöwer mattress to a running subcutaneous suture because if an infection develops, a limited number of sutures can be removed
- *Running subcutaneous stitch:*
  - When used by skilled surgeon, provides the best cosmetic results.
  - Reserve for wounds under low tension where infection is unlikely.
- *Buried corner suture (Zoltan):*
  - Used in Z-plasty, flats and grafts to avoid compromising vascular supply of a tip.

  – Similar to Allgöwer stitch, but the tip is incorporated with a horizontal sub-
    cutaneous passage.
- **Ligatures:**
  - Ligatures are designed to stop bleeding from a vessel by "strangulating" it. In or-
    dinary surgery, they can be tied over a clamp.
  - When larger vessels are ligated, as during phlebologic surgery, then the ligature
    can be passed on a round noncutting needle to insure that the vessel is correctly
    captured but not damaged. Usually material is polyglactin (Vicryl) 3/0 or 4/0.
  - *☑ Caution:* Avoid tugging or exerting excess pressure when placing ligatures, es-
    pecially on larger vessels. If the vessel is torn, then two ligatures must be placed
    in a bloody field—often a hard task.
- **Suture removal:**
  - *◻ Note:* Removal of sutures at the earliest safe moment is the surest way to insure
    a good cosmetic result and avoid the "railroad track" markings that arise when
    sutures are left in place too long. The surgeon should establish the date and
    clearly inform the patient.
  - Rough guidelines are:
    – Face: 4–9 days.
    – Scalp and trunk: 10–14 days.
    – Hands and feet: 7–10 days.

45.3 Closure Techniques

Overview

- An excision must be planned considering the relaxed tension lines, the skin tension of the patient, the orientation of the lesion, and the skills of the surgeon. Thus
  every procedure is unique; none can be copied exactly out of a book.
- The best method of closure is the one that accomplishes the best functional and
  aesthetic result in the shortest period of time. Some of the more common methods
  are shown in Fig. 45.**4**.
- Flaps are usually done with local anesthetic without epinephrine; otherwise it is
  difficult to notice flap ischemia.
- The surgeon must master both the geometry of flaps as well as a minimally traumatic approach to tissue handling to maximize success. Temporary sutures are a
  more gentle way to retract tissue during mobilization than skin hooks; forceps
  should be completely avoided.
- When in doubt, provide wound drainage. On the face, flat drains custom-cut out of
  sterile surgical gloves are often useful.
- The wound dressing should not exert excessive pressure, because this can threaten
  a flap. A clear dressing makes it easier to check the vascular status of the flap.
- The exact lines of a flap are usually determined during the operation, with the
  placement of Burow triangles reserved for the end.
- Sometimes the surgical site must be kept absolutely at rest; for example, with facial surgery a ban on speaking and the provision of liquid diet to avoid chewing are
  sometimes necessary.
- A satisfactory cosmetic result can only be obtained when the skin sutures are free
  of tension and loosely tied.

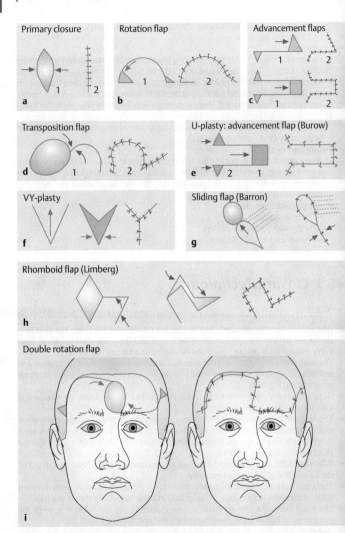

Fig. 45.4 · Methods of wound closure. **a** Primary closure. **b** Rotation flap. **c** Advancement flap. **d** Transposition flap. **e** U-plasty (advancement flap). **f** VY-plasty. **g** Sliding flap. **h** Rhomboid flap. **i** Double rotation flap. **j** Axe flap (rotation flap with back cut). **k** U-plasty (advancement flap). **l** H-plasty.

Axe flap (rotation flap with back cut)

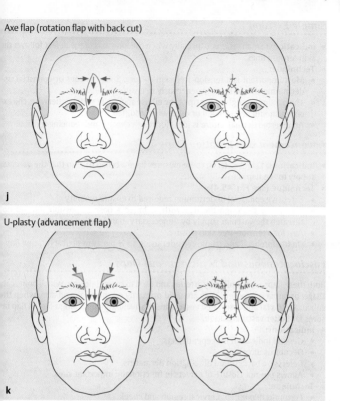

j

U-plasty (advancement flap)

k

H-plasty

l

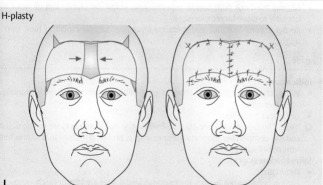

Simple Excision

► **Indications:** Small lesions, especially when the long axis of the defect follows the skin tension lines.
► **Technique:**
  • Most important is a tension-free skin closure. Subcutaneous or epifascial undermining should be used generously to ensure this.
  • The maximum angle of the tip of the ellipse should be < 30°. Otherwise, the excision should be extended or otherwise modified.
  • An inverted dermal suture is ideal for rough closure and reducing tension.

Advancement and Rotation Flaps

► **Indications:** Larger defects; these closures have a broad base so that the vascular supply to the flap is usually stable.
► **Technique (see Fig. 45.4):**
  • Extensive epifascial undermining required to ensure mobility.
  • Always try to design the flap with as broad a base as possible and do not threaten the vascular supply by unnecessary manipulation or force.
  • Aim for a tension-free skin closure.
  • On the forehead and trunk, consider using an *H-plasty* or *double rotation flap*.

Fasciocutaneous and Myocutaneous Flaps

Both these flaps are supplied by arteries and used to cover defects in which bone, cartilage, or fascia is exposed. They are used primarily on the thigh and arm, when the subcutaneous fat and associated vessels are relatively thin; including a fascial flap insures far better vascularization.
► **Indications:**
  • General indication is deeper defects.
  • Decubitus ulcers.
  • Defects on background of radiation dermatitis.
  • Allows prompt closure of defects in functionally important sites.
► **Technique:**
  • *Pectoralis major flap:* Cervical region and cheek.
  • *Gluteus maximus flap:* Sacral, especially for decubital ulcers; can be done bilaterally to close larger ulcers.
  • *Rectus femoris flap and tensor fasciae latae flap:* Lateral aspect of hips, upper thighs.

Grafts

► **Indications:**
  • When closure with a flap appears impossible, or associated with increased operative risk.
  • To correct ectropion.
  ◘ *Note:* The best results are obtained when the donor site is close to the defect and has comparable properties. For example, pre- or retroauricular skin is best suited for facial grafts.
► **Split-thickness graft:**
  • *Technique:*
    – Skin is harvested using a dermatome. Usual sites are lateral thigh, buttocks, and scalp. Desired thickness 0.3–0.8 mm. Cover donor site with inert polyurethane membrane dressing for 5–10 days.
    – Graft is tacked using nonfilament sutures or metal clips.

⚠ Caution: When covering chronic venous ulcers, which generally are at risk of infection, sutures should be avoided.
- Wound is dressed with nonadherent dressing, immobilized, and first re-examined after 5–7 days.
- If minimal local infection develops, wet dressings soaked in Octenisept solution are useful.

- *Mesh graft:* Cutting the graft with a mesh cutter can provide up to a 6-fold increase in coverage. Mesh grafts are well-suited for leg ulcers and other infected wounds, as they automatically allow for drainage.

► **Full-thickness graft:**
- These grafts consist of epidermis and dermis; they require a well-vascularized wound, but do not shrink, thus producing better cosmetic results than split-thickness grafts.
- *Technique:*
  - Usual donor sites are pre- or postauricular, supraclavicular, medial upper arm, or inguinal region.
  - Donor site is closed primarily.
  - Graft must be completely defatted.
  - Graft is fixed with monofilament sutures, which are left long so that they can be tied over a dressing so that it exerts a gentle pressure immobilizing the graft.
  - Dressing first changed after 5–7 days.

▣ Note: With full-thickness graft, hair follicles are also transferred. This must be anticipated in planning the graft.

► **Composite graft:**
- *Technique:* Usual procedure is to take a piece of ear containing cartilage and use it to correct nasal defect. The graft should be a bit larger than the defect, as shrinkage is inevitable.

⚠ Caution: In areas with scarring (previous surgery) or radiation dermatitis, grafts are at greater risk because of reduced vascular supply.

45.4 Other Techniques

Cryotherapy

► **Principle:** Solid tissue freezing using liquid nitrogen (-196°C) induces tissue necrosis. Patients must be warned about the pain, blister formation, and slow healing.

► **Indications:**
- Routine indications are actinic keratoses and warts. Other lesions that can be treated include hypertrophic scars, keloids, superficial malignancies (early squamous cell carcinoma, Bowen disease, superficial basal cell carcinoma), and leukoplakia (after histological diagnosis), small hemangiomas, Kaposi sarcoma.
- Experienced physicians may use deep cryotherapy with thermoprobe for treating basal cell carcinoma in selected locations in patients who are not good operative risks.

► **Technique:**
- Ordinary treatment involves using a spray unit or contact probe. Length of exposure depends on thickness of lesion. Actinic keratoses can be treated for 5–10 seconds; warts should be frozen until the entire lesion and a tiny peripheral rim appear white. In other lesions, individual adjustment is required.

- Actinic keratoses need only be frozen once; other lesions should be frozen at least twice, allowing for adequate thawing in between.
- ▶ *Note:* If cotton-tipped applicators are used, then a generous applicator, such as a vaginal swab, is required. Traditional small applicators (cotton buds) do not transfer enough cold to produce effects.
- When an invasive tumor is treated, a thermoprobe is needed to insure that the base of the tumor is frozen solid to a predefined temperature (usually −25 °C); such procedures should be left for experts in cryotherapy.

Dermabrasion

▶ **Principle:** Superficial removal of skin using high-speed (>25 000 rpm) diamond fraise or brush. Irregular features are exchanged for a smoother, flatter scar.

▶ **Indications:**
- Rhinophyma, large congenital nevi in first months of life.
- Uses have become more limited in recent years with increasing emphasis on lasers and chemical peeling. In the past, dermabrasion was widely used for tattoos, but is now replaced entirely by lasers. Severe acne scarring is still an indication, although mild scarring is almost exclusively treated with chemical peels.
- Extensive actinic keratoses of the scalp may also respond well.

▶ **Technique:**
- Usually done under sedation with nerve block or local anesthetic. General anesthesia required for infants with congenital nevi.
- Preoperative coverage with antibiotics and antiviral agents is necessary for widespread procedures. Prophylaxis against herpes simplex virus is particularly important for whole-face dermabrasions.
- The skin is stretched taut by the assistant and the fraise moved across the skin at a right angle to its axis of rotation. Only light pressure and a uniform motion are required; otherwise it is easy to penetrate the dermis.
- Gauze pads dipped in physiologic saline solution are used to remove abraded tissue and provide cooling. They must be kept out of the way of the fraise.
- ▮ *Caution:* Extreme caution must be exerted around the mouth and eyes. Skin can be caught on the fraise and rolled away or otherwise damaged.
- Acne dermabrasions using a wire brush require a special Freon 114 (1,2-dichlorotetrafluoroethane) spray, which is used to harden the skin making the tissue removal easier. Other chlorofluorocarbons and liquid nitrogen are too cold, and produce extensive tissue damage.
- The usual depth is into the papillary dermis until punctate bleeding points are seen.

▶ **Postoperative care:**
- *Small lesions:* Cover with hydrocolloid gels.
- *Larger areas, such as large nevi:* Cover with nonadherent dressing and gauze soaked in an antiseptic solution.

Circumcision

▶ **Principle:** The foreskin is excised in a circular fashion. Electrosurgical resection is no longer practiced because of problems with necrosis and scarring.

▶ **Indications:** Phimosis, following emergency surgery for paraphimosis, lichen sclerosus (often associated with phimosis), chronic balanitis, recurrent condylomata acuminata under foreskin, tumors of foreskin, deviation caused by foreskin.

▶ **Technique:**
- Administer penis block using 2% prilocaine and provide additional circular block on ventral surface.
- Marker clamps at 12, 6 (frenulum), 3, and 9 o'clock positions to insure no torsion is introduced between the inner and outer parts of the foreskin during suturing.
- Incision of foreskin with scissors and circular resection with immediate adaption with rapidly absorbed polyfilament sutures (Vicryl 3/0 or 4/0).
- Watch for frenular artery and use ligature or fine electrocautery. Sometimes useful to reposition frenulum if deviation has been a problem.
- When treating lichen sclerosus, do not be too aggressive in removing foreskin but leave a bit in case tissue is needed for a foreskin plasty.

▶ **Postoperative care:**
- Dressing with antiseptic ointments and solutions.
- Immobilization for 3 days.
- Elevation of penis to reduce edema.

▶ **Medications:**
- Subcutaneous heparin.
- Diazepam 10 mg p.o. t.i.d. for prophylaxis against erections.
- NSAIDs usually suffice for pain.

Liposuction

▶ **Principle:** Removal of fatty tissue with high-pressure suction devices.
▶ **Indications:**
- Extensive lipomas, lipomatosis, lipodystrophy.
- Aesthetic indications for body remodeling, especially for hips and thighs.
- To obtain tissue for autologous fat transplantation.

▶ **Instruments:**
- Manually manipulated cannulas.
- *Ultrasonographic liposuction:* Fat broken apart by sound waves; makes rapid removal possible but carries risk of overheating.
- *Vibration liposuction:* Tip of canula vibrates rapidly, freeing fragments of fat for suction. Minimizes blood loss and trauma.

▶ **Technique:**
- The extent of the procedure and the patient's general health determine whether procedure is done on an inpatient or outpatient basis.
- Area marked with waterproof marker while patient is standing.
- Tumescence anesthesia is introduced, using the following mixture:
  - 50 mL prilocaine 1%.
  - 3 mL sodium hydrogen carbonate 8.4%.
  - 0.5 mL epinephrine 1:1000.
  - 500 mL lactated Ringer solution.
- Wait at least 50 minutes for anesthesia to take effect.
- Regular symmetrical passage of canula through fatty tissue. Always hold opening down (away from skin surface) to avoid creating folds or furrows in remodeled area.
- Always monitor amounts of fluid and fat removed.

▶ **Postoperative care:**
- Large absorbent dressings are applied to capture remaining anesthesia fluid, which will slowly leak out. For this reason, cannula holes are not closed.
- Use compression garments for 2–3 months.

▢ **Note:**
- Especially in aesthetic procedures, document the preoperative discussion and subsequent informed consent in detail. Preoperative photographs are essential.
- Warn the patient about the risk of hemorrhage, dysesthesias, edema, irregular skin surface, and asymmetry.
- Emphasize the possible need for reduction plasties to remove excessive skin, depending on age of patient and elasticity of skin.
- Complications include anaphylaxis, thrombosis, embolus, increased or decreased sensation in overlying skin, hemorrhage, necrosis and penetration into body cavities.

Nail Surgery

▢ **Note:** Nail surgery should only be done by experienced physicians, because of the the risk of loss of function with subsequent medico-legal problems.

▶ **Nail extraction:**
- *Indications*: Ingrown nail, chronic paronychia, exposing nail bed for surgical procedure.
- *Technique*: Finger block plus tourniquet (rubber drain fixed with hemostat). Separate nail from nail bed with nail elevator and then extract with hemostat. Antiseptic ointment and dressing.

▶ **Emmert procedure:**
- *Indications*: Ingrown nail, chronic lateral nail bed inflammation.
- *Technique*: Nail block and tourniquet. Wedge excision of edge of nail and nail bed down to periosteum; removal of lateral and proximal nail matrix: Use monofilament nonabsorbable Prolene 2/0 or 3/0 with transungual approach to close. Antiseptic ointment and dressing.

45.5 Laser Therapy

Principles

▶ **Function:**
- LASER = **l**ight **a**mplification by **s**timulated **e**mission of **r**adiation.
- Various media (gases, solids, liquids) can be stimulated to produce coherent (same frequency and wavelength) bundles of high energy light in UV, visible, or infrared range.
- Laser systems are named according to the medium, the method of stimulation, and whether they generate continuous wave (cw) or pulsed energy. There are many variation on pulsing, including Q-switching (QS), and a variety of scanners and shuttering devices.

▶ **Mechanism of action:**
- Laser radiation is absorbed by chromophores in the skin. Melanin, other skin pigments (carotenoids), hemoglobin, and water are damaged by thermal effects or scattered by pressure waves.
- The depth of penetration is proportional to the wavelength of the laser, so that highly selective sites of action can be chosen. Longer wavelength lasers (red, infrared) provide greater penetration.
- Lasers can be used as a fine destructive "knife" (CO_2 laser), for coagulation (argon, Nd:YAG, copper vapor) and for selective photothermolysis (dye laser, QS-ruby laser).

- The essence of selective photothermolysis is that laser energy is delivered to a chromophore structure at intervals greater than the cooling time for the material, so that the thermolysis is confined to the structure such as a vessel and does not involve adjacent tissue.
- The longer the impulse, the greater the thermal effects. When treating pigmented lesions, the impulse duration should be less than 100 ns.

Laser Safety

▶ In Europe, lasers are classified as class I–IV based on the intensity of their beam. All dermatologic lasers as class IV. Different safety standards are established for each class of laser.

▶ Before a laser is put into use, it should be registered both with the facility's and physician's insurance firms and with the local safety regulation officers.

▶ A qualified technician, often a physicist, should be appointed with responsibility for the technical status of the laser. Regular inspections of the device are required. This is technically independent of routine maintenance.

▶ Any area where lasers are in use must be marked. The doors should have warning signs or lights and should be locked so that only authorized personnel have access.

▶ Eyes must be protected. Physicians, nurses. and technicians should wear special laser protective glasses. Patients should have eye shields.

▶ All surfaces that could be hit by the laser beam should have diffuse-reflecting surfaces.

▶ Laser plume should be evacuated; viable human papillomavirus (HPV) particles can be found in the smoke plume.

Instruments

▶ The medically important lasers are summarized in Table 45.**3**.

▶ **Intense pulsed light source (IPL):**
- Not a laser, but similar indications.
- Intense light over a wide range (5550–1200 nm) with pulses of 2–20 ms.
- Main indications are epilation (larger field size than laser), superficial vascular lesions, and nonablative treatment of skin aging.

Indications

▶ The indications are shown in Table 45.**4**.

☒ *Note:* Laser therapy is destructive; the diagnosis must always be clinically or (in the case of tumors) histologically established before treatment.

Laser Phototherapy

▶ **Indications:** Psoriasis, vitiligo, other forms of hypopigmentation.

▶ **Lasers:** Excimer or IPL.

▶ **Mechanism of action:** Intense high-dose UVB energy at 308 nm is delivered directly to the psoriatic plaque, sparing the surrounding skin. In the case of vitiligo, the annoying tanning of the adjacent skin is avoided.

▶ **Side effects:** Burns, just as with UVB therapy.

Vascular Lesions

▶ **Indications:** Vascular lesions are generally amenable to laser treatment. The choice of laser depends on the size of the vessels, color of lesion, and location. Sometimes longer wavelengths are better, to avoid competitive absorption by melanin and increase depth of penetration.

Operative Dermatology

Table 45.3 · **Medically important lasers**

Laser	Wavelength (nm)	Continuous wave (cw) power (W)	Pulsed fluence (J/cm²)	Indications
Argon	514 488 + 514	< 1	–	Coagulation of superficial vascular lesions
Frequency–doubled (fd) Nd:YAG (KTP)	532	–	< 20	Coagulation of superficial vascular lesions
Flashlamp pulsed dye laser (FPDL)	500–630	–	< 20	Nevus flammeus at 585nm
Ruby	694	–	Q-switched: < 12 Normal mode: < 60	Q-switched: pigment removal Long–pulsed: epilation
Alexandrite	755	–	Q-switched: < 7 Long pulsed: < 60	Q-switched: pigment removal Long–pulsed: epilation
Nd:YAG-cw	1064	< 100	Q-switched: < 12 Pulsed: < 250 Long pulsed: < 60	cw: coagulation, cutting Q-switched: pigment removal Pulsed: vascular lesions Long pulsed: epilation
Erbium:YAG	2940	–	Pulse energy up to 2J	Athermal ablation
CO₂	10600	< 50	Pulse energy up to 1J	Cutting, ablation
Excimer	308	–	5mJ	Psoriasis, vitiligo

► **Mechanism of action:** The major effect is absorption of energy by hemoglobin.
► **Side effects:**
  • Scarring, hypo- and hyperpigmentation.
  • *Pain:* All procedures are painful, roughly in the order dye < argon < copper vapor < Nd:YAG, with the last being most troublesome. Larger lesions must be treated with lidocaine/prilocaine (EMLA) or local infiltration; in infants with hemangiomas, general anesthesia is needed.

Pigmented Lesions
The pigmented lesions can be divided into congenital and acquired lesions, as well as tattoos. A variety of lasers are available.
► **Congenital and acquired lesions:**
  • These lesions contain melanin, which absorbs at a maximum of 520nm. Examples include nevi of Ota and Ito, as well as lentigines, ephelides, and café-au-lait macule.

Table 45.4 · Indications for different lasers

Laser	Indications
Dye laser	Superficial and deep vascular lesions
	Facial erythema
Argon laser	Superficial vascular lesions
Copper vapor laser	Facial erythema
	Xanthelasma
CO_2 laser	Xanthelasma
	Warts
	Epidermal nevus
	Rhinophyma
	Flat seborrheic keratoses
	Neurofibromas
	Syringomas
Q-switched solid phase lasers	Café-au-lait macule
	Nevus spilus
	Nevus of Ota and Ito
	Ephelides
	Senile lentigines
	Tattoos
Erbium:YAG laser	Senile lentigines
	Flat seborrheic keratoses
	Superficial tumors (trichoepitheliomas, angiofibromas)
	Leukoplakia
	Acne scars
	Skin resurfacing
	Actinic keratoses
Long-pulsed solid lasers, IPL	Epilation
Excimer laser	Psoriasis
	Vitiligo
	Hypopigmentation

- Melanocytic nevi are generally best removed surgically so that material is available for histologic examination.

Operative Dermatology

▶ **Tattoos:**
- Lasers have replaced dermabrasion and other scarring methods for the removal of tattoos.
- The pigment particles are attacked by a laser chosen to match the absorption of the tattoo color and vaporized so they can be engulfed by macrophages.
- Multiple procedures are usually required.
- Side effects include hypo- and hyperpigmentation, scarring, changes in tattoo color, dermatitis changes, and rarely pyogenic granuloma.

Miscellaneous Lesions
▶ **Indications:**
- Once the diagnosis has been established, a wide variety of lesions can be ablated with a laser. The list includes warts, condylomata, seborrheic keratoses, actinic keratoses, actinic cheilitis, xanthelasma, multiple adnexal tumors (syringomas, trichoepitheliomas), neurofibromas, and angiofibromas.
- In special cases, malignant tumors may also be destroyed with a laser. Examples include superficial basal cell carcinoma and Kaposi sarcoma, as well as palliative treatment of inoperable or metastatic tumors.

▶ **Lasers:**
- A CO_2 *laser* is often chosen for ablation; usually used in short-pulsed mode with very short (ns) impulse duration and high energy, often coupled with a scanner device. The tissue is vaporized and coagulated; it can be removed carefully in layers as the level of penetration is only 0.01–0.1 mm.
- An *erbium:YAG laser* is useful for very superficial lesions such as actinic keratoses, in which case it does not have a coagulatory effect.
- ◻ *Note:* When lasers are used for tissue ablation, an effective plume or smoke removal system is needed. The odor can be most unpleasant. In addition, when viral lesions are treated, infectious HPV particles are found in the smoke. Special protective glasses are also required.

Epilation
▶ **Indications:** Hypertrichosis, hirsutism, cosmetic indications, transsexual changes.
▶ **Lasers:**
- Long-pulsed solid lasers such as alexandrite, Nd:YAG, or ruby.
- IPL.
▶ **Mechanism of action:** Destruction of follicle with high-energy light. Only possible for pigmented hairs. Treatment must be repeated several times; at least six sessions required.
◻ *Note:* The skin should be cooled to reduce epidermal damage.

Skin Rejuvenation
▶ **Synonyms:** Laser skin resurfacing, laser skin regeneration.
▶ **Indications:** Photoaging, solar elastosis, wrinkles; perhaps prophylaxis against actinic keratoses and squamous cell carcinomas on face.
▶ **Lasers:** CO_2, erbium:YAG for ablative rejuvenation; Nd:YAG with cooling, diode, and erbium glass for nonablative dermal remodeling; pulsed dye laser at low fluence.
▶ **Mechanism of action:** All have wavelengths that are primarily absorbed by water, sparing melanin and hemoglobin. Superficial ablation is a "laser peeling," or removal of the most superficial layers. Nonablative lasers cause dermal shrinking and thus tighten the skin.
▶ **Side effects:** Hypo- and hyperpigmentation; scarring (with ablative lasers).

46 Wound Healing

Disturbances in Wound Healing

Both the disease process itself and inappropriate treatment can impair wound healing. Both local and also systemic factors play significant roles.

▶ **Factors that enhance wound healing:**
- *General:* Youth, good general condition, good nutritional status.
- *Local:* Sterile wound, good circulation, maintenance of normal body temperature, tension-free suture repair, elevation or immobilization of wound (not of patient).

▶ **Factors that retard wound healing:**
- *General:* Inadequate treatment of underlying disease, advanced age, systemic disorders (metabolic diseases, anemia, arteriosclerosis, malignancy), impaired immunity, malnutrition, vitamin, protein and trace element deficiencies —for example, vitamin C, iron, or zinc), infections, medications (corticosteroids, cytostatic agents), allergies (suture materials, topical medications), bed rest, smoking.
- *Local:* Infection, necrosis, exudates, foreign bodies, drying out, cold, hematoma, edema, previous damage to tissue (ionizing irradiation, previous surgery, chronic venous insufficiency), neuropathy, focal disturbances in circulation (one artery occluded), tumors (ulcerated basal cell carcinoma does not heal as ulcer), suture repair under tension, wound not immobilized.

Treatment of Underlying Diseases

▣ *Note:* Treatment of chronic wounds, primarily ulcers, is futile if the underlying disease is not addressed.

▶ **Chronic venous ulcer:** Compression, mobilization, treat associated varicosities (p. 560).

▶ **Diabetic foot ulcer:** Reduce pressure, special shoes and foot care, maximize control of blood sugar levels.

▶ **Decubitus ulcer:** Reduce pressure, special beds or mattresses, partial mobilization.

▶ **Arterial ulcer:** Endovascular or vessel replacement therapy to restore arterial supply, rheologic therapy.

Rheologic Therapy

Attempts to improve circulation are an essential part of wound healing. If patients have peripheral arterial occlusion, a number of agents may be helpful. They include:

▶ **Rheologic agents:** Pentoxifylline 400 mg b.i.d.–t.i.d. to decrease blood viscosity; side effects include gastrointestinal problems, retinal bleeding, and leukopenia.

▶ **Musculotropic vasodilators:** Naftidrofuryl 100–200 mg t.i.d. to dilated vessels; side effects include disorientation and dizziness.

▶ **Calcium channel blockers:** Nifedipine 10–20 mg daily; diltiazem 120 mg daily. Side effects include edema, dizziness, and cardiovascular problems.

▶ **Prostaglandins:** Alprostadil i. v. 60 μg in 250 mL 0.9% NaCl solution over 2 hours. Usually given for 14–21 days, or for 7 days every month. Many side effects including edema, increased pain in extremities without adequate circulation, nausea, vomiting, and headache; can ameliorate by slowing rate of administration; pulmonary edema in patients with cardiac failure.

Topical Therapy

Modern wound therapy is adjusted to the severity of the wound, considers economic aspects and incorporates new understanding of the science of wound healing.

▶ **Cleansing or exudative phase:** Débridement is the key step. There are many possibilities:
- *Mechanical:* Débride with forceps, scalpel, or curette. Usually can be done with lidocaine/prilocaine (EMLA) anesthesia. Removal of necrotic tissue minimizes risk of infection, allows granulation to develop more luxuriously.
- *Biosurgery:* Sterile maggots can be used to meticulously groom a wound.
- *Autolytic:* Interactive dressings (alginates, hydrocolloids, polyurethane foams, hydrogels, activated charcoal, various membranes): All "trap" neutrophils over wound and encourage autolysis of necrotic tissue; painless but time-consuming.

▶ **Granulation phase:** Clean, well-vascularized wound base develops.
- Encourage granulation with appropriate dressings (alginates, hydrocolloids, hyaluronic acid) and nonsensitizing agents such as sterile sand or dextrose.
- Apply wound healing factors such as granulocyte macrophage colony stimulating factor (GM-CSF); platelet-derived growth factor (PDGF); transforming growth factor (TGF) β2, basic fibroblast growth factor (bFGF); or epidermal growth factor (EGF).
- ⚠ *Caution:* All these biologicals are very expensive and, although promising, their effectiveness has not been overwhelming.
- Vacuum seal technique (wound is placed under low vacuum pressure with sealed system).

▶ **Epithelialization phase:** Re-epithelization occurs at this point.
- Moist wound dressings stimulate re-epithelization. The wound must be protected; good choices include hydrogel and hydropolymer dressings.
- Pinch, split skin, or keratinocytic culture grafts can be used.

▶ **Other factors:**
- Dressing changes should be done under sterile conditions.
- Wounds can be rinsed with lactated Ringer solution, physiologic saline, or tap water.
- Antiseptics are preferred to antibiotics because of problems with resistance. Excellent choice is Octenisept solution, which is only minimally cytotoxic. Most useful in exudative phase to reduce bacteria.
- Antibiotics are generally avoided and should always be chosen carefully on the basis of culture and sensitivity results.
  - *Topical:* Fusidic acid is useful for the usual Gram-positive mixed infections; if MRSA or resistant mixed infections are present, mupirocin.
  - *Systemic:* Ciprofloxacin 500 mg p.o. b.i.d. for 10 days is a good choice for widespread local disease or systemic spread (lymphangiitis).
  - If culture results indicate resistance, then adjust accordingly.

47 Dermatologic Emergencies

Emergency Equipment

► **Emergency set:** Every practice and clinic should have the following immediately available:
- *Epinephrine* 1:1000 ampoule for subcutaneous use. Dilute 1:10 for i.v. use, giving final concentration of 1:10000.
- *Antihistamine*, for example diphenhydramine 50 mg ampoule.
- *Corticosteroids*, for example hydrocortisone 500 mg or methylprednisolone 125 mg for intravenous use.
- The set should also include laryngoscope, endotracheal tubes, resuscitator bag, and ideally a defibrillator.
- ▣ *Note:* The above equipment is necessary but not sufficient. All personnel must be trained in resuscitation. Both scheduled practice sessions and surprise drills should be held and documented. The telephone number of the appropriate emergency service should be posted prominently.

► **Prophylactic kit for patient:** Every patient who has had an anaphylactic reaction to Hymenoptera toxin should carry a kit containing an autoinjection device for epinephrine, as well as solutions of antihistamines and corticosteroids.

Anaphylactic Shock

► The most common cause for anaphylaxis in dermatologic patients is hyposensitization. Only those individuals trained in resuscitation should carry out hyposensitization procedures. In high-risk situations, such as testing for venom response, an intravenous line should be placed.

► The administration of the allergen should be stopped if possible; a tourniquet can be placed proximal to the site of inject to stop venous return and the area cooled to slow absorption. The appropriate measures, depending on the severity of the reaction, are shown in Table 47.**1**.

Table 47.1 · **Treatment of anaphylaxis**

Grade	Clinical features	Therapy
I	Pruritus, erythema, edema	Stop exposure Antihistamines i.v. (diphenhydramine 50 mg) Monitor cardiovascular status
II	Early bronchospasm, tachycardia, hypotension, nausea, vomiting	As above, +: Oxygen (nasal tube) Intravenous access with 500 – 1000 ml Ringer solution Corticosteroids i.v. (hydrocortisone 500 mg i.v.) Inhaled bronchodilators for bronchospasm
III	Shock, severe bronchospasm, coma	As above, +: See anaphylactic shock below
IV	Cardiopulmonary arrest	Cardiopulmonary resuscitation

► **Treatment for anaphylactic shock:**
  • Carefully monitor vital signs. Be prepared to intubate or do a tracheotomy.
  • Epinephrine 0.3–0.5 mg (0.3–0.5 mL of 1:1000 solution) subcutaneously; may be repeated at 20 minute intervals. If shock is severe, the epinephrine may be given i.v. but then using 3–5 mL of 1:10000 solution). Other possible routes are sublingual, inhaled, endotracheal, or via i.v. drip.
  • Further steps should be coordinated with intensive medicine or anesthesia, and follow local guidelines.

Acute Urticaria (p. 169)

Acute urticaria can become an emergency when angioedema or cardiovascular signs and symptoms develop.
► **Mild mucosal swelling:** Admit, i.v. fluids, antihistamines, and corticosteroids.
► **More severe mucosal swelling:** See anaphylaxis above. Admit, subcutaneous epinephrine, corticosteroids, antihistamines; careful monitoring.
► **Bronchospasm:** Beta-agonists (metaproterenol or albuterol as inhalant) or terbutaline 0.25 mg subq.
► **Hereditary angioedema** (p. 174):
  • C1-esterase inhibitor 500–100 IU i.v.; effects seen after 20–30 minutes.
  • Danazol 200–800 mg p.o. can also be given (more effective for prophylaxis).
  ▷ *Note:* Corticosteroids, epinephrine, and antihistamines are generally ineffective.
  • Be prepared to intubate or do tracheostomy; often difficult because of swelling.

Toxic Epidermal Necrolysis (TEN) (p. 185)

⚠ *Caution:* TEN has a high mortality rate (25–40%) and should be treated with the same urgency as a severe burn.
► **Diagnosis:**
  • **Skin biopsy with frozen section** (Call the pathologist out at night!): Distinguish between the full-thickness epidermal involvement of TEN and the superficial peeling of staphylococcal scalded skin syndrome (SSSS), which appears quite similar but more often in children. SSSS requires less aggressive therapy.
  • **Drug history:** Almost all TEN is drug-induced; look for high-risk drugs and stop all medications that are not essential.
  • Immediate admission, with consultation with intensive medicine. Room must be warm; be careful in summer with air-conditioned rooms. Patient should be in isolation, with regular monitoring for bacterial infections.
► **Systemic therapy:**
  • Careful attention to fluids and electrolytes.
  • Use of systemic steroids is controversial; follow local guidelines.
  • Local burn unit standards for prophylactic antibiotics.
  • Intravenous immunoglobulins 0.2–0.75 mg/kg daily for 4 days appears to block Fas-mediated keratinocyte death; most promising treatment.
  • Plasmapheresis is another alternative, but less well established than intravenous immunoglobulins.
► **Topical therapy:**
  • Use nonadherent dressings or if widespread denudation, use a burn bed.
  • Remove necrotic skin; puncture blisters.
  • Topical antibiotics such as fusidic acid or silver sulfadiazine.
  • Local anesthetics for oral lesions to facilitate eating.
  ⚠ *Caution:* Always get ophthalmologic consultation; there is a risk of erosions and scarring.

Paraphimosis

Phimosis is the condition where the foreskin cannot be contracted back over the glans; it may be congenitally tight or affected by lichen sclerosus, trauma, or infections. In *paraphimosis*, the foreskin becomes partially retracted, edematous, and exerts pressure on the glans, potentially leading to necrosis. In Germany, patients with paraphimosis may present to dermatologists rather than urologists.

▶ **Initial measures:**
  • Attempt to reduce edema by manual pressure, milking fluid from distal to proximal aspect of penis.
  • Then try the "door bell trick"; hold penis between middle and index fingers and press glans with thumb, aiming to push it back under the foreskin.
  • If unsuccessful, try cold bath (10–15 °C) or multiple needle punctures to allow fluid to drain.

▶ **Operative approach:**
  • If the foreskin cannot be reduced, then surgical intervention is required to avoid necrosis.
  • The foreskin should be split via a dorsal longitudinal incision and urology consulted. Once the swelling is resolved, circumcision is needed.

  ⚠ *Caution:* Patients with paraphimosis should always be hospitalized and the nursing staff warned to check frequently until definitive treatment can be provided.

Facial Furuncle/Carbuncle (p. 25)

⚠ *Caution:* There are two major risks—lid edema and cavernous sinus thrombosis.

▶ **Initial measures:**
  • Admission, bed rest, prohibit talking and chewing.
  • Culture and sensitivity studies.
  • Local disinfectants.

▶ **Systemic therapy:**
  • Penicillinase-resistant penicillin (dicloxacillin 500–1000 mg t.i.d.–q.i.d. i. v.) or cephalosporins (cephalexin 250–500 mg q.i.d.).
  • Adjust antibiotics based on culture.

Erysipelas (p. 78)

▶ Patients should be admitted, especially with facial erysipelas.
▶ High-dose penicillin i. v.; raise limb; cool compresses.
▶ Later, attempt to address portal of entry; consider compression, prophylactic antibiotics.

Necrotizing Fasciitis (p. 80)

▶ **Definition:** Severe destruction soft tissue infection caused by mixed infection (type I) or *Streptococcus pyogenes* (type II); recent cases from community-based methicillin-resistant *Staphylococcus aureus*. In addition, bullous erysipelas may evolve into necrotizing fascitis.

▶ **Initial measures:**
  • Admission, bed rest.
  • Aspiration or incision for culture and sensitivity; exclude clostridial infection with wound smear.
  • Baseline laboratory tests and then follow for leukopenia, hypocalcaemia (fat necrosis), and elevated creatinine (muscle necrosis).

- Surgical consultation.
- Imaging studies (MRI).
► **Surgical management:**
- Extensive debridement.
- Fasciotomy.

  ⚡ Caution: Mortality without surgical intervention is 99%; in the best of hands, 30%.

► **Internal therapy:**
- Fluid replacement.
- Broad-spectrum antibiotic coverage following local guidelines; usually includes penicillin, an aminoglycoside and either metronidazole or clindamycin for Gram-negative organisms.
- Adjust antibiotics on the basis of culture and sensitivity.
- Watch for shock.

Deep Vein Thrombosis

► **Diagnosis:** With slightest suspicion, order D-dimer and compression sonography. Doppler ultrasonography and impedance plethysmography are only reliable for pelvic vein thrombosis. If tests are negative, repeat in a few hours or do phlebography.

► **Isolated calf vein thrombosis:** Ambulatory care possible, low molecular weight heparin once daily, compression therapy, and consider for coumarin therapy. Some advise initially monitoring because only 20% of calf vein thromboses extend and risk of emboli is very small. Follow local guidelines.

► **Thigh or pelvic vein thrombosis:** No controversy; complete anticoagulation with heparin and then coumarin.
- Heparin 5000–10000 IU as i.v. bolus; then either by i.v. drip (25–50000 IU daily) or subq. injection (15000 IU b.i.d.).
- Measure activated partial thromboplastin time (aPTT) before starting heparin; aim for value 1.5–2.0× normal value (usually then 50–80 seconds). Monitor b.i.d.
- Simultaneously start coumarin and aim for INR of 2–3.
- Watch for heparin-induced thrombocytopenia and coumarin necrosis.
- Fibrinolytic therapy with urokinase, streptokinase, or tissue plasminogen activator (tPA) may be indicated in selected patients; consult with cardiology.
- Surgical thrombectomy may be indicated in femoroiliac thrombosis less than 1 week old; consult with cardiovascular surgery.

Burns

► **Definition:** Tissue damage caused by thermal energy
► **Clinical features:**
- In most instances, diagnosing a burn is easy but grading it to assess risk and plan treatment can be difficult. The classification of burns is shown in Table 47.**2**.
- Scalds are usually less deep than burns from flames, hot surfaces, or electrical current. Chemical burns vary with agent, but tend to progress over days.
- The other important task is to assess the extent of the burns. It is not always possible to do this immediately. The *Rule of Nines* (Table 47.**3**) is generally employed as shown. One adds the values for areas burned to estimate the percentage of total surface area which is affected. Another rough measure is that the palm of the hand represents 1% of the body surface in all age groups.

Table 47.2 · Severity of burns

Degree	Clinical features	Color	Painful	Depth	Scarring
I	Superficial	Erythema, later peeling	Red	+	Upper epidermis	None
II	Partial thickness	Blisters	Red	+	Epidermis, upper dermis	None; re-epithelializes from adnexal structures
III	Full thickness	Necrosis	White, brown, black	–	Epidermis, dermis, appendages, deeper structures	Scars; grafting required

Table 47.3 · Rule of nines

Region	Newborn	Infant	Child	Adult
Head	21	19	15	9
Chest	16	16	16	18
Back	16	16	16	18
Arm	9.5	9.5	9.5	9
Leg	14	15	17	18
Genitalia	1	1	1	1

► **Therapy:**
  ◘ *Note:* The initial management of all burns is cooling; it relieves pain and reduces the extent of damage.
  • Children with more than 10% or adults with more than 15% second-degree burns should be admitted. If in doubt, admit.
  • All patients should receive analgesics and tetanus immunization as needed.
  • Those who are admitted should have an intravenous line, fluid replacement. and be monitored for shock.
  • *First-degree burns:* No special care needed; soft dressing; polidocanol ointment or topical corticosteroids.
  ◘ *Note:* Topical anesthetics of the benzocaine family are widely sold over the counter for first-degree burns but carry a high risk of sensitization and then allergic contact dermatitis.
  • *Second-degree burns:*
    – Débridement.
    – Topical disinfectants or antibiotics and soft dressings.
    – Silver sulfadiazine.
    – Mafenide.
    – Povidone-iodine.
    – Biosynthetic membrane dressings also useful.

- *Third-degree burns:* Specialized burn care, surgical debridement, temporary coverage with skin substitutes; later coverage with skin grafting, cultured keratinocytes, or other bioengineered dressings. Meticulous monitoring for infections. Pressure garments for prophylaxis against keloids.
► **Special cases:**
- *Electrical burns:* Usually deep, often subtle burns—at the sites of entry and exit; watch for myoglobinuria, renal failure, and compartment syndrome.
- *Lightning burns:* Cutaneous injuries may be subtle; sometimes fern figures seen; biggest risks are cardiac conduction defects and neurological problems.

Chemical Burns

► **Clinical features:** Chemical burns result when strong alkali or acid materials are spilled on the skin. The exact nature of the chemical is important in determining the degree and nature of injury.
- *Acid burns* tend to be dry as the liquid immediately kills and fixes the skin, producing superficial, sharply bordered lesions.
- *Alkali burns* are liquefactive, as the bases continue to dissolve the skin causing deeper, more necrotic ulcers.
- In either case, systemic resorption may occur.
► **Therapy:**
- Immediate and extensive rinsing; either with tap water or with antidote solutions if available.
- Balance of management depends on nature of chemical.
- ◪ *Note:* Hydrofluoric acid burns are particularly destructive; the lesions should be injected with calcium gluconate 10% and mepivacaine solution mixed 1:1. In more extensive burns, i.v. calcium gluconate is required with monitoring by anesthesiology. The calcium salts form harmless calcium fluoride.

Cold Injury

► **Hypothermia:** Diffuse cooling of the body, caused by exposure to cold, snow, cold water; core temperature < 35 °C; major medical emergency.
► **Frostbite:** Defined as cold injury caused when skin temperature drops below 0 °C. Also divided into three classes:
- *First degree:* Blanching, following by re-warming with painful erythema.
- *Second degree:* More extensive, with edema and blisters.
- *Third degree:* Deep tissue damage, with vascular injury and necrosis.
► **Therapy:**
- ⚠ *Caution:* No rubbing; no attempt at re-warming until in hospital.
- Re-warm with total body bath at 40 °C; hot tap water is usually too warm.
- If less severe, use a lower temperature because of risk of shock.
- Rest of management is just like burn care, except that as necrosis delineates itself, amputation is often needed.
- In second and third degree frostbite, limb remains very sensitive to cold.
► **Immersion foot:**
- *Definition:* Cold damage caused by prolonged exposures at temperature > 0 °C; no true freezing.
- Common military injury, also known as *trench foot*.
- Initially painful with erythema, livedo, ulcerations; can progress to gangrene.
- Limb remains very sensitive to cold.

Traumatic Tattoos

► **Clinical features:** Several common causes for particles to be embedded in the skin, including exploding fireworks, accidents using black gunpowder, traumatic road accidents with sand and dirt particles.

  ☑ *Caution:* Treatment should be undertaken within 24 hours; otherwise it is very difficult to remove dermal particles.

► **Initial measures:**
  • Ophthalmology consult: Corneal injury?
  • Otorhinolaryngology consult: Ruptured tympanic membrane?
  • Perhaps radiologic evaluation.

► **Removal of particles:**
  • Adequate preoperative analgesia, such as:
    – Ibuprofen 800 mg.
    – Tramadol drops (20 drops = 0.5 mL = 50 mg).
    – Diazepam 10 mg.
    – Topical anesthetic such as EMLA.
  • Topical spray disinfection.
  • Remove larger particles with fine forceps; finer ones with hard toothbrush (perhaps dipped in topical anesthetic).
  • Still deeper particles can be removed with 2 mm biopsy punch.
  • Postoperative therapy with topical retinoids can create additional peeling and discharge of residual particles, as well as helping with healing.
  • Laser therapy for residual hyperpigmentation.

  ▣ *Note:* Dermabrasion in this setting has a considerable risk of scarring and is best avoided.

Tick Bite (p. 93)

▣ *Note:* It is far easier to avoid ticks than to risk the difficulties of identification and removal, and the worry. Use insect repellents, ideally with high concentration of DEET; wear long sleeves and trousers in woods, stuff trousers into socks; clothes be can impregnated with insecticide or permethrin.

► **Removal of tick:** Stretch skin tight, and remove tick either with rapid flick of curette or fine forceps, grasping anterior part of tick mouth parts as close to skin surface as possible.

  ☑ *Caution:* Trying to suffocate or burn the tick, or squeezing its engorged body, carries the risk of additional regurgitation of infectious material into the skin.

► **Potential infections:** Know what ticks in your area are likely to carry. In Europe, there are two major problems:
  • *Borreliosis:*
    – In endemic areas, 5–50% of ticks may have *Borrelia burgdorferi*. Transfer occurs in 10% of bites, with clinical disease in less than half. Usually tick must be attached for more than 24 hours. Thus daily tick checks in high-risk areas or professions (farmer, forest worker).
    – Only treat if clinical features or serology indicates infection.
    – Prophylactic antibiotics not indicated (although often used).
  • *Tick-borne encephalitis:*
    – Caused by flaviviruses.
    – Endemic areas in Central Europe, including many parts of Germany; more virulent form in Russia.
    – About 1–5% of ticks infected; even with transfer, only 10% of patients symptomatic, so risk very low.

- Immunization available; should be used by those in endemic areas with frequent exposure.
- Onset of disease 1–4 weeks after bite; if tick removed in endemic area, refer to primary physician for monitoring.
- Treatment is symptomatic.
- *Other tick-borne diseases that can be potential emergencies:*
  - Rocky Mountain spotted fever in parts of USA (especially Oklahoma, North Carolina); caused by *Rickettsia rickettsii.* Treatment: doxycycline.
  - Babesiosis or Nantucket fever, caused by *Babesia microti,* a protozoan; particular problem in splenectomized patients. Treatment complex: clindamycin and quinine or other antimalarial agents.
  - Human monocytic ehrlichiosis caused by *Ehrlichia chaffeensis,* primarily in Midwestern USA and also in Europe. Treatment: doxycycline.
  - Human granulocytic ehrlichiosis, caused by *Anaplasma phagocytophila* and *Ehrlichia ewingii,* in USA and Europe. Treatment: doxycycline.

⚠ *Caution:* In endemic areas, ticks may carry more than one pathogen; always consider mixed infections when clinical course of borreliosis is atypical or acute. On Cape Cod and Nantucket Island, ticks may have *Borrelia burgdorferi, Babesia microti,* and *Anaplasma phagocytophila.*

Appendix I Common Systemic Medications

■ **Note:** The following list includes most of the systemic medications described in this book, for quick reference. Some medications are used in quite different dosages for different dermatologic indications. We have tried to insure uniformity, but if differences are found, always rely on the manufacturers' guidelines and latest prescribing information available online.

■ **Caution:** Note that no information has been provided on adjusting dosage for renal impairment. In addition, chemotherapy agents, many analgesics, and psychotropic agents have been omitted. Refer to latest sources for detailed information.

Table I.1 · Common systemic medications

Medication	Use	Dose
Acetaminophen	NSAID	1.5–4.0 g daily
Acitretin	Disorders of keratinization, psoriasis	0.2–1.0 mg/kg p.o. daily (lower doses for disorders of keratinization)
Acyclovir	Herpes simplex Zoster In immunosuppressed	200 mg 5 × p.o. daily 800 mg 5 × p.o. daily 5–10 mg/kg i.v. q8h
Albendazole	Anthelminthic	400 mg p.o. daily for 1–3 days
Amoxicillin	Antibiotic	500–1000 mg p.o. t.i.d. 1–2 g i.v. q8h
Amoxicillin + clavulanate	Antibiotic	500 mg amoxicillin/125 mg clavulanic acid 1–2 tab p.o. t.i.d. 1 g amoxicillin/250 mg clavulanic acid i.v. q6–8h
Amphotericin B	Antifungal	0.25 mg/kg i.v. daily over 4–6 h ■ **Caution:** Liposomal form preferred; complex protocols; see other sources
Ampicillin	Antibiotic	250–500 mg p.o. t.i.d.–q.i.d. 500 mg–3.0 g i.v. q4–6h
Ampicillin + sulbactam	Antibiotic	1.5–3.0 g i.v. q6h
Aspirin	Analgesic Anticoagulant	325–650 mg p.o. q4–6h 165 mg p.o. daily
Azathioprine	Immunosuppressive	1–3 mg/kg p.o daily; can use q.o.d.

Continued Table I.1 ▶

Table I.1 · Continued

Medication	Use	Dose
Azelastine	Antihistamine	2 mg p.o. b.i.d.
Azithromycin	Antibiotic	250 mg p.o. daily; 1.0 g as single dose for gonorrhea; 1.0 g as single dose for chancroid
Bexarotene	Retinoid	100–300 mg/m² p.o. daily
Brivudin	Herpes zoster	125 mg p.o. daily
Buprenorphine	Central analgesic	0.2–0.4 mg sublingual q6–8 h 0.15–0.3 mg i.v. or i.m. q6–8 h
Calcitonin	Polypeptide hormone	100 IU i.v. or via nasal spray daily ■ *Note:* Off-label use for Raynaud syndrome
Carbamazepine	Anticonvulsant, antineuralgic	100–200 mg p.o. b.i.d.; can increase to 1.2 g daily; lower doses for neuralgia; serum level 3–8 mg/L ⚡ *Caution:* High risk of drug reactions!
β-Carotene	Vitamin	75–100 mg daily
Caspofungin	Antifungal	50 mg i.v. daily
Cefazolin	1st generation cephalosporin	500–1000 mg i.v. q6–8 h
Cefixime	2nd generation cephalosporin	200 mg p.o. b.i.d. or 400 mg p.o. daily; 400 mg p.o. in single dose for gonorrhea
Cefotaxime	3rd generation cephalosporin	1–2 g i.v. q8–12 h
Cefotiam	2nd generation cephalosporin	1–2 g i.v. q8–12 h
Ceftriaxone	3rd generation cephalosporin	1–2 g i.v. or i.m. daily or in 2 divided doses; 250 mg i.m. in single dose for gonorrhea
Cefuroxime	2nd generation cephalosporin	0.75–1.5 g i.v. q8–12 h
Cephalexin	1st generation cephalosporin	500 mg p.o. b.i.d.; higher doses for severe infections

Table I.1 · Continued

Medication	Use	Dose
Cephalothin	1st generation cephalosporin	500–1000 mg i.v. q4–6 h; 2.0 g i.m. in single dose for gonorrhea
Cetirizine	Antihistamine	10 mg p.o. daily or b.i.d.
Chlorambucil	Immunosuppressive	0.1–0.2 mg/kg p.o. daily; often 4 mg p.o. daily
Chlormadinone	Anti-androgen	2 mg p.o. daily
Chloroquine	Antimalarial	250 mg daily
Chlorpheniramine	Antihistamine	2–4 mg p.o. q4–6 h
Cidofovir	Antiviral	5 mg/kg i.v. once weekly
Cimetidine	Antihistamine (H2 blocker)	300 mg p.o. q.i.d., 400 mg p.o. b.i.d., or 800 mg p.o. HS; also used i.v.; consult other sources
Ciprofloxacin	Antibiotic	250–500 mg p.o. b.i.d. 200–400 mg i.v. q12 h
Clarithromycin	Antibiotic	250 mg p.o. b.i.d.
Clemastine	Antihistamine	1–2 mg p.o. b.i.d. 1–2 mg i.v. in single dose
Clindamycin	Antiobiotic	150–450 mg p.o. q6–8 h 200–600 mg i.v. q6–8 h
Clofazimine	Antiobiotic	100 mg p.o. daily–t.i.d
Clomipramine	Antidepressant	50–100 mg p.o. daily
Codeine	Analgesic	15–30 mg p.o. 4–6 × daily
Colchicine	Anti gout	0.5–2.0 mg p.o. daily
Co-trimoxazole	Antibiotic	Sulfamethoxazole: 400–800 mg/ trimethoprim 80/160 mg 1 double-strength tab p.o. b.i.d.
Cromolyn	Antiasthmatic; anti-allergic	2 sprays q.i.d.; also available as eye drops, nose drops
Cyclophosphamide	Immunosuppressive	1–3 mg/kg p.o. daily; pulse 7.5–15.0 mg/kg p.o. or 500–1000 mg/m² i.v. once monthly

Continued Table I.1 ▶

Table I.1 · Continued

Medication	Use	Dose
Cyclosporine	Immunosuppressive	2.5–5 mg/kg p.o.; also available i.v.; serum level 100–300 µg/L
Cyproheptadine	Antihistamine	4 mg p.o. q4–6 h
Cyproterone acetate	Antiandrogen	Usually used with ethinyl estradiol; can also be used to supplement ethinyl estradiol; dose 2.5–5.0 mg p.o. daily
Danazol	Androgen	200–600 mg daily
Dapsone	Immunomodulator	50–100 mg daily; can go to 150 mg; watch for hemolysis, methemoglobinemia
Dimethindene	Antihistamine	1–2 mg p.o. t.i.d. 4 mg i.v. in single dose or b.i.d.
Desloratadine	Antihistamine	5 mg p.o. daily
Dexamethasone	Corticosteroid	0.75–9.0 mg p.o. or i.v. daily in divided doses
Diazepam	Sedative	2–10 mg p.o. t.i.d.–q.i.d. 5–10 mg i.v. t.i.d. 2–20 mg p.o. or rectal in single dose
Diclofenac	NSAID	50 mg p.o. t.i.d.
Dicloxacillin	Antibiotic	0.5–1.0 g p.o. q6–8 h
Diltiazem	Antihypertensive	30 mg p.o. t.i.d.–q.i.d.; wide range upwards
Diphenhydramine	Antihistamine	25–50 mg p.o. q4–6 h
Doxepin	Tricyclic antidepressant, antihistamine	10–20 mg p.o. q.i.d.
Doxycycline	Antibiotic	100 mg p.o. daily; loading dose 200 mg; for acne 50 mg p.o. daily
Ebastine	Antihistamine	10 mg p.o. daily or b.i.d.
Erythromycin	Antibiotic	250–500 mg p.o. t.i.d.–q.i.d.
Ethambutol	Antituberculosis	15–25 mg/kg p.o. daily

Table I.1 · Continued

Medication	Use	Dose
Famciclovir	Antiviral	250 mg p.o. t.i.d.
Flucloxacillin	Antiobiotic	1 g i.v. 3 x daily
Fexofenadine	Antihistamine	60 mg p.o. b.i.d. or 60–180 mg p.o. daily
Fluconazole	Antifungal	50 mg p.o. daily for dermatophytes; 150 mg p.o. weekly for onychomycosis; 200–800 mg p.o. daily for systemic candidiasis
Flucytosine	Antifungal	50–150 mg/kg i.v. daily divided q6 h
Foscarnet	Antiviral	60 mg/kg i.v. over 1 hour q8 h ⚠ *Caution:* Complex regimens; check other sources
Fumaric acid	Antipsoriatic	Detailed dosages (p. 635)
Gentamicin	Antibiotic	2–5 mg/kg i.v. daily in 2 or 3 divided doses
Griseofulvin	Antifungal	500–1000 mg p.o. daily (microsize); 330–375 mg p.o. daily (ultramicrosize); children 10–20 mg/kg p.o. daily
Hydroxychloroquine	Antimalarial	200–400 mg p.o. daily
Hydroxyzine	Antihistamine	10–50 mg p.o. q6–8 h; 50 mg p.o. HS
Ibuprofen	NSAID	200–600 mg p.o. q8–12 h
Indomethacin	NSAID	25–50 mg p.o. q8–12 h
Interferon-α2a and α2b	Immunomodulator	3–10 million IU subq or IM 3× weekly
Isoniazid	Anti-tuberculosis	5 mg/kg p.o. daily
Isotretinoin	Acne	0.5 mg/kg p.o. daily
Itraconazole	Antifungal	100–200 mg p.o. daily; other regimens for onychomycosis
Ivermectin	Anthelminthic	150–400 µg/kg; scabies is treated with 1–2 doses; see literature for anthelminthic therapy

Continued Table I.1 ▶

Table I.1 · Continued

Medication	Use	Dose
Ketotifen	Antihistamine	2 mg p.o. b.i.d.
Ketoconazole	Antifungal	200–400 mg p.o. daily
Levocetirizine	Antihistamine	5 mg p.o. daily or b.i.d
Loratadine	Antihistamine	10 mg p.o. daily
Mebendazole	Anthelminthic	Pinworms: 100 mg p.o. in single dose Others: 100 mg p.o. b.i.d. × 3 days
Methotrexate	Immunosuppressive	7.5–25 mg p.o. or i.m. weekly
Methotrimeprazine	Analgesic	10–20 mg i.m. q4–6 h
Methylprednisolone	Corticosteroid	4–48 mg p.o. daily 10–40 mg i.v. as single dose
Metronidazole	Antibiotic	500–750 mg p.o. b.i.d. for anaerobic infections
	Antiprotozoal	2.0 g in single dose for trichomoniasis
Mizolastine	Antihistamine	10 mg p.o. daily
Morphine	Opiate analgesic	5–30 mg p.o. q4 h PRN 4–15 mg i.v. or i.m. q4 h PRN
Mycophenolate mofetil	Immunosuppressive	1.0–2.0 g p.o. daily
Nafcillin	Antiobiotic	500 mg p.o. q.i.d.; 500–1000 mg i.v. q4–6 h
Naftidrofuryl	Vasodilator	100–200 mg p.o. t.i.d.
Nicotinamide	Vitamin	0.2–1.2 g p.o. daily
Nifedipine	Antihypertensive	5–10 mg p.o. t.i.d.; wide range upwards
Norfloxacin	Antibiotic	400 mg. b.i.d.
Nystatin	Antifungal	2 tab p.o. t.i.d. (1 tablet = 500 000 IU)
Ofloxacin	Antibiotic	400 mg p.o or i.v. q12 h
Omeprazole	Proton pump blocker	20 mg p.o. daily

Table I.1 · Continued

Medication	Use	Dose
Ondansetron	Serotonin antagonist	8 mg p.o. or i.v. 30 minutes before chemotherapy; repeat after 30 and 60 min
Penicillin-Benzathine	Antibiotic	1.2–2.4 million IU i.m. in single dose
Penicillin-G	Antibiotic	400–500 000 IU p.o. q8–12 h 0.5–10 million IU i.v. q4–6 h
Penicillin-V	Antibiotic	125–500 mg p.o. q6 h
Penicillamine	Immunomodulator	250 mg b.i.d.–t.i.d.
Pentoxifylline	Rheologic	400–600 mg p.o. b.i.d.–t.i.d.
Praziquantel	Anthelminthic	40 mg/kg p.o. in single dose or 20 mg/kg p.o. q8 h × 3
Prazosin	Antihypertensive	1–6 mg p.o. daily
Prednisolone	Corticosteroid	5–60 mg p.o. daily Emergencies: 250–1000 mg i.v.
Prednisone	Corticosteroid	5–60 mg p.o. daily
Promethazine	Antihistamine	12.5 mg p.o. t.i.d.–q.i.d.; 25 mg p.o. HS
Pyrantel pamoate	Anthelminthic	10 mg/kg p.o. in single dose
Pyrazinamide	Anti-tuberculosis	1.5–2.0 g p.o daily or 3 × weekly
Quinacrine	Antimalarial	100 mg p.o. daily
Ranitidine	Antihistamine (H2 blocker)	150–300 mg p.o. HS
Rifampicin	Antibiotic	600 mg p.o. 1–2 × daily
Spectinomycin	Antibiotic	2.0 g i.m. in single dose for gonorrhea
Streptomycin	Anti-tuberlosis	1.0 g i.m. daily
Sulfasalazine	Anti-inflammatory	500–1000 mg p.o. b.i.d.; start with lower dose and work up
Terbinafine	Antifungal	250 mg daily; other regimens for onychomycosis

Continued Table I.1 ▶

Table I.1 · Continued

Medication	Use	Dose
Thalidomide	Antileprosy	100–200 mg p.o. q.i.d. ⚠ *Caution:* Pregnancy precautions, highly variable dosages
Thiabendazole	Anthelmintic	500 mg p.o. b.i.d. for 3–4 days
Tilidine + naloxone	CNS analgesic	50–100 mg p.o. q6–8h Tablet = 50 mg tilidine + 4 mg naloxone
Tramadol	Analgesic	50–100 mg p.o., i.v. or subq. q6–8h
Tripelennamine	Antihistamine	25–50 mg p.o. q4–6h
Tropisetron	Serotonin antagonist	5 mg p.o. or i.v.
Valacyclovir	Herpes simplex Zoster	500–1000 mg p.o. b.i.d. 1000 mg p.o. t.i.d.
Vancomycin	Antiobiotic	500 mg i.v. q6h
Verapamil	Antihypertensive	80–120 mg p.o. t.i.d.
Voriconazole	Antifungal	200–400 mg p.o. or i.v. daily

Appendix II   Favorite Compounding Recipes

Overview

Compounding is no longer as essential to dermatologic practice as it was 50 years ago when every dermatologist had a list of favorite prescriptions (Table II.1). In general, the commercially available products cover the entire spectrum of topical treatment, are more stable than compounded products, and are tested to insure that the active ingredients are delivered to the skin. Nonetheless there are situations where compounding is still very useful. They include:

► Allergies to preservatives or other additives in commercial vehicles.
► Lack of availability of certain combinations of vehicles and active ingredients.
► Lack of flexibility as when dithranol concentration is slowly increased.
► Expense—in many instances, the compounded product is far cheaper.

Practical Approach

► It is best to rely on tested formulations available in a variety of sources such as national formularies. Any changes in such prescriptions should be checked with a pharmacist or colleague experienced in compounding, as even minor changes can influence the effectiveness and stability of the final product. For example, a study in Germany showed that many of the extemporaneously compounded erythromycin solutions were neither stable nor active.
► The effectiveness of the vehicle in dermatologic therapy cannot be underestimated. The choice of the vehicle depends on the acuity and location of the disease, the properties of the skin and chemical nature of the active ingredient.
► It is better to compound from scratch than to add an active ingredient to a commercial product. For example, most corticosteroid creams are fairly finely tuned mixtures; when an antibiotic is added to them, often neither the corticosteroid or the antibiotic is effectively available.
► Compounded products almost always have a shorter shelf life than commercial products. If a large supply is provided, patients should be instructed to transfer the contents stepwise to a smaller jar to minimize the risk of contaminating the main supply.
🗷 *Caution:* Resist the temptation to compound creatively; more than two active ingredients usually means incompatibility or decreased effectiveness.

Table II.1 · Favorite formulations

Name and ingredients[a]	Concentration (%)	Indications
Anal dermatitis paste		
	Vehicle: Hydrocarbon gel	Anal dermatitis
Ammonium bitumino-sulfonate	5.0	
Acid. tannic	2.0	
(Polidocanol)	3.0	
Pasta Zinci DAB	ad 100.0	
Arning tincture (former NRF 11.13.)		
		Antimicrobial; acute dermatitis, especially weeping or super-infected; fissures
Anthrarobin	3.0	
Ammonium bituminosulfonate	3.0	
Propylene glycol	6.0	
Isopropyl alcohol	40.0	
Ether	ad 100.0	
ASS lotion		
		Postherpetic neuralgia
Acetylsalicylic acid	5.0	
Emulsifying cetearyl alcohol (type A)	2.0	
White clay	10.0	
Titanium dioxide	5.0	
Propylene glycol	15.6	
Water	ad 100.0	
Betamethasone valerate hydrophilic cream (0.025, 0.05 or 0.1%) (NRF 11.37.)		
	Vehicle type: ambiphilic cream	Acute and subacute dermatitis
Bethamethasone-17 valerate	0.025 | 0.05 | 0.1	
Triglyceride (medium chain)	0.5	
Citric acid solution 0.5%	2.5	
Sodium citrate solution 0.5%	2.5	
Basiscreme DAC	ad 100.0	

Table II.1 · Continued

Name and ingredients[a]	Concentration (%)	Indications

Betamethasone valerate hydrophilic emulsion (0.025, 0.05 or 0.1%) (NRF 11.47.)

Name and ingredients[a]	Concentration (%)	Indications
	Vehicle type: Non-ionic O/W lotion	Acute scalp dermatitis, mucosal lichen planus
Low-fat easily washable emulsion		
Bethamethasone-17 valerate	0.025 | 0.5 | 0.1	
Hydrophilic skin emulsion (NRF S. 25.)	ad 100.0	

Capsaicin cream (0.025, 0.05, or 0.1%) (NRF 11.125.)

	Anionic O/W cream	Postherpetic neuralgia, intense pruritus
Ethanolic capsaicin solution 1%	2.5 | 5.0 | 10.0	
Basiscreme DAC	50.0	
Propylene glycol	10.0	
Water	ad 100.0	

Clioquinol cream A

		Infected acute or subacute dermatitis
Clioquinol	1.0 | 2.0	
Anionic hydrophilic cream SR DAC (NRF S. 27.)	ad 100.0	

Clioquinol cream B

Clioquinol	2.0	
Hydrous liniment SR DAC (NRF 11.93.)	ad 100.0	

Clioquinol Lotio Cordes

	Vehicle type: Non-ionic O/W lotion	Herpes simplex, zoster; acute dermatitis
Clioquinol	1.0 | 2.0	
Lotio Cordes	ad 100.0	

Continued Table II.1 ▶

Table II.1 · Continued

Name and ingredients[a]	Concentration (%)	Indications
Clobetasol or betamethasone in white petrolatum		
	Vehicle type: hydrocarbon gel	Short-term therapy of dermatitis; not face; clobetasol class IV; betamethasone class III
Clobetasol-17-proprionate or	0.05	
Betamethasone-17-valerate	0.1	
White petrolatum	ad 100.0	
Dermatitis ointment		
		Chronic dermatitis
Leukichthol[b] or	3.0 – 5.0	
Betamethasone-17-valerate[b]	0.1	
Citric acid solution 0.5%	2.5	
Sodium citrate solution 0.5%	2.5	
Basiscreme DAC	ad 100.0	
Dexamethasone liniment		
	Vehicle type: Anionic O/W cream	Acute and subacute dermatitis
Dexamethasone	0.05	
Hydrous liniment SR DAC (NRF 11.93.)	ad 100.0	
Dithranol–Macrogol[b] ointment (0.25, 0.5, 1 or 2%)(NRF 11.53.)		
		Psoriasis; easily washable; especially suited for scalp
Dithranol	0.25 | 0.5 | 1.0 | 2.0	
Salicylic acid	3.0 | 3.0 | 3.0 | 3.0	
Propylene glycol	24.2 | 24.1 | 24.0 | 23.75	
Macrogol 400	24.2 | 24.1 | 24.0 | 23.75	
Macrogol 1500	24.2 | 24.1 | 24.0 | 23.75	
Macrogol 4000	ad 100.0	

Table II.1 · Continued

Name and ingredients[a]	Concentration (%)	Indications
Eosin alcoholic solution (0.5, 1, or 2%) (NRF 11.94.)		
Eosin dinatrium	0.5 | 1.0 | 2.0	
Ethanol 96%	20.0	
Anhydrous citric acid	0.02 | 0.04 | 0.08	
Water	ad 100.0	
Eosin aqueous solution (0.5, 1 or 2%) (NRF 11.95.)		
Eosin dinatrium	0.5 | 1.0 | 2.0	
Anhydrous citric acid	0.01 | 0.0175 | 0.025	
Water	ad 100.0	
Erythromycin hydrophilic cream (0.5, 1, 2 or 4%) (NRF 11.77.)		
	⚠ **Caution:** Very unstable; never combine erythromycin with other active ingredients.	Acne vulgaris; impetigo and impetiginized dermatitis
Erythromycin base	0.55 | 1.1 | 2.2 | 4.4	
Anhydrous citric acid	0.015 | 0.04 | 0.06 | 0.07	
Propylene glycol	10.0	
Basiscreme DAC	50.0	
Water	ad 100.0	
Erythromycin tincture (0.5, 1, 2 or 4%) (NRF 11.78.)		
		Acne, folliculitis
Erythromycin base	0.55 | 1.1 | 2.2 | 4.4	
Anhydrous citric acid	0.038 | 0.076 | 0.154 | 0.3	
Ethanol 96%	45.0	
Water	ad 100.0 If too dry, also add octyldodecanol q. sat.	
Estrogen scalp tincture for men		
17-β-Estradiol benzoate	0.005	
Isopropyl alcohol 70%	ad 100.0	

Continued Table II.1 ▶

Table II.1 · Continued

Name and ingredients[a]	Concentration (%)	Indications
Estrogen scalp tincture for women		
		Androgenetic alopecia, telogen effluvium in women
17-β-estradiol benzoate	0.015–0.040	
Isopropyl alcohol 70%	ad 100.0 | ad 300.0	
Ichthyol ointment		
	Vehicle type: Hydrocarbon gel or water-absorbent ointment (W/O type)	Psoriasis, chronic dermatitis, prurigo nodularis
Leukichthol	3.0–10.0	
White petrolatum or Ungt. alcohol. lanae DAB	ad 100.0	
Keratolytic ointment		
	Vehicle type: water absorbent ointment (O/W type)	Hyperkeratotic lesions
Acid salicyl.	5.0	
Kerasal Basissalbe (ointment)	ad 100.0	Contains 10% urea
Lactic acid cream		
	Vehicle type: O/W cream	Chronic dermatitis
Acid. lact.	1.0	
Sodium lactate 50%	4.0	
Abitima cream	ad 100.0	
Lipid-poor corticosteroid lotion		
	Vehicle type: Non-ionic O/W lotion	Non-comedogenic, cooling corticosteroid lotion
Triamcinolone acetonide	0.025–0.1	
Hydrophilic skin emulsion (NRF S. 25.)	ad 100.0	
Lipid-rich corticosteroid Lotion		
	Vehicle type: W/O lotion	For very dry skin; contains 4% urea
Triamcinolone acetonide	0.2	
Excipial U Lipolotio	ad 200.0	

Table II.1 · Continued

Name and ingredients[a]	Concentration (%)	Indications
Menthol lotion		
	Vehicle type: Non-ionic O/W cream paste	Arthropod bites and stings; urticaria
Menthol	0.25	
Zinc oxide shake lotion 25% SR (NRF 11.109.)	ad 100.0	
Methylrosaniline chloride solution (0.1 or 0.5%) (NRF 11.69.)		
	Known in English as methyl violet	Topical antiseptic and antifungal; interdigital dermatophytosis, candidal intertrigo, gramnegative toe web infection
Methylrosaniline chloride ethanol solution 10% (NRF S. 16.)	1.0 | 5.0	
Water	ad 100.0	
Metronidazole hydrophilic cream (1 or 2%) (NRF 11.91.)		
	Vehicle type: Non-ionic O/W cream ◨ **Note:** Store 1% cream in refrigerator.	Rosacea
Metronidazole	1.0 | 2.0	
Non-ionic hydrophilic cream SR DAC (NRF S. 26.)	49.0 | 48.0	
Potassium sorbate	0.7	
Anhydrous citric acid	0.035	
Water	ad 100.0	
Minoxidil scalp tincture (2 or 5%)		
	◨ **Note:** Minoxidil is dissolved in the mixture of propylene glycol and ethanol with heating; after cooling add water	Androgenetic alopecia
Minoxidil	2.0 | 5.0	
Propylene glycol	15.0	
Water	15.0	
Ethanol 96%	ad 100.0	

Continued Table II.1 ▶

Table II.1 · Continued

Name and ingredients[a]	Concentration (%)	Indications
Nail removal paste 40% urea (NRF 11.30.)		
		Removal of dystrophic or ony-chomycotic nails
Urea	40.0	
Thick paraffin	15.0	
White petrolatum	20.0	
Bees wax, white	5.0	
Wool wax	20.0	
Nystatin zinc paste		
		Candida intertrigo, angular cheilitis
Nystatin	10 million IU	
Olive oil	5.0	
Zinc paste DAB	ad 100.0	
Rhagade ointment		
		Chronic hand dermatitis
Betamethesone-17-valerate	0.1	
Salicylic acid	5.0	
Leukichthol	20.0	
Ungt. alcohol. lanae DAB	ad 100.0	
Salicylic acid scalp oil (2, 5, or 10%) (NRF 11.44.)		
	▶ **Note:** Salicylic acid is hard to keep in solution; thus complex formulations	To loosen scales in psoriasis, severe seborrheic dermatitis.
Salicylic acid	2.0 | 5.0 | 10.0	
Refined castor oil	0 |0 | 45.0	
Thick paraffin	73.0 | 0 | 0	
Octyldodecanol	25.0 | 95.0 | 45.0	
Salicylic acid scalp oil, washable 10% (NFA)		
		Washable scalp oil to loosen scales in psoriasis, severe seborrheic dermatitis
Salicylic acid	10.0	
Ethanol 96%	10.0	

Table II.1 · Continued

Name and ingredients[a]	Concentration (%)	Indications
Salicylic acid scalp oil, washable 10% (NFA)(continued)		
Macrogol-8-stearate	10.0	
Isopropyl myristate	35.0	
Peanut oil	35.0	
Skin care lotion		
	Vehicle type: anionic O/W lotion	Slightly greasy lubricating lotion
Emulsifying cetearyl alcohol (type A)	4.0	
Glycerol monostearate	2.2	
Potassium sorbate	0.14	
Citric acid	0.07	
Triglyceride (medium chain)	5.0	
Peanut oil	5.0	
Water	ad 100.00	
Tar paste, soft		
	Vehicle type: Hydrocarbon gel	Psoriasis, chronic dermatitis, prurigo nodularis
Pix lithanthracis (tar)	5.0	
Soft zinc paste DAB	ad 100.0	
Tar scalp cream		
		Psoriasis, severe seborrheic dermatitis of scalp; can also be used on psoriasis on rest of body
Liquor carbonis detergens	5.0	
Salicylic acid	5.0	
Ungt. emulsificans aquosum	ad 100.0	
Thiabendazole cream		
	Vehicle type: hydrophobic W/O cream	
Thiabendazole	10.0	
Hydrous wool alcohol ointment DAB	ad 100.0	

Continued Table II.1 ▶

Table II.1 · Continued

Name and ingredients[a]	Concentration (%)	Indications
Thiabendazole lipophilic gel 10% (NRF 11.130.)		
	Vehicle type: oleo gel	
Thiabendazole	10.0	
Hydrophobic Basisgel DAC	ad 100.0	
Thiabendazole ointment		
	Vehicle type: hydrophobic ointment	
Thiabendazole	15.0	
(Salicylic acid)	(3.0)	
White petrolatum	ad 100.0	
Thiabendazole solution		
Thiabendazole	2.0	
Water	10.0	
DMSO	ad 100.0	
Thioglycollate epilation cream		
		Removing unwanted hairs; apply, leave on 10 minutes or until hair appears damaged
Emulsifying cetearyl alcohol (Type A)	10.0	
Oleyl oleate	6.0	
Thioglycolic acid solution 80%	6.0	
Calcium hydroxide	8.0	
Calcium carbonate	15.0	
Fragrance	1.0	
Water	ad 100.0	
Urea and lactic acid cream		
	Vehicle type: ambiphilic cream	Ichthyosis vulgaris, long-term care of dermatitis
Urea pura	5.0 – 10.0	
Lactic acid	1.0	
Sodium lactate 50%	4.0	
Basiscreme DAC	ad 100.0	

Table II.1 · Continued

Name and ingredients[a]	Concentration (%)	Indications
Urea lotion		
	Vehicle type: W/O lotion	For very dry skin
Urea	10.0	
Lactic acid	2.0	
Sodium lactate 50%	8.0	
Water	10.0	
Lipoderm lotion	ad 200.0	
Urea ointment		
	Vehicle type: lipogel	Chronic dermatitis
Urea	5.0 | 10.0	
Liquor carbonis detergens	(5.0 – 10.0)	
Excipial Mandelölsalbe (almond oil ointment)	ad 100.0	
Zinc oxide paste for Unna boot (ex-NRF 11.19.)		
		Gauze wrap impregnated with paste is used to wrap leg when treating chronic venous ulcers, lichen simplex chronicus, artifacts; dries to create a firm, cast-like device
Zinc oxide	10.0	
Glycerol 85%	40.0	
Gelatin	15.0	
Water	ad 100.0	
Zinc oxide paste, antimycotic		
	Vehicle type: W/O cream paste	Intertriginous dermatophyte or candidal infections; inflamed lichen sclerosus
Clotrimazole	1.0	
(Triamcinolone acetonide)	(0.1)	
Zinc oxide	30.0	
Eucerin cum aqua (50% water)	ad 100.0	

Continued Table II.1 ▶

Table II.1 · Continued

Name and ingredients[a]	Concentration (%)	Indications
Zinc oxide paste, aqueous (FH Z.3.)		
	Vehicle type: hydrophilic paste	Acute dermatitis
Zinc oxide	15.0	
Talcum	15.0	
Propylene glycol	15.0	
Bentonite (Veegum)	5.0	
Water	ad 100.0	
Zinc oxide paste, cooling		
	Vehicle type: pseudo-W/O cream paste	Acute dermatitis
Soft zinc paste DAB	50.0	
Ungt. leniens DAB	50.0	
Zinc oxide paste, hard (zinc paste DAB)		
	Vehicle type: hydrocarbon gel	Protective paste; low sensitizing potential; not easily removed
Zinc oxide	25.0	
Corn starch	25.0	
White petrolatum	ad 100.0	
Zinc oxide paste, lipophilic 30% (NRF 11.111.)		
		Protective paste
Zinc oxide	30.0	
Beeswax, white	30.0	
White petrolatum	40.0	
Zinc oxide paste, soft (DAB)		
	Vehicle type: Hydrocarbon gel	Protective paste
Zinc oxide	30.0	
Thick paraffin	40.0	
White petrolatum	20.0	
Beeswax, white	10.0	

Table II.1 · Continued

Name and ingredients[a]	Concentration (%)	Indications
Zinc oxide shake emulsion (NRF 11.49.)		
	Vehicle type: emulsifier-stabilized shake lotion	Acute dermatitis
Emulsifying cetearyl alcohol (Type A)	3.0	
Zinc oxide	18.0	
Talc	18.0	
Glycerol 85%	18.0	
Ethanol 70%	18.0	
Water	ad 100.0	

DAB = Deutsches Arzneibuch, DAC = Deutsches Arzneimittel Codex, NRF = Neues Rezeptur Formularium, FH = Formularium Helveticum, NFA = Neues Formularium Austriacum, SR = Standardrezepturen (former German Democratic Republic).

a   Ingredients indicated in parentheses are optional; the remainder is adjusted.

b   Use either leukichthol (ammonium bituminosulfonate) without buffer solution or betamethasone with buffer solution.

c   Macrogol is also known as polyethylene glycol.

d   Mixture of cetearyl alcohol and sodium cetearylsulfate.

Note: We realize most readers will use other formularies and references. We cite these sources because they are standardized and well-established.

Appendix III Dermatologic Differential Diagnosis

How to Use This Chapter

In the tables below, a variety of different approaches to dermatologic differential diagnosis are offered, hopefully making it easier to identify a single disease or a small number of diseases out of the vast number of skin conditions with which we are confronted.

Differential diagnostic possibilities are presented on the basis of the type, shape, color, consistency, and distribution of skin lesions, as well as on common subjective complaints. Sites of predilection and typical patterns of distribution are also listed.

▶ *Note:* These lists cover topics that we find particularly difficult or interesting. We have made no attempt to include all the primary and secondary lesions or body sites: Many scenarios such as "papules on trunk" are simply too large, covering most of dermatology.

Differential Diagnostic Lists

Vesicles and Bulla

Table III.1 · Differential diagnosis of vesicles and bullae

Diagnosis	Clues	See
Acute contact dermatitis (allergic, toxic)	Rapid appearance of poorly circumscribed erythema, papulovesicles, blisters, often weeping areas	p. 195
Acute photodermatitis (allergic, toxic)	Erythema and then blisters minutes to hours after sun exposure	p. 297
Arthropod bite or sting	Tense blister on exposed surface, often other bites nearby; secondary to edema.	p. 130
Bullous pemphigoid	Large tense blisters, often preceded by pruritus or urticarial lesions, elderly patients.	p. 235
Burn	History provides the answer	p. 676
Dermatitis herpetiformis	Intensely pruritic blisters which are usually destroyed by scratching and not seen by physician; knees, elbows, buttocks; patients with gluten-sensitive enteropathy	p. 214
Dyshidrotic dermatitis	Deep-seated small pruritic vesicles on hands and feet, sometimes with fine scale	p. 200

Table III.1 · Continued

Diagnosis	Clues	See
Eczema herpeticatum	Disseminated herpes simplex in atopic patient; worse in areas of dermatitis such as face and neck but can be widespread	p. 58
Epidermolysis bullosa	Easily-induced mechanical blisters on palms and soles, or widespread; present at birth or later (depends on variant)	p. 351
Epidermolysis bullosa acquisita	Often resembles bullous pemphigoid, but has other patterns; can be associated with inflammatory bowel disease	p. 239
Erysipelas	Circumscribed erythema with fever and chills, facial lesions often symmetrical; can evolve to blisters and necrosis; may be bullous when severe	p. 78
Erythema multiforme	Target lesions on extremities, palms and soles; blue-violet center with white intermediate zone and erythematous rim	p. 281
Erythema multiforme-like drug reaction	Lesions similar to erythema multiforme, but usually truncal, iris features less well-developed, often not bullous	p. 282
Fixed drug eruption	Red-brown patch or plaque; history of recurrence in exactly the same site with ingestion of same drug; rarely bullous	p. 182
Friction blister	Large blister with peripheral erythema at site of friction, thus usually palms or soles	
Herpes simplex	Grouped blisters on erythematous base, rapidly become pustular, painful, history of recurrences	p. 57
Impetigo	Honey-colored crusts develop rapidly from blisters and pustules, small children, exposed areas	p. 77
Linear IgA disease of childhood	Blisters grouped in rosette-fashion; often buttocks or facial	p. 240
Lymphangioma	Dilated lymphatics, resembles frog eggs, often congenital, not a true blister	p. 451
Miliaria	Grouped small papules and vesicles on trunk, neck, intertriginous areas; caused by heat, sweating and occlusion	p. 88
Pemphigoid gestationis	Resembles bullous pemphigoid but in 2nd–3rd trimester; favors abdomen and extremities	p. 238
Pemphigus vulgaris	Fragile blisters, usually presents as erosions with crusting, oral involvement, rarely pruritic.	p. 229
Porphyria cutanea tarda	Fragile skin and blisters backs of hands, hypertrichosis on face	p. 312

Continued Table III.1 ▶

Table III.1 · Continued		
Diagnosis	**Clues**	**See**
Staphylococcal scalded skin syndrome (SSSS)	Diffuse erythema with superficial peeling, in small children, looks like burn; some lesions may be bullous	p. 75
Stevens–Johnson syndrome	Painful mucosal erosions (mouth, eyes), malaise, fever, sudden appearance; associated with erythema multiforme–like drug reactions.	p. 184
Toxic epidermal necrolysis (TEN)	Diffuse skin loss as maximal variant of erythema multiforme–like drug reaction; drug-induced; patients sick with fever, fluid loss, requires burn care	p. 185
Varicella (chickenpox)	Vesicles on erythematous base, lesions in different stages at same anatomic site, pruritic, mouth and scalp involved, palms and soles free	p. 60
Zoster	Grouped blisters on erythematous base, rapidly become pustular, dermatomal, rarely crosses midline; may be preceded by pain	p. 61

Pustules

Table III.2 · Differential diagnosis of pustules		
Diagnosis	**Clues**	**See**
Follicular pustules		
Acne	Inflamed papules and pustules along with comedones; face, chest, upper back	p. 530
Acne inversa	Pustules, nodules, sinus tracts and fistulas; axillary or inguinal; not primarily bacterial	p. 531
Demodex infestation	Pustules either associated with rosacea or arising on normal facial skin	p. 536
Dermatophyte infection	Round or polycyclic, slightly scaly lesion with raised border, central clearing; occasionally pustules	p. 106
Folliculitis	Small pustules with erythematous base	p. 74
Furuncle, carbuncle	Tender red nodule with superficial pustule; neck, face, axillae, groin, upper back	p. 74
Malassezia folliculitis	Closely group follicular pustules and inflammation on trunk and back; often in atopic patients	p. 158
Perioral dermatitis	Tiny papules and pustules in perioral region with classic zone of sparing around mouth; also periorbital but can involve entire face	p. 535
Pseudofolliculitis barbae	Ingrown hair adjacent to follicle causes pustule; seen primarily in blacks	

Table III.2 · Continued		
Diagnosis	**Clues**	**See**
Rosacea	Papules, telangiectases and small pustules; almost exclusively on face; triggered by alcohol, nicotine, spices, heat.	p. 533

Nonfollicular pustules

Acrodermatitis continua (Hallopeau)	Pustular psoriasis located on fingertips, often with nail involvement	p. 265
Acute generalized exanthematous pustulosis (AGEP)	Large pustules, widespread exanthem, drug reaction with systemic symptoms	p. 186
Behçet syndrome	Recurrent aphthae, genital ulcers; common in Asia and Middle East; rarely pustules, sometimes at site of trauma (pathergy)	p. 256
Candidiasis	Macerated epidermis with crusts, typically pustules at periphery	p. 112
Herpes simplex	Grouped blisters on erythematous base, rapidly become pustular, painful, history of recurrences	p. 57
IgA pemphigus	1–2 cm pustules, often arranged in patterns, truncal (formerly known as Sneddon–Wilkinson disease)	p. 234
Impetiginized dermatitis	Pustules and crusts in area of dermatitis	
Impetigo	Honey-colored crusts develop rapidly from blisters and pustules, small children, exposed areas	p. 77
Palmoplantar pustulosis	Small pustules on palms and soles, often confluent, may be triggered by infections and smoking	p. 265
Pustular psoriasis	Highly variable depending on type; pustules either alone or associated with psoriatic lesions	p. 265
Pyoderma gangrenosum	Large deep rapidly spreading ulcers; heal with cribriform scar; earliest lesion is sterile pustule, also induced by trauma (pathergy)	p. 250
Scabies	Pruritus, burrows, excoriations and secondary pyoderma with pustules	p. 127
Vasculitis	Palpable purpura, pustules, necrosis	p. 247
Zoster	Grouped blisters on erythematous base, rapidly become pustular, dermatomal, rarely crosses midline; may be preceded by pain	p. 61

Hives

▶ *Note:* The scientific word for a single hive is urtica; the condition with multiple hives is urticaria.

Table III.3 · Differential diagnosis of hives

Diagnosis	Clues	See
Acute exanthem with urticarial features	Virus? Drugs? Multiple small lesions in contrast to classic urticaria with larger lesions	
Angioedema	Acute appearance of subcutaneous facial swelling; laryngeal edema, gastrointestinal problems; rare familial forms (HANE)	p. 173
Arthropod bite or sting	History, involvement of exposed surfaces, lesions often grouped	p. 130
Bullous pemphigoid	Prebullous phase often has pruritus and urticarial lesions; later tense stable large blisters	p. 235
Dermatitis herpetiformis	Intensely pruritic urticarial lesions and blisters which are usually destroyed by scratching and not seen by physician; knees, elbows, buttocks; patients with gluten-sensitive enteropathy	p. 241
Urticaria	Generalized hives, pruritus	p. 167
Urticaria pigmentosa	Red-brown papules and nodules which urticate on manipulation; mast cell proliferation	p. 466
Urticarial vasculitis (and other forms of vasculitis)	Hives persist for more than 24 hours; heal with hyperpigmentation, classic form associated with arthritis	p. 248

Telangiectases

▶ **Telangiectases** are permanently dilated small vessels.
▶ **Poikiloderma** refers to the combination of telangiectases, atrophy, and hyper- or hypopigmentation.

Table III.4 · Differential diagnosis of telangiectases

Diagnosis	Clues	See
Basal cell carcinoma	Glassy papules or nodule with prominent peripheral rim rich in telangiectases; often central ulceration	p. 433
Cushing disease	Facial erythema with telangiectases	p. 318
Erythema ab igne	Localized reticular hyperpigmentation and telangiectases caused by local, long-term exposure to heat	p. 383
Generalized essential telangiectasia	Acquired or congenital; widespread telangiectases	p. 452

Appendix III Dermatologic Differential Diagnosis

Table III.4 · Continued

Diagnosis	Clues	See
Genodermatoses with poikiloderma	Bloom syndrome	p. 306
	Xeroderma pigmentosum	p. 304
	Ataxia-telangiectasia	p. 453
	Rothmund–Thomsen syndrome	p. 306
Hereditary hemorrhagic telangiectasia (Osler–Weber–Rendu syndrome)	Young patients, telangiectases on face, nasal and oral mucosa, frequent nose bleeds, pulmonary arteriovenous fistulas predispose to brain abscesses	p. 452
Necrobiosis lipoidica	Circumscribed atrophic yellow patch, usually on shins, with prominent telangiectases; associated with diabetes mellitus	p. 293
Nevus araneus (spider nevus)	1–2 cm papule with radial telangiectases, usually on face or décolleté, can be sign of liver disease	p. 451
Radiation dermatitis	Poikiloderma following ionizing radiation; history should give answer	p. 615
Starburst veins	Microvaricosities, medial shins and anterior thighs	p. 553
Telangiectases secondary to actinic damage, topical or systemic corticosteroid therapy	Localization and history	
Telangiectases with collagen-vascular disorders (systemic sclerosis—CREST, lupus erythematosus, dermatomyositis)	History, search for other stigmata.	p. 203
Telangiectasia macularis eruptiva perstans (form of mastocytosis)	Red-brown macules with prominent telangiectases, disseminated, urticate when rubbed; other types of mastocytoses less often have telangiectases.	p. 467

Erythema and Flushing

▶ **Erythema** is a persistent flat red area, usually caused by vasodilation or increased blood flow but without the requirement of visible permanently dilated vessels.
  • *Figurate erythemas* have a pattern, often annular and occasionally migratory.
▶ Flushing is a transient erythema caused by acute dilation of cutaneous blood vessels.

Table III.5 · Differential diagnosis of erythema and flushing

Diagnosis	Clues	See
Erythema		
Systemic lupus erythematosus	Butterfly rash—symmetric erythema and edema of cheeks, initially transient, later permanent	p. 209

Continued Table III.5 ▶

Table III.5 · Continued

Diagnosis	Clues	See
Annular erythema of Sjögren syndrome	Common in Japanese patients; occasionally in whites	p. 225
Erythema annulare centrifugum	Slowly expanding annular erythema, sometimes with scale	p. 285
Erythema chronicum migrans	Slowly expanding annular erythema without scale; often with central tick bite; sign of borreliosis	p. 93
Erythema gyratum repens	Erythema with scale in "wood grain" pattern, on trunk, paraneoplastic sign	p. 486
Erythema marginatum (rheumaticum)	Transient, rapidly moving erythematous bands in rheumatic fever	p. 224
Erythromelalgia	Painful acute erythema of the digits, often triggered by heat or stress	p. 484
Necrolytic migratory erythema	1–4 cm crusted erythematous patches with central necrotic blisters; marker for pancreatic glucagonoma	p. 486
Palmar erythema	Search for underlying disease (liver disease, hyperthyroidism, rheumatoid arthritis, pregnancy, oral contraceptives, systemic lupus erythematosus, diabetes mellitus, hereditary)	
Rosacea	Erythema often first sign; later papules, telangiectases and small pustules; almost exclusively on face; triggered by alcohol, nicotine, spices, heat	p. 533
"Slapped cheeks"	Erythema of cheeks with nose and mouth free; sign of erythema infectiosum	p. 573

Flushing

Carcinoid syndrome	Attacks of red-blue discoloration of upper trunk and arms with heat flashes and diarrhea; later pellagra-like changes	p. 320
Drug-induced	Fumaric acid therapy for psoriasis; rarely others (mast cell degranulators, hormones, chemotherapy agents, nicotinic acid, IL-2)	
Mastocytosis	Red-brown macules and papules, sometimes with telangiectases; occasionally flushing	p. 466
Menopause	Hot flashes; history usually obvious	
Pheochromocytoma	Increased blood pressure, tachycardia; attacks for flushing	p. 319
Rosacea	Some patients present with flushing with no other signs; later papules, telangiectases and small pustules; almost exclusively on face; triggered by alcohol, nicotine, spices, heat	p. 533

Distribution of Lesions

Frequently the distribution or localization of a lesion provides an important clue for the correct diagnosis. Figures 50.**1** and 50.**2** provide information on this topic.

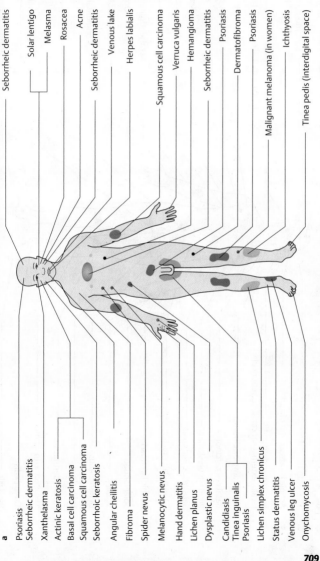

Fig. 50.**1** · **a**, **b** Homo dermatologicus: typical locations of many common skin diseases.

Appendix III Dermatologic Differential Diagnosis

Appendix III Dermatologic Differential Diagnosis

b

Trichilemmal cyst

Squamous cell carcinoma (in bald-headed men)

Psoriasis (scalp, external ear canal, retroauricular)

Acne

Dysplastic nevus

Keratosis pilaris

Melanoma

Psoriasis

Acral lentiginous melanoma

Onychomycosis

Dyshidrotic dermatitis

Congenital melanocytic nevus

Candidiasis
Tinea inguinalis
Pruritus ani
Lichen simplex chronicus
Psoriasis

Plantar wart, clavus (corn)

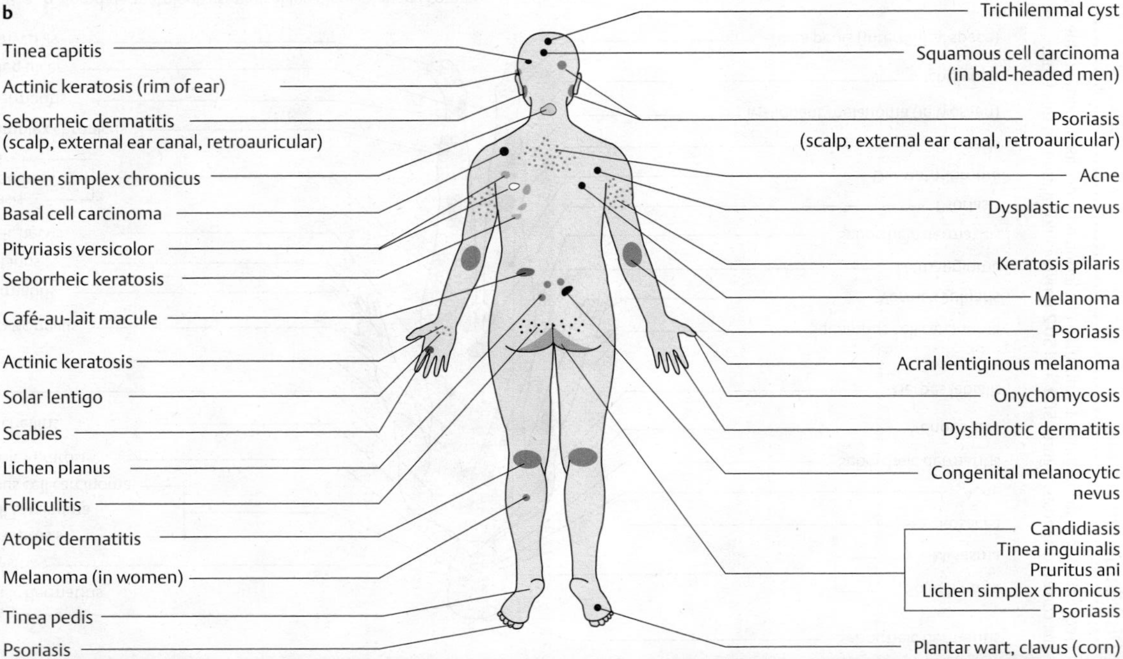

Tinea capitis

Actinic keratosis (rim of ear)

Seborrheic dermatitis (scalp, external ear canal, retroauricular)

Lichen simplex chronicus

Basal cell carcinoma

Pityriasis versicolor

Seborrheic keratosis

Café-au-lait macule

Actinic keratosis

Solar lentigo

Scabies

Lichen planus

Folliculitis

Atopic dermatitis

Melanoma (in women)

Tinea pedis

Psoriasis

Fig. 50.**1** · **b**

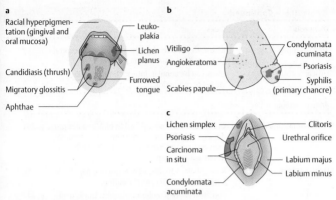

Fig. 50.**2** · **Common diseases. a** Mouth. **b** Male genitalia. **c** Female genitalia.

Special Patterns

Sometimes the pattern of a disease allows a rapid diagnosis or at least allows you to limit the number of possibilities.

Table III.6 · Special patterns

Diagnosis	Clues	See
Annular with scale		
Disseminated superficial actinic porokeratosis (DSAP)	1–2 cm plagues, look atrophic but have sharp fine hyperkeratotic border; usually on forearms, shins	p. 343
Erythema annulare centrifugum	Slowly expanding annular erythema, sometimes with scale	p. 285
Erythema chronicum migrans	Slowly expanding annular erythema without scale; often with central tick bite; sign of borreliosis	p. 93
Psoriasis	Silvery scales on erythematous base; favors scalp, gluteal cleft, knees, elbows; rarely annular	p. 262
Reiter syndrome	Annular erosions of glans with white border (circinate balanitis); skin lesions resemble psoriasis; sometimes associated arthritis, urethritis or bowel disease	p. 275
Seborrheic dermatitis	Petaloid variant on chest may be circular or annular	p. 276
Subacute cutaneous lupus erythematosus	Subacute form often psoriasiform or annular	p. 207

Continued Table III.6 ▶

Table III.6 · **Continued**		
Diagnosis	**Clues**	**See**
Tinea corporis	Ring with peripheral erythema and scale; central clearing; KOH examination positive	p. 107
Urticaria	Hives can be annular, intersecting, in various stages of regression.	p. 167
Annular without scale		
Granuloma annulare	Grouped small flesh-colored to pink papules producing ring with central clearing; no scale; common on backs of hands and feet; often misdiagnosed as tinea corporis	p. 292
Lichen planus	Rare annular variants; either grouped papules or large plaques with central clearing.	p. 286
Lichen sclerosus	Porcelain white papules or plaques; trunk, genitalia	p. 217
Morphea	Circumscribed sclerotic plaque with violet ring at periphery; maybe quite large	p. 216
Mycosis fungoides	Cutaneous T-cell lymphoma; patches and plaques which are sometimes annular	p. 474
Polycyclic	▶ *Note:* All the annular lesions can occasionally evolve into polycyclic patterns	
Erythema gyratum repens	Erythema with scale in "wood grain" pattern, on trunk, paraneoplastic sign	p. 486
Erythema marginatum (rheumaticum)	Transient, rapidly moving erythematous bands in rheumatic fever	p. 224
Iris, target, or cockade		
Cockade nevus	Melanocytic nevus with rings of inflammation (variant of halo nevus)	p. 388
Erythema multiforme	Target lesions on extremities, palms and soles; blue-violet center with white intermediate zone and erythematous rim	p. 281
Erythema multiforme–like drug reaction	Lesions similar to erythema multiforme, but usually truncal, iris features less well-developed, often not bullous.	p. 282
Subacute cutaneous lupus erythematosus	Annular form occasionally has dramatic rings	p. 207
Urticaria	Hives with concentric patterns	p. 167
Dermatoses which follow vessels		
Mondor disease	Phlebitis of large subcutaneous veins of lateral chest	p. 557
Temporal arteritis	Painful, indurated temporal artery; severe headaches, can lead to blindness; giant cells in vessel wall on biopsy	

Table III.6 · Continued

Diagnosis	Clues	See
Thrombophlebitis	Painful subcutaneous cords; if recurrent, exclude pancreatic carcinoma and clotting disorder	p. 557
Varicosities	Usually on legs; look for signs of chronic venous insufficiency	p. 553

Dermatoses which follow lymphatics

Diagnosis	Clues	See
Lymphangiitis	Linear ascending red streak from area of cellulitis or other infection	
Sclerosing lymphangiitis	Nonvenereal, post-traumatic inflammation of penile lymphatics	p. 549
Sporotrichoid infections	Sporotrichosis, nocardiosis, atypical mycobacteria, and others spread from inoculation site via lymphatics, dotting the path of the lymphatic vessel with nodules	

Bizarre or unnatural patterns

Diagnosis	Clues	See
Artifacts	Lesions caused by patient or someone else (spouse, parent)—sometimes for special gain (workman's compensation, sometimes for psychiatric reasons)	p. 581
Contact dermatitis (irritant or allergic)	Erythema, scale, papulovesicles; appropriate history	p. 195
Dermatoses in scars	Sarcoidosis, psoriasis, lichen planus in scars (Koebner phenomenon); years later, squamous cell carcinoma or basal cell carcinoma; hyperpigmentation when ACTH/MSH levels elevated	
Radiation dermatitis	Confined to radiation fields, so often rectangular or unnatural; may ulcerate	p. 615
Trauma	Physical or chemical damage; history tells story—burns, lightening strikes, chemical spills and the like.	

Spared areas

Diagnosis	Clues	See
Arthropod bites or stings	Usually not in areas covered by clothing	p. 130
Excoriations	Area of mid-back which cannot be reached by hands is usually spared	
Papuloerythroderma Ofuji	Confluent papules spare skin folds on abdomen (deck chair sign)	
Perioral dermatitis	Striking spared area directly adjacent to lips— "periperioral" dermatitis is better name	p. 535
Pityriasis rubra pilaris	Diffuse scaly erythema with follicular hyperkeratotic papules; salmon color; palmoplantar keratoderma; nappes claires (areas of sparing)	p. 278
Vasculitis	Often area under pressure—tight socks—relatively spared	p. 247

Painful Tumors and Other Lesions

Only a handful of skin tumors are often painful. They are typically vascular or neural in nature. A limited number of other conditions also frequently present with pain.

▶ *Note:* A mnemonic for painful tumors is **ANGEL**: **a**ngiolipoma, **n**eural tumors, **g**lomus tumor, **e**ccrine tumors, **l**eiomyoma.

Table III.7 · Painful tumors

Diagnosis	Clues	See
Angiolipoma	Subcutaneous fat tumor with numerous vessels, sometimes thrombi; no clinical clues to separate from other lipomas	p. 447
Neural tumors	Many neural tumors, especially traumatic neuromas, are painful; most common are neurofibroma and neurilemmoma	p. 463
Glomus tumor	Blue-gray nodule Solitary: often painful, frequently subungual Multiple: compressible, not painful	p. 458
Eccrine tumors	Eccrine tumors often contain myoepithelial cells; this may explain their painful nature	p. 426
Leiomyoma	1–2 cm skin-colored to red-brown papules around hair follicles (arms) or plaques on scrotum or nipple; painful when stroked	p. 445

Table III.8 · Other painful lesions

Diagnosis	Clues	See
Adiposis dolorosa (Dercum disease)	Multiple painful lipomas in women; rare and controversial	p. 447
Aphthae	Gray mucosal ulcers with erythematous periphery; recurrent; both oral and genital involvement in Behçet syndrome	p. 494
Atrophie blanche	Superficial painful ulcers in chronic venous insufficiency	p. 559
Bullous autoimmune diseases	Mucosal involvement with erosions can be quite painful, interfere with eating	p. 229
Chancroid	Painful dirty genital ulcer with ragged edges	p. 150
Chondrodermatitis nodularis helicis	Painful nodule on helix which is tender and symptomatic when sleeping	
Erysipelas	Circumscribed erythema with fever and chills, facial lesions often symmetrical; can evolve to blisters and necrosis	p. 78
Erythema nodosum	Bruise-like tender deep nodules on shins; never ulcerate; usually sign of acute infection or drug reaction	p. 540
Erythropoietic protoporphyria	Painful burning or urticarial erythema following minor sun exposure	p. 311

Table III.8 · Continued

Diagnosis	Clues	See
Fissures—anal, palmoplantar, lips, retroauricular	Chronic dermatitis, especially periorificial, leads to painful splits and tears	
Herpes simplex	Grouped blisters on erythematous base, rapidly pustular, painful, history of recurrences	p. 57
Lichen planus	Erosions in mouth; look for other signs of lichen planus elsewhere	p. 286
Livedo vasculitis	Net-like vascular patterns, vasculitis, ulcers	p. 258
Pyoderma gangrenosum	Large deep rapidly spreading ulcers; heal with cribriform scar; earliest lesion is sterile pustule, also induced by trauma (pathergy)	p. 250
Stevens–Johnson syndrome	Painful mucosal erosions (mouth, eyes), malaise, fever, sudden appearance; associated with erythema multiforme-like drug reactions	p. 184
Temporal arteritis	Painful, indurated temporal artery; severe headaches, can lead to blindness; giant cells in vessel wall on biopsy	
Ulcers	Most ulcers are painful; exceptions listed in Table III.9	
Zoster	Grouped blisters on erythematous base, rapidly become pustular, dermatomal, rarely crosses midline; may be preceded by pain	p. 61

Painless Ulcers

The occasional painless ulcer should help you narrow down the differential diagnostic considerations.

Table III.9 · Differential diagnosis of painless ulcers

Diagnosis	Clues	See
Neoplastic ulcers	Ulcerated tumors, usually squamous cell carcinoma or basal cell carcinoma	
Neuropathic ulcers	Located overlying bony structures with excessive mechanical load because of loss of warning	
	Peripheral neuropathies (alcohol, drugs)	
	Diabetes mellitus	p. 319
	Leprosy	p. 101
	Syringomyelia	
Venous leg ulcers	Usually surprisingly painless, considering their size and chronicity	p. 560
Chancre	Firm hard, button-like lesion with superficial erosion; usually painless	p. 136

Scalp Lesions

Table III.10 · Differential diagnosis of scalp lesions		
Diagnosis	**Clues**	**See**
Exudative and erosive lesions		
Langerhans cell histiocytosis	Tiny hemorrhagic papules, tend to erode, may become confluent producing dermatitic plaques and ulcers	p. 467
Pediculosis capitis	Weeping dermatitis of nape; nits on hairs	p. 126
Pemphigus vulgaris	Painful erosions of the mouth, but also scalp and face; other bullous autoimmune diseases may also affect scalp	p. 229
Zoster	Grouped blisters on erythematous base, rapidly become pustular, dermatomal, rarely crosses midline; may be preceded by pain	p. 61
Papules and plaques		
Actinic keratoses	Rough scaly papules, often easier to feel than see, on sun-exposed skin	p. 417
Folliculitis decalvans	Family of non-infectious scalp disorders; all rare; sometimes associated with acne inversa	p. 508
Lichen simplex chronicus	Persistently rubbed plaque with exaggerated skin markings, usually on nape, back of hands or feet; often in atopics	p. 330
Nevus sebaceus	Yellow-orange, usually hairless plaque on scalp or forehead, present at birth	p. 411
Seborrheic keratoses	Hyperkeratotic papules or plaques 0.2–6 cm diameter. Warty to smooth or polished surface, looks like it could be easily peeled off	p. 414
Nodules		
Acne keloidalis nuchae	Keloids on nape in blacks, caused by ingrown hairs	
Basal cell carcinoma	Glassy papules or nodule with prominent peripheral rim rich in telangiectases; often central ulceration	p. 433
Cylindroma (turban tumor)	Solitary or multiple skin-colored to red papules and nodules; when numerous, have been compared to a turban	p. 428
Lipoma	Soft lobular subcutaneous tumor, often on nape; smaller lesions on forehead are deeper (subgaleal lipoma)	p. 447

Table III.10 · Continued		
Diagnosis	**Clues**	**See**
Nodules (Continued)		
Metastases	Quickly growing dermal or subcutaneous nodules; scalp is favored site for metastases presumably because it is so vascular	
Squamous cell carcinoma	Asymmetrical red scaly or crusted tumor, often with adjacent actinic keratoses	p. 419
Trichilemmal cyst	Firm, marble-like cyst, often multiple, almost exclusively on scalp	p. 408

Alopecia

Alopecia is covered in detail under hair disorders, but reviewed here.

Table III.11 · Differential diagnosis of alopecia		
Type of alopecia	**Clues**	**See**
Alopecia areata	One or many round areas of complete hair loss; nail changes	p. 503
Anagen effluvium	Follows chemotherapy, poisoning: sudden loss of growing hairs, while resting hairs are retained	p. 499
Androgenic alopecia	Thinning of hair: men frontal and top; women, diffuse on top	p. 500
Scarring alopecia	Many different causes including: Inflammation (lupus erythematosus, lichen planus, sarcoidosis, morphea, bullous dermatoses) Infections (deep dermatophyte infections, furuncles) Folliculitis decalvans, folliculitis capitis abscedens et suffodiens—peculiar scarring inflammatory reactions that appear to be not primarily infectious Tumors (lymphoma, follicular mucinosis, metastases) Physical damage (radiation therapy, scars) Pseudopelade of Brocq—probably end stage of many inflammatory disorders	p. 506
Syphilitic alopecia	Moth-eaten hair loss in secondary syphilis	p. 138
Telogen effluvium	Severe illness, pregnancy, emotional distress may shift hairs into resting cycle; increased hair loss occurs 2–4 months later	p. 498
Tinea capitis	Multiple areas of broken-off hairs and inflammation; primarily in children	p. 108
Trichotillomania	Focal hair loss with breakage and stubble (never as complete as alopecia areata); patients remove hairs themselves	p. 506

Facial Lesions

Table III.12 · Differential diagnosis of facial lesions

Diagnosis	Clues	See
Acneiform follicular lesions		
Acne vulgaris	Inflamed papules and pustules along with comedones	p. 530
Adenoma sebaceum	1–2 mm red-violet smooth papules; chin and nasolabial folds; marker for tuberous sclerosis; early lesions often mistaken for acne	p. 365
Comedones	Early lesions of acne; also sign of solar damage on cheeks of elderly (Favre–Racouchot disease); plugged hair follicles; also known as whiteheads and blackheads	p. 530
Demodex folliculitis	Deep pustules usually with rosacea but can occur on normal skin	p. 536
Gram-negative folliculitis	Pustules, no comedones (except in acne patients); diagnosis made on culture	p. 534
Perioral dermatitis	Tiny papules and pustules in perioral region with classic zone of sparing around mouth; also periorbital but can involve entire face	p. 535
Pseudofolliculitis barbae	Perifollicular pustules and scars from ingrown hairs; on neck primarily in blacks	
Rosacea	Papules, telangiectases and small pustules; almost exclusively on face; triggered by alcohol, nicotine, spices, heat	p. 533
Sebaceous hyperplasia	Yellow 1–4 mm papules with central puncta	p. 429
Scaly lesions		
Actinic keratoses	Rough scaly papules, often easier to feel than see, on sun-exposed skin	p. 417
Atopic dermatitis	Pruritic dermatitis; facial and diffuse in children, flexural in adolescents, acral and excoriated in adults; history of atopic diathesis (asthma, rhinitis, conjunctivitis)	p. 190
Chronic cutaneous lupus erythematosus	Discoid plaques with follicular hyperkeratoses, on sun-exposed skin	p. 205
Contact dermatitis (irritant or allergic)	Erythema, scale, papulovesicles; appropriate history	p. 195

Table III.12 · Continued		
Diagnosis	**Clues**	**See**
Lichen simplex chronicus	Persistently rubbed plaque with exaggerated skin markings, usually on nape, back of hands or feet; often in atopics	p. 330
Psoriasis	Silvery scales on erythematous base; favors scalp, gluteal cleft, knees, elbows	p. 262
Seborrheic dermatitis	Greasy yellow scales on erythematous base, scalp, hairline, nasolabial folds, eyebrows and external ear	p. 276
Tinea faciei	Inflamed scaly, pruritic patches and plaques; usually in individuals who sleep with pets	p. 109

Lip Swelling

Lip swelling can portend a medical emergency, as it may be the first sign of angioedema with airway obstruction.

Table III.13 · Differential diagnosis of lip swelling		
Diagnosis	**Clues**	**See**
Angioedema	Acute appearance of subcutaneous facial swelling; laryngeal edema, gastrointestinal problems; rare familial forms (HANE)	p. 173
Contact dermatitis (cheilitis)	Erythema, scale, papulovesicles; appropriate history	p. 195
Erysipelas	Circumscribed erythema with fever and chills, facial lesions often symmetrical; can evolve to blisters and necrosis	p. 78
Furuncle	Painful firm nodule; often starts from hair follicle or sebaceous gland at vermilion border	p. 74
Granulomatous cheilitis	Edematous swelling of upper lip; initially waxes and wanes; later persistent.	p. 489
Melkersson–Rosenthal syndrome	Granulomatous cheilitis plus facial nerve paralysis and fissured tongue	p. 291
Trauma	History	

Other Lip Lesions

Many of the lesions found on the lips are clinically difficult to identify because they are developing on transitional epithelium that is often moist and traumatized.

Table III.14 · Differential diagnosis of lip lesions

Diagnosis	Clues	See
Actinic cheilitis	White discoloration of lower lip, sometimes with erosions or crusts; lip equivalent of actinic keratosis	p. 491
Angular cheilitis (perlèche)	Erythema, rhagades	p. 489
Free sebaceous glands	Tiny yellow papules on lips (Fordyce glands); harmless	p. 429
Herpes simplex	Grouped blisters on erythematous base, rapidly pustular, painful, history of recurrences	p. 57
Impetigo	Honey-colored crusts develop rapidly from blisters and pustules, small children; frequently starts just adjacent to lip.	p. 77
Labial melanotic macules	Tan macules on lips; also occur on genitalia; harmless but often worrisome	p. 376
Lichen planus	White lacy network on lips; intraoral painful erosions; look for other skin findings	p. 286
Lick dermatitis	Erythema and scaling in area reached by tongue or teeth (biting lower lip)	
Mucocele	Submucosal nodule, often with glassy sheen, frequently beneath labial mucosa	p. 410
Other forms of dermatitis	Adult atopics often have lip dermatitis; history for allergic contact dermatitis	
Squamous cell carcinoma	Exaggeration of actinic cheilitis with erosions, crusts and induration ▶ *Note:* Any nonhealing lip erosion should be biopsied to exclude squamous cell carcinoma	p. 419
Venous lake	Blue-gray compressible papule or nodule	p. 451
Wart	Hyperkeratotic papillomatous papules with punctate bleeding; surface usually white on lip	p. 491

Typical Lesions of the Oral Mucosa

On the oral mucosa, almost all lesions are white because of the persistent moisture. In addition, the epithelium is normally parakeratotic in many areas such as the palate. Erosions and ulcerations are common because the epithelium is thin and often traumatized, but usually heals readily.

Table III.15 · Differential diagnosis of oral mucosal lesions

Diagnosis	Clues	See
White lesions		
Candidiasis	Thrush: white plaques that can be rubbed off; other variants are erosive or atrophic	p. 112
Florid oral papillomatosis	HPV-induced papillomatous plaques; variant of verrucous squamous cell carcinoma	p. 421
Leukoplakia	White mucosal patch that will not rub off; many causes—congenital, trauma, HPV, carcinoma—if verrucous or multicolored (speckled leukoplakia), always biopsy	p. 490
Lichen planus	White lacy network on buccal mucosa; white papules on tongue	p. 286
Morsicatio buccarum	Bite lines; white ridges on buccal mucosa where it is traumatized by teeth	
Mucosal warts	White papules; usually in children or immuno-suppressed patients; often transferred by chewing from digital warts	p. 491
Nicotine stomatitis (smokers' palate)	Gray-white papules on the palate with a red central puncta; associated with smoking, especially pipes	
White sponge nevus	White-gray, sharply bordered, folded or complex plaques; present at birth	p. 491
Erosions		
Herpetic gingivostomatitis	First infection with herpes simplex virus; usually infants, erosions, hemorrhagic crusts, foul odor, feeding problems	p. 58
Stevens–Johnson syndrome	Painful mucosal erosions (mouth, eyes), malaise, fever, sudden appearance; associated with erythema multiforme-like drug reactions	p. 184
Lichen planus	Painful erosions plus white lacy network on buccal mucosa; white papules on tongue	p. 286
Pemphigus vulgaris, cicatricial pemphigoid	Erosions, crusts on lips; two autoimmune bullous diseases most likely to affect mucosa	
Geographic tongue	Erythematous patches admixed in map-like pattern with more white areas; not true erosions	p. 492

Continued Table III.15 ▶

Diagnosis	Clues	See

Table III.15 · Continued

Erosions (Continued)

Diagnosis	Clues	See
Herpangina	Tiny gray papulovesicular lesions on hard palate; usually in small children; associated with fever and malaise	p. 66
Hand-foot-and-mouth disease	Triad of small oral (mainly palatal) ulcers, papules and vesicles on palms and soles and exanthem; viral symptoms	p. 65
Stomatitis secondary to chemotherapy	Appropriate history; usually widespread and painful erosions; often secondary candidiasis	

Ulcers

Diagnosis	Clues	See
Acute necrotizing ulcerative gingivitis (ANUG)	Mixed bacterial infection, common in immunosuppressed hoists (HIV/AIDS) and in those who neglect oral care	
Extranodal NIC/T-cell lymphoma, nasal type	Old name of lethal midline granuloma says it all; aggressive tumor often with palatal ulcerations	p. 479
Aphthae (major type)	Large necrotic ulcer with white fibrinous coating	p. 494
Behçet disease	Recurrent aphthae, genital ulcers; common in Asia and Middle East	p. 256
Chancre	Hard painless ulcer; when oral, usually on lip or palate; take sexual history when oral ulcer is not readily explained	p. 136
Langerhans cell histiocytosis	Localized version (eosinophilic granuloma) common in mouth; floating (loose) teeth, periodontal ulcerations	p. 467
Squamous cell carcinoma	Ulcerated tumor; smoking and alcohol abuse are risk factors	p. 419
Traumatic ulcer	Burns, electrical burns (chewing on electric cable), chemical burns and trauma all produce similar effects on mucosa; history is the answer	
Wegener granulomatosis	Form of destructive vasculitis; may have gingival erosions or oral ulcers	p. 253

Lesions of the External Ear

Ear lesions may been painful when slept upon, and are frequently manipulated.

Table III.16 · Differential diagnosis of external ear lesions

Diagnosis	Clues	See
Actinic keratosis	Rough scaly papules, often easier to feel than see, on sun-exposed skin	p. 417
Allergic contact dermatitis	Allergy to nickel in jewelry; papulovesicles, erythema.	p. 196
Basal cell carcinoma	Glassy papule or nodule with prominent peripheral rim rich in telangiectases; on ear usually on upper part of helix while chondrodermatitis nodularis helicis is closer to edge of helix	p. 433
Chondrodermatitis nodularis helicis	Painful nodule on helix which is tender and symptomatic when sleeping	
Chronic cutaneous lupus erythematosus	Discoid plaques with follicular hyperkeratoses, which in ear may be mistaken for comedones	p. 205
Comedones	Plugged hair follicles; also known as whiteheads and blackheads; common in acne patients	p. 530
Cutaneous horn	Focal hyperkeratotic horn; always biopsy since any of the above tumors, as well as warts, can be at base	p. 417
Elastotic nodule	Tiny papules on edge of helix; diagnosis usually made on histology; form of solar degeneration. Weathering nodule is same clinically, but shows no elastosis.	
Gouty tophus	White papules and nodules on antihelix; can be large or ulcerated	p. 322
Granuloma annulare	Grouped small flesh-colored to pink papules producing ring with central clearing; no scale	p. 292
Keloid	Excessive scar tissue extending beyond original injury; earlobe following piercing is very common site	p. 441
Keratoacanthoma	Solitary nodule with central crusted plug, rapid growth, usually on sun-exposed skin; variant of squamous cell carcinoma	p. 421
Lymphadenosis cutis benigna	Swollen red plaques; face, especially nose and ear lobes, nipples. Swollen red plaques; face, especially nose and ear lobes, nipples	p. 94
Necrotizing otitis externa	External ear infection with *Pseudomonas aeruginosa*; diabetics and immunosuppressed patients; also known as malignant otitis externa	
Otitis externa	Inflammation of outer ear canal with drainage, which can cause secondary dermatitis; causes include bacteria, rarely fungi (otomycosis), moisture (swimmer's ear) and allergic contact dermatitis to ear drops	

Continued Table III.16 ▶

Table III.16 · Continued

Diagnosis	Clues	See
Psoriasis	Silvery scales on erythematous base; favor scalp, gluteal cleft, knees, elbows; rarely limited to ears	p. 262
Relapsing polychondritis	Tender ears; autoimmune damage to cartilage; also involves nose, airways	
Seborrheic dermatitis	Greasy yellow scales on erythematous base, scalp, hairline, nasolabial folds, eyebrows; sometimes limited to ears	p. 276
Squamous cell carcinoma	Asymmetrical red scaly or crusted tumor, often with adjacent actinic keratoses	p. 419

Lesions of the Palms and Soles

The skin of the palms and soles is markedly thickened, even containing some keratin molecules different than those found at other body sites. Almost every lesion is hyperkeratotic, which is often confusing as reactive hyperkeratotic changes accompany an array of underlying problems.

Table III.17 · Differential diagnosis of lesions of the palms and soles

Diagnosis	Clues	See
Inflammatory-hyperkeratotic palmoplantar lesions		
Dyshidrotic dermatitis	Deep-seated small pruritic vesicles on hands and feet, sometimes with fine scale. Deep-seated small pruritic vesicles on hands and feet, sometimes with fine scale	p. 200
Hyperkeratotic palmoplantar dermatitis	Combination of dermatitis, hyperkeratotic plaques, and rhagades	p. 200
Tinea pedis	Variable patterns—interdigital maceration, dry hyperkeratotic scale, erythematous patches with fine scale, papulovesicular lesions	p. 109
Psoriasis	Silvery scales on erythematous base; favor scalp, gluteal cleft, knees, elbows; may present with palmoplantar disease	p. 262
Lichen planus	Polygonal violet flat-toped papules, lacy white network; on palms and soles, often painful hyperkeratotic lesions	p. 286
Pityriasis rubra pilaris	Diffuse scaly erythema with follicular hyperkeratotic papules; salmon color; Nappes claires (areas of sparing); frequently involves palms and soles	p. 278

Table III.17 · Continued

Diagnosis	Clues	See
Inflammatory-hyperkeratotic palmoplantar lesions (Continued)		
Keratoderma blennorrhagicum	Erythematous palmoplantar macules that become thick and crusted; associated with Reiter disease (reactive arthritis, circinate balanitis, signs of psoriasis)	p. 275
Hereditary palmoplantar keratodermas	Long list of diffuse, punctate, and linear forms of congenital keratoderma; family history. Some appear inflamed; others, verrucous	p. 345
Juvenile plantar dermatitis	Symmetrical erythema and scale of soles in child wearing occlusive footwear; snowmobilers' feet	p. 191
Sézary syndrome	Erythroderma, pruritus, lymphadenopathy, frequent involvement of palms and soles.	p. 477
Palmoplantar pits	True pits are only seen in nevoid basal cell carcinoma syndrome, but all the other lesions are clinically almost identical.	
Punctate keratoderma of palmar creases	Normal variant; more common in blacks; do not treat as warts	p. 347
Nevoid basal cell carcinoma syndrome	Multiple basal cell carcinomas, macrocephaly, medulloblastoma, skeletal anomalies	p. 435
Cowden syndrome	Multiple hamartomas, breast cancer, macrocephaly	p. 366
Darier disease	Tiny palmar hyperkeratoses; 1–2 mm dirty brown papules in seborrheic areas, linear nail streaks, oral cobblestoning	p. 341
"Warts" of the soles		
Arsenical keratoses	Multiple plantar keratoses; other stigmata (pigmentary changes and increased malignancies) and appropriate history	p. 418
Callus (tylosis)	More diffuse reactive hyperkeratosis; also caused by rubbing without underlying bony pressure point.	
Corn (clavus)	Local hyperkeratotic response to pressure; usually underlying bony protuberance; very painful; hard corns are lateral or plantar—soft corns are interdigital.	
Mal perforant	Neurotropic plantar ulcer; early lesions resemble clavi but with central defect	p. 140
Pitted keratolysis	Tiny punched-out lesions in mosaic pattern; more common in athletes, especially swimmers, and those unable to change shoes frequently (infantry soldiers).	

Continued Table III.17 ▶

Table III.17 · Continued

Diagnosis	Clues	See
"Warts" of the soles		
Plantar warts	Only slightly raised keratotic papules on soles; distinct bleeding points; various forms (solitary, mosaic, giant)	p. 69
Syphilitic clavi	Blue-red to red-brown oval scaly 1–2 papules; look for other signs of secondary syphilis	p. 137
Verrucous carcinoma	Chronic, slow-growing HPV-induced squamous cell carcinoma; formerly known on foot as epithelioma cuniculatum; a large chronic wart that fails to respond to treatment deserves a biopsy	p. 421
Papules or plaques on the hands and feet		
Actinic keratoses	Gray-brown discrete papules with adherent scale; often easier to feel than to see	p. 417
Bowen disease	Circumscribed hyperkeratotic plaque with variable scaling; squamous cell carcinoma in situ; often mistaken for dermatitis	p. 418
Chilblain lupus erythematosus	Blue-red plaques and nodules; looks like pernio but more permanent	p. 207
Common warts	Hyperkeratotic papillomatous papules with punctate bleeding	p. 68
Erysipeloid	Uncommon bacterial infection; often on fingers of butchers, farmers, veterinarians; blue-red plaque with minimal systemic symptoms	p. 90
Erythema multiforme	Target lesions on extremities, palms and soles; blue-violet center with white intermediate zone and erythematous rim	p. 281
Granuloma annulare	Grouped small flesh-colored to pink papules producing ring with central clearing; no scale; often misdiagnosed as tinea; back of hands and feet most common sites	p. 292
Lichen planus	Polygonal violet flat-toped papules, lacy white network; most common sites are flexor aspect of wrist and dorsal foot	p. 286
Palmoplantar pustulosis	Deep-seated, sometimes painful pustules, secondary scale; associated with smoking	p. 265
Pernio	Blue-red infiltrates; not painful; develops after long exposure to moderately low temperature	p. 309
Plane warts	Small papules which are often tan; face and backs of hands in children, young adults, spread by scratching with linear streaks	p. 69

Table III.17 · Continued

Diagnosis	Clues	See
Papules or plaques on the hands and feet (Continued)		
Psoriasis	Silvery scales on erythematous base; favor scalp, gluteal cleft, knees, elbows; may present with patches on hands or feet, as well as palmoplantar pustules	p. 262
Pustular palmoplantar lesions	▣ *Note:* Palmoplantar pustules are rarely infectious; almost always reactive	
Psoriasis	Palmoplantar pustules usually accompany obvious psoriasis elsewhere; on occasion, only sign of disease—search for other clues	p. 262
Scabies	Burrows especially between digits; intense pruritus worse at night; secondary dermatitis and pyodermas. In infants, feet are common place for burrows; intense pruritus; infants also may have face and scalp disease	p. 127

Lesions of the Shins

Table III.18 · Differential diagnosis of shin lesions

Diagnosis	Clues	See
Cellulitis	Painful soft tissue swelling; extends deeper than erysipelas and often associated with trauma	p. 80
Erysipelas	Circumscribed erythema with fever and chills; can evolve to blisters and necrosis; may be bullous when severe	p. 78
Erythema induratum (Bazin)	Indurated plaques on calves, favor middle-aged women; often ulcerated; sign of tuberculosis	p. 541
Erythema nodosum	Bruise-like tender deep nodules on shins; never ulcerate; usually sign of acute infection or drug reaction	p. 540
Kaposi sarcoma, classic variant	Red-brown to red-blue macules, nodules or plaques; symmetrical on lower legs and feet; usually older men; not HIV-associated	p. 460
Necrobiosis lipoidica	Circumscribed atrophic yellow patch with prominent telangiectases; associated with diabetes mellitus	p. 293
Pernio	Reticular blue-red infiltrates; not painful; develops after long exposure to moderately low temperature	p. 309

Continued Table III.18 ▶

Table III.18 · Continued

Diagnosis	Clues	See
Post-bypass cellulitis	Mild, chronic cellulitis in patients following vein removal for cardiac surgery; entry site invariably chronic interdigital tinea pedis	
Pretibial myxedema	Swollen red plaques on shin, often with overlying peau d'orange change	p. 318
Thrombophlebitis	Painful subcutaneous cords; if recurrent, exclude pancreatic carcinoma and clotting disorder	p. 557

Leg Ulcers

The approach to leg ulcers is also considered under phlebology, as almost all ulcers are related to chronic venous insufficiency (p. 560).

Table III.19 · Differential diagnosis of leg ulcers

Diagnosis	Clues	See
Arterial leg ulcer	More often lateral malleolus or distal; painful; reduced pulses, clammy feet	
Ecthyma	Punched-out ulcer with peripheral erythema, 0.5–3.0 cm; usually streptococcal	p. 78
Hematologic disorders	Sickle cell anemia (in blacks), cryoglobulinemia (check hepatitis serology)	
Iatrogenic ulcers	Sclerotherapy—history	
Livedo vasculitis	Extremely painful ulcers on background of livedo racemosa and atrophie blanche	p. 258
Necrobiosis lipoidica	Circumscribed atrophic yellow patch, usually on shins, with prominent telangiectases; associated with diabetes mellitus; when ulcerated, extremely slow to heal	p. 293
Polyarteritis nodosa	Red-blue 1–2 cm dermal papules, often associated with livedo racemosa; associated with systemic vasculitis or rarely limited to skin	p. 255
Post-traumatic	Burn, trauma, radiation—the answer is in the history. Chronic lesions have risk of malignant degeneration—development of squamous cell carcinoma	
Tropical ulcer	Variety of infectious causes in returning tourists: leishmaniasis and mixed bacterial infections most common	
Ulcerated panniculitis	Red to red-blue subcutaneous nodules with drainage; most common ulcerated form is α1-antitrypsin deficiency (liquefying panniculitis)	

Table III.19 · **Continued**		
Diagnosis	**Clues**	**See**
Ulcerated tumor	Any tumor can ulcerate—most common on leg are squamous cell carcinoma and amelanotic melanoma; surprisingly painless.	
Venous leg ulcer	Accounts for over 90% of all leg ulcers. Usually medial malleolus and surprisingly painless; other signs of chronic venous insufficiency	p. 560

Intertrigo

Intertrigo refers to any dermatitis involving opposed skin surfaces and thus by definition is usually flexural, except in obese individuals where rolls of skin rub upon one
another. Some consider intertrigo only a sign; we consider it a disease when there is
no evidence for infection or underlying disease, but just for friction.

Table III.20 · **Differential diagnosis of intertriginous lesions**		
Diagnosis	**Clues**	**See**
Acanthosis nigricans	Velvety dark patches in axilla and groin; para-neoplastic marker in adults; otherwise associated with obesity, diabetes mellitus and lipodystrophy	p. 485
Acne inversa	Inflammatory papules and nodules with fistula formation; axillary, inguinal and perianal	p. 531
Candidiasis	Macerated patches with erosions and peripheral pustules	p. 112
Contact dermatitis (allergic or toxic)	Erythema, scale, papulovesicles; appropriate history	p. 195
Diaper dermatitis	Limited to covered, occluded areas; often combination of candidiasis and irritant dermatitis; increasingly more common in elderly people	p. 199
Erythrasma	Red-brown superficial fine patches in axillae and groin; fluoresce coral red on Wood's light examination	p. 83
Fox–Fordyce disease	Skin-colored axillary papules; intensely pruritic when sweating	p. 529
Hailey–Hailey disease	Weeping plaques with fissures; likened to a dusty road drying out after a rainstorm	p. 342
Inverse psoriasis	Red macerated plaques without characteristic silvery scale; sometimes limited to penis; very difficult to diagnose without other signs of psoriasis	p. 265
Langerhans cell histiocytosis	Tiny hemorrhagic papules, tend to erode, may become confluent producing dermatitic plaques and ulcers	p. 467

Continued Table III.20 ▶

Table III.20 · Continued

Diagnosis	Clues	See
Lichen simplex chronicus	Area of persistent rubbing, exaggerated skin markings; common with vulvar dermatitis	p. 330
Pemphigus vegetans	Variant of pemphigus with red juicy (vegetating) plaques in axilla and groin	p. 232
Skin tags	Small stalked papules; very common in axillae, groin, especially in obese individuals; easily macerated	p. 439
Tinea inguinale	Involves medial thigh, not scrotum or labia; scaly patch with prominent erythematous border	p. 111
Trichomycosis axillaris	Small orange-yellow bacterial colonies attached to axillary, pubic hairs; unpleasant odor	p. 84

Cutaneous Signs of Systemic Disease

One of the fascinating aspects of dermatology is the ability of an experienced practitioner to examine the skin and suggest the possibility of underlying systemic diseases, often with an astounding degree of accuracy. Table III.21 is simply a beginning. The degree of association varies from almost 100% to quite low, but in our opinion, still worth looking at and trying to remember!

Table III.21 · Cutaneous signs of systemic disease

Skin findings	Associated systemic disease	
Acanthosis nigricans	Carcinoma (usually gastrointestinal), insulin-resistance, diabetes mellitus, obesity	p. 485
Acrokeratosis (Bazex)	Carcinoma (often bronchial or gastrointestinal)	
Alopecia areata	Autoimmune diseases (Hashimoto thyroiditis, vitiligo, pernicious anemia, lupus erythematosus)	p. 503
Alopecia, androgenetic in women	Androgen-producing tumors, iron or ferritin deficiency (increased androgen sensitivity), hyperprolactinemia, hyperandrogenism syndromes (polycystic ovary syndrome (Stein–Leventhal)	p. 500
Alopecia, scarring	Lupus erythematosus, systemic sclerosis, metastases, lichen planus, sarcoidosis, amyloidosis, lymphoma	p. 506
Alopecia, loss of axillary and chest hairs	Cirrhosis, endocrine disorders	
Amyloidosis	Multiple myeloma, other gammopathies, chronic infections, autoimmune diseases	p. 322

Table III.21 · Continued

Skin findings	Associated systemic disease	
Anal dermatitis	Hemorrhoids, anal tags, worms, anal polyps, anal fissure, anal fistula, rectal carcinoma, extramammary Paget disease	p. 544
Angiofibromas, multiple	Tuberous sclerosis, MEN1 with risk of Zollinger–Ellison syndrome and other endocrinopathies	p. 365
Angiokeratomas	Fabry disease and other even rarer metabolic disorders	p. 454
Aphthae, oral ulcers	Behçet syndrome, Stevens–Johnson syndrome	p. 256
Arachnodactyly	Marfan syndrome, homocystinuria	p. 356
Bacillary angiomatosis	HIV/AIDS	p. 155
Basal cell carcinomas, multiple	Nevoid basal cell carcinoma syndrome with risk of medulloblastoma and ovarian tumors	p. 435
Beau lines	Severe illness, poisoning, drug reaction dating back several months	p. 525
Bullous skin diseases		
Paraneoplastic pemphigus	Lymphoma, thymoma, sarcoma	p. 234
Epidermolysis bullosa acquisita	Diabetes mellitus, Crohn disease, ulcerative colitis, multiple myeloma, amyloidosis, thyroid disease, tuberculosis	p. 239
Bullous disease of diabetes	Diabetes mellitus	p. 319
Candidiasis	Diabetes mellitus, immunosuppression (HIV, leukemia, lymphoma, chemotherapy, hypothyroidism	p. 112
Chicken skin	Pseudoxanthoma elasticum with cardiac and ocular complications	p. 358
Circinate balanitis	Reiter syndrome with arthritis	p. 275
Clubbed fingers	Chronic pulmonary diseases (carcinoma, COPD, chronic bronchitis, pulmonary fibrosis), subacute bacterial endocarditis, cardiac disease with cyanosis, hyperthyroidism, virtually any chronic disease	p. 526
Cutis verticis gyrata, acquired	Carcinoma (bronchial), mesothelioma, myxedema, amyloidosis	p. 526
Dermatitis herpetiformis	Celiac disease (gluten-sensitive enteropathy)	p. 241
Dermatomyositis (adult form)	Carcinoma (breast, ovarian, uterine, pulmonary, gastric)	p. 213
Ear lobe folds	Correlation with cardiovascular disease	
Effluvium (acute hair loss)	Endocrine diseases, severe illness, pregnancy, malnutrition, chemotherapy, hyperprolactinemia, virilizing tumors, hepatic disease, HIV/AIDS	

Continued Table III.21 ▶

Table III.21 · Continued

Skin findings	Associated systemic disease	
Eosinophilic folliculitis	HIV/AIDS, severe immunosuppression, idiopathic	p. 161
Epidermoid cysts, multiple	Gardner syndrome (colon polyposis, carcinoma)	p. 368
Erythema		
Cheeks	Lupus erythematosus (butterfly rash), Cushing syndrome (full moon face with red cheeks)	
Palmar	Cirrhosis, pregnancy	
Erythema gyratum repens	Underlying malignancy often with ectopic hormone production, rarely idiopathic	p. 486
Erythema marginatum	Rheumatic fever (watch for carditis, arthritis, glomerulonephritis, chorea)	p. 224
Necrolytic migratory erythema	Glucagonoma	p. 486
Erythema nodosum	Infections (tuberculosis, yersiniosis, streptococcal and staphylococcal disease, deep fungal), acute sarcoidosis, Crohn disease, ulcerative colitis, drugs	p. 540
Erythroderma	Sézary syndrome, other malignancies, drug reactions, exacerbation of underlying skin diseases (atopic dermatitis, psoriasis, seborrheic dermatitis, pityriasis rubra pilaris), ichthyoses in infants	p. 282
Eyebrows, lateral thinning	Hypothyroidism, panhypopituitarism, secondary syphilis, poisoning, atopic dermatitis, trichotillomania	
Fibrofolliculomas, multiple	Birt–Hogg–Dubé syndrome with risk of renal carcinoma and spontaneous pneumothorax	p. 367
Fistulas	Tuberculosis, Crohn disease, ulcerative colitis, actinomycosis, osteomyelitis, deep abscesses, malignant tumors, congenital anomalies	
Folliculitis, recurrent	Diabetes mellitus, immunosuppression, HIV/AIDS	p. 319
Flush	Carcinoid syndrome, systemic mastocytosis, pheochromocytoma, carcinoma (gastric, pulmonary, thyroid), drugs	p. 222
Gangrene	Diabetes mellitus, thromboangiitis obliterans, vasculitis, arterial emboli, arteriosclerosis, cryoglobulinemia	

Table III.21 · Continued

Skin findings	Associated systemic disease	
Hyperpigmentation, diffuse	Addison disease (primary or tumor secreting ectopic hormone), Cushing syndrome, malignant melanoma with circulating melanin, hemochromatosis, argyrosis, chrysiasis, pellagra, cirrhosis, malabsorption, some forms of porphyria, chronic renal disease	
Hypertrichosis		p. 513
Localized	Porphyria cutanea tarda (cheeks), under cast (most common cause), other trauma, Becker nevus, faun tail, hair nevus	
Generalized	Drugs (cyclosporine, minoxidil, corticosteroids), acromegaly, anorexia nervosa, mucopolysaccharidoses	
Hypertrichosis lanuginosa acuisita	Carcinoma	p. 486
Hypopigmentation		p. 733
Localized	Vitiligo, poliosis, nevus depigmentosus, nevus anemicus, pinta, leprosy, tuberous sclerosis	
Generalized	Albinism, Chediak–Higashi syndrome, Hermansky–Pudlak syndrome, many other syndromes	
Ichthyosis, acquired	Drugs, carcinoma, lymphoma, sarcoidosis	
Janeway lesion (palmoplantar hemorrhagic macules)	Subacute bacterial endocarditis	p. 81
Kaposi sarcoma	HIV/AIDS, immunosuppression	p. 161
Keratoacanthoma, multiple	Muir–Torre syndrome (carcinomas of colon, lungs, other organs)	p. 369
Koilonychia	Iron deficiency, endocrine disease, polycythemia, hemochromatosis	p. 526
Lentigines, multiple		
Oral, perioral	Peutz–Jeghers syndrome	p. 369
Axillary	Neurofibromatosis (Crowe sign)	p. 362
Diffuse	Carney complex, LEOPARD syndrome	p. 385
Lichen, myxedematous	Gammopathy	p. 320
Scleromyxedema	Gammopathy	p. 320
Lipodystrophy, lipoatrophy	Drugs (protease inhibitors in HIV), complement deficiency, glomerulonephritis, diabetes mellitus, variety of syndromes,	p. 538
Livedo racemosa	Vasculitis (livedo vasculitis, polyarteritis nodosa, thromboangiitis obliterans	p. 258

Continued Table III.21 ▶

Table III.21 · Continued

Skin findings	Associated systemic disease	
Lymphedema	Filariasis, tumor infiltrates, status post-lymph node dissection, retroperitoneal fibrosis, other forms of pelvic instruction, idiopathic (congential and acquired)	p. 450
Mal perforant	Diabetes mellitus, neurosyphilis, syringomyelia, other peripheral neuropathies	p. 140
Milia (especially nonfacial)	Porphyria cutanea tarda, epidermolysis bullosa acquisita	p. 407
Angular cheilitis (perlèche)	Vitamin and mineral deficiencies, diabetes mellitus, candidiasis, improperly fitting dentures, nursing, staphylococcal infections (children)	p. 489
Myxedema		
Pretibial	Usually hyperthyroidism (Graves syndrome)	p. 318
Diffuse	Usually hypothyroidism	p. 318
Nail fold capillaries		
Thickened dilated giant capillary loops	Dermatomyositis, systemic sclerosis	p. 213, 219
Capillary loops twisted and irregular but not thickened or dilated	Systemic lupus erythematosus	p. 209
Neuromas, multiple mucosal	MEN2B syndrome with risk of medullary thyroid carcinoma and pheochromocytoma	p. 367
Onycholysis	Drugs, psoriasis, ischemia, hyperthyroidism	p. 525
Osler nodes (fingertip nodules)	Subacute bacterial endocarditis	p. 81
Palmoplantar keratoderma		
Congenital with leukoplakia	Howel–Evans syndrome with almost 100% risk of esophageal carcinoma	p. 346
Acquired	Weak marker for variety of carcinomas (gastric, pulmonary, esophageal)	p. 345
Panniculitis (especially if above waist or ulcerated)	Carcinoma of pancreas	p. 542
Paronychia, chronic	Diabetes mellitus, hypothyroidism, chronic mucocutaneous candidiasis, drugs (retinoids, protease inhibitors)	p. 520
Poikiloderma	Congenital (many syndromes), graft-versus-host disease, radiation dermatitis, mycosis fungoides, connective tissue disease	p. 360
Polyarteritis nodosa	Hepatitis C (and B)	p. 255
Prurigo nodularis	Chronic renal disease, diabetes mellitus, other causes of pruritus	p. 330

Appendix III Dermatologic Differential Diagnosis

Table III.21 · Continued		
Skin findings	**Associated systemic disease**	
Pruritus ani	Hemorrhoids, anal tags, worms, anal polyps, anal fissure, anal fistula, rectal carcinoma, intestinal candidiasis	p. 545
Psoriasiform lesions (but definitely not psoriasis)	Acrodermatitis enteropathica, acquired zinc deficiency, malnutrition, syphilis (especially under the microscope), early pityriasis rubra pilaris	
Purpura		
Palpable	Palpable purpura = vasculitis. Always biopsy palpable purpura to rule out vasculitis See p. 247 for differential diagnosis	
Nonpalpable	Clotting disturbance (thrombopenia, coagulopathy, disseminated intravascular coagulation), vessel wall defect (scurvy, amyloidosis, lupus erythematosus, erythropoietic protoporphyria) or "leakage" (pigmented purpuras, p. 246)	
Pyoderma gangrenosum	Crohn disease, ulcerative colitis (rarely precedes), IgA gammapathy (almost always precedes), rheumatoid arthritis, Behçet syndrome, leukemia, chronic active hepatitis	p. 250
Raynaud phenomenon	Collagen-vascular disorders (systemic sclerosis, dermatomyositis, lupus erythematosus), hyperviscosity syndrome, arteriosclerosis, thromboangiitis obliterans, thoracic outlet syndrome, neurological disorders; idiopathic is diagnosis of exclusion and waiting	p. 226
Scleredema adultorum	Diabetes mellitus	p. 320
Sclerosis	Systemic sclerosis, dermatomyositis, porphyria cutanea tarda, scleromyxedema, scleredema	p. 222
Spider nevi	Hepatic disease, Osler–Weber–Rendu syndrome	p. 451
Striae	Pregnancy, Cushing syndrome, corticosteroids (systemic, topical or inhaled), body building (anabolic steroids, sudden weight gain), Marfan syndrome	
Sweet syndrome	Various forms of leukemia, especially hairy cell leukemia; also multiple myeloma	p. 249
Telangiectases	Sun-damage, rosacea, CREST syndrome, systemic lupus erythematosus, dermatomyositis, Cushing syndrome (cheeks), telangiectasia macularis eruptiva perstans (mast cell disease), Osler–Weber–Rendu syndrome, essential telangiectasia, carcinoid syndrome, radiation dermatitis, diabetes mellitus (necrobiosis lipoidica), hepatic disease, poikiloderma (see there)	p. 452

Continued Table III.21 ▶

Table III.21 · Continued

Skin findings	Associated systemic disease	
Thrombophlebitis, migratory (not in area of chronic venous insufficiency)	Carcinoma of the pancreas, pancreatitis, mesothelioma	p. 557
Tongue changes		
Hairy tongue	HIV, chronic diseases; usually normal variant	p. 161
Geographic tongue	Psoriasis	p. 492
Fissured tongue	Melkersson–Rosenthal syndrome	p. 492
Macroglossia	Down syndrome, amyloidosis, acromegaly, hypothyroidism	
Glossitis	Vitamin or mineral deficiency, anemia	
Trichilemmomas, multiple	Cowden syndrome with high risk of breast carcinoma, increased risk of thyroid and gastrointestinal carcinomas	p. 366
Vascular malformations	Underlying cerebral, ocular, musculoskeletal or cardiovascular problems (Sturge–Weber syndrome, Klippel–Trenaunay–Weber syndrome)	p. 449
Xanthomas	Exclude elevated cholesterol or triglyceride levels	p. 314
Normolipemic	Apolipoprotein variants, plant sterols, storage disorders, trauma, paraneoplastic markers (diffuse normolipemic plane xanthoma), macrophage disorders (papular xanthoma, xanthoma disseminatum)	p. 315
Xerostomia (dry mouth)	Drugs, Sjögren syndrome, systemic sclerosis, vitamin deficiencies, anemia, uremia, infections with fever	p. 225
Yellow skin	Diabetes mellitus, myxedema	p. 319
With yellow sclerae	Hepatitis (viral, toxic), biliary obstruction	p. 66
Yellow-brown	Hemochromatosis (bronze diabetes)	p. 316

Index

Quick Check B—Diagnosis not clear? What next?

Have you considered these diagnoses?

- Artifacts
- Borreliosis
- Bullous dermatoses
- Contact dermatitis to not obvious allergens—sunscreens, corticosteroids, nail polish
- "Dermatitis"—DD: Psoriasis, tinea, atopic dermatitis, seborrheic dermatitis, nummular dermatitis, allergic or irritant contact dermatitis
- Erythema multiforme
- Genodermatoses
- Herpes simplex
- HIV/AIDS associated dermatoses
- Langerhans cell histiocytosis
- Leprosy
- Lupus erythematosus
- Mastocytosis
- Mycosis fungoides
- Nevi of different types
- Normal variations
- Occupational dermatoses
- Paget disease (mammary/extra-mammary)
- Paraneoplastic markers
- Parapsoriasis
- Polymorphous light eruption
- Porphyria
- Psoriasis—inverse, pustular
- Pyoderma gangrenosum
- Reticulated erythematous mucinosis (REM)
- Sarcoidosis
- Skin signs of internal disease
- Sweet syndrome
- Syphilis
- Tinea versicolor
- Urticarial vasculitis
- Vasculitis

Possible etiologies

- Allergy
- Arthropod assault (insect bite or sting)
- Artifact
- Autoimmune disease
- Bacterial infections (including tuberculosis, leprosy, atypical mycobacteria, *Neisseria gonorrhoeae* and chlamydia)
- Drug reaction
- Endocrine disease
- Foreign body
- Fungi (including subcutaneous and deep infections)
- Genetic defect
- Granulomatous process
- Infestation (scabies)
- Malignancy—cutaneous or underlying
- Metastasis
- Nutritional disorder
- Parasites (including tropical disorders)
- Photosensitivity
- Psychosomatic disorder
- Spirochetes (borreliosis, syphilis)
- Toxic-irritant processes
- Vasculitis
- Viral infections